S0-BQM-126

Prevention and
Detection of Cancer

Prevention and Detection of Cancer

Part I (*in two volumes*): Prevention
Volume 1: Etiology
Volume 2: Etiology; Prevention Methods
Part II (*in two volumes*): Detection
Volume 1: High Risk Markers; Detection Methods and Management
Volume 2: Cancer Detection in Specific Sites

*Proceedings of the Third International
Symposium on Detection and Prevention of Cancer
New York, April 26 to May 1, 1976*

Sponsored by
The International Study Group for the Detection and Prevention of Cancer (DePCa)

Co-Sponsored by
International Agency for Research on Cancer of the World Health Organization (IARC)
American Cancer Society
Mount Sinai School of Medicine of The City University of New York

Editor
H. E. Nieburgs, M.D.
Mount Sinai School of Medicine of The City University of New York, New York,
New York, U.S.A.

Associate Editor
V. E. O. Valli, D.V.M., Ph.D.
Guelph University, Guelph, Canada

Assistant Editor
S. A. Kay, B.A., B.L.S.
International Study Group for the Detection and Prevention of Cancer (DePCa),
New York, New York, U.S.A.

Members of the Editorial Board
J. G. Bekesi, M.D.
Mount Sinai School of Medicine of The City University of New York,
New York, U.S.A.

Henry Colcher, M.D.
Lahey Clinic Foundation, Boston, Massachusetts, U.S.A.

Murray M. Copeland, M.D.
University of Texas System Cancer Center, M. D. Anderson Hospital and Tumor
Institute, Houston, Texas, U.S.A.

Franco Rilke, M.D.
Istituto Nazionale per lo Studio e la Cura dei Tumori, Milan, Italy

Philip Strax, M.D.
Guttman Institute, New York, New York, U.S.A.

Lorenzo Tomatis, M.D.
International Agency for Research on Cancer of the World Health Organization (IARC),
Lyon, France

International Symposium on Detection and Prevention of Cancer

Prevention and Detection of Cancer

PART I. PREVENTION
Volume 1. Etiology

Edited by Herbert E. Nieburgs

Mount Sinai School of Medicine
of The City University of New York
New York, New York

RC 268
I57
pt. 1:1
1977

MARCEL DEKKER, INC.   New York and Basel

347006

Library of Congress Cataloging in Publication Data

Main entry under title:

Prevention and detection of cancer.

CONTENTS: v. 1 Prevention. pt. 1 Etiology.
1. Cancer-Prevention. 2. Cancer-Diagnosis.
3. Carcinogenesis. I. Nieburgs, Herbert E.
RC 268.P73   616.9'94'05   77-87546
ISBN 0-8247-6491-9 (v. 1, pt. 1)

COPYRIGHT © 1977 by MARCEL DEKKER, INC. ALL RIGHTS RESERVED.

Neither this book nor any part may be reproduced or transmitted in any form or by
any means, electronic or mechanical, including photocopying, microfilming, and
recording, or by any information storage and retrieval system, without permission
in writing from the publisher.

MARCEL DEKKER, INC.
270 Madison Avenue, New York, New York 10016

Current printing (last digit):
10 9 8 7 6 5 4 3 2 1

PRINTED IN THE UNITED STATES OF AMERICA

THE SYMPOSIUM

The Third International Symposium on Detection and Prevention of Cancer was held in New York City from April 26 through May 1, 1976. The Symposium was sponsored by The International Study Group for the Detection and Prevention of Cancer (DePCa) and organized by the Program Committee under the patronage of the Symposium's President, Mrs. Albert D. Lasker. Advice and assistance to the Secretary-General, H. E. Nieburgs, was also received from the International Scientific Advisory Committee members. The Symposium was cosponsored by the International Agency for Research on Cancer of the World Health Organization, American Cancer Society, and the Mount Sinai School of Medicine of The City University of New York.

Clinicians and researchers from 56 countries participated in the Third International Symposium on Detection and Prevention of Cancer, presenting over 800 papers in 115 sessions. The abstracts of these papers were published by DePCa. The information contained in the abstracts is available around the world through the International Cancer Research Data Bank of the National Cancer Institute, CANCERLINE information services.

Special contributions were received from the following: Cancer Research Institute, Inc., and The Earle and Bessie Whedon Cancer Detection Foundation; American Express Company, Hoffmann La-Roche, Inc., Olivetti Corporation of America, Olympus Corporation of America, Picker Corporation, S and S X-Ray Products, Inc., and Springer-Verlag New York, Inc.

Partial support was awarded by institutes of the U.S. Department of Health, Education and Welfare: The National Cancer Institute of the National Institutes of Health and The National Institute for Occupational Safety and Health of the Public Health Service.

President
Mrs. Albert D. Lasker

Secretary-General
Herbert E. Nieburgs

Program Committee

N. J. M. Aarts Netherlands	M. M. Copeland USA	A. Meisels Canada	L. Tomatis IARC
R. R. Bates USA	R. A. Good USA	H. E. Nieburgs USA (ex officio)	V. E. O. Valli Canada
H. Colcher USA	E. C. Hammond USA	P. Strax USA	U. Veronesi Italy

International Scientific Advisory Committee

J. Arias Stella Peru	I. Elsebai UAR	A. F. Montoro Brazil	L. Santi Italy
N. N. Blokhin USSR	C. M. Gros France	J. J. Murray South Africa	K. Shanmugaratnam Singapore
D. P. Burkitt United Kingdom	T. Hirayama Japan	M. L. Nasiell Sweden	J. Svoboda Czechoslovakia
J. Clemmesen Denmark	H. Holzner Austria	K. Oota Japan	H. J. Tagnon Belgium
P. Correa Columbia	T. Koszarowski Poland	I. Padovan Yugoslavia	G. Terzano Argentina
W. Davis IARC	J. P. Mach Switzerland	A. J. Phillips Canada	D. W. Van Bekkum Netherlands
A. Delachaux Switzerland	I. Martinez Puerto Rico	K. Ranadive India	G. L. Wied USA
L. Dmochowski USA	O. Melander Sweden	F. Rilke Italy	A. O. Williams Nigeria
S. Eckhardt Hungary	D. Metcalf Australia	G. Riotton Switzerland	J. Zajicek Sweden
T. Elicano, Jr. Philippines	M. Montero Van R. Chile	L. Sachs Israel	A. Zubiri Spain

PREFACE

Throughout the world, attempts are being made to reduce morbidity from cancer through primary prevention, by eliminating occupational and environmental carcinogens, and by protection of individuals who are exposed to carcinogenic hazards. Secondary prevention is aimed at reduction of mortality from cancer by detection and treatment of tumors in early stages of development.

Primary and secondary prevention are not entirely separate entities. Much experimental and epidemiologic data related to primary prevention serves as a basis for secondary prevention. Biologic characterization of human tumors, the etiology and natural history of neoplastic diseases, the epidemiologic identification of cancer hazards, and of populations at risk, are essential parameters for screening and surveillance of susceptible groups of individuals.

There is increasing evidence that cancer is a multitude of neoplastic diseases arising from a variety of endogenous and exogenous etiologic factors that may interact in various combinations, either simultaneously or at different times. Susceptibility for tumor development may exist as a result of genetic or acquired abnormalities that have the potential to change normal tissue architecture into malignant neoplasms. Sequence and duration of exposure to carcinogenic factors, the age, and sex seem to be related to site predilection and type of tumor growth. Resistance to oncogenesis, depending upon various host factors, may protect individuals from cancer.

The vast amount of data rapidly added to the world literature requires periodic reviews and correlation of new and old findings to extrapolate meaningful information for cancer control. The Third International Symposium on Detection and Prevention of Cancer, held in New York, April 26 to May 1, 1976, offered a forum for an international exchange of relevant information for review on the prevention and detection of cancer. Over 800 papers were presented and more than 600 manuscripts were submitted for publication in The Proceedings. Careful appraisal by the Editorial Board led to the acceptance of 403 manuscripts for publication in the four volumes of *Prevention and Detection of Cancer*. Regretfully, many worthy papers had to be omitted because of space limitations.

Prevention and Detection of Cancer provides a comprehensive review of our current state of knowledge on the role of experimental and human oncogenesis and of host and environmental factors for primary and secondary prevention. The four volumes constitute a multidisciplinary approach to cancer control that bridges fundamental research and clinical oncology.

Part I: Prevention (in two volumes) is devoted to recent progress in experimental oncology, offering to the researcher a valuable and extensive overview and providing the clinician with important basic information for the practice of cancer prevention and detection. The 29 chapters contain reports on the multiplicity of etiologic factors and their interaction; genetic and acquired susceptibility; the role of predisposing diseases and of potentially malignant lesions; the natural history of cancer; genetic, biochemical, and morphological markers of human neoplasms; identification of environmental and occupational hazards; methods of professional and public education.

Part II: Detection (in two volumes) is devoted to cancer detection methods in general, diagnostic and prognostic procedures, and detection of asymptomatic tumors in specific sites. Relevant experimental findings are integrated with clinical oncology. Various cancer detection methods are evaluated according to sensitivity and specificity, and feasibility of use for different sites. The final volume deals with specific sites and provides information on diagnostic methods and on management of detected cases. All chapters include numerous carefully selected reports. Breast and uterine cervix are extensively described, as are head and neck, respiratory system, stomach, colon-rectum, liver, pancreas, kidney, urinary bladder, ovaries, prostate, and lymphoma-leukemia.

Acknowledgment for the preparation of *Prevention and Detection of Cancer* is made to the leading experts throughout the world who have contributed from the various fields of oncology. Their reprots of original studies and contribution of overview articles permitted the editors of these four volumes to present integrated data pertaining to different disciplines for the experimental oncologist and practicing clinician.

I would like to express my appreciation to the Editorial Board and the Symposium's Program Committee and International Scientific Advisory Committee, for their editorial assistance in the reviewing of abstracts and manuscripts. The Secretaries of each Symposium session deserve special mention for their excellent summaries of the presentations. The summaries were invaluable to the Editorial Board as they began the enormous task of organizing over 7,000 pages of manuscripts. Dr. V. E. O. Valli deserves special recognition for the time that he generously gave to assist me in the organization of the volumes, chapter by chapter.

Acknowledgment is also due to my colleagues at Mount Sinai School of Medicine for their valuable advice: to Drs. J. G. Bekesi and C. A. Laing, for their editorial assistance in the organization of the chapters on immunology and virology; to Drs. K. K. Kay and I. J. Selikoff for their assistance in planning the Symposium's program on occupational and environmental exposures that resulted in the excellent chapters on this problem; and to Dr. A. S. Teirstein with whom I consulted in the preparation of the chapter on respiratory disease.

Finally, thanks is due to Mr. Marcel Dekker and his staff for their interest and unending patience that made it possible for so many worthy papers to be published; and to the Symposium's staff, including Mr. Steven Rosenberg who assisted in preparing the abstracts and manuscripts for editorial review.

Herbert E. Nieburgs
New York

CONTENTS

Volume 1: Etiology

1. MOLECULAR BIOLOGY

2. GENETICS AND MUTAGENESIS

3. VIROLOGY AND ONCOGENESIS

4. IMMUNOLOGY

Section 1. Fundamental Immunology

Section 2. Cell Mediated Immunity

6. NUTRITION

7. SMOKING

8. RADIATION

9. OCCUPATIONAL HAZARDS

10. ENVIRONMENTAL CARCINOGENESIS

CONTENTS OF VOLUME 2

22. ENVIRONMENTAL AND OCCUPATIONAL EXPOSURE

PREVENTION AND CONTROL OF OCCUPATIONAL EXPOSURES:
  AN OVERVIEW, T. F. Mancuso

ENVIRONMENTAL FACTORS AND CANCER PREVENTION, M. A. Schneiderman

HEALTH PROBLEMS ASSOCIATED WITH SELECTED PETROCHEMICALS:
  BENZENE, CHLORINATED HYDROCARBONS, AND STYRENE-BUTADIENE RUBBER,
  R. A. Lemen, D. P. Brown, R. A. Rinsky, R. J. Young, T. J. Meinhardt

INORGANIC CARCINOGENS, R. W. Rawson

ON THE POSSIBLE FORMATION OF BIS(CHLOROMETHYL) ETHER FROM FLAME
  RETARDANTS, G. Loewengart, B. L. Van Duuren

IDENTIFICATION OF CARCINOGENIC HAZARDS FROM AROMATIC AMINE EXPOSURES
  AND MEASURES FOR CONTROL, H. G. Parkes

A PROSPECTIVE MEDICAL SURVEILLANCE PROGRAM FOR THE DETECTION AND
  PREVENTION OF INDUSTRIALLY RELATED CANCER, R. A. Greenberg,
  C. H. Tamburro, C. E. Kupchella

INDIVIDUAL AGENT VERSUS INDUSTRY CONTROL IN SETTING STANDARDS,
  D. V. Lassiter

23. CARCINOGEN IDENTIFICATION

SCREENING TECHNIQUES FOR IDENTIFICATION OF CARCINOGENS:
  AN OVERVIEW, P. N. Magee

VOLATILE CARCINOGENS: OCCURRENCE, FORMATION AND ANALYSIS,
  D. Hoffmann, I. Schmeltz, S. S. Hecht, K. D. Brunnemann,
  E. L. Wynder

SEPARATION AND ANALYSIS OF VARIOUS CARCINOGENIC AROMATIC AMINES
  AND THEIR METABOLITES, E. K. Weisburger, P. H. Grantham, T. Benjamin

ANALYTICAL METHODS FOR POLYNUCLEAR AROMATIC HYDROCARBONS, I. Schmeltz,
  K. D. Brunnemann, D. Hoffmann

FURTHER EVALUATION OF A HAMSTER EMBRYO CELL CARCINOGENESIS BIOASSAY,
  R. J. Pienta, J. A. Poiley, W. B. Lebherz III

THE *SALMONELLA*/MICROSOME TEST FOR DETECTION OF CARCINOGENS AS
  MUTAGENS, B. N. Ames, J. McCann

PRELIMINARY REPORT ON THE POSSIBLE USE OF NEURONAL TISSUE CULTURE
  IN CARCINOGENESIS *IN VITRO*, B. M. Boulos

RAPID DETECTION OF DNA DAMAGE BY CARCINOGENIC AGENTS USING
  IMMUNOFLUORESCENCE AND ULTRACENTRIFUGATION, S. Neubort,
  D. Liebeskind, A. Leifer, R. Bases

A COMPARISON OF SHORT TERM BIOASSAY RESULTS WITH CARCINOGENICITY
  OF EXPERIMENTAL CIGARETTES, P. K. Basrur, S. McClure, B. Zilkey

ANALYTICAL BIOCHEMISTRY IN CANCER RESEARCH AND THERAPY, J. Roboz

THE PROBLEMS IN COLLABORATIVE STUDIES ON ANALYSIS OF CHEMICAL
  CARCINOGENS, E. A. Walker

24. CHEMICAL STRUCTURE AND PREDICTION OF CARCINOGENICITY

STRUCTURAL PROGNOSTICATION OF CARCINOGENICITY AND TUMOR-ENHANCING
  ACTIVITY IN VARIOUS CHEMICALS, B. L. Van Duuren

29.   EDUCATION AND LEGISLATION

CIRCULATING DNA AND ONCONGENESIS

Philippe Anker*, Maurice Stroun**, and Pierre Maurice*

*Division of Oncohaematology, Department of Medicine,
        Hôpital Cantonal, Geneva, Switzerland
**Department of Plant Physiology, Faculty of Science,
        University of Geneva, Switzerland

I INTRODUCTION

Does DNA circulate between cells in higher organisms ? Perhaps is it pertinent to ask first : "Is there a spontaneous release of DNA by eukaryote cells ?"

It is known that bacteria in culture spontaneously release DNA. In transformable bacteria, it has been shown that this extracellular DNA is genetically active since it can as such induce transformation (12, 19).

We have demonstrated that DNA is also released from eukaryote cells and have suggested that it represented a general phenomenon since the same excretion mechanism was found in amphibian organs (1, 6, 24, 26) as well as in human cells (4, 5).

In the present study we shall report some special characteristics of this released DNA. We shall then discuss the possibility of intercellular DNA circulation, taking into account results showing that eukaryote cells can also take up spontaneously released DNA (2, 22, 23, 25, 26, 27, 28).

Finally a possible role of circulating DNA in oncogenesis will be postulated.

II PROCEDURES AND MATERIALS USED

A. Biological Material

In experiments with whole organs, frog auricles were used since in Ringer solution they can easily live on their own for more than two days and have no blood vessels where coagulated blood could remain trapped. Human blood lymphocytes were used as single cell suspensions in TC 199 medium.

B. Auricle and Lymphocyte Cultures, Separation of the Supernatants

Suspension of sterily isolated frog auricles (100-200/80 ml of Ringer solution) or human lymphocytes (10^6/ml in 200 ml of TC 199 medium)

3

isolated by Ficoll Isopaque gradient, were cultured for different periods of time under sterile conditions. In some experiments the medium was regularly renewed. The auricles were removed by hand, while the lymphocytes were gently centrifuged (1,000 g) and both supernatants were centrifuged : first at 12,000 rpm and then at 50,000 rpm for at least 2 hr in order to remove any cellular debris, the complex containing the released nucleic acids remaining in the supernatant.

C. Control of Cell Viability, Sterility Test and Cell Counting

Cell viability of the frog auricles was controled by determining the pulsation rate at the beginning and at the end of the experiments. Control auricles were also labeled with ^{3}H uridine during the last hour of a 24 hr culture and labeled cells counted on autoradiographs showing that 100 % of the cells were labeled. Moreover, the pellet of the supernatant was examined after centrifugation for the presence of cell or cell fragments, revealing no complete cell and only very few fragments. Even if each fragment was counted as a cell, they could not account for more than 1×10^{-6} of the total cell population.

Cell recovery of the lymphocytes was checked after incubation and their viability tested by trypan blue exclusion. Moreover, control series were examined for their capacity to synthesize DNA under mitogen induced stimulation at the end of the various incubation periods, showing a fully maintained functional integrity.

Sterility of the supernatants was controlled at the beginning and at the end of incubation.

D. Labeling

Methyl ^{3}H thymidine (26 Ci/mmole, 10 μCi/ml) was added for various periods of time to the cell suspension. Possible acellular synthesis was investigated by adding ^{3}H thymidine triphosphate (^{3}H TTP) (47 Ci/mmole, 1μCi/ml) or one of the other 3 tritiated deoxytriphosphates to the acellular medium. In experiments designed for nearest neighbour analysis the cell free supernatant was labeled with α^{32}P thymidine triphosphate (α^{32}P TTP) (50 Ci/mmole, 1 μCi/ml).

In some experiments the following hydrolases and DNA synthesis inhibitors were added to the cell free supernatant before labeling : 200 μg/ml of DNase II, 100 μg/ml of RNase, 1 mg/ml of pronase, 0.7 μg/ml or 30 μg/ml of Actinomycin D.

E. DNA Extraction

DNA was isolated from the cells and from the supernatants by chloroform extraction (16) for the frogs and by phenol treatment (4) for the lymphocytes. The different solutions were then loaded on hydroxyapatite columns (9) and the eluted double stranded DNA was pelleted by centrifugation for 16 hr at 45,000 rpm. Extracellular DNA was always more difficult to purify than cellular DNA.

F. DNA Characterization

The following studies were performed on the DNA extracted from the cells and from the supernatants. (a) Their amount was determined by UV absorption and by deoxyribose colorations (11, 13). (b) The DNA was subjected to treatments with DNase I, DNase II, pancreatic RNase and pronase. (c) The molecular weight was estimated by zonal centrifugation on linear gradients of 5 to 20 % sucrose. (d) The buoyant density of the DNA was determined by CsCl density-gradient centrifugation. (e) The tritiated DNA were hybridized against an excess (ratio 1 : 1000) of non labelled cellular DNA. Moreover, renaturation kinetics of the same labeled DNA were compared. The C_0t curves were performed according to the method of Britten and Kohne (10).

II. RESULTS

A. Quantitative Determination of the released DNA

Table 1 & Table 2 show that the amount of DNA released did not depend on incubation time. When the incubation medium was renewed several times, similar amounts of DNA were released each time. However resuspension of the cells in an unrenewed medium was not followed by any additional DNA release. In the case of lymphocytes, no relation was found between cell loss or cell death and amount of released DNA. The same observation was made with frog auricles cut in three which did not release more DNA than whole auricles.

B. Characterization of DNA Released

1. NATURE, SIZE AND SPECIFICITY OF RELEASED DNA

The material released from frog auricles as well as from lymphocytes presented all DNA characteristics : (a) it had a typical UV absorption, a maximum at 258 nm and a minimum at 230 nm; (b) its amount, determined by UV absorption was fully confirmed by deoxyribose reactions; (c) while more than 95 % of it was digested by DNase, it remained insensitive to RNase and pronase.

The molecular weight of the released DNA was not as homogenous as that of the cellular DNA. Whereas the cellular DNA had 1 peak over 18 S, the extracellular DNA had 2 main peaks of about 12S and 7S. Separation on CsCl gradient indicated that the general AT/GC ratio was the same for the cellular and the extracellular DNA. The specific activity of the DNA released from labeled cells was higher than that of the cellular DNA. The renaturation curve of the cellular DNA (Fig. 1 A and B) starts to fall at C_0t 1 already while the released ^{3}H DNA (Fig. 1 A and B) falls down only when 30 to 50 % of the cellular DNA is already renatured. The hybridization curves (Fig. 1 C and D) indicate that both released and newly synthesized cellular ^{3}H DNA present an important homology with non labeled cellular DNA. However, the released ^{3}H DNA curve reaches a plateau after ½ C_0t

5

whether the mass ratio of labeled released DNA to unlabeled cellular DNA was 1 : 100 or 1 : 1.000.

2. SPONTANEOUS EXTRACELLULAR SYNTHESIS OF THE RELEASED DNA

a. Precursor Incorporation

The ^{32}P DNA which had been labeled with α^{32}P TTP in the absence of cells, was digested with splenic DNase and splenic phosphodiesterase and yielded upon chromatography all four 3' monophosphates carrying radioactivity.

The extracellular DNA was labeled when one of the four specific triphosphate precursors was added to the cell free supernatant. In addition, the specific activity of the DNA was not decreased by the presence of an excess of unlabeled triphosphate precursor carrying a different base for instance ^{3}H TTP with a 1 x 10^4 fold excess of unlabeled dGTP.

The extracellular DNA had the same specific activity whether the incubation lasted 2 or 24 hr. When the auricles had been killed or the lymphocytes lysed by distilled water, the amount of DNA recovered from the supernatant was about the same as the amount found in the supernatant of a normal culture while the precursor incorporation was about two times lower.

Extracellular precursor incorporation was inhibited by DNase II, RNase and pronase and in the case of lymphocytes by Actinomycin D (0,7 µg/ml).

b. Characterization of ^{3}H DNA Synthesized in the Cell Free Medium

The purified ^{3}H DNA was sensitive to both pancreatic and splenic DNase. After 12 hr of digestion, over 90 % of the acid insoluble radioactivity became acid soluble. With venom phosphodiesterase the acid insoluble radioactivity became gradually soluble (50 % after 12 h) while with pancreatic DNase a plateau at 90 % was rapidly reached. On the other hand, pronase or RNase had no effect on the purified molecules. After centrifugation in sucrose gradient the DNA synthesized in the cell free medium banded unhomogenously with two mains peaks from 4 S to 12 S.

The renaturation curves (Figure 1, A and B) of the acellularly labeled DNA remain stable while an important part of the cellular DNA is already renatured. The extracellularly labeled DNA hybridizes with unlabelled cellular DNA only at high C_0t (fig. 1, C and D).

III. DISCUSSION

A. The DNA is Released by Living Cells

The release of DNA from frog auricles as well as from human lymphocytes is not due to a DNA loss from damaged, dying or dead cells. This is

evidenced by the fact that : (a) Cell death or cell recovery rate has no
effect on the amount of extracellular DNA found in the supernatant of
lymphocytes. In the case of frog auricles, a similar argument can be
raised from the series of auricles which have been cut in three. These
auricles, still alive but beating slowly, do not release more DNA than
whole auricles.(b) Similar quantities of DNA (about 2 % of cellular DNA)
are present in the medium whether the incubation has been short or long,
instead of the increase with time which would be expected if DNA release
were due to dying cells.(c) There is a constant renewal of extracellular
DNA with each change of medium which suggests an active homeostatic
mechanism. This repeated release of DNA appears to depend on some kind of
hommeostasy rather than to be caused by mechanical injuries since there is
no significant increase of extracellular DNA when the cells are taken out
of their medium and put back in the same medium. (d) The DNA released
seems qualitatively different from the bulk of the cellular DNA. This is
shown by the C_ot curves which will be discussed later and by the specific
activity. Indeed values far exceeding cellular DNA specific activity were
observed on extracellular DNA samples.

B. Characterization of the Released DNA

1. NATURE SIZE AND SPECIFICITY OF THE RELEASED MATERIAL

The released material which has been shown to be DNA is formed of
unhomogenous fractions which can be quite important in size : over
5×10^6 daltons. As indicated by CsCl density gradients, the released DNA
has the same GC content as the bulk cellular DNA a finding which rules out
a mitochondrial origin.
The differences in the renaturation curves of the cellular DNA and of
the released DNA show that the reiterated sequences of the newly synthesized cellular DNA are absent in the medium at least in the form of
multiple copies. A preferential release of unique DNA is also indicated by
the hybridization between unlabeled cellular DNA and ^{3}H DNA released from
labeled cells. Indeed the hybridization curve appears to follow a second
order kinetics with a high half C_ot value, indicating that the released
^{3}H DNA is highly complex and is not composed of numerous copies of simple
sequences. The fact that the hybridization curve of the released ^{3}H DNA
reaches a plateau before the cellular ^{3}H DNA wether the mass ratio of
labeled DNA to unlabeled DNA is 1 : 100 or 1 : 1.000 can be explained if
one assumes that 50 % of the released DNA consist of sequences rarely
present in the cell genome. The complexity of the released DNA shown by
the C_ot curves rules out a direct microbial contamination.

2.   THE DNA IS RELEASED AS A COMPLEX

Several facts indicate that the DNA is released in a complex : (a)
The purification of the extracellular DNA is much more difficult than that
of the cellular DNA. (b) The released DNA is quite resistant to DNase in

the medium before purification. (c) The DNA is not only complexed to protein but also to some light components since before purification, the DNA in the medium cannot be pelleted even after 12 hr of centrifugation at 50,000 rpm.

3. A PORTION OF THE RELEASED DNA IS SPONTANEOUSLY SYNTHESIZED OUTSIDE THE CELLS

a. Precursor Incorporation Reflects true Synthesis

That the released DNA is accompanied by proteins including enzymes is also shown by the spontaneous extracellular synthesis observed in the culture media of frog auricles (6, 24) and of human lymphocytes (5).

The results obtained by nearest neighbour analysis when $\alpha^{32}P$ TTP is added to the medium demonstrate that the precursor has really been incorporated and that a simple adsorption process can be excluded.

b. Dying or Dead Cells are not the Cause of the Acellular Synthesis

The low incorporation observed in the extracellular DNA could suggest that this low synthesis is due to traces of enzymes and DNA released into the medium from damaged cells. This trivial explanation is ruled out by the same arguments as those presented for DNA release. (a) The extracellular DNA has the same specific activity whether the auricles or the lymphocytes were cultured for 2 or 24 hr before the acellular labeling. If the acellular synthesis were due to leakage of enzymes by dying cells one would expect an increase with time of the specific activity. (b) Moreover, when the auricles have been killed or the lymphocytes lysed by distilled water, the amount of DNA recovered from the supernatant is about the same as the amount found in the supernatant of a normal culture while the precursor incorporation is about two times lower. (d) Finally the renaturation and the hybridization curves show that the DNA synthesized in the cell free medium is qualitatively different from the DNA synthesized in the cells and from the DNA released from previously labeled cells.

c. Characterization of the Acellularly Synthesized DNA

We seem to be in presence of a preferential extracellular synthesis of unique sequences of the cell genome. This hypothesis is supported by the absence of reiteration observed in the renaturation curve of the extracellular ^3H DNA labeled in the cell free supernatant and could explain the low hybridization observed between cellular DNA and extracellularly labeled DNA. It thus appears that only a small part of the released DNA which was shown to present an important homology with the cellular DNA is synthesized in the cell free supernatant. As for the released DNA, the possibility of a direct microbial contamination is ruled out by the complexity of the DNA synthesized acellularly.

Although the exact kind of synthesis cannot be determined at this stage, inhibition experiments and C_0t curve results eliminate some possibilities. An unscheduled DNA synthesis as described in DNA repair processes appears unlikely since this kind of synthesis is not sensitive to a low concentration of Actinomycin D (in any case for the lymphocytes) nor to our knowledge to RNase. The possibility of a terminal transferase system in which an enzyme would merely add a nucleotide at the end of the chain can also be excluded. Indeed if the labeled nucleotides were added at the end of the chain, a much larger amount of radioactivity would be found in the acid-soluble fraction after the first hours of digestion with phosphodiesterase. Actinomycin and RNase sensitivity also militate against a terminal transferase. The inhibition of precursor incorporation by RNase suggests either some sort of replicative synthesis where an initiator RNA is required or an RNA directed synthesis. The presence of RNA in the medium is not surprising since we have previously shown that a polyribonucleotide is released by eukaryotic cells (1, 3). Release of RNA has also been reported by another laboratory (14). Inhibition by Actinomycin D (which is observed in lymphocyte systems) rather suggests a DNA directed DNA synthesis with the help of an initiator RNA.

The release of DNA seems to be a general phenomenon ruled by a common homeostatic mechanism observed in bacterial (24), amphibian (24, 26) and human systems (4). It thus appears that the phenomenon is not restricted to lymphoid cells as postulated by other authors who have reported DNA release by stimulated lymphocytes (18, 20, 21).

C. DNA Released by Bacteria is Taken up by Eukaryote Cells where it is Transcribed

DNA being released in a complex by eukaryote cells, the next obvious question is "can this spontaneously released complex be taken up by other cells".

No work has yet been done showing spontaneous transfer of released DNA by eukaryote cells to other eukaryote cells. However, since 1969 it has been reported that the DNA spontaneously released by bacteria could enter cells of higher organisms (plants or animals) during bacterial infection and subsequently be transcribed (2, 22, 23, 25, 27, 28). The transcription is realized with the help of the bacterial DNA-dependant RNA polymerase which accompanies the released DNA (22, 23). This spontaneous transfer of bacterial DNA and its subsequent transcription in host cells has been called "transcession". It should be mentioned that the DNA released by bacteria is also released in a complex similar to that observed with eukaryote cells, and that the mechanism of excretion, at least for stagnant bacteria follows the same homeostasy (24). We therefore have good ground to assume that the spontaneous transfer of DNA from bacteria to higher organisms during bacterial infection might reflect a general biological process which probably occurs between eukaryote cells in normal conditions. In other words transcession might be a general phenomenon in living organisms.

Whatever the biological role of transcession might be, it is known that the transcription of the DNA spontaneously released by the bacteria Agrobacterium tumefaciens can, after being transcribed in the plant cells, play a pathological role since it induces a vegetal cancer called Crown Gall (28).

9

D. Possible Role of Circulating DNA in Oncogenesis

The plant cancer Crown Gall can give rise to metastases. Such metastases have been observed with bacteria-free primary tumors and therefore cannot be due to migrating bacteria. Since tumors are obtained with phage free bacteria and since no viruses have been detected in the metastases, a viral etiology seems to be ruled out. Now, plant cells are held together by the network of their pectocellulosic walls which prevent the migration of the transformed cells. Thus, in the case of plants at least, metastatization is more probably due to a migrating molecule. As in Crown Gall the bacterial nucleic acids are at the origin of tumor formation, it is very likely that these molecules are also responsible for metastatization.

In the case of mammals it is generally accepted that metastases are due to migrating malignant cells. However, DNA extracted from malignant cells can induce experimentally a malignant transformation in normal cells (8, 29). The fact that DNA is released and circulates in animals implies that the hypothesis of a role of circulating nucleic acids in secondary tumor formation deserves investigation. Along these lines one should also bear in mind the possibility that a circulating DNA, which may not be necessarily transformant, might be involved in other modifications such as malignancy associated changes which have been found in almost all tissues of patients suffering from diverse malignant tumors (17).

IV SUMMARY

Amphibian organs and human lymphocytes release DNA which consists of newly synthesized cellular DNA composed mainly of unique sequences. This release is not due to damaged cells and is governed by a precise homeostatic mechanism. The DNA is released in a complex containing proteins amongst which the enzymes necessary for a partial extracellular synthesis of the released DNA. This acellular synthesis is a true synthesis as shown by nearest neighbour analysis.

This general biological event is related to the uptake by eukaryote cells of spontaneously released bacterial DNA, thus suggesting the existence of circulating DNA. In view of the malignant transformations obtained with DNA the oncogenic role of circulating DNA is postulated.

ACKNOWLEDGEMENTS

We thank Mrs. J. Henri and Mrs. C. Lederrey for their excellent technical assistance.
This work was supported by grants from the O.J. Isvet fund, La Ligue Suisse contre le Cancer, and by Hoffmann-La Roche.

Table I. Amount of DNA extracted from lymphocytes and from their
supernatants after various periods of incubation in culture
medium with or without serum

Incubation time	Cell DNA (µg)	Medium DNA (µg) (%)	Cell recovery (%)	deaths (%)
With 20 % serum				
A. 8 hr	941	21.7 (2.2)	98	0.9
B. 2 hr (1st incub)		21 (2.1)	99	1.5
2 hr (2nd incub)		19 (1.9)	100	2
2 hr (3rd incub)		23 (2.3)	97	0.6
2 hr (4th incub)	974	24 (2.4)	98	0.6
C. 4 successive 2 hr incubations in the same medium	847	26 (3)	100	3.5
Without serum				
A. 8 hr	778	24.5 (3)	100	9
B. 2 hr (1st incub)		23.5 (2.6)	100	11
2 hr (2nd incub)		20 (2.2)	81	10
2 hr (3rd incub)		11 (1.2)	81	23
2 hr (4th incub)	900	21.5 (2.4)	73	45

Table II. Amount of DNA extracted from frog auricles and from their
culture medium after various incubation periods

Incubation time	Auricle DNA (µg)	Medium DNA (µg) (%)
A. 24 hr	1.360	27 1.9
B. 4 hr (1st incubation)		26 1.7
4 hr (2nd incubation)		23.5 1.9
4 hr (3rd incubation)		24.9 1.6
4 hr (4th incubation)		17.8 1.2
4 hr (5th incubation)		16.5 1.1
4 hr (6th incubation)	1.491	19.3 1.3
C. 6 successive 4 hr incubations in the same medium	1.430	32 2.2
D. 4 hr (auricles cut in three)	1.391	11.1 0.8

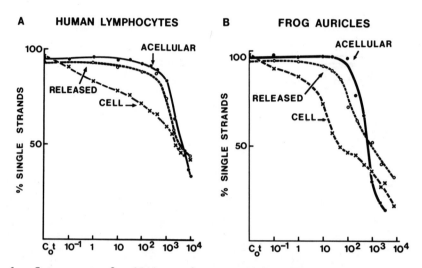

FIG. 1. $C_o t$ curves of cellular and extracellular DNA of frog auricles or human lymphocytes. (A) Comparison of the renaturation kinetics of lymphocyte [^{3}H]DNA, of [^{3}H]DNA released from previously labeled cells and of extracellular [^{3}H]DNA labeled in the cell free supernatant. (B) Comparison of the renaturation kinetics of frog auricle [^{3}H]DNA, of [^{3}H]DNA released from previously labeled cells and of extracellular [^{3}H]DNA labeled in the cell free supernatant. (C) Comparison of $C_o t$ curves of lymphocyte [^{3}H]DNA, [^{3}H]DNA released from previously labeled cells, and extracellular [^{3}H]DNA labeled in the cell free supernatant hybridized with an excess of nonlabeled cellular DNA (mass ration of 1:1.000). (D) Comparison of $C_o t$ curves of frog auricle [^{3}H]DNA, [^{3}H]DNA released from previously labeled cells, and extracellular [^{3}H]DNA labeled in the cell free supernatant and hybridized with an excess of nonlabeled cellular DNA (mass ration of 1:1.000). Cellular [^{3}H]DNA or released [^{3}H]DNA were obtained after lymphocytes or frog auricles had been labeled for 8 hr with [^{3}H] thymidine.

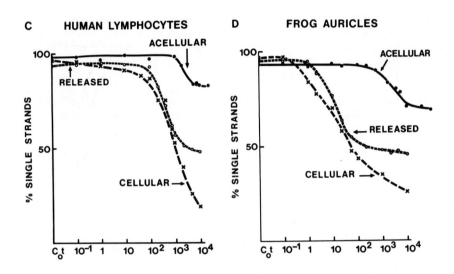

Acellular [³H]DNA was obtained from cell free supernatants labeled with
[³H]TTP for 8 hr. The DNA were sheared to 7S size and separated in different aliquots. They were denatured in a silicone oil bath at 120 for
15 min and cooled rapidly on ice. DNA solutions previously maintained in
0.03 M phosphate buffer were adjusted to 0.12 M of the same buffer and incubated in sealed disposable micropipets at 60 . The sealed tubes were
removed at desired intervals and frozen at 20 until processed. Percentage
of renaturation or hybridization was determined by applying each sample to
an individual 1 cm water-jacketed column containing 2 cm of hydroxyapatite
maintained at 60 . The samples were eluted with 16 successive 1 ml fractions of 0.12 M phosphate buffer followed by 16 successive 1 ml fractions
of 0.48 M phosphate buffer. The radioactivity of each fraction was counted
by liquid scintillation. Data are plotted as percentage of single strands
of ³H DNA vs. C_0t (moles/liter x sec).

VII. REFERENCES

1. Anker, P., and Stroun, M. Spontaneous Release of Nucleic Acids by
   Living Bacteria and Cells of Higher Organisms, Abstracts of the
   VIIIth International Congress of Cell Biology, Brighton, 3, 1972.

2. Anker, P., and Stroun, M. Bacterial Ribonucleic Acid in the Frog
   Brain after a Bacterial Peritoneal Infection.Science, 178 : 621-623,
   1972.

3. Anker, P., Stroun, M., Deshusses, J., Cattaneo, A., and Henri, J.,
   Cell free Extracellular Synthesis of a Polyribonucleic Fraction (PRN)
   after the Spontaneous Release of Nucleic Acids by Living Bacteria and
   by Cells of Frogs and Mammals. Biochem. Soc. Trans. London, 4 : 890-
   892, 1973.

4. Anker, P., Stroun, M., and Maurice, P. Spontaneous Release of DNA by
   Human Blood Lymphocytes as Shown in an In Vitro System. Cancer Res.,
   35 : 2375-2382, 1975.

5. Anker, P., Stroun, M., and Maurice, P. Spontaneous Extracellular
   Synthesis of DNA Released by Human Lymphocytes. Cancer Res., in press.

6. Anker, P., Stroun, M., and Bernardi, A. Spontaneous Extracellular
   Synthesis of DNA Released by Frog Auricles. In preparation.

7. Becker, A., and Hurwitz, J. Current Thoughts on the Replication of DNA.
   In Prog. Nucleic Acid Res. Mol. Biol. Ed: J.N. Davidson and W.E. Cohen.
   Academic Press New York and London, 11 : 423-459, 1971.

8. Bendich, A., Borenfreund, E., and Honda, Y. DNA-Induced Heritable
   Alteration of Mammalian Cells. In Informative Molecules in Biological
   Systems. Ed. : L.G.H. Ledoux. North-Holland Publ. Co. Amsterdam,
   80-86, 1971.

9. Bernardi, G. Chromatography of Nucleic Acids on Hydroxyapatite. Nature,
   206 : 779, 1965.

10.Britten, R.J., and Kohne, D.E. Repeated Sequences in DNA. Science, 161:
   529-540, 1968.

11.Ceriotti, G.A. Microchemical Determination of Deoxyribonucleic Acid.
   J. Biol. Chem., 198 : 297-303, 1952.

12.Borenstein, A., and Ephrati-Elizur, E. Spontaneous Release of DNA in
   Sequential Genetic Order by Bacillus Subtilis. J. Mol. Biol., 45 :
   137-152, 1969.

13.Giles, K.W., and Myers, A. An improved Diphenylamine Method for the
   Estimation of DNA. Nature, 206 : 93, 1965.

14

14. Kolodny, G.M., Culp, L.A., and Rosenthal, L.J. Secretion of RNA by Normal and Transformed Cells. Exptl. Cell Res :, 73 : 65-72, 1972.

15. Kornberg, A. The Enzymatic Synthesis of DNA. Wiley, London, p. 21-26, 1961.

16. Marmur, J.A. Procedure for the Isolation of Deoxyribonucleic Acid from Micro-organisms. J. Mol. Biol., 3 : 208-218, 1961.

17. Nieburgs, H.E. Recent Progress in the Interpretation of Malignancy Associated Changes (MAC). Acta Cytol., 12 : 445-453, 1968.

18. Olsen, I and Harris, G. Uptake and Release of DNA of Lymphoid Tissue and Cells. Immunology, 27 : 973-987, 1974.

19. Ottolenghi, E., and Hotchkiss, R.D. Release of Genetic Transforming Agent from Pneumococcal Cultures during Growth and Disintegration. J. Exptl. Med., 116 : 491-519, 1962.

20. Rogers, J.C., Bold, D., Kornfeld, S., Skinner, A., and Valeri, P. Excretion of Deoxyribonucleic Acid by Lymphocytes Stimulated with Phytohemagglutinin or Antigen. Proc. Nat. Acad. Sci. USA, 69 : 1685-1689, 1972.

21. Sarma, D.S.R., and Zubroff, J. Synthesis and Fragmentation of DNA in Phytohaemagglutinin Stimulated Human Peripheral Blood Lymphocytes. Immunol. Commun., 2 : 277-285, 1973.

22. Stroun, M. On the Nature of the Polymerase Responsible for the Transcription of Released Bacterial DNA in Plant Cells. Biochem. Biophys. Res. Comm., 44 : 571-578, 1971.

23. Stroun, M., Anker, P. Bacterial Nucleic Acid Synthesis in Plants Following Bacterial Contact. Molec. Gen. Genet., 113 : 92-98, 1971.

24. Stroun, M., and Anker, P. In vitro Synthesis of DNA. Spontaneously Released by Bacteria or Frog Auricles. Biochimie, 54 : 1443-1452, 1972.

25. Stroun, M., and Anker, P. Transcription of Spontaneously Released Bacterial Deoxyribonucleic Acid in Frog Auricles. J. Bacteriol., 114 : 114-120, 1973.

26. Stroun, M., Anker, P., and Gahan, P. Spontaneous Release of DNA from Animal Organs. In preparation.

27. Stroun, M., Gahan, P., and Sarid, S. Agrobacterium tumefaciens RNA in Non-Tumorous Tomato Cells. Biochem. Biophys. Res. Commun. 37 : 652-657, 1969.

28. Stroun, M., Anker, P., Gahan, P., Rossier, A., and Greppin, H.
    Agrobacterium tumefaciens Ribonucleic Acid Synthesis in Tomato Cells
    and Crown Gall Induction. J. Bacteriol., 106 : 634-639, 1971.

29. Szybalska E.H., and Szybalski, W. Genetics of Human Cell Lines, IV.
    DNA-mediated Heritable Transformation of a Biochemical Trait. Proc.
    Nat. Acad. Sci. U.S.A., 48 : 2026-2034, 1962.

DNA POLYMERASE REACTIONS IN HUMAN BLADDER TUMOR CELLS IN CULTURE: CHARACTERIZATION OF THE RNA-ASSOCIATED PRODUCT

A. R. Davis, B. S. Vayuvegula, and D.P. Nayak

Department of Microbiology and Immunology
University of California School of Medicine
Los Angeles, California 90024

INTRODUCTION

RNA tumor viruses contain RNA-directed DNA polymerase (reverse-transcriptase). After the discovery of this unique enzyme (1, 29) a search was undertaken in both normal (17) and neoplastic cells (see review by Green and Gerard, 15) for this or a similar enzyme. Various methods have been used to analyze human cancer cells and tissues for this enzyme. Principal examples of these are: (1) characteristic response to artifical templates (22); (2) co-fractionation with known virus reverse transcriptase upon purification of the enzymes (10); (3) detection of high-molecularweight complexes (35-70S) of the nascent DNA of endogenous in vitro DNA polymerase reactions occurring in sub-cellular fractions (23); (4) hybridization of the DNA product to the RNA of known oncornaviruses (2, 3, 11); (5) observation of a DNA polymerase activity in a particle or structure with a density characteristic of known oncornaviruses (19), and (6) immunological relatedness of DNA polymerase enzymes from human cancer cells to known oncornavirus reverse-transcriptase (30).

In this paper we describe and partially characterize a ribonuclease-sensitive endogenous DNA polymerase activity obtained in the cytoplasmic pellet fraction of cultured cells of transitional cell carcinoma of the bladder. This enzyme produces RNA-associated DNA as one of its early products. It is suggested that such products are RNA-DNA hybrids, one of the most rigorous criteria for establishing the presence of reverse-transcriptase (9, 12, 20, 24).

PROCEDURES AND MATERIALS USED

Cell Culture

T-24, a cell line derived from human urinary bladder carcinoma, was maintained in Eagle's minimal essential medium supplemented with 10% fetal bovine serum (Rehatuin, Phoenix, Ariz.), 100 U/ml penicillin, 100 ug/ml streptomycin, 0.25 ug/ml fungizone, 60 ug/ml tylocine, and 2 mM glutamine. Cells were examined routinely for the characteristic morphology and karotype of the original isolate (6). WI-38, a diploid cell line of human lung was obtained from L. Hayflick, Stanford University, and cultured as described above.

Preparation of Sub-Cellular Fractions and Synthesis of (^{3}H)-DNA

Cells were removed from culture by trypsinization, washed once with PBS, and treated with sufficient lima bean trypsin inhibitor (Worthington Biochemical Corp.,

Freehold, N.J.) to neutralize 10% of the trypsin originally added. Cells were swollen 10 min at 0°C in RSB (0.01 M tris-HCl (7.4), 0.01 M KCl, 0.0015 M $MgCl_2$) and ruptured with 30-40 strokes of a Dounce homogenizer. Nuclei were removed by centrifugation at 4000 g for 10 min at 4°C and mitochondria were removed by two cycles of centrifugation at 10,000 g for 10 min at 4°C. The supernatant was then layered over 15 ml 20% glycerol in TNE buffer (0.01 M tris-HCl (pH 8.3), 0.15 M NaCl, 0.001M EDTA, brought to 0.1% Nonidet P-40 (Particle Data Laboratories, Ltd., Elmhurst, Ill.) and 0.01M dithiothreitol, and incubated at 0°C for 15 min. DNA was synthesized for 5 min at 37°C in a reaction mixture containing tris-HCl (pH 8.3), 50mM; $MgCl_2$, 6 mM; NaCl, 20 mM; dithiothreitol, 5 mM; dATP, dGTP, dCTP, 1.6 mM each, and ^{3}H-dTTP, 6 uM (20,340 cpm/pmole).

Purification of Product Nucleic Acids

When product nucleic acids were to be recovered, the ^{3}H-dTTP concentration was increased to 18 uM (20, 340 cpm/pmole) and actinomycin D (50 ug/ml) was included in the reaction mixture. After incubation at 37°C for 5 min, the reaction was adjusted to 0.2 M NaCl and 1% SDS, deproteinized by phenol extraction, and the nucleic acids recovered by ethanol precipitation. These were dissolved in 0.01M tris-HCL (7.4), 0.001M EDTA, passed through a 1.5 x 26 cm column of Sephadex G 50 fine (Pharmacia Fine Chemicals, Uppsala, Sweden) equilibrated with 0.01 M tris-HCl (pH 7.4), 0.4 M NaCl, 0.001 M EDTA, and the material eluting in the void volume recovered. This material was precipitated with ethanol and stored at -20°C.

Cs_2SO_4 Equilibrium-Density Centrifugation

Samples were made to a density of 1.51 g/ml with Cs_2SO_4 (optical quality, Calbiochem., San Diego, Calif.) and centrifuged in pollyallomer tubes in a SW50.1 rotor at 35,000 rpm for 65 h at 5°C. Densities were measured by refractive index and trichloroacetic-acid precipitable cpm in each fraction were determined.

S-1 Nuclease Assays

S-1 nuclease was prepared according to the method of Sutton (26). The starting material was crude amylase from Aspergillus oryzae (Sigma Chemical Co., St. Louis, Mo.). Samples to be tested were dissolved in 2 ml of a reaction mixture containing sodium acetate buffer (pH 4.5), 0.03 M; $ZnSO_4$, 5 x 10^{-3}M; NaCl, 0.3 M; salmon sperm DNA, 20 ug/ml; and S-1 enzyme, 200 ug/ml. Samples were divided into two 1 ml portions, one unincubated (0 min) and the other incubated 30 min at 37°C. Trichloroacetic-acid precipitable cpm in each sample were determined.

Synthesis of (^{3}H)-DNA Using AMV

Avian myeloblastosis virus was kindly provided by J. Beard, Life Sciences Research Laboratories, St. Petersburg, Fla. The virus was further purified on a linear 20-65% sucrose gradient in 0.01 M tris-HCl (7.4), 0.1 M NaCl, 0.001 M EDTA at 26,000 rpm for 2.5 h in a SW27 rotor. Synthesis of (^{3}H)-DNA was performed for 30 minutes at 37°C in a reaction mixture containing tris-HCl (pH 7.6), 100 mM; magnesium acetate, 2 mM; dithiothreitol, 30 mM; dATP, dGTP, dCTP, 1 x 10^{-4} M each; actinomycin D, 50 ug/ml; ^{3}H-dTTP, 18 uM (20,340 cpm/pmole); and triton-X-100, 0.0225%. Product nucleic acids were recovered, purified, and analyzed on Cs_2SO_4 gradients as described above.

RESULTS

Kinetics of T-24 Endogenous DNA Polymerase Reactions

Particulate cytoplasmic fractions of T-24 (5,6) cultured bladder tumor cells have been found to catalyze endogenous DNA polymerase reactions. Pre-treatment of the cytoplasmic pellet with RNase reduces the activity 3-fold. Reaction kinetics are linear for 5 min only. Similar reaction kinetics were observed using the cytoplasmic pellet of human leukemic cells in culture (19).

Although endogenous reverse-transcriptase reactions of known RNA tumor viruses are sensitive to pre-incubation with ribonuclease (1,12,24,29) such sensitivity is not sufficient evidence to describe a reverse-transcriptase reaction. RNase sensitivity may derive at least in part from a dependency on RNA as a primer, analogous to DNA replication in Escherichia coli (25).

Nucleic-Acid Analysis of the Products of DNA Polymerase Reactions of Cytoplasmic Nuclear, and Mitochondrial Fractions

Endogenous DNA synthesis by RNA tumor viruses is known to generate DNA-RNA hybrids (9,12,20,24). Such hybrids are composed of short lengths of newly synthesized DNA associated with a longer, single-chain RNA template and therefore have a buoyant density approximately equal to that of single-stranded RNA. The products of 5 min endogenous DNA polymerase reactions from the cytoplasmic pellet, nuclear, and mitochondrial fractions of T-24 cells were therefore prepared and analyzed by cesium sulfate equilibrium-density gradient centrifugation. Only in the product prepared from the cytoplasmic pellet did a significant percentage (38%) of the nascent DNA migrate as RNA (Fig. 1). In products prepared from nuclei and mitochondria less than 1% of the total DNA migrated with the density of RNA. When DNA synthesis is carried out using the cytoplasmic pellet of another cell line of human urinary bladder carcinoma, J-82, 47% of the nascent DNA migrates as RNA (data not shown), while in products prepared from the cytoplasmic pellet of WI-38, a normal human diploid cell line, less than 1% of the nascent DNA migrates as RNA (Fig.1). Approximately 80% of the DNA polymerase reaction product of detergent disrupted AMV migrates as RNA (Fig. 1). These results show that the cytoplasmic pellet fractions of T-24 and J-82 cells contain a unique DNA polymerase activity that produces an RNA-associated DNA product co-fractionating with that produced by viral reverse-transcriptase. This DNA polymerase activity apparently does not arise from contamination, during cell fractionation, of the cytoplasmic pellet with the nuclear and mitochondrial fractions since the latter do not possess such an activity.

Characterization of the RNA-Associated DNA Product

Aggregation of RNA in Cs_2SO_4 (31) may cause entrapment of small DNA pieces in the RNA region of the gradients. To test this possibility single-stranded ^{32}P-DNA was included in the cytoplasmic-pellet (^3H)-DNA polymerization reaction and the product analyzed on a Cs_2SO_4 gradient. While 10% of the (^3H)-DNA synthesized migrated as RNA (total 3H cpm = 1339) less than 0.5% of the ^{32}P cpm migrated as RNA (total ^{32}P cpm = 1944). This shows that DNA is not entrapped in the RNA region of the gradients nor does the reaction produce artifactual association of this DNA with the RNA present.

The RNA-associated DNA product was further analyzed by treatment of the total product with nucleases followed by analysis on Cs_2SO_4. In this method two types of nucleases have been used: ribonucleases A and $T-1$ which degrade only single-stranded RNA in medium of high ionic strength but digest all RNA in medium of low ionic strength (20) and S-1 nuclease, which digests any single-stranded nucleic acid (26). When the total product is treated with ribonuclease in high-salt and analyzed in Cs_2SO_4 (Fig. 2B) no nascent DNA is seen migrating as RNA. In addition, a small amount of the product migrates in the hybrid region of the gradient (1.48 - 1.54 gm/ml), suggesting the conversion of a hybrid molecule composed of long chains of RNA and short chains of DNA to one where the proportion of RNA and DNA are nearly the same. Ribonuclease treatment in low salt also results in the disappearance of DNA migrating in the RNA region and is accompanied by a small increase in the amount of single-stranded DNA (Fig. 2C). Again, after treatment with S-1 nuclease (Fig. 2D) none of the product migrates as RNA. In addition some of the product again migrates in the hybrid region of the gradient (1.46 - 1.54 gm/ml).

Preliminary attempts have been made to recover the RNA region from Cs_2SO_4 gradients and analyze its structure with the use of nucleases. It can be seen that 24-51% of the material recovered from the RNA region is resistant to nuclease S-1 (Table 1) suggesting that 24-51% of the material migrating in this region is in the form of a DNA-RNA hybrid and 49-76% is single-stranded DNA. When a complex of AMV-(^{3}H)-DNA and 50-60S RNA is similarly recovered from the RNA region of a Cs_2SO_4 gradient approximately 65% is found to be resistant to S-1 nuclease (Table 1). Substantial amounts of single-stranded DNA have been found previously in the RNA-DNA hybrid intermediates of oncornaviral DNA synthesis (4,20). It has been suggested (28) that this single-stranded DNA arises from the prompt hydrolysis of the RNA template of a circular intermediate in the DNA transcription (27) by the RNase H activity resident in the polymerase. We have, however, encountered problems in recovery of the RNA region from Cs_2SO_4 gradients and have observed substantial losses of material from the RNA region. The use of guanidinium-CsCl density gradients (8) has allowed up to 80% recovery of the RNA region (Davis, Vayuvegula, and Nayak; unpublished observations) and should facilitate such analysis.

Denaturation of the DNA Region

It has been reported (21) that the high speed cytoplasmic pellet fraction of phytohemagglutinin-stimulated normal blood lymphocytes catalyze DNA-directed and RNA primed DNA synthesis. After heat denaturation 95% of the nucleic-acid product of these reactions appears in the RNA region of Cs_2SO_4 gradients, indicating that small RNA molecules (primers) covalently attached to even shorter fragments of nascent DNA were hydrogen bonded to much larger pieces of pre-existing DNA.

The possibility that such reactions were occurring when the cytoplasmic pellet fraction of T-24 cells was used for DNA polymerization was tested. The DNA region of Cs_2SO_4 gradients of the nucleic acid products was isolated, heat denatured, and re-analyzed on Cs_2SO_4 gradients (data not shown). Heat denaturation shifts the DNA to the single-stranded density yet yields less than 0.3% of the material migrating as RNA. This result along with the partial S-1 resistance of the RNA-associated DNA product suggests that the reaction occurring in phytohemagglutinin-stimulated lymphocytes may be different than the one described here.

DISCUSSION

Known RNA tumor viruses catalyze endogenous DNA polymerization, the early products of such reactions being RNA-DNA hybrids (9, 12, 20, 24). Although the presence of reverse-transcriptase has been looked for in human neoplastic cells and tissues by both the simultaneous detection test (3) and the hybridization of the DNA product of the endogenous polymerization reaction to known RNA tumor virus RNA (11) these studies do not clearly demonstrate the presence of an RNA DNA hybrid as a reaction product. Indeed it has been found that 70% of 40 milk samples from normal cancer-free women were positive by simultaneous detection (14) and that known RNA tumor viruses may encapsulate cellular RNA (7, 13, 26) that may hybridize to DNA transcripts produced using these tumor cells.

In this paper we examine an endogenous DNA polymerase reaction from the cytoplasmic particulate fraction of human bladder tumor cells in culture. This synthesis is partially sensitive to ribonuclease. Partial sensitivity may be accounted for either 1) by true incomplete sensitivity of the reaction to pre-incubation with ribonuclease or 2) by the presence of more than one enzyme only one of which is sensitive to ribonuclease. Such a distinction will require further purification of this activity. Although the reaction in inhibited 80% by actinomycin D at least some portion of the synthesis is resistant to this antibiotic. The non-linear kinetics of the reaction could be due to the presence of nucleases in the crude cytoplasmic particulate fraction. Such a possibility is now being tested by looking for inhibition of the polymerization activity of known oncornaviruses. Only polymerization reactions from the cytoplasmic pellet fraction produce significant quantities of RNA-associated DNA (Fig. 1). This observation suggests that this activity is of cytoplasmic origin and probably does not arise from contamination of the cytoplasmic fractions with nuclear or mitochondrial polymerases. Detectable quantities of RNA-associated DNA are not produced using the cytoplasmic pellet of normal human diploid cells (WI-38).

The nature of the cytoplasmic-pellet DNA polymerase product has been investigated. An RNA-associated DNA product is not found after treatment of the total product with RNase in either high or low salt or with S-1 nuclease. Under conditions where hybrid structures are maintained (RNase in high-salt and S-1 nuclease) a small proportion of the product migrates in a region more dense than single-stranded DNA, suggesting conversion to a hybrid structure with equal amounts of DNA and RNA.

A more direct determination of the structure of the RNA-associated DNA product has been difficult. Because of aggregation in the RNA region of Cs_2SO_4 gradients (31) recoveries of the region have been low. In preliminary experiments (Table 1) 24-51% of the cpm in the RNA region are resistant to S-1 nuclease, suggesting that part of the RNA-associated DNA product is RNA-DNA hybrid and that part is single-stranded DNA not in hybrid form. This single-stranded DNA could from part of a replicative complex as suggested for RNA tumor viruses (28).

The RNA-associated DNA detected here could also result from RNA primed DNA synthesis (18,25). Indeed such a synthesis has been detected in the microsomal and mitochondrial fractions of phytohemagglutinin-stimulated normal human blood lymphocytes (21). In these experiments, however, heat denaturation of nucleic acid product from in vitro polymerization resulted in 95% of the product banding as RNA whereas only 65% of the undenatured product bands as RNA. This experiment indicates that the RNA-associated portion of this product was originally hydrogen-bonded to and thus templated by DNA. When the DNA region of the DNA product from T-24 cytoplasmic pellets is heat denatured no material is seen migrating as RNA. Thus, coupled with the results described above, it appears that the DNA polymerase product from cytoplasmic pellets of bladder tumor cells may be different from that of normal human lymphocytes.

21

SUMMARY

Particulate cytoplasmic fractions of cultured human bladder tumor cells (T-24 and J-82) have been found to catalyze endogenous DNA polymerization reaction. Such polymerization is partially sensitive to actinomycin D and ribonuclease. Analysis of the DNA product of 5 min reactions, prepared in the presence of actinomycin D, by cesium sulfate equilibrium-density gradient centrifugation reveals nucleic acid product migrating as 10-47% RNA (density = 1.63) and 30-70% DNA (density = 1.39-1.42). Less than 1% of the product prepared under the same reaction conditions from either T-24 nuclei or mitochondria or from the cytoplasmic pellet fraction of WI-38, a normal human diploid cell line, migrates as RNA. The label in the RNA region of the Cs_2SO_4 gradients no longer migrates as RNA after treatment of the total product with ribonuclease in high or low salt or S-1 nuclease. Under conditions where hybrids are maintained (high-salt ribonuclease and S-1) small amounts of material are seen migrating in the hybrid region of the gradients. Nascent (^{3}H)DNA recovered from the RNA region of the gradient is found to be partially resistant to S-1 nuclease.

Known RNA tumor viruses catalyze the transcription of RNA to DNA via reverse transcriptase, the early products of such reactions being RNA-DNA hybrids. The DNA polymerase reaction product migrating as RNA as well as other properties of this reaction may indicate that such an enzyme is present in these cells.

Acknowledgement

This investigation was supported in part by PHS Grant CA 16880 from the National Cancer Institute through the National Bladder Cancer Project. A.R. Davis is a fellow of the Leukemia Society of America, Inc.

TABLE 1

STRANDEDNESS OF NUCLEIC ACID REGIONS RECOVERED FROM Cs_2SO_4 GRADIENTS OF T-24 ENDOGENOUS REACTION PRODUCTS[a]

Region	Treatment	Trichloroacetic-acid precipitable cpm			S-1 Resistance %		
		Exp 1	Exp 2	Exp 3	Exp 1	Exp 2	Exp 3
RNA[b]	0 min	70.6	242.9 230.6	136.2 150.9	--	--	--
RNA	S-1	35.7	54.8 57.7	55.2 43.6	50.6	23.8	34.4
DNA[c]	0 min	134.8	522.7 524.0	320.6 322.5	--	--	--
DNA	S-1	125.4	444.4 439.4	274.9 273.1	93.0	84.4	85.2
AMV (RNA region)[d]	0 min	147.0 139.2			--		
AMV (RNA region)	S-1	91.6 94.6			65.1		
ss DNA[e]	0 min	142.3			--		
ss DNA	S-1	6.9			4.8		
ds DNA[e]	0 min	128.8			--		
ds DNA	S-1	129.2			100		

[a] A T-24 cytoplasmic DNA-polymerase reaction product was prepared and fractionated on Cs_2SO_4. The RNA and DNA regions of the gradient were pooled, dialyzed exhaustively against NTE (0.01M tris-HCl (pH 7.4), 0.1M NaCl, 0.001M EDTA), and recovered by ethanol precipitation. Each region was then tested for resistance to S-1 nuclease.

[b] 1.57 - 1.76 g/ml.

[c] 1.27 - 1.41 g/ml.

[d] An endogenous DNA polymerase reaction was carried out using purified AMV as described in Procedures and Materials Used. The product was isolated and fractionated on a linear 5-20% sucrose gradient. ^{3}H-DNA migrating with 50-60S RNA was isolated, fractionated on a CS_2SO_4 gradient, and the 1.55 - 1.76 density region was pooled and recovered for S-1 assay as described.

[e] A portion of ^{3}H-labeled mammalian cell DNA was denatured by heating 5 min at 100°C and a portion remained untreated. Single-stranded ^{3}H-DNA was prepared by hydroxyapatite fractionation of the heat denatured sample and double-stranded DNA by hydroxyapatite fractionation of the untreated DNA.

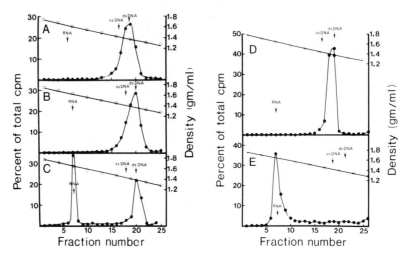

FIG. 1. Cs$_2$SO$_4$ equilibrium density-gradient analysis of the DNA polymerase nucleic acid products. T-24 and WI-38 cells were fractionated as described in Materials and Procedures, and nuclear, mitochondrial, and cytoplasmic pellets obtained. Detergent pretreatment and DNA polymerase reactions were carried out on each fraction as described in Materials and Procedures except the nuclear pellet was first sonicated 30 sec at full power using an Insonator (Ultrasonics Systems, Inc., Farmingdale, N.Y.). A DNA polymerase reaction using purified AMV was carried out as described in Procedures and Materials. Product nucleic acids were purified and analyzed on Cs$_2$SO$_4$ gradients. (A) Mitochondrial product, 2390 total cpm. (B) Nuclear product, 11,620 total cpm. (C) Cytoplasmic product, 1249 total cpm. (D) WI-38 cytoplasmic product, 28, 764 total cpm. (E) AMV endogenous DNA polymerase product, 1826 total cpm. The arrows indicate the densities of marker RNA and DNAs.

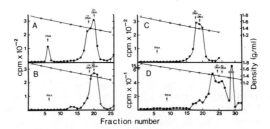

FIG. 2. Analysis of the nucleic acid products of DNA polymerase reactions of T-24 cytoplasmic particulates by nuclease treatment followed by analysis on Cs$_2$SO$_4$ gradients. A DNA polymerase reaction was carried out using the cytoplasmic fraction of T-24 cells. The purified products were divided into four equal aliquots, subjected to nuclease treatment, and analyzed directly on Cs$_2$SO$_4$ gradients. (A) Untreated. (B) Ribonuclease treatment in high-salt (30 min at 37°C in 0.12 M sodium phosphate). (C) Ribonuclease treatment in low-salt min at 37°C in 0.01 M tris-HCl (7.4), 0.01 M NaCl(20) with ribonuclease A, 20 ug/ml and ribonuclease T-1, 10 units/ml). (D) S-1 nuclease treatment.

REFERENCES

1. Baltimore, D. Viral RNA-Dependent DNA Polymerase. Nature, 226:1209-1211 1970.
2. Baxt, W.G. Sequences Present In Both Human Leukemic Cell Nuclear DNA And Rauscher Leukemia Virus. Proc. Natl. Acad. Sci. U.S.A., 71:2853-2857, 1974.
3. Baxt, W., Hehlman, R., and Spiegelman, S. Human Leukemic Cells Contain Reverse Transcriptase Associated With A High Molecular Weight Virus-Related RNA. Nature New Biology, 240:72-75, 1972.
4. Bishop, S.H.L., Ruprecht, R., Simpson, R.W., and Spiegelman, S. Deoxyribonucleic Acid Polymerase Of Rous Sarcoma Virus: Reaction Conditions And Analysis Of The Reaction Product Nucleic Acid. J. Virol., 8:730-734, 1971.
5. Bloom, E.T., Ossorio, R.C., and Brosman, S.A. Cell-Mediated Cytotoxicity Against Human Bladder Cancer. Int. J. Cancer, 14:326-334, 1974.
6. Bubernik, J., Baresova, M., Viklicky, V., Jakoubkova, J., Sainerova, H., and Donner, J. Established Cell Line Of Urinary Bladder Carcinoma. Int. J. Cancer, 11:765-773, 1973.
7. Dahlberg, J.E., Sawyer, R.C., Taylor, J.M., Faras, A.J., Levinson, W.E., Goodman, H.M., and Bishop, J.M. Transcription Of DNA From The 70S RNA Of Rous Sarcoma Virus. I. Identification Of A Specific 4S RNA Which Serves As Primer. J. Virol., 13:1126-1133, 1974.
8. Enea, V., and Zinder, N.D. Guanidinium-CsCl Density Gradients For Isopycnic Analysis of Nucleic Acids. Science, 190:584-585, 1975.
9. Fanshier, L., Garapin, A., McDonnell, J., Faras, A., Levinson, W., and Bishop, J.M. Deoxyribonucleic Acid Polymerase Associated With Avian Tumor Viruses: Secondary Structure Of The Deoxyribonucleic Acid Product. J. Virol., 7:7786, 1971.
10. Gallo, R.C., Gallagher, R.E., Miller, N.R., Mondal, H., Saxinger, W.C., Mayer, R.J., Smith, R.G., and Gillespie, D.H. Relationships Between Components In Primate RNA Tumor Viruses And In The Cytoplasm Of Human Leukemic Cells: Implications To Leukomogenesis. Cold Spring Harbor Symp. Quant. Biol., 39:933-961, 1974.
11. Gallo, R.C., Miller, N.R., Saxinger, W.C., and Gillespie, D. Primate RNA Tumor Virus-Like DNA Synthesized Endogenously By RNA-Dependent DNA Polymerase In Virus-Like Particles From Fresh Human Acute Leukemic Blood Cells. Proc. Natl. Acad. Sci. U.S.A., 70:3219-3224, 1973.
12. Garapin, A., McDonnell, J.P., Levinson, W., Quintrell, N., Fanshier, L., and Bishop, J.M. Dexoyribonucleic Acid Polymerase Associated With Rous Sarcoma Virus And Avian Myeloblastosis Virus: Properties Of The Enzyme And Its Product. J. Virol., 6:589-598, 1970.
13. Garapin, A.C., Varmus, H.E., Faras, A.J., Levinson, W.E., and Bishop, J.M. RNA-Directed DNA Synthesis By Virions Of Rous Sarcoma Virus: Further Characterization Of the Templates And Extent Of Their Transcription. Virology, 52:264-274, 1973.
14. Gerwin, B.I., Elert, P.S., Chopra, H.C., Smith, S.G., and Kvedar, J.P. DNA Polymerase Activities Of Human Milk. Science, 180:198-201, 1973.
15. Green, M. and Gerard, G.F. RNA-Directed DNA Polymerase-Properties And Functions In Oncogenic RNA Viruses And Cells. Prog. In Nucl. Acid Res. And Mol. Biol., 14:187-334, 1974.
16. Ikawa, Y., Ross, J., and Leder, P. An Association Between Globin Messenger RNA And 60S RNA Derived From Friend Leukemia Virus. Proc. Natl. Acad. Aci. U.S.A., 71:1154-1158, 1974.
17. Kang, C., and Temin, H. Endogenous RNA-Directed DNA Polymerase Activity

In Uninfected Chicken Embryos. Proc. Natl. Acad. Sci. U.S.A., 69:1550-1554, 1972.

18. Keller, W. RNA-Primed DNA Synthesis In Vitro. Proc. Natl. Acad. Sci. U.S.A. 691560-1564, 1972.

19. Mak, R.W., Manaster, J., Howatson, A.F., McCullogh, E.A., and Till, J.E. Particles With Characteristics Of Leukoviruses In Cultures Of Marrow Cells From Leukemic Patients In Remission And Relapse. Proc. Natl. Acad. Sci. U.S.A., 71:4336-4340, 1974.

20. Manly, K.F., Smoler, D.F., Bromfeld, E., and Baltimore, D. Forms Of Deoxyribonucleic Acid Produced By Virions Of Ribonucleic Acid Tumor Viruses. J. Virol., 7:106111, 1971.

21. Reitz, M.S., Smith, M.G., Roseberry, E.A., and Gallo, R.C. DNA-Directed And RNA-Primed DNA Synthesis In Microsomal And Mitochondrial Fractions Of Normal Human Lymphocytes. Biochem. Biophys. Res. Comm., 57:934948, 1974.

22. Robert, M.S., Smith, R.G., Gallo, R.C., Sarin, P., and Arbell, J.W. Viral and Cellular DNA Polymerase: Comparison Of Activities With Synthetic And Natural Templates. Science, 176:798-800, 1972.

23. Schlom, J., and Spiegelman, S. Simultaneous Detection Of Reverse Transcriptase And High Molecular Weight RNA Unique To Oncogenic RNA Viruses. Science, 174:840-843, 1971.

24. Spiegelman, S., Burny, A., Das, M.R., Keydar, J., Schlom, J., Travnicek, M., and Watson, K. Characterization Of The Products Of RNA-Directed DNA Polymerases In Oncogenic Viruses. Nature, 227:563-567, 1970.

25. Sugino, A., Susumu, H., and Okazaki, R. RNA-Linked Nascent DNA Fragments In Escherichia Coli. Proc. Natl. Acad. Sci. U.S.A., 69:1863-1867, 1972.

26. Sutton, W.D. A Crude Nuclease Preparation Suitable For Use In DNA Reassociation Experiments. Biochim. Biophys. Act., 240:522-531, 1971.

27. Taylor, J.M., and Illmensee, R. Site On The RNA Of An Avian Sarcoma Virus At Which Primer Is Bound. J. Virol., 16,553-558, 1975.

28. Taylor, J.M., Illmensee, R., Trusal, L.R., and Summers, J. Transcription Of Avian Sarcoma Virus RNA, in press.

29. Temin, H.M., and Mizutani, S. RNA-Dependent DNA Polymerase In Virions Of Rous Sarcoma Virus. Nature, 226:1211-1213, 1970.

30. Todaro, G.J., and Gallo, R.C. Immunological Relationship Of DNA Polymerases From Human Acute Leukemia Cells And Primate And Mouse Leukemic Virus. Nature, 244:206-209, 1973.

31. Williams, A.E., and Vinograd, J. The Buoyant Behavior Of RNA And DNA In Cesium Sulfate Solutions Containing Dimethylsulfoxide Biochim. Biophys. Acta., 228:423-439, 1971.

RNA TURNOVER AFTER TRYPTOPHAN OR NICOTINAMIDE LOADING IN BLADDER CANCER PATIENTS

Henrik Rist Nielsen and
Hans Wolf

Department of Clinical Chemistry,
Sundby Hospital and Department of
Urology, Gentofte Hospital,
Copenhagen, Denmark

INTRODUCTION

Many cancer patients including patients with bladder cancer have elevated urinary excretion of nucleic acid catabolites such as β-aminoisobutyric acid (β-AIB) (12), originating from both DNA- and tRNA-thymine (11, 12), as well as methylated purines and pseudo-uridine (Ψrd) (9), which are found in RNA and particularly abundant in tRNA. The methylated bases such as 7-methylguanine (m^7G) as well as Ψrd are synthesized after the macromolecule is formed, and are not reincorporated after the metabolic breakdown of the macromolecule (2), but are excreted unchanged in the urine (4, 16). Thus the excretion of these substances reflects RNA turnover.

In some bladder cancer patients it has been demonstrated that abnormalities of tryptophan metabolism occur (18). Urinary catabolites of tryptophan such as kynurenine, acetylkynurenine and 3-hydroxyanthranilic acid, representing endogenous aromatic amines, have been suggested to play a role in bladder carcinogenesis (17). During a comparative study of tryptophan metabolism, including loading with tryptophan, and urinary excretion of nucleic acid catabolites in bladder cancer patients, an unexpected decrease of Ψrd excretion was observed after tryptophan loading, see fig. 3 (13).

In the present communication, this original finding is extended to m^7G. In addition, data obtained before and after loading with nicotinamide, a catabolite of tryptophan, are reported as an approach to the evaluation of the effect of tryptophan loading on RNA turnover.

II. MATERIALS AND METHODS

A. Urine Collection

Twenty-four-hr urine samples were collected for quantitative determination of nucleic acid catabolites. The urine samples were stored without a preservative at -2o°C until examination. No dietetic restrictions were imposed. Samples were collected on two consecutive basal days, on two 24-hr periods before and after an oral L-tryptophan load of 2 g, and also following an oral nicotinamide load of 5o mg q.i.d. There was at least 2 weeks between each collection period.

B. Patients

Twelve patients with bladder cancer were included in these studies, 11 of these had recurrent low grade bladder tumors treated surgically. One patient had received radiotheraphy more than 6 months before study. Seven of these patients had abnormally high urinary excretion af nucleic acid catabolites, and when studied on more than one occasion, the increased urinary excretion remained high on all occasions.

C. Urinary β-AIB, Ψrd, m^7G and Urate

β-AIB was isolated by thin-layer chromatography on silica gel of the dinitrophenylderivate and quantitated spectrophotometrically (1o). Ψrd and m^{7}G were isolated by 2-dimensional thin-layer chromatography on silica gel with fluorescein indicator and quantitated UV-spectrophotometrically as described elsewhere (12). The assay of m^{7}G was modified by application of 1oo μl instead of 5o μl and by using micro-cuvette resulting in 4 times higher concentration in the sample compared to the original method. The excretion of urate was determined by using a uricase-UV method modified from the originally described method (14).

III. RESULTS

In table I the 24-hr urinary excretion of β-AIB, Ψrd, m^{7}G and urate on two consecutive basal days and before and after tryptophan or nicotinamide loading is presented. Changes in β-AIB and urate excretion following tryptophan or nicotina-mide loading did not differ significantly compared to the variation of β-AIB and urate excretion on two control days. However, as illustrated in figs. 1 and 2 it was found that Ψrd and m^{7}G were excreted in significantly lower levels following tryptophan or nicotinamide loading compared to the consecutive control days. This may indicate decreased RNA turnover as mentioned above.

IV. DISCUSSION

Loading doses of tryptophan or nicotinamide, a catabolite of tryptophan, were both shown to decrease urinary excretion of Ψrd and m^{7}G, indicating decreased RNA turnover following tryptophan or nicotinamide administration. The unchanged excretion of β-AIB and urate after tryptophan or nicotinamide loading, may be due to the fact that their precursors, thymine and purines respectively are present in both RNA and DNA, and may be reutilized, whereas Ψrd and m^{7}G are present in RNA only and can not be reutilized.
In a preliminary report (13), we have demonstrated (fig. 3) that the decrease in urinary Ψrd following tryptophan load

29

was only seen in patients with elevated Ψrd excretion on the basal day. This was also found in the present study (table I). Dietary tryptophan or nicotinamide as well as loading doses of tryptophan or nicotinamide are partly converted to N-methylnicotinamide and N-methyl-2-pyridone-5-carboxamide (2-pyridone). The methyl groups for N-methylnicotinamide and 2-pyridone formation originate from the SAM-pool (5), which also is the methyl donor for the methylation of bases of RNA (8). Thus, it is possible that increased formation of N-methylnicotinamide and 2-pyridone following tryptophan or nicotinamide load may interfere with methylation of RNA by depleting the SAM-pool probably resulting in a methyl-deficient RNA being synthesized. In addition to the elevated excretion of RNA components, such as methylated purines and Ψrd as well as β-AIB from tRNA thymine, in tumor bearing animals and cancer patients, tRNA methyltransferase activities have been shown to be elevated in a wide range of tumors of both human and animal origin (1). Furthermore, a competing enzyme system, glycine-N-methyltransferase, has been shown to be very low or absent in a number of tumor tissues (6, 7). Other workers found absence of an inhibitor of tRNA methyltransferases from Walker 256 carcinoma, and this inhibitor was shown to be nicotinamide (5), which inhibited tRNA methyltransferases in crude extracts from a number of rodent and human tumors (3).

On the other hand it has been shown that dietary tryptophan deficiency results in a change in the ribosome profile from polysomes towards monosomes (15). The reverse is seen with administration of tryptophan (15). However, the available data have no indication of the possible effect on RNA degradation.

Therefore, with our present data no definite resolution can yet be made as to the causal mechanism for the observed

decrease in urinary Ψrd and m^{7}G excretion following tryptophan or nicotinamide loading in bladder cancer patients,
whether this observation is due to a decreased turnover of
tRNA and/or other RNA's.

V. SUMMARY

In a comparative study of tryptophan metabolism and urinary
excretion of nucleic acid derivatives, including β-aminoisobutyric acid, 7-methylguanine, pseudouridine and urate in 12
male bladder cancer patients, it was found that the excretion
of pseudouridine and 7-methylguanine decreased significantly
following an oral dose of 2 g L-tryptophan. Since urinary
pseudouridine and 7-methylguanine are reflecting RNA turnover,
these data may indicate a decreased RNA turnover after
tryptophan load in bladder cancer patients. Several intermediary metabolites are formed from tryptophan including
nicotinamide, which is further converted to N-methylnicotinamide and N-methyl-2-pyridone-5-carboxamide. A similar
decrease as following the tryptophan load was observed after
an oral nicotinamide load of 5o mg q.i.d., indicating a
possible common mode of action of tryptophan and nicotinamide.
However, from the present data no definite resolution can be
made as to the causal mechanism for the observed decrease in
RNA turnover.

ACKNOWLEDGMENT

This investigation was supported by grants from Danish
Medical Research Council j. nr. 512-4336.

patient	day	μmoles/24hr m^{7}G	mmoles/24hr ψrd	β-AIB	Urate
B	I				
	II				
C	I				
	II				
D	I	155	0.22	0.05	3.13
	II	141	0.08	0.08	4.04
E	I	67	0.27	0.16	2.68
	II	60	0.33	0.11	1.41
F	I	88	0.24	0.34	1.92
	II	104	0.31	0.32	2.11
G	I	61	0.28	0.26	2.82
	II	76	0.26	0.24	3.92
H	I				
	II				
I	I	88	0.14	0.14	2.86
	II	86	0.29	0.12	2.88
K	I	5	0.57	0.38	2.67
	II	25	0.54	0.37	2.67
M	I				
	II				
O	I	36	0.09	0.10	3.29
	II	42	0.11	0.13	3.16
P	I	60	0.09	0.17	4.65
	II	77	0.13	0.16	2.32

Table I[a]

I	BASAL DAY			I	BASAL DAY		
II	AFTER L-TRYPTOPHAN 2 g			II	AFTER NICOTINAMIDE 50 q.i.d.		

| μmoles/24hr | mmoles/24hr | | | μmoles/24hr | mmoles/24hr | | |
m^7G	ψrd	β-AIB	Urate	m^7G	ψrd	β-AIB	Urate
74	1.00	0.59	3.44	76	0.85	0.37	3.19
55	0.58	0.53	2.86	25	0.66	0.41	3.11
50	1.06	0.12	3.69	148	0.50	0.14	1.55
10	0.64	0.14	3.77	43	0.14	0.13	2.87
	0.25	0.11	2.66	40	0.22	0.09	3.22
	0.25	0.11	2.59	41	0.27	0.07	3.16
49	0.41	0.28	2.60	58	0.36	0.08	2.44
36	0.41	0.27	3.50	59	0.30	0.07	4.51
70	0.61	0.35	2.76	91	0.34	0.52	3.46
34	0.31	0.34	2.92	54	0.20	0.33	2.62
68	0.45	0.25	3.04	58	0.44	0.16	2.83
60	0.25	0.23	2.74	37	0.26	0.23	3.74
27	0.27	0.87	2.18	75	0.16	0.60	2.82
35	0.36	0.90	2.12	61	0.24	0.75	3.08
	0.27	0.14	3.06	63	0.22	0.10	2.59
	0.15	0.16	2.46	36	0.12	0.10	2.79
80	0.58	0.73	2.62	47	0.94	0.76	1.74
38	0.53	0.69	2.03	44	0.86	0.66	2.80
49	0.56	0.33	4.20	88	0.47	0.41	3.01
16	0.23	0.24	3.15	80	0.32	0.28	3.38

[a]Abbreviations used: m^7G, 7-methylguanine; ψrd, pseudouridine; β-AIB, β-aminoisobutyric acid.

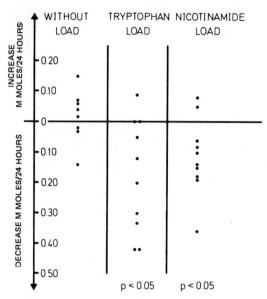

FIG. 1. Changes in urinary excretion of pseudouridine expressed as mmoles/
24 hr on two consecutive days (without load) compared with changes in
urinary excretion of pseudouridine expressed as mmoles/24 hr before and
after an oral loading dose of 2 g L-tryptophan (tryptophan load), and
before and during the administration of an oral dose of 50 mg nicotinamide
q.i.d. (nicotinamide load) in 12 male bladder cancer patients. P-Values
are calculated according to the Wilcoxon rank sum test.

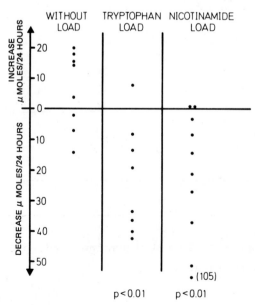

FIG. 2. Changes in urinary excretion of 7-methylguanine expressed as
μmoles/24 hr on two consecutive days (without load) compared with changes
in urinary excretion of 7-methylguanine expressed as μmoles/24 hr before
and after an oral loading dose of 2 g L-tryptophan (tryptophan load), and
before and during the administration of an oral dose of 50 mg nicotinamide
q.i.d. (nicotinamide load) in 12 male bladder cancer patients. P-Values
are calculated according to the Wilcoxon rank sum test.

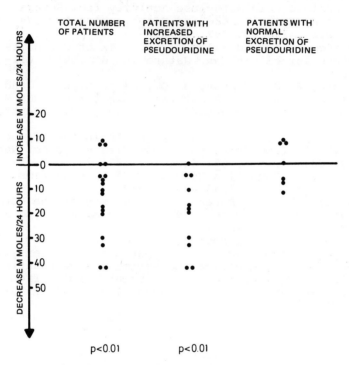

FIG. 3. Changes in urinary excretion of pseudouridine expressed as mmoles/ 24 hr after an oral loading dose of 2 g L-tryptophan in 11 male bladder cancer patients with increased basal excretion (> 0.33 mmoles/24 hr) and in 7 male bladder cancer patients with "normal" basal excretion (> 0.33 mmoles/24 hr). P-Values are calculated according to Wilcoxon's test for pair differences.

REFERENCES

1. Borek, E. Introduction to Symposium: Transfer RNA and Transfer RNA Modification in Differentiation and Neoplasia. Cancer Res., 31: 596-597, 1971.
2. Borek, E. and Kerr, S. J. Atypical Transfer RNA's and Their Origin in Neoplastic Cells. Adv. Cancer Res., 15: 163-19o, 1972.
3. Buch, L., Streeter, D., Halpern, R. M., Simon, L. N., Stout, M. G. and Smith, R. A. Inhibition of Transfer Ribonucleic Acid Methylase Activity from Several Human Tumors by Nicotinamide and Nicotinamide Analogs. Biochemistry, 11: 393-397, 1972.
4. Dlugajczyk, A. and Eiler, J. J. Lack of Catabolism of 5-Ribosyluracil in Man. Nature (Lond.), 212: 611-612, 1966.
5. Halpern, R. M., Chaney, S. Q., Halpern, B. C. and Smith, R. A. Nicotinamide: A Natural Inhibitor of tRNA Methylase. Biochem. Biophys. Res. Commun., 42: 6o2-6o7, 1971.
6. Kerr, S. J. Absence of a Natural Inhibitor of the tRNA Methylases from Fetal and Tumor Tissues. Proc. Nat. Acad. Sci. (U.S.), 68: 4o6-41o, 1971.
7. Kerr, S. J. Competing Methyltransferase Systems. J. Biol. Chem., 247: 4248-4252, 1972.
8. Mandel, L. R. and Borek, E. The Source of the Methyl Group for the Thymine of RNA. Biochem. Biophys. Res. Commun., 6: 138-14o, 1961.
9. Mrochek, J. E., Dinsmore, S. R. and Waalkes, T. P. Analytic Techniques in the Separation and Identification of Specific Purine and Pyrimidine Degradation Products of tRNA: Application to Urine Samples from Cancer Patients. J. Natl. Cancer Inst., 53: 1553-1563, 1974.
1o. Nielsen, H. R. Variability in Urinary β-Aminoisobutyric Acid and Creatinine in a Human Control Group. Dan. Med. Bull., 19: 144-147, 1972.
11. Nielsen, H. R., Borek, E., Sjølin, K.-E., and Nyholm, K. Dual Origin of β-Aminoisobutyric Acid, a Thymine Catabolite. Acta Path. Microbiol. Scand., 8o A: 687-688, 1972.
12. Nielsen, H. R., Nyholm, K. and Sjølin, K.-E. Relationship between Urinary β-Aminoisobutyric Acid and Transfer RNA Turnover in Cancer Patients. Cancer Res., 34: 3428-3432, 1974.
13. Nielsen, H. R. and Wolf, H. The Effect of Tryptophan Load on Transfer RNA Turnover in Bladder Cancer Patients. (Abstract) Scand. J. Clin. Lab. Invest., 35, suppl. 143: 73, 1975.
14. Praetorius, E. An Enzymatic Method for the Determination of Uric Acid by Ultraviolet Spectrophotometry. Scand. J. Clin. Lab. Invest., 1: 222-23o, 1949

15. Sidransky, H., Verney, E. and Sarma, D. S. R. Effect of Tryptophan on Polysomes and Protein Synthesis in Liver. Amer. J. Clin. Nutr., 24: 779-785, 1971.
16. Weissman, S., Eisen, A. Z., Lewis, M. and Karon, M. Pseudouridine Metabolism. III. Studies with Isotopically Labeled Pseudouridine. J. Lab. Clin. Med., 6o: 4o-47, 1962.
17. Wolf, H. Studies on the Role of Tryptophan Metabolites in the Genesis of Bladder Cancer. Acta Chir. Scand. Suppl., 443: 154-168, 1973.
18. Wolf, H., Brown, R. R. and Nyholm, K. K. Studies on Tryptophan Metabolism in Danish Bladder Cancer Patients. Acta Vitaminol. (Milano) in press.

DNA REPAIR IN CONDITIONS ASSOCIATED WITH MALIGNANCY: AGING AND ACTINIC KERATOSIS.

Ulrik Ringborg[1], Bo Lambert[2] and Gunnar Swanbeck[3]

Radiumhemmet[1], Department of Clinical Genetics[2]
and Department of Dermatology[3],
Karolinska Hospital,
S-104 01 Stockholm 60, Sweden

INTRODUCTION

With a decreased capacity for DNA repair, the cell appears to be more susceptible to external chemical and physical factors which are capable of introducing somatic mutations. With the discovery that in the genetic disease Xeroderma pigmentosum (2), there was a defect in DNA repair following UV-induced damage, a molecular interpretation of the genetic predisposition for malignancy appeared. It is understandable that other defects in the repair process could also give rise to the same clinical syndrome (14,9). In fact, several DNA repair mechanisms have been described (8) and defects in different steps may give rise to similar pathological lesions.

In two other genetic diseases, Fanconi's anemia (12) and Down's syndrome (10) a decreased capacity for DNA repair has been described. Both diseases are associated with an increased frequency of malignancy.

In attempting to clarify the relationship between a decreased capacity for DNA repair and malignant disease, we have studied the UV-induced DNA excision-repair process in two conditions associated with malignancy: aging and actinic keratosis. Age and malignancy are in some way linked, since most malignant diseases appear in older individuals. It has also been found that malignant disease secondary to exposure to X-rays was more frequent in higher age groups (5).

An actinic keratosis is a premalignant lesion of the epidermis in which extensive exposure of the skin to sun light is an important etiological factor *(11)*. About 12 o/o of the patients, if left untreated will develop invasive squamous cell carcinoma *(7)*.

We shall now report on a decrease in DNA excision-repair in response to UV-light that correlates with age and with the presence of actinic keratoses.

PROCEDURES AND MATERIALS

Peripheral leucocytes from 48 healthy individuals 13-94 years old were used for the study of DNA repair synthesis during aging.

Ten patients, five men and five women, 53-81 years old, with actinic keratoses were analysed. Multiple epidermal lesions were required for diagnosis and punch biopsies for histology confirmed the diagnosis in each case. Except for the presence of actinic keratoses the patients were considered healthy. Ten healthy individuals, five men and five women, in the age-range 53-80 years were control subjects.

The UV-induced DNA repair synthesis was measured according to Evans and Norman (1968). Peripheral leucocytes were obtained from 10-20 ml of fresh, heparinized venous blood. White cells from each donor were washed in phosphate buffered saline (PBS), resuspended in the same solution and aliquoted into 7 plastic Petri dishes at a cell density of about 5-10 x 10^6 cells/ 5 ml of PBS. The Petri dishes numbered 2-6 were exposed to UV-light at four doses between 3.2 - 19.2 J/m^2 while being slowly agitated to allow optimal dispersion of the cells. The Petri dishes 1 and 7 were left on the bench during the irradiation but were not exposed, and served as controls for background incorporation. The UV-light was delivered by two parallel, low-pressure Mercury vapour lamps (Philips, TUV 6 W) which produced a dose of 0.64 J/m^2/sec. Immediately after irradiation, the cells were centrifuged, and the cell pellets resuspended in 1 ml of Parker-199 medium (Flow laboratories) supplemented with 25 o/o of fetal calf serum, 125 µg of streptomycin and 125 IE of bensyl penicillin. Samples from each tube were taken for cell counting. Hydroxyurea was added to five of the tubes, including one unexposed control, for a final concentration of 10^{-2}M. Two tubes, including one unexposed control and one sample which was given 9.6 J/m^2, did not receive any hydroxyurea.

All tubes were pre-incubated for 30 minutes at 37°C before addition of ^{3}H-thymidine (5 Ci/mM, 1 mCi/ml, The Radiochemical Centre, Amersham, England) for a final concentration of 10 μCi/ml. The incubation continued for two hours and was interrupted by the addition of 1 ml of cold 10 o/o TCA to each tube. Extraction of free nucleotides took place for 30 minutes at +4°C. Two more washes in cold 5 o/o TCA were carried out. The cell pellet was then resuspended in 70 o/o ethanol and collected on a glass-fibre filter. After drying the filter at 60°C for two hours or over night, the filters were placed in scintillation vials and treated with solubiliser to release the radioactivity. Ten ml of scintillation fluid was added and the vials analysed for radioactivity in a Packard liquid scintillation spectrometer at an efficiency of about 30 o/o and a background of 20 cpm.

White cell counts from all the different individuals were within the normal range and no differences were found between the different age groups or between patients and control subjects.

RESULTS

UV-induced DNA excision-repair and aging

The effect of hydroxyurea on the incorporation of ^{3}H-thymidine into human leucocytes is shown in Table I. Hydroxyurea depressed the spontaneous DNA synthesis to about the same extent in the age groups 13-59 years and 60-94 years (9.1 versus 8.1 o/o). The difference in spontaneous DNA synthesis in the two groups was not statistical significant.

To estimate the capacity for DNA excision-repair, dose dependence of UV-induced DNA repair synthesis was studied. Leucocytes were irradiated with four different UV-doses and incubated with ^{3}H-thymidine in the presence of hydroxyurea. In Fig.1 dose-response curves for four different individuals in the age-range 20-39 years are shown. The curves level off at UV-doses above 9.6 J/m^2. The maximal incorporation shows great differences among the individuals.

The mean value for the UV-induced DNA repair synthesis at 9.6 and 19.2 J/m^2 when the background of hydroxyurea-treated, non-irradiated cells was substracted, has been used as a measure of the DNA repair capacity. In Table II the method variation is estimated by making 10 measurements on one individual. The standard deviation was 12.4 o/o of the mean value. When the same calculation was done on 48 different subjects the standard deviation was 39.5 o/o of the mean value. The difference in standard deviations was statistically significant and indicates variation in the capacity for DNA excision-repair in individuals.

In Table III the UV-induced DNA excision-repair among individuals younger than 60 years old is compared to that of individuals older than 60 years. For the UV-doses 6.4, 9.6 and 19.2 J/m^2 individuals 60-94 years old showed a statistically significant decrease in DNA repair synthesis compared to individuals 13-59 years old.

In Fig.2 a correlation analyses of the UV-induced DNA excision-repair synthesis by age is seen (r =-0.41, p$<$0.005). The average DNA repair capacity decreases by about 30 o/o between 20- 90 years of age.

UV-induced DNA excision-repair in patients with actinic keratosis.

Leucocytes from patients with actinic keratoses and from healthy controls of the same age-range were irradiated with four different UV-doses, and incubated in the presence of 10^{-2}M hydroxyurea and ^{3}H-thymidine for two hours. The incorporated radioactivity at each dose level for all subjects is shown in Fig. 3 together with the group mean values. In both groups the incorporation levels off at UV-doses above 9.6 J/m^2. The average amount of incorporated radioactivity is 25-30 o/o less for patients with actinic keratoses compared to the control subjects at all UV-doses given. The individual variation is great, however, and there is a considerable overlap in repair activities between subjects of the two groups.

For statistical analyses of differences between DNA excision-repair synthesis in patients with actinic keratoses and control subjects, the UV-induced DNA repair synthesis was calculated for each individual. The values and the results of the statistical treatment are shown in Table IV. According to both t-test and the Wilcoxon parameter-free rank test the UV-induced DNA repair synthesis is significantly lower (p$<$ 0.02) in leucocytes from patients with actinic keratoses when compared to normal subjects.

DISCUSSION

Great variations in DNA excision-repair synthesis were found when
48 healthy subjects in the age-range 13-94 years were studied. By repeated measurements on one individual, an estimation of the methodo-
logical variation showed a standard deviation of 12.4 o/o of the value.
Since the variation among individuals was considerably greater, we conclude it to be of biological origin.

A decreased capacity for DNA excision-repair synthesis was found
in higher ages, the capacity at 90 years being about 30 o/o less when
compared to that at 20 years. The peripheral leucocytes are a heterogeneous cell population with small, but variable amounts of cells in S-
phase. Since UV-light inhibits the replicative DNA synthesis as well as
induces repair synthesis, it is essential to exclude the replicative
DNA synthesis for proper estimation of the repair synthesis. This was
effectively done with hydroxyurea, which inhibits the replication synthesis (4).

An estimation of the relative amount of lymphocytes in the leucocyte preparation used did not reveal any differences between the age
groups or between patients with actinic keratoses and normal subjects.
We also plotted the DNA repair synthesis against the lymphocyte counts,
but no correlation was found. We therefore conclude that the decrease of
DNA excision-repair synthesis with increasing age and in patients with
actinic keratoses is not dependent on heterogeneity in cell populations,
but rather on different activity of DNA repair enzymes.

Reduced DNA repair synthesis in UV-induced lesions has been
found in fibroblasts and lymphocytes of patients with Xeroderma pigmentosum (3, 1), in fibroblasts of patients with Fanconi's anemia (12) and
in lymphocytes of patients with Down's syndrome (10). These conditions
are also associated with an increased incidence of malignant disease,
suggesting a possible relationship between a decreased capacity for DNA
repair and malignancy. If damage introduced into the DNA is not effectively repaired, an accumulation of DNA lesions should lead to an increased risk of somatic mutations and malignant transformation. The results in this paper are in accord with this hypothesis.

Whether a reduction of 30 o/o in the capacity for DNA repair would increase the susceptibility for somatic mutations very much is impossible to answer. The way the lesions are introduced is probably of great importance. If a decrease in proper DNA repair is an etiological factor for malignancy in general, one would expect minor deviations from the normal repair capacity to increase the risk for neoplastic transformation. Since about 25 o/o of the population aquire neoplastic diseases, about 25 o/o of the investigated 48 healthy individuals are candidates for malignant diseases. The DNA repair values for these individuals, however, cannot be less than about 50 o/o of the mean value.

We have studied only one part of the DNA repair mechanisms. On the other hand, excision repair is regarded as a defense against mutation and probably also against carcinogenesis (13). As a working hypothesis we suggest, that the decreased DNA repair capacity with age is responsible for the increased risk for malignancy in higher ages. For most neoplastic diseases the incidence is proportional to the fifth or sixth power of the age with an increase of the incidence of 2^5 or 2^6 when the age is doubled (5). Such a relationship may be caused by an accumulation of somatic mutations during a long time or an increased frequency of somatic mutations by age. Our results give some support for the latter possibility.

We also consider the reduced DNA repair synthesis to be an important etiological factor in the development of actinic keratoses along with other factors like individual pigmentation and degree and duration of sun exposure.

SUMMARY

The UV-induced DNA excision-repair synthesis was measured in human leucocytes from 48 healthy individuals in the age-range 13-94 years. Great variations among individuals were observed and considered to be biological in origin. The DNA repair synthesis was significantly lower in individuals 60-94 years old when compared to that in individuals 13-54 years old. About a 30 o/o decrease in the repair synthesis was observed between 20-90 years of age.

Ten patients with actinic keratoses were compared to ten healthy subjects of corresponding age with regard to UV-induced DNA repair synthesis in peripheral leucocytes. The patients with actinic keratoses showed a 30 o/o decrease in the capacity for DNA repair synthesis when compared to the controls.

Most malignant diseases develop in higher age groups and about 12 o/o of the untreated patients with actinic keratoses will develop invasive, squamous cell carcinoma. The possibility that the reduced capacity for DNA repair in these two conditions predisposes an individual to malignant diseases is discussed.

ACKNOWLEDGEMENT

We thank Eva Grafström and Kerstin Hansson for excellent technical assistance, and Monica Antonsson and Ingrid Volny for preparing the illustrations. The work was supported by grants from King Gustav V Jubilee Fund, Stockholm, the Swedish Medical Research Council and Finsen Stiftelsen.

Table I.

THE EFFECT OF HYDROXYUREA (HU) ON THE INCORPORATION OF ^{3}H-THYMIDINE INTO NON-IRRADIATED HUMAN LEUCOCYTES IN INDIVIDUALS 13-59 AND 60-94 YEARS OLD.

SUBJECTS	Incorporation of ^{3}H-thymidine (cpm/10^{6} cells $\pm$ SD)	
	No HU	10^{-2}M HU
13-59 years (n=30)	1043 $\pm$ 518	95 $\pm$ 41
60-94 years (n=17)	830 $\pm$ 438	67 $\pm$ 25

Table II.

EXAMINATION OF THE VARIATION IN DNA EXCISION-REPAIR SYNTHESIS AMONG INDIVIDUALS.

	UV-INDUCED DNA REPAIR SYNTHESIS (cpm/10^{6} leucocytes)
Mean value $\pm$ SD for 48 subjects	994 $\pm$ 393
Mean value $\pm$ SD for 10 repeated measurements on one individual	893 $\pm$ 111

$p < 0.001$ according to analyses of variance quotients (F-test)

Table III.

COMPARISON OF THE UV-INDUCED DNA EXCISION-REPAIR SYNTHESIS IN HUMAN LEUCOCYTES FROM INDIVIDUALS 13-59 AND 60-94 YEARS OLD.

Age	Number	Incorporation of ^{3}H-thymidine (cpm/10^6 leucocytes $\pm$ SD) at different UV-doses (J/m^2)				
		3.2	6.4	9.6	19.2	mean value of 9.6 and 19.2
13-59 years	30	828 ± 293	970 ± 343	1101 ± 444	1114 ± 399	1108 ± 415
60-94 years	18	676 ± 241	731 ± 287	767 ± 272	873 ± 305	805 ± 269
T-test		t = 1.85	t + 2.48	t = 2.88	t = 2.49	t = 2.76
		p < 0.1	p < 0.02	p < 0.01	p < 0.02	p < 0.01

Table IV.

UV-INDUCED DNA REPAIR SYNTHESIS IN LEUCOCYTES FROM PATIENTS WITH ACTINIC KERATOSES AND CONTROL SUBJECTS: STATISTICAL ANALYSIS.

Subjects		UV-induced DNA-repair synthesis (cpm/10^6 cells)[*]		Rank
Sex	Age	Controls	Actinic keratoses	No
f	58	1 560		1
m	71		1 145	2
f	61	1 028		3
m	80	1 025		4
m	62	991		5
m	59	971		6
f	62	872		7
m	60		862	8
f	81		852	9
m	77	820		10
m	62	774		11
f	53	761		12
f	62	692		13
f	78		672	14
f	68		668	15
f	53		605	16
m	70		568	17
m	67		516	18
m	74		409	19
f	53		389	20

Mean incorporation
$\pm$ S.D.   949 $\pm$ 245   669 $\pm$ 231
                        $0.01 < p < 0.02$[**]

Sum of rank numbers   72   138
                        $0.01 < p < 0.02$[***]

[*]Mean of the incorporated activity at the two highest UV-doses (9.6 and 19.2 J/m^2) minus the hydroxyurea-inhibited background activity (0 J/m^2).

[**] Level of significance according to t-test.

[***]Level of significance according to Wilcoxon's rank test.

48

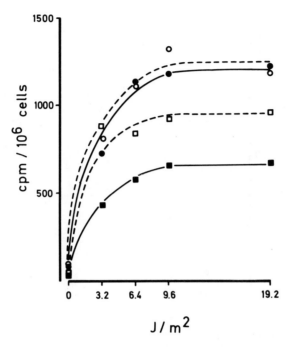

FIG. 1. UV-induced DNA excision-repair synthesis in human leucocytes.
Dose-response curves for four different individuals in the age range
20-39 years. The cells were irradiated with different UV-doses, preincubated for 30 min with 10^{-2} M hydroxyurea, and subsequently incubated for
2 hr in the presence of 10 μCi/ml of [^{3}H]thymidine and hydroxyurea.

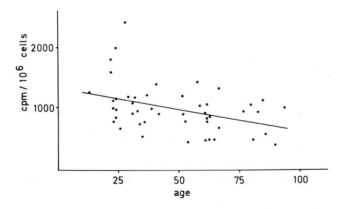

FIG. 2. A correlation analysis of UV-induced DNA excision-repair synthesis
in human leucocytes and age of the donors. (r = -0.41, n = 48, p > 0.005).

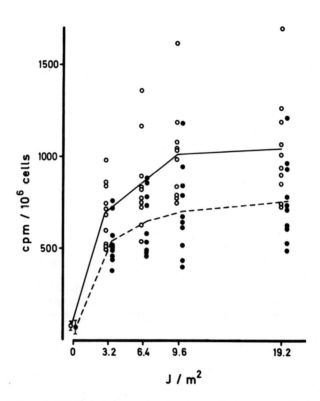

FIG. 3. UV-induced DNA repair synthesis in peripheral leucocytes from patients with actinic keratoses (●) and from control subjects (o). The cells were irradiated at various UV-doses, preincubated for 30 min with 10^{-2} M hydroxyurea, and subsequently incubated for 2 hr in the presence of 10 μCi/ml of [^{3}H]thymidine and hydroxyurea. The solid line connects the group mean values of controls at each UV-dose, and the broken line represents the group mean values of patients with actinic keratoses.

50

REFERENCES

1. Burk,P.G.,Yuspa,S.H.,Lutzner,M.A., and Robbins,J.H. Xeroderma pigmentosum and DNA repair. Lancet 1:601, 1971.

2. Cleaver,J.E. Defective repair of DNA in Xeroderma pigmentosum. Nature 218:652-656, 1968.

3. Cleaver,J.E. Xeroderma pigmentosum: a human disease in which an initial stage of DNA repair is defective. Proc.Natl.Acad.Sci.,USA 63:428-435, 1969.

4. Cleaver,J.E. Repair replication of mammalian cell DNA: Effects of compounds that inhibit DNA synthesis or dark repair. Radiat.Res. 37:334-348, 1969.

5. Doll,R. Age differences in susceptibility to carcinogenesis in man. Brit.J.Radiol. 35:31-36, 1962.

6. Evans,R.G., and Norman,A. Radiation stimulated incorporation of thymidine into the DNA of human lymphocytes. Nature 217:455-456, 1968.

7. Graham,J.H., and Helwig,E.B. Premalignant cutaneous and mucocutaneous diseases. In: Dermal Pathology. Eds.: J.H.Graham, W.C. Johnsson and E.B.Helwig. New York, pp 561-624, 1972.

8. Howard-Flanders,P. DNA repair and recombination. Brit.Med.Bull. 29:226-235, 1973.

9. Kraemer,K.H.,Coon,H.G.,Petinga,R.A.,Barrett,S.F.,Rahe,A.E., and Robbins,J.H. Genetic heterogeneity in Xeroderma pigmentosum: complementation groups and their relationship to DNA repair rates. Proc. Natl.Acad.Sci.,USA 72:59-63, 1975.

10. Lambert,B.,Hansson,K.,Bui,T.H.,Funes-Cravioto,F.,Lindsten,J.,Holmberg, M., and Strausmanis,R. DNA repair and frequency of X-ray and UV-light induced chromosome aberrations in leucocytes from patients with Down's syndrome. Ann.Hum.Genet.,London 39:393-403,1975.

11. Pinkus,H. Epithelial neoplasms and precancerous lesions. In: Derma-
    tology of General Medicine. Eds.: Th.B. Fitzpatrick, K.A. Arndt, W.
    H. Clark, A.Z. Eisen, E.J. van Scott and J.H. Vaughan. New York,
    pp 399-407, 1971.

12. Poon,P.K.,O'Brien,R.L., and Parker,J.W. Defective DNA repair in
    Fanconi's anemia. Nature 250:223-225, 1974.

13. Strauss,B.S. Repair of DNA in mammalian cells. Life Sciences 15:1685
    -1693,1975.

14. de Weerd-Kastelein,E.A.,Keijzer,W., and Bootsma,D. Genetic hetero-
    geneity of Xeroderma pigmentosum demonstrated by somatic cell hybri-
    dization. Nature New Biology 238:80-83, 1972.

ALTERED CONTROL OF TRANSCRIPTION DURING TUMOR PROGRESSION

Ruth Whisler Shearer
Issaquah Group for Health
and Environmental Research
Issaquah, Washington

I. INTRODUCTION

Eucaryotic DNA consists largely of short sequences of repetitive DNA interspersed between longer sequences of unique-sequence DNA (Lewin, 1975; Pays and Ronsse, 1975). Repetitive DNA consists of families of genes of related but not identical base sequence which can recognize each other as complements in the molecular hybridization assay done in conditions of specificity such that there is no cross-reaction between mammalian and bacterial DNA. Each molecule of the large pre-messenger RNA of eucaryotic nuclei contains tran- scripts of both repetitive and unique-sequence DNA, as does polysomal RNA (Spradling, et al, 1974). RNA transcripts of the repetitive fraction are thought to be involved in the regulation of the transcripts of the single-copy genes which code for proteins (Georgiev, 1969).

Cancer is a disorder of cellular control mechanisms at the molecular level. Since no structurally abnormal gene product has been associated with malignant transformation (Anderson and Coggin, 1974), it is necessary to look for changes in the regulatory genes which could cause the observed reprogramming of the synthesis of various structurally-normal proteins.

No repression or derepression of repetitive gene families in primary rat hepatomas or their early transplants can be detected (Shearer, 1974; Shearer and Smuckler, 1971) using the competitive hybridization assay which is a sensitive detector of qualitative differences between RNAs transcribed from different gene families. However, that technique does

not assay differences within the families of related and
cross-hybridizing base sequences.

II.   PROCEDURES AND MATERIALS USED

A.   Theory

Differences in the fraction of members of the active
gene families which are being transcribed can be detected by
a new "Walking T_m" technique, which utilizes the reversibility
of the hybridization reaction of RNA with related but noniden-
tical DNA sequences. A very small amount of isolated repetitive DNA labeled to very high specific activity is incubated
with a large amount of RNA for a short time, and the hybrid
is isolated to free it of unreacted DNA (inactive genes,
complementary strands of active genes). The hybrid is then
incubated with RNA until its melting temperature ceases to
rise. During this incubation, the hybrid molecules dissociate
and reassociate into progressively more perfectly matched
combinations because the poorest matches are the least stable
and dissociate fastest.

If all members of a gene family are active, eventually
all of its DNA sequences will be covered with perfectly
complementary RNA sequences and the melting temperature will
be about three degrees below that of sheared native DNA (the
difference between RNA/DNA and DNA/DNA duplexes). If only
one member of a gene family is active, its transcripts will
cover all members of that gene family, but no amount of further
incubation will increase the stability because no better
matching RNA is available. If a fraction of the members of a
gene family are active, the melting temperature will rise a
fraction of the distance toward the melting temperature of
perfect hybrids, then plateau. The rate of reaction in the
second incubation is limited by the dissociation rate of the
mismatched duplexes.

B.   Cells

Human colon adenocarcinoma and normal human colon mucosa
were from the same patient and were obtained fresh from
surgery and immediately processed for RNA. The section of
colon within four centimeters of the tumor was not used.

Human DNA was obtained from a culture of newborn foreskin fibroblasts.

Rat liver was obtained from a four-month-old male Buffalo rat. Hepatomas were induced by chronic feeding of 0.06% 3'methyl-4-dimethylaminoazobenzene (DB tumors) or 0.03% N-2-fluorenylacetamide (FB tumor). Rat DNA was from a culture of hepatoma DB-1(5). Hepatoma DNA has been shown to be indistinguishable from liver DNA by two different hybridization assays (Shearer, 1971, Markov and Ivanov, 1975).

C.   RNA

Human RNAs were isolated from total cells. Rat RNAs were from crude preparations of nuclei. RNAs were purified by the hot phenol method (Shearer and McCarthy, 1967) and polysaccharides were removed by centrifuging at 35,000g for 40 min. Purity was determined from the spectrum of absorbance of ultraviolet light, as described previously (Shearer and Smuckler, 1971).

D.   Isotope-labeled DNA fragments

Cells in culture were labeled with 200 μCi{^{3}H}Thymidine in 10ml medium/75cm^2 of monolayer for 16 hours. Cells were removed from the flasks by scraping in cold saline, and DNA was isolated by chloroform-octanol extraction and digested with boiled RNAse. Purified DNA (250 μg/ml) was sheared by sonifying it at 4° at setting 70 on a Bronwill BP IIA with standard tip 10 seconds x 10 at 1 min intervals.

E.   Isolated DNA of active gene families

Human: Sheared DNA in 0.3M NaCl at 2.5 mg/ml was boiled 10 min and incubated at 60° for 6.5 hours. Double-stranded fragments of repetitive DNA were isolated on a hydroxylapatite column (Bio-Gel HTP, Bio·Rad) at 60° in 0.12 M phosphate buffer, eluted with 0.4 M phosphate buffer, and freed of bound bits of hydroxylapatite by batch extraction with Chelex 100 (Bio·Rad). 0.5μg of this DNA (116,500 cpm) and 5.0mg of RNA in 2.0 ml of 0.3 M NaCl were boiled, cooled to 60°, and incubated for four hours at that temperature. RNA/DNA hybrid molecules were isolated on hydroxylapatite, purified on Chelex, and dialyzed into 0.3 M NaCl. Rat:

Sheared DNA in 0.3 M NaCl at 250 µg/ml was boiled 10 min and
then incubated at 60° for 17 hours. Double-stranded fragments
of repetitive DNA were isolated and purified with hydroxylapatite and Chelex as above. 0.45 µg of this DNA (45,500 cpm)
and 4.5mg of RNA in 0.54ml of 0.3 M NaCl were boiled, cooled
to 60°, and incubated for two hours. Double-stranded molecules
were isolated by digestion with S1 nuclease (see below) and
RNAse-1 (Worthington Biochemical Corp.), and purified by warm
phenol extraction in 1% sodium dodecylsulfate.

F. Exhange of RNA in the hybrid molecules
Human: 5.0mg of RNA was added to the hybrid in 0.3M
NaCl, an equal volume of formamide (J.T. Baker Chemical Co.)
was added, and the mixture was incubated at 37° for nine
weeks. RNA concentration was 0.27mg/ml. Rat: 1.0 mg of RNA
was added to the hybrid molecules and the mixture was precipitated with two volumes of ethanol. The pellet was dried
with N_2 and resuspended in 1.0ml of 0.3 M NaCl plus 1.0ml of
formamide, and the mixture was incubated at 37°. RNA concentration was 0.5 mg/ml.

G. Thermal denaturation of hybrid molecules
Aliquots were taken during incubation and melted in 0.1M
phosphate buffer on hydroxylapatite columns. Temperatures
at five degree intervals were maintained for five minutes
with the column stopped, then 10ml of buffer was allowed to
wash through. Fractions were precipitated with trichloroacetic acid after addition of carrier RNA, filtered onto
glass-fiber filters (GF/C, Whatman Biochemicals Ltd.) and
counted in a Beckman LS-100 scintillation counter using BBOT
fluor (Beckman).

H. Saturation of unique-sequence DNA with RNA
Sheared, single-stranded, labeled rat hepatoma DNA was
eluted from hydroxylapatite in 0.12 M phosphate buffer at 60°
after incubating for 17 hr at 250 µg/ml in 0.3 M NaCl at 60°.
0.4µg of this DNA (40,000 cpm) was mixed with 4.0mg RNA in
0.43ml of 0.3 M NaCl plus 0.43ml of formamide, boiled, cooled
to 37°, and incubated at that temperature in autoclaved vials
with tight screw-caps for 54 days. 50 µl aliquots were taken
at intervals, diluted into 2.0 ml 0.3 M NaCl pH 4.6 and

digested with S1 nuclease. Double-stranded hybrid molecules remaining were precipitated with trichloroacetic acid after addition of carrier RNA, filtered onto glass-fiber filters and counted.

I. S1 nuclease preparation

S1 nuclease was prepared by a modification of the method of Vogt (Vogt, 1973). After loading the DEAE-cellulose column (DE-52, preswollen, Whatman Biochemicals Ltd.), elution was by stepwise gradient rather than linear. The column was rinsed with 100ml buffer B (Vogt, 1973), then 100ml buffer D (Like buffer B but with 0.18 M NaCl). Elution was begun with 100 ml buffer E (Like buffer B but with 0.22 M NaCl), collecting 10ml fractions, and was completed with 50ml buffer F (Like buffer B but with 0.3 M NaCl). Fractions were assayed for nuclease activity against 5,000cpm of DB-1(5) hepatoma DNA and 5000cpm of single-stranded unique-sequence DNA of DB-2E(1) hepatoma. Single-strand nuclease activity was present in all fractions of buffers E and F, but double-strand activity was also present in the first 8 fractions. The last two fractions in buffer E and all of buffer F were pooled and used as S1 nuclease.

J. S1 nuclease assay

Up to 0.1ml of the hybridization mixture to be assayed (in NaCl plus formamide or in NaCl alone) was put into 1.0ml of 0.3 M NaCl pH 4.6 containing 1 mM $ZnSO_4$. 0.2ml of S1 nuclease was added and the mixture incubated 10 minutes at 45°. Then a second 0.2ml of S1 nuclease was added and the incubation repeated. The reaction was stopped by addition of 1 drop of 0.1 M EDTA, the solution was chilled, carrier DNA was added, trichloroacetic acid was added to 5%, and the precipitate filtered onto glass-fiber filters and counted.

K. DNase assay

Pancreatic DNase I (DPFF) was purchased from Worthington Biochemical Corp. and was used in 0.01 M Tris 0.01 M $MgCl_2$ pH 7.8.

L. RNAse-H assay

Ribonuclease H (E. Coli JG112) was purchased from Miles Laboratories, Inc. 50,000 units was diluted to 1.0 ml with

0.01 M Tris 0.01M $MgCl_2$ pH 7.8.   0.1ml of hybrid in 0.3 M NaCl and formamide was diluted to 1.0ml with the same Tris-$MgCl_2$ buffer, 20µl of 0.1 M $MnCl_2$ and 5 units of RNAse-H were added, and the mixture incubated at 37° for 20 min.   The digest was diluted to 10ml with 0.12 M phosphate buffer and passed through a hydroxylapatite column at 60°.   After rinsing the column with 20ml of the same buffer, remaining double-stranded nucleic acids were eluted with 10ml of 0.4 M phosphate buffer. Carrier DNA was added to all fractions, they were precipitated with TCA, filtered and counted.

III.   RESULTS

Figure 1 demonstrates that in human colon mucosa and colon adenocarcinoma all members of the active gene families are being transcribed into RNA coordinately.   During the second incubation, the melting temperature of the hybrids increases progressively until it is at the level expected for perfectly matched hybrids, 2.5^O to 3.5^O below the level of the DNA/DNA duplexes.   Native DNA melted 0.5^O below the sheared DNA duplexes (not shown).   This probably reflects a difference in base composition between total DNA and isolated repetitive DNA.   The low melting shoulder shown at the early time points disappears later, indicating a difference in the frequency distributions of the members of different gene families.   The 1^O Tm difference between colon and tumor RNAs is unexplained.

The technique was improved to allow a higher concentration of reactants and therefore a shorter incubation time on the second incubation.   Then the experiment was repeated using rat liver and hepatoma RNAs, with the surprising result seen in Figure 2.   The melting temperature of the liver RNA/DNA hybrid continues to rise after 18 days of incubation, at which time it is 5.2^O below that of sheared native DNA, but the hepatoma RNA/DNA hybrid reaches a maximum by 13 days, 10.8^O below that of DNA, indicating that a significant fraction of the members of the gene families have been repressed.   Many more time-points were analyzed in the experiments of Figures 1 and 2, but in the interest of clarity only representative curves are shown.

The gross discrepancy in results between the human and rat tumors was puzzling, so it was decided to test a number of different hepatomas to see if only the one was unusual, since it had been transplanted 12 times. The results are shown in Figure 3. The primary hepatoma RNA melts slightly higher than the normal liver, as did the human primary colon tumor. After only two transplants, another hepatoma shows a decrease in melting temperature. After four transplants, the former primary tumor shows a decrease in melting temperature of 4.7^O, indicating that some members of the active gene families become repressed during serial transplant.

It has been suggested that the observed repression might occur much earlier, but be disguised by the presence of normal cells in the primary tumor. This is not plausible because by the second transplant any normal cells would already be diluted by a factor of at least 10^4 (0.1 ml grown to 10 ml twice), yet the second transplant does not show a gross change from the primary.

Another possible interpretation of the walking T_m is that both strands of DNA within a gene family are being transcribed, so both are present in the second incubation, and the RNA is progressively dissociated in favor of more stable DNA/DNA duplexes. This has been ruled out in both human colon and rat liver systems by enzyme sensitivity tests. The duplexes with the highest T_m are completely resistant to DNaseI and are 80 to 88% sensitive to RNAse-H, which specifically degrades the RNA strand of RNA/DNA hybrid molecules.

The low-melting shoulders evident in Figures 2 and 3 indicate that about 20% of the active repetitive DNA families in liver transcribe fewer than all of their members, or transcribe many fewer copies of some members than most. The significance of this is unknown at present. It is possible that further incubation of the liver and primary tumor RNAs would obliterate this shoulder as in the human tumor experiment.

The results of the rat liver experiments described here cannot be attributed to the presence of unique-sequence DNA attached to the repetitive DNA in the 22% isolated as double-stranded after reannealing the sheared, denatured DNA. The time of incubation with RNA ($R_{o}t$ 200) is only 1/100th of that needed to saturate the unique-sequence DNA with RNA ($R_{o}t$ 20,000, see Figure 4), so these sequences will remain single-stranded and be destroyed by the S1 nuclease step.

39% of the human DNA was isolated as repetitive. This is similar to the 35% reported by others (Saunders, et al, 1972; Grouse, et al, 1973). Since S1 nuclease was not used, this repetitive DNA could contain some attached unique-sequence DNA in the final incubation. Hybrids with this DNA could not mask the presence of incompletely transcribed gene families if such existed, but could decrease the apparent fraction of such gene families.

If the members of a repetitive gene family regulate transcription of the adjacent single-copy genes, then altered transcription of repetitive DNA should result in concomitant alteration of transcription of unique-sequence DNA. This is supported by the data of Figure 4 which show that over half of the single copy genes active in the normal liver are not being transcribed in the 12th passage hepatoma. Liver nuclear RNA saturates 10.8% of the sheared, denatured unique-sequence DNA while hepatoma DB-2E(12) nuclear RNA is complementary to only 3.3%.

Nuclear and cytoplasmic RNAs of the 12th-passage hepatoma saturate the same fraction of the unique-sequence DNA, indicating that none of the single-copy-gene transcripts are restricted to the nucleus in this tumor; RNAs which are normally nucleus-restricted are found in the tumor cytoplasm except for those which are not transcribed in the tumor. Since this tumor has already been shown to have lost the normal ability to restrict transcripts of repetitive DNA to the nucleus (Shearer and Smuckler, 1972), this is also consistent with the hypothesis that interspersed repetitive and unique-sequence DNAs are transcribed in a single large RNA molecule in which the repetitive fraction regulates the subsequent fate of the adjacent unique-sequence fraction (Georgiev, 1974).

IV. DISCUSSION

The finding that all members of a gene family transcribe the same strand of DNA is consistent with a role for each family member in recognizing the same regulator molecule in order to activate or inactivate a battery of single-copy genes coordinately (Coggin and Anderson, 1974).

This evidence that inactivation of RNA transcription is an early event in tumor progression emphasizes the desirability of using primary tumors for studying the mechanism of carcinogenesis. Previous data showed that Novikoff hepatoma, which had been transplanted hundreds of times, has lost whole gene families from transcription so that the repression is detectable by the competitive hybridization assay (Shearer and Smuckler, 1971). This may indicate random loss of functions not needed by the tumor cells for self-perpetuation, with selection for those cells which have lost more differentiated functions and can therefore devote a larger fraction of their energy and materials to rapid cell division.

Early changes during malignant transformation involve reappearance of gene products characteristic of an earlier stage of development (Manes, 1974), and can be explained by the release of stage-specific messenger RNAs from the cell nucleus in an uncontrolled manner. Changes in tumor progression involve loss of gene products normal to the mature cells, such as enzymes (Weinhouse, et al, 1972), cell surface components (Hakomori, 1975), and hormone receptors (Jensen et al, 1972), and can be explained by the repression, or failure of transcription, of many species of pre-messenger RNA.

V. SUMMARY

This study was designed to look for correlations between the pattern of transcription of unique-sequence and repetitive DNA in normal cells and tumors. A newly-developed assay of the fraction of members of active gene families which are being transcribed into RNA was used, along with an improved technique of saturation of complementary DNA sites by RNA.

61

In human colon and primary colon carcinoma, all members of the active gene families are being transcribed coordinately. This is also true of the majority of active gene families in rat liver and primary hepatoma, but transcription of members within active gene families is lost progressively during serial transplant of hepatomas.

Analysis of transcription of unique-sequence DNA in hepatomas indicates a rapid decrease in the number of single-copy genes being transcribed during serial transplant. This implies a close correlation between transcription of repeated and single-copy genes which is consistent with the known interspersion of these sequences in DNA, nuclear pre-messenger RNA, and polysomal RNA.

VI. ABBREVIATIONS

DNA: Deoxyribonucleic acid

$R_o t$: RNA concentration (moles of nucleotide/liter) x time of incubation (seconds).

$R_o t$=1 at 83 μg/ml x 1 hour

RNA: Ribonucleic acid

T_m: temperature at which 50% of double-stranded molecules have melted

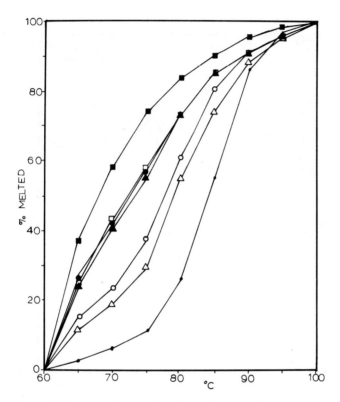

FIG. 1. Melting of human colon and colon adenocarcinoma RNAs hybridized to
isolated repetitive DNA. 0.5 μg labeled human fibroblast repetitive DNA
and 5.0 mg RNA from human colon mucosa or tumor in 2.0 ml of 0.3 M NaCl
were boiled, cooled to 60°, and incubated 4 hr. Double-stranded molecules
were isolated on hydroxylapatite, purified on Chelex, dialyzed into 0.3 M
NaCl, mixed with 5.0 mg RNA and an equal volume of formamide, and incubated at 37°. In the second incubation, RNA concentration was 0.27 mg/ml.
Melting was done in 0.1 M phosphate buffer on hydroxylapatite columns.
Recovery of repetitive DNA in double-stranded form before melting was
10.44 ± 0.86% for the mucosa and 10.65 ± 0.89% for the tumor RNA. T_{mi} of
sheared native DNA was 89°. Open symbols: mucosa. Closed symbols: tumor.
Incubation time: □ ■ 5 days; ○ ● 6 weeks; Δ ▲ 9 weeks. Dots: sheared,
boiled DNA was used instead of RNA.

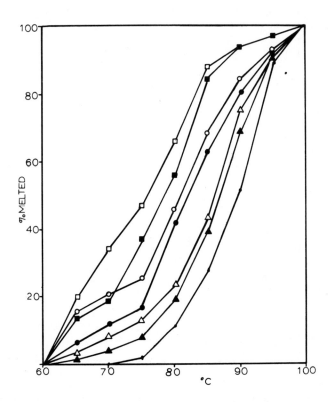

FIG. 2. Melting of rat liver and hepatoma DB-2E(12) RNAs hybridized to isolated repetitive DNA. 0.45 g labeled rat hepatoma repetitive DNA and 4.5 mg RNA from rat liver or tumor in 0.54 ml of 0.3 M NaCl were boiled, cooled to 60°, and incubated 2 hr. Double-stranded molecules were isolated by digestion with S1 nuclease and RNAse-I, and purified by warm phenol extraction in 1% sodium dodecylsulphate and precipitation from ethanol after addition of 1.0 mg of RNA. The precipitate was suspended in 1.0 ml 0.3 M naCl plus 1.0 ml formamide and incubated at 37°. Melting was done in 0.1 M phosphate buffer on hydroxylapatite columns. Open symbols: liver. Closed symbols: tumor. Incubation time: □ ■ 6 days; o ● 13 days; Δ ▲ 18 days. Dots: melt of sheared, native DNA.

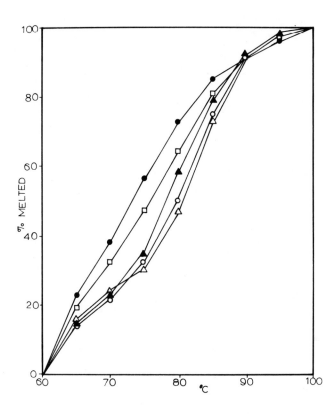

FIG. 3. Melting of rat liver and hepatoma RNAs hybridized to isolated
repetitive DNA. Conditions of Fig. 2, 18-day incubation. Recovery of
DNA in double-stranded form before melting was between 7.0 and 8.7%. T_{mi}
of sheared native DNA was 84.2°. RNAs: o liver, ● tumor DB-2E(12); □
tumor DB-6B(4); ▲ tumor FB-3(2); Δ tumor DB-6B. Numbers in ( ) indicate
number of transplants. DB tumors were induced by 3'methyl-4-dimethylamino-
azobenzene. FB tumor was induced by N-2-fluorenylacetamide.

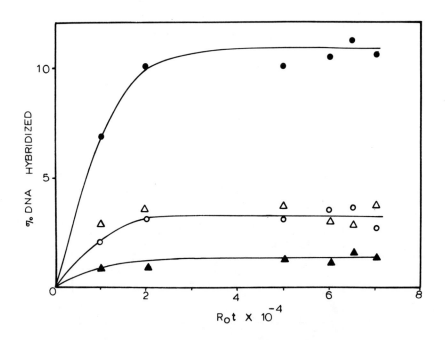

FIG. 4. Saturation of rat unique-sequence DNA with nuclear and cytoplasmic RNAs of liver and 12th-passage hepatoma. R_0t 6×10^4 was 45 days. RNAs: ● Liver nuclear, o DB-2E(12) nuclear, ▲ Liver cytoplasmic, Δ DB-2E(12) cytoplasmic.

REFERENCES

1. Anderson, N.G., and Coggin, J.H. Introduction to third conference on embryonic and fetal antigens in cancer. Cancer Res., 34: 2032-2033, 1974.

2. Coggin, J.H., and Anderson, N.G. Cancer, differentiation, and embryonic antigens: some central problems. In: Adv. in Cancer Res. Eds.: Klein, G., Weinhouse, S., and Haddow, A. Academic Press Inc., New York, 19: 105-165, 1974.

3. Georgiev, G.P. On the structural organization of operon and the regulation of RNA synthesis in animal cells. J. Theoret. Biol., 25: 473-490, 1969.

4. Georgiev, G.P. Precursor of mRNA (pre-mRNA) and ribonucleoprotein particles containing pre-mRNA. In: The Cell Nucleus. Ed.: Busch, H. Academic Press Inc., New York, Vol. III: 67, 1974.

5. Grouse, L., Omenn, G.A., and McCarthy, B.J. Studies by RNA-DNA hybridization of transcriptional diversity in human brain. J. Neurochem, 20: 1063-1073, 1973.

6. Hakomori, S. Structures and organization of cell surface glycolipids; dependency on cell growth and malignant transformation. Biochem. Biophys. Acta., 417: 55-89, 1975.

7. Jensen, E.V., Block, G.E., Smith, S., Kyser, K. and DeSombre, E.R. Estrogen receptors and hormone dependency. In: Estrogen Target Tissues and Neoplasia. Ed.: Dao, T.L. Univ. of Chicago Press, Chicago,: 23-57, 1972.

8. Lewin, B. Units of transcription and translation: sequence components of heterogeneous nuclear RNA and messenger RNA. Cell, 4: 77-93, 1975.

9. Manes, C. Phasing of gene products during development. Cancer Res., 34: 2044-2052, 1974.

10. Markov, G.G., and Ivanov, I.G. DNA and tumor progression. C.R. Acad. Bulg. Sci., 28: 1261-1264, 1975.

11. Pays, E., and Ronsse, A. Interspersion of repetitive sequences in rat liver DNA. Biochem. Biophys. Res. Commun., 62: 862-867, 1975.

12. Saunders, G.F., Shirakawa, S., Saunders, P., Arrighi, F.E., and Hsu, T.C. Populations of repeated DNA sequences in the human genome. J. Mol. Biol., 63: 323-334, 1972.

13. Shearer, R.W. DNA of rat hepatomas: Search for gene amplification. Biochem. Biophys. Res. Commun., 43: 1324-1328, 1971.

14. Shearer, R.W. Specificity of chemical modification of ribonucleic acid transport by liver carcinogens in the rat. Biochem., 13: 1764-1767, 1974.

15. Shearer, R.W., and Smuckler, E.A. A search for gene derepression in RNA of primary rat hepatomas. Cancer Res., 31: 2104-2109, 1971.

16. Shearer, R.W., and Smuckler, E.A. Altered regulation of the transport of RNA from nucleus to cytoplasm in rat hepatoma cells. Cancer Res., 32: 339-342, 1972.

17. Spradling, A., Penman, S., Camp, M.S., and Bishop, J.O. Repetitious and unique sequences in the heterogeneous nuclear and cytoplasmic messenger RNA of mammalian and insect cells. Cell, 3: 23-30, 1974.

18. Vogt, V.M. Purification and further properties of single-strand-specific nuclease from Aspergillus oryzae. Eur. J. Biochem., 33: 192-200, 1973.

19. Weinhouse, S., Shatton, J.B., Criss, W.E., Farina, F.A., and Morris, H.P. Isozymes in relation to differentiation in transplantable rat hepatomas. In: Isozymes and Enzyme Regulation in Cancer. Eds.: Weinhouse, S., and Ono, T. University Park Press, Baltimore: 1-17, 1972.

CELL CYCLE KINETICS AND CONTROL OF SOLID TUMORS IN MICE BY FRACTIONATED X-IRRADIATION

F.A. Tewfik, T.C. Evans, and E.F. Riley

Radiation Research Laboratory, University of Iowa
Iowa City, Iowa 52242

INTRODUCTION

The aim of radiotherapy, of course, is to kill the greatest number of tumor cells while sparing the normal tissues as much as possible, i.e., to increase the therapeutic ratio. To study the effects of X-irradiation on tumor growth as well as on the surrounding normal tissues, we have developed an experimental animal model for solid tumors. After injecting Ehrlich ascites carcinoma cells intramuscularly into the thigh of mice, we could irradiate the tumor bearing limb while shielding the rest of the body and then evaluate the effects produced. This model closely simulates the human radiation therapy situation.

Some pilot studies had been done in our laboratory to determine the minimal dose and the optimal time between fractionated exposures to get: (1) maximal tumor control and (2) minimal normal tissue damage. These pilot studies indicated that 2400 R was the lowest total exposure that satisfied the two conditions. The aim of the present study was to utilize a total exposure of 2400 R and to compare the influence of different exposure increments and different intervals between fractionated exposures on both normal tissues and tumor control.

PROCEDURES AND MATERIALS

Experimental Animals and the Induction of Tumors

Ehrlich carcinoma was maintained in the ascitic form by weekly intraperitoneal injections of 4.0×10^6 tumor cells into Swiss female mice from our closed colony. CF_1 female mice between the ages of 8 and 12 weeks were used to induce Ehrlich carcinoma in the solid form by injecting 1.6×10^6 cells intramuscularly into the right thigh. After injection, mice were numbered by toe clipping.

Tumor growth was determined by daily measurements of the tumor bearing limb using vernier calipers. The skin reactions of the irradiated feet were also recorded daily after the first dose of radiation and continued until the end of the experiment.

Irradiation Procedures

Irradiation of tumor bearing limbs was carried out with a G.E. Maxitron 250 operated at 250 kVp, 30 mA, with 1/4 mm Cu and 1.0 mm Al added filtration (HVL = 1.0 mm Cu). The distance from the target to the tumor was 55 cm. The exposure rate in air, measured with a Victoreen condenser R-meter and thimble chanber, was approximately 80 R/minute.

Groups of 10 mice were irradiated 2-3 days after tumor implantation. A jig was custom made to reproducibly irradiate each group. It consisted of 10 small lead boxes arranged in a circle on a board. Each box had a small hole on one side. One mouse was placed in each box, the right leg was pulled out through the hole, and the foot was taped to the board. The jib was then placed on a turntable and rotated during irradiation. Mice were not anesthetized for the irradiation procedures. Control groups were sham irradiated. Exposures of 2400 R were given to the tumor bearing leg as follows:

    (a) 6 exposures of 400 R each (400 R x 6) given every 6, 12, 24, or 48 hours

    (b) 4 exposures of 600 R each (600 R x 4) given every 6, 12, or 24 hours

    (c) 3 exposures of 800 R each (800 R x 3) given every 24 hours

    (d) a single exposure of 2400 R (2400 R x 1)

Kinetics of Tumor Cells

To study DNA synthesis, tritiated thymidine (^{3}H-TdR, Amersham/Searle, 5 Ci/mmole) was given intratumorly using a microliter syringe. At the appropriate time after ^{3}H-TdR injection, animals were sacrificed, tumors were excised and sectioned in two perpendicular planes, and the cut surfaces were used to make touch prints on subbed slides (3). Slides were then fixed 5 minutes in 3:1 methanol:acetic acid, rinsed in distilled water for 5 minutes, and allowed to air dry. If slides were to be used for scoring mitotic index, the touch prints were then stained in Harris-Lillie hematoxylin and coverslipped using Permount. For the determination of labeling index or the percent labeled mitoses, autoradiographs were prepared by dipping the slides in liquid photographic emulsion (Eastman Kodak NTB). After exposure for 3 weeks in light-tight boxes at 4°C, slides were developed using Kodak D-11. The prints were then stained as described before.

A minimum of 1000 cells were counted to determine the mitotic index (MI) or the labeling index (LI) for each animal. One hundred mitotic figures were scored per animal for each determination of the percent labeled mitoses (PLM). To derive PLM data, 15 μCi of ^{3}H-TdR were injected once immediately after irradiation. The mice were then sacrificed to get samples of tumors at regular intervals of 1-4 hours thereafter. To determine the LI at various times after irradiation, 3 mice were pulse labeled (15 μCi of ^{3}H-TdR) at each 2 hour interval from 0 to 30 hours post-irradiation and sacrificed 2 hours later (7, 9).

RESULTS

Growth Characteristics of Solid Tumors

Ehrlich carcinoma cells grown intramuscularly have very reproducible growth properties in our laboratory. The tumor grown exponentially in the first week after implantation and then slows down with time (8). Cell cycle parameters were determined by the percent labeled mitoses technique (10). Experimental data were analyzed by a computer, using a polynomial regression equation, to derive the curve that best fit the experimental data. In the solid form, the average duration of the cell cycle, G_1, S, G_2, and M periods were 16, 2, 10, 3, and 1.5 hours, respectively. The slowing down of tumor growth with time was mainly due to a decrease in the growth fraction and an increase in cell loss. Tannock (11) and Frindel et al. (5) reported that the duration of G_1, S, G_2, and M remained relatively constant regardless of the size of the tumor.

For our tumor model, tumor weight could be determined from a calibration curve correlating the tumor weight with the diameter of the tumor bearing limb.

Table I shows the tumor response to various schemes of irradiation using the same total exposure and varying the dose increments and time interval between fractionated exposures.

The 400 R x 6 given every 24 hours gave the best tumor control (0% tumor survival). It was found that the mean skin reaction decreases as the time interval between exposures increases.

The growth rate of the individual tumors in each group following 0 R, 2400 R x 1 or 400 R x 6 every 6, 12, or 24 hours is shown in Figs. 1-5 respectively. The arrows indicate the time of exposures.

During the first week of treatment, the tumors in the control group continued to grow and reached an average weight equal to about 1.7 times the average weight at the start of the treatment. Three control tumors regressed during the second and third weeks and then resumed growth during the fourth week.

When the treatment was applied as a single exposure or every 6 hours, a small weight decrease was observed during the first and second week. Growth was resumed in the third week after treatment in those tumors that survived. Another tumor started to grow in the single exposure group on day 45.

When the treatment was applied every 12 or 24 hours, the tumor continued to grow slowly during the first 2 weeks. Then a distinct tumor regression was observed during the third week. All of the tumors regressed completely by the end of the third week except one tumor in the 12 hour group that did not respond to X-irradiation and a second tumor that began to grow about 4 weeks post-irradiation.

Fig. 6 summarizes the percent tumor survival as a function of the time interval between fractionated exposures. When the time interval between fractions was increased to 48 hours, the tumor survival showed an increase. In fact, it was greater than the single exposure group (Table I).

71

In an attempt to explain why this scheme, 400 R x 6 every 24 hours, gave the best tumor control, mitotic and labeling indices were determined after 400 R to the tumor bearing limb. The mitotic activity dropped to zero 1.5 hours after irradiation (Fig. 7) and the mitotic inhibition lasted for a period of about 4 hours. At about 8 hours, the mitotic activity returned to control values and at 24 hours after irradiation, the mitotic activity was almost double the control values.

Fig. 8 shows that the percent labeling index did not change immediately after irradiation. There was a significant drop of the number of labeled cells at 12 hours following irradiation; the drop lasted for about 4 hours. However, the changes in ^{3}H-TdR cell labelind index did not seem to be related to variation in the effectiveness of different fractionation schedules.

DISCUSSION

In our present study, the results demonstrated that the response of a tumor to fractionated exposures is critically dependent on the time interval between radiation treatments.

Withers (12) emphasizes the importance of redistribution of cells within the cell cycle in multifraction irradiation. Following moderate exposure, i.e. 300-400 R, there will be a shift in the distribution of viable cells within the sensitive and resistant phases of the cell cycle. This redistribution results from a higher relative survival of cells that were in the radioresistant phase of the cell cycle and a partial synchronization by mitotic arrest. Fig. 7 demonstrated that relatively few cells were in the radiosensitive "M" phase of the cell cycle at 6 hours after 400 R. On the other hand, 24 hours after irradiation there was a high proportion of the population in the sensitive phase. This accounts for the fact that tumor control was best when intervals of 24 hours were utilized.

Several investigators have emphasized the importance of reoxygenation on the radiosensitivity of tissue. Barendsen and Broese (1), reported that daily doses of X-rays of about 300 rads are the most effective in producing damage to the tumor and a tolerable level of damage to normal tissue. This might be due to the presence of resistant hypoxic cells which require rather long time intervals for reoxygenation.

In experiments with animals breathing air and where oxygenation could occur between fractions, Cheshire and Lindop (2) found that the largest therapeutic gain was achieved with 24 hours between fractions. They suggested that the differential effect on the tumor and the overlying normal tissues is the result of:
(1) increasing recovery (sublethal damage) in normal tissues up to 24 hours, and
(2) an increasing radiosensitivity of tumor cells with increasing reoxygenation that was maximal with 24 hour intervals.

Repopulation attains more importance as the time between fractions is increased. Howes and Suit(6) reported that the increase in 50% tumor control dose (TCD$_{50}$) with increasing intervals of more than one day between fractions was due to repopulation of viable tumor cells. DuSault (4), found that when 400 R x 20 was given every day, the cure rate was

72

double that obtained when the treatment was given 5 times a week. She explained that this was the result of tumor repopulation or regrowth during a two day interval without treatment.

This agrees with our observation that the highest tumor survival was when we spaced the exposures 48 hours apart.

SUMMARY

Ehrlich carcinoma, grown intramuscularly in the thigh of CF_1 female mice, has been irradiated with single or fractionated exposures of 250 kVp X-rays. All treatments consisted of a total exposure of 2400 R given at different time intervals and with various dose increments. A regimen of 400 R x 6 given every 24 hours was the best fractionation schedule, i.e., the scheme that gave 100% tumor control. This optimal regimen seems to be correlated with changes in mitotic activity after irradiation. Changes in the labeling index after irradiation did not seem to be related to the effectiveness of different fractionation schedules.

ACKNOWLEDGMENT

This research was partially supported by Grant DT-30-0 from the American Cancer Society, Inc.

Table I

Percentage of Tumors Surviving 50 Days Following 2400 R.

Fractionation Schemes	Time Between Exposures, Hours				
	0	6	12	24	48
400 R x 6	50%	40%	20%	0%	60%
600 R x 4	50%	60%	50%	40%	-
800 R x 3	50%	-	-	20%	-

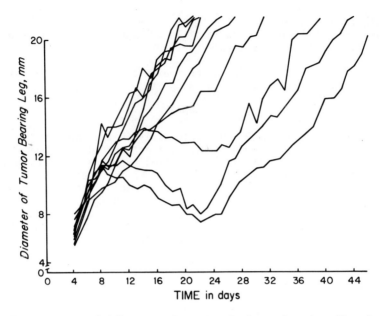

FIG. 1. Growth of tumors in control mice, sham irradiated.

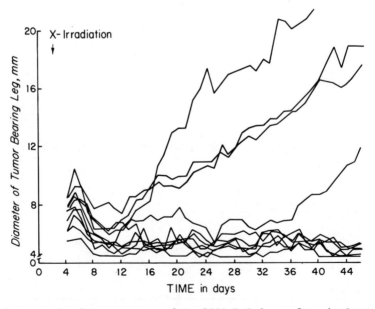

FIG. 2. Growth of tumors exposed to 2400 R 2 days after implantation.

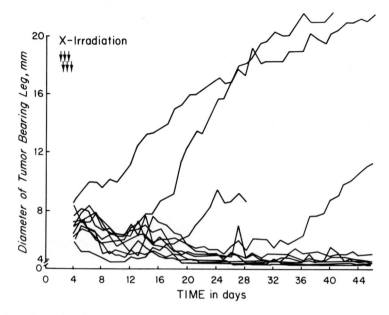

FIG. 3. Growth of tumors given 6 exposures of 400 R at 6-hr intervals.

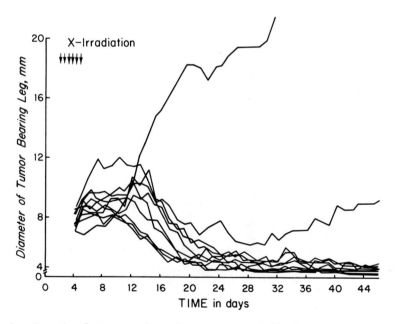

FIG. 4. Growth of tumors given 6 exposures of 400 R at 12-hr intervals.

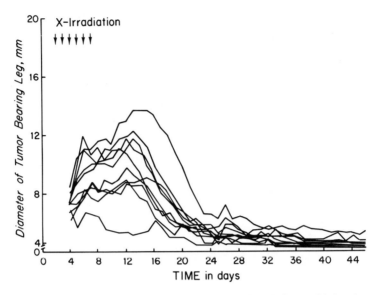

FIG. 5. Growth of tumors given 6 exposures of 400 R at 24-hr intervals.

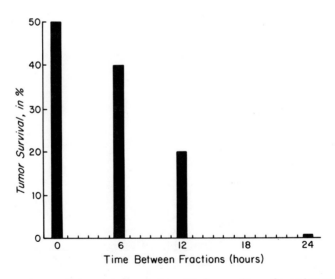

FIG. 6. Percentage of tumors surviving 50 days after fractionated exposures totaling 2400 R.

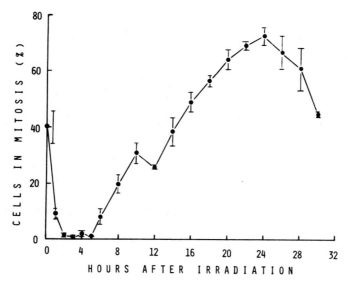

FIG. 7. Variation in mitotic index (percent of cells in mitosis) after 400 R.

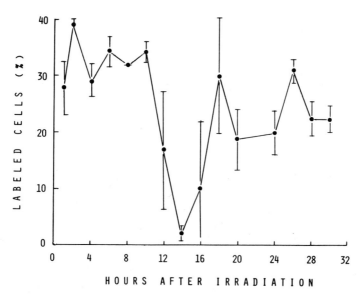

FIG. 8. Variation in labeling index (percent of cells labeled with tritiated thymidine) after 400 R.

REFERENCES

1. Barendsen, G.W., and Broerse, J.J., Experimental Radiotherapy for a Rat Rhabdomyosarcoma with 15 MeV Neutron and 300 kVp X-rays. II. Effects of Fractionated Treatment, Applied 5 Times a Week for Several Weeks. Europ. J. Cancer, 6:89-109, 1970.

2. Cheshire, P.J., and Lindop, P.J., The Influence of Intracellular Recovery and Hypoxic Cells on the Radiation Response of Mammary Tumours and Skin in C3H Mice. Brit. J. Radiology, 42:215-223, 1969.

3. DeGowin, R.L., Miller, S.H., and Grund, F.M., Studies of Recovery of Erythropoiesis after Irradiation as a Function of the Cellularity of the endocolonized spleen. J. Lab. Clin. Med., 77:219-227, 1971.

4. DuSault, L.A., Dose-Response at Each Fraction in a Radiotherapy Series. Front. Radiation Ther. Onc., 3:36-45, 1968.

5. Frindel, E., Malaise, E., Alpen, E., and Tubiana, M., Kinetics of Cell Proliferation of an Experimental Tumor. Cancer Res., 27:1122-1131, 1967.

6. Howes, A.E., and Suit, H.D., The Effect of Time Between Fractionation on the Response of Tumors to Irradiation. Rad. Res., 57:342-348, 1974.

7. Kim, J.H., and Evans, T.C., Effects of X-irradiation on the Mitotic Cells of Ehrlich Ascites Tumor Cells. Rad. Res., 21:129-143, 1964.

8. Laird, A.K., Dynamics of Tumour Growth: Comparison of Growth Rates and Extrapolation of Growth Lines to One Cell. Brit. J. Cancer, 19:278-291, 1965.

9. Lindgren, A.L., and Riley, E.F., Use of the Wound Response to Demonstrate Latent Radiation Damage and Recovery in X-irradiated Intermitotic Cells of the Rat Lens Epithelium. Rad. Res., 54:411-430, 1973.

10. Quastler, H., and Sherman, F.G., Cell Population Kinetics in the Intestinal Epithelium of the Mouse. Exptl. Cell. Res., 17:420-438, 1959.

11. Tannock, J.F., A Comparison of Cell Proliferation Parameters in Solid and Ascites Ehrlich Tumors. Cancer Res., 29:1527-1534, 1969.

12. Withers, R.H., Cell Cycle Redistribution as a Factor in Multifraction Irradiation. Radiology, 114:199-202, 1975.

FLOW-SYSTEMS ANALYSIS AND CHARACTERIZATION OF PROTEIN CONTENTS AND PROLIFERATING KINETICS IN ASCITES AND SOLID TUMORS

H. A. Crissman, R. J. Kissane, P. L. Wanek, M. S. Oka, and J. A. Steinkamp

Biophysics and Instrumentation Group, Los Alamos Scientific Laboratory
University of California, Los Alamos, New Mexico 87545 U.S.A.

I. INTRODUCTION

Analysis of the cellular DNA and protein content in malignant tumors provides useful kinetic information for characterizing the dynamics of tumor cell growth and proliferation. Kinetic data have been used in the design of rational schedules for chemotherapy (1) and for determining the effects of various potential drug agents on cycle progression (2,3). However, obtaining cell kinetic information by conventional biochemical methods is often quite tedious and time-consuming. It would be extremely useful to have an analytical system available which could rapidly provide detailed information for characterization of tumors at various stages of development. Flow microfluorometery (FMF) has been shown to be a rapid and reliable approach for simultaneous determination of both DNA and protein in single-cell populations (4,5), thus providing information on both cell proliferation and cell growth. Since the methodology does not rely on cellular incorporation of ^{3}H-thymidine, the technique is especially useful for analysis of slowly traversing or arrested cells such as encountered in many tumor systems. Furthermore, the FMF system has the unique advantage of providing complete accountability of the proportion of cells at various stages in the cell cycle.

In this report, we present the initial results of our attempts to characterize the mouse L1210 ascites and Lewis lung carcinoma tumor systems using FMF analysis of cytochemically stained tumor cell populations. Time-sequence sampling and flow analysis were used to detect fluctuations in proliferation kinetics of tumor cell populations associated with tumor age and development. Other kinetic information relating to cell death and cell loss, as well as analysis of proliferating and nonproliferating compartments, obviously is necessary to characterize completely these model systems. However, FMF techniques, coupled with standard biochemical techniques, should provide additional detailed information for assaying the dynamics of tumor growth.

II. PROCEDURES AND MATERIALS USED

A. Tumor Systems

1. L1210 ASCITES

The L1210 leukemia was chosen as the standard model tumor reference system for screening and evaluation of chemotherapeutic drugs during the 1974 World Conference on Drug Screening held in Geneva, Switzerland (6).

The tumor originated in 1948 in the spleen and lymph nodes of mice whose skin had been painted with methylcholanthrene (7). The tumor is propagated in vivo in DBA/2 mice, and BDF_1 mice (C57B1/6 x DBA/2) are commonly used for drug testing. In the present study, L1210 ascites were grown in DBA/2 mice following an initial intraperitoneal inoculum of 10^5 cells. Under these conditions, hemorrhaging was noticeable in the peritoneal cavity on about days six or seven and extensive at death (days eight to ten).

2. LEWIS LUNG CARCINOMA

The Lewis lung carcinoma (LLC) is a solid tumor system that has also been used for drug screening. Tumors are propagated as subcutaneous (sc) implants in C57B1/6 mice, and tests are generally performed with BDF_1 mice serving as host animals. Primary (sc) tumors grow rapidly and eventually metastasize to the lung and other organs. This presents an interesting system for studying growth kinetics of the tumor under differing in vivo environmental conditions. In these studies, the LLC were grown initially as solid (sc) tumors in C57B1/6 mice.

B. Cell Dispersal, Fixation, and Staining

DBA/2 mice were sacrificed at daily intervals beginning on day two after L1210 cell inoculation. Cells were harvested by aspiration, washed once in saline GM (balanced salt solution lacking calcium and magnesium) containing 0.5 m$\underline{M}$ EDTA, and fixed in 70% ethanol for subsequent DNA staining with mithramycin (100 μg/ml in normal saline containing 15 m$\underline{M}$ $MgCl_2$) (8). For staining both DNA and protein, L1210 cells were centrifuged from the ethanol fixative, resuspended in RNase (1 mg/ml, pH 7.0, Worthington, beef pancreatic RNase, code R), and incubated for 30 minutes at 37°C in a water bath. Following RNase hydrolysis, the cells were washed once in water and stained for total protein using fluorescein isothiocyanate (FITC in 0.5 $\underline{M}$ $NaHCO_3$ adjusted to pH 8.0, J. T. Baker), rinsed once in PBS, and then stained for DNA with propidium iodide (PI, CalBiochem, 0.1 mg/ml in PBS). Cells were rinsed in PBS and then resuspended in normal saline for analysis (5).

The solid Lewis lung carcinoma, primary and metastatic, as well as the spleen from nontumor-bearing mice, were forced through a 500-micron Teflon mesh into cold saline GM. The tumor material was pipetted 20-30 times through a 5-ml pipette and then filtered first through a 120-micron filter and then a 62-micron nylon filter to remove the larger tumor material. Cells were pelleted by centrifugation, washed once in a large volume of saline GM, and fixed in cold 70% ethanol. Cell staining for both DNA and protein was as described for L1210 ascites cells.

C. Flow-Systems Analysis

Simultaneous analysis of the DNA and protein contents of PI-FITC stained cells was performed using the multiparameter analysis and cell sorting system (9) previously described (5) using a 488-nm wavelength laser excitation source. The DNA content distribution of mithramycin-stained cells was obtained using a 457-nm laser line for excitation. Descriptions of the design and operational features of the single-parameter (10,11) and the multiparameter analysis and cell sorting systems (8,12) have been discussed elsewhere.

Cells were sorted from the 2C and 4C-8C regions of the LLC DNA distribution and analyzed microscopically as previously described (13). The relative proportions of cells in G_1, S, and G_2 + M were derived from the DNA distribution profiles using the Dean and Jett (14) computer program. Computer analysis was used to obtain the density contours for DNA-protein profiles of the L1210 ascites and the primary and lung metastases of the Lewis lung carcinoma.

III. RESULTS

A. Analysis of L1210 Ascites Cells

Typical DNA distribution patterns obtained for mithramycin-stained populations of L1210 cells obtained on days three, four, six, and seven following an inoculum of 10^5 cells are shown in Fig. 1. Comparison of these DNA distributions to those of normal (diploid) spleen cells (not shown) indicates that G_1 cells of L1210 have a 2C DNA content. The percentage of cells in G_1, S, and G_2 + M for days two through eight is provided in Table I. These data and data obtained from other experiments in our Laboratory clearly reveal changes in proliferation kinetic patterns that are concomitant with increased cell density or tumor age.

There is an initial lag in tumor growth as indicated by the low percentage of cells in S phase on day two; however, a rapid increase in cell proliferation is apparent by days four and five, followed by a precipitous decrease in proliferating cells on day six. This dramatic decrease in cell progression capacity could possibly be caused by release of cytotoxic substances during hemorrhaging which is quite apparent by day six. The percentage of cells in S phase remains unchanged on day seven; however, there is a significant increase in the G_2 + M fraction.

Simultaneous analysis of DNA and protein provides useful information relating to the biosynthetic capacity of cells at specific phases of the cell cycle (4,5). Since a gross imbalance in DNA/protein ratio will eventually lead to cell death, analysis of the quantitative relationship of these parameters can be useful for elucidating the occurrence of ensuing phase-specific cell death. Figure 2 shows the single-parameter and two-parameter DNA-protein profiles for L1210 ascites cells. The protein content distribution is similar to that obtained for cultured L1210 cells (not shown).

The DNA-protein contour profiles for L1210 ascites cells harvested on days three, four, six, and seven are shown in Fig. 3. Computer-generated density contour lines were obtained for arbitrary threshold settings of 20, 100, 200, 500, and 700 cells. These profiles reflect the same DNA distribution patterns (x axis) seen in Fig. 1; however, the protein distributions reveal a subpopulation of cells having a lower protein content than the bulk of the population. This subpopulation is most apparent on days three and four but is significantly decreased by days six and seven. Although these cells have not been sorted and morphologically identified at this time, it is speculated that, on the basis of cell volume studies performed in this Laboratory, this subpopulation of cells represents normal 2C diploid cells in the peritoneal cavity which are harvested along with tumor cells. These diploid cells initially represent a small but substantial proportion of the total cell population; however, as the tumor cell density increases rapidly, normal cells become less apparent. Figure 3 also

81

illustrates the rapid increase in proportion of cells having a large protein mass. All of the profiles show the accumulation of cell clumps which may be noted at the extreme right of each distribution.

B. Analysis of Primary and Lung Metastases of Lewis Lung Carcinoma

DNA and protein contour profiles of a primary tumor and lung metastases of the Lewis lung carcinoma from C57B1/6 mice are shown in Fig. 4. Computer-generated density contours were obtained at threshold settings of 50, 100, 150, 200, 350, and 500 cells. Based on results obtained in both cell sorting experiments and DNA content analysis of diploid spleen cells, the portion of cells designated 2C in the DNA profile (x axis) shown in Fig. 4 represents normal cells and the remaining portion of the profile G_1 (4C), S, and G_2 + M (8C) populations of the tumor cells, respectively. The percentages of cells in G_1, S, and G_2 + M were 38.7, 54.9, and 6.4, respectively, for the primary tumor and 58.8, 32.0, and 9.2 for the metastatic population. Single-parameter DNA and protein distributions have been presented elsewhere (15).

It may be noticed that, in general, tumor cells have a greater protein mass than most but not all normal cells. Also, the protein profiles of the primary and lung metastases appear to be quite different, particularly through the S and G_2 + M regions. In particular, the primary tumor appears to contain cells having a wider range in protein content through these regions.

IV. DISCUSSION

The DNA distribution patterns obtained for L1210 ascites cells clearly reveal the fluctuations in cycle kinetic patterns associated with increased cell density or tumor age. Based on studies presented in this report, there is an initial lag phase reflected by the low percentage of cells in S phase on day two, followed by a rapid increase in cell proliferation (i.e., days four and five) and then a decrease in proliferation just prior to death of the host animal. The growth and proliferation patterns presented here are similar to those observed for L1210 cells in culture. In fact, the percentages of cells in G_1, S, and G_2 + M at the peak of growth on day five (Table I) are quite comparable to values obtained previously in our Laboratory for exponentially growing L1210 cells in vitro (i.e., percentages in G_1, S, and G_2 + M are 29.2, 65.5, and 8.3, respectively).

The DNA distribution patterns presented for L1210 ascites cells (Fig. 1) also contain the subpopulation of normal diploid cells revealed by the DNA-protein contour profiles (Fig. 2). Since normal cells have different ranges in protein content levels than tumor cells, it would be possible to strip the true DNA distribution of tumor cells from the normal cell population. For example, by gating on the protein content (green fluorescence) range of tumor cells, it is possible to analyze only the DNA (red fluorescence) of tumor cells. Analysis of the corrected DNA distributions would reflect more accurately the cycle distribution of cells than do the data in Table I, particularly for days two, three, and four where normal cells probably represent a small but significant proportion of the population. Gated analysis techniques are being employed in more recent studies.

Simpson-Herren et al. (16) have recently presented results of autoradiographic studies which demonstrate differences in proliferation of the primary and lung metastases of the Lewis lung carcinoma. The fraction of

cells in S phase for the lung metastases is in good agreement with the
pulse-labeling index (36%) obtained by Simpson-Herren et al. (16) in
spontaneous metastatic lung tumors 17 days post-implant of the primary (sc)
tumors. However, these investigators found a much lower labeling index
(25%) for primary tumors than the 54% S fraction obtained in our studies.
Several significant differences in experimental design of both studies
make it difficult to compare the results directly.

Differences observed in protein content levels of metastatic and primary
Lewis lung carcinoma must await further studies for verification, since
these represent only initial studies of this nature with this tumor system.
It is possible that the metastatic tumor has certain characteristic properties, among which is a more rigid protein content range during specific
portions of the cell cycle. On the other hand, the differences in protein
content range may be caused by differences in the in vivo environment.
This is to infer that differences in nutrient supply are available to the
tumor in lung tissue, as opposed to the subcutaneous region of the mouse.

Normal cells are present in most solid tumors where they function in
various aspects of nutrition (i.e., provide adequate blood supply) or aid
in providing a framework system for tumor architecture. In spite of the
fact that the numbers and types of normal cells must change during the
various stages of tumor development, little attempt has been made to
exploit this phenomenon for characterizing the developmental stages of
tumor growth and proliferation. In the context of drug evaluation, the
effects of various chemical agents on normal cells are often as important
as the effects on the tumor cell population. In either instance, the use
of techniques demonstrated here should be extremely useful. Cell sorting
based on DNA content measurements can provide a concentrated population
composed of large numbers of normal cells for microscopic analysis, while
the protein content analyses of normal and tumor cells would be useful for
determining the physiological condition of cells during drug testing experiments.

V. SUMMARY

Flow microfluorometric analysis of the DNA and protein content of mouse
ascites and solid tumor cell populations grown in vivo has provided
information on protein distribution of cells in various phases of the cell
cycle, as well as age-associated changes in proliferation kinetics of these
tumor systems. L1210 ascites cells and solid Lewis lung carcinomas were
dispersed, fixed, and stained for both DNA and protein, respectively, using
the fluorochromes propidium iodide (red) and fluorescein isothiocyanate
(green). Simultaneous DNA and protein determinations were performed using
a flow system in which rapid two-color analysis of stained cells was
achieved at approximately 10^3 cells/second. Analysis of the DNA distributions of L1210 cells on days three, four, six, and seven following
implantation of 10^5 cells revealed changes in cycle kinetic patterns concomitant with increased cell density or tumor age. DNA distribution
patterns for Lewis lung tumors showed a 2C peak and a cell proliferation
pattern extending between the 4C and 8C peaks. Cells sorted electronically
from the 2C and 4C-8C contents of the DNA spectrum were identified morphologically as normal and tumor cells, respectively. Tumor cells exhibited
elevated protein distributions compared to normal cells; however, tumor
cells were quite heterogeneous in cell size and morphology. Analysis of
cellular DNA and protein in various tumor systems permits characterization

of the growth kinetics at various stages of tumor development, and such information is of predictive value in chemotherapeutic regimen scheduling. Cell analysis and sorting provide a method for detection and visual inspection of tumor cell populations.

ACKNOWLEDGMENTS

The authors thank J. H. Jett, G. C. Salzman, and A. Stevenson for help in computer analysis of the data; S. R. McLaughlin for technical assistance in flow analysis; P. F. Mullaney for helpful criticism of the manuscript; J. Grilly for photography; and C. Oldenborg and E. Sullivan for manuscript preparation. We also thank the Pfizer Company for generously supplying the compound mithramycin used for cell staining in these studies and the A. D. Little Company of Boston, Massachusetts, for supplying the animals and tumor material.

This work was performed under the joint sponsorship of the U. S. Energy Research and Development Administration and the Division of Cancer Treatment (interagency agreement YO1-CM-40102, R214) and the Division of Cancer Biology and Diagnosis (interagency agreement YO1-CB-10055, R030) of the National Cancer Institute.

TABLE I

Cell-Cycle Distribution of L1210 Ascites Cells

on Various Days following Inoculation[a]

| Day | Percentage of cells | | |
	G_1	S	$G_2 + M$
2	71.0	15.8	13.2
3	40.6	50.0	9.4
4	32.9	59.2	7.9
5	30.1	63.7	6.2
6	45.1	46.7	8.2
7	38.8	46.9	14.3
8	48.7	36.6	14.7

[a]Represents averages of at least three samples.

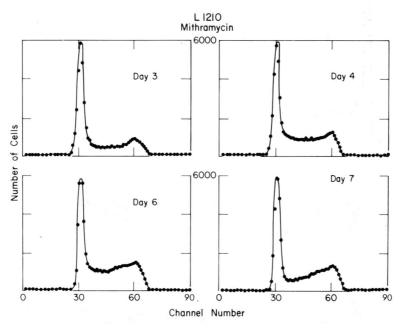

FIG. 1. DNA content distributions of mithramycin-stained L1210 ascites cells grown in DBA/2 mice and harvested on days 3, 4, 6, and 7.

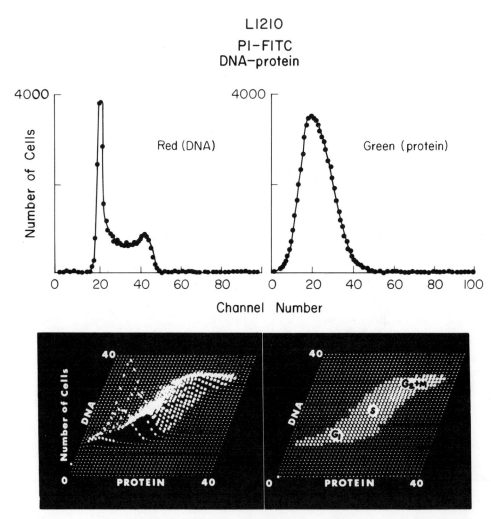

FIG. 2. Single-parameter and dual-parameter analysis of DNA and protein in PI-FITC stained L1210 ascites cells.

L1210   Ascites

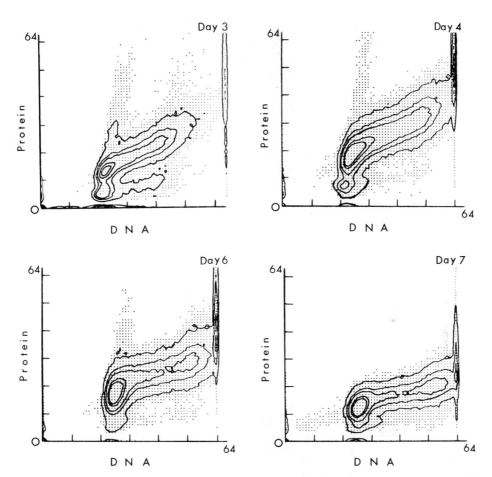

FIG. 3. Computer-generated contour profiles of DNA and protein content of
PI-FITC stained L1210 ascites cells grown in DBA/2 mice and harvested on
3, 4, 6, and 7.   The contour density lines are at 20, 100, 200, 500, and 700
cells.

Lewis Lung Carcinoma

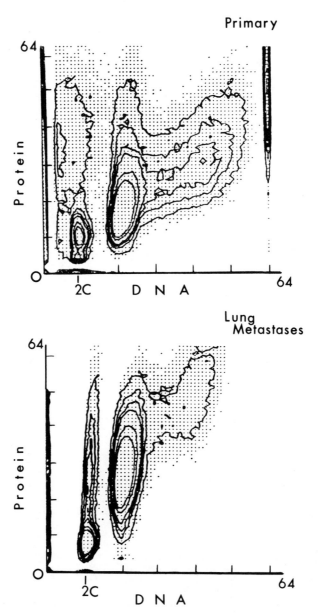

FIG. 4. Computer-generated contour profiles of DNA and protein content of PI-FITC stained primary and lung metastases of the Lewis lung carcinoma. The contour lines are at 50, 100, 150, 200, 350, and 500 cells.

REFERENCES

1. Schabel, F. M., Jr. The Use of Tumor Growth Kinetics in Planning "Curative" Chemotherapy of Advanced Solid Tumors. Cancer Res., 29:2384-2389, 1969.

2. Tobey, R. A., and Crissman, H. A. Use of Flow Microfluorometry in Detailed Analysis of the Effects of Chemical Agents on Cell Cycle Progression. Cancer Res., 32:2726-2732, 1972.

3. Tobey, R. A., Oka, M. S., and Crissman, H. A. Differential Effects of Two Chemotherapeutic Agents, Streptozotocin and Chlorozotocin, on the Mammalian Cell Cycle. Eur. J. Cancer, 11:433-441, 1975.

4. Crissman, H. A., Mullaney, P. F., and Steinkamp, J. A. Methods and Applications of Flow Systems for Analysis and Sorting of Mammalian Cells. In: Methods in Cell Biology. Ed.: D. M. Prescott. Academic Press Inc., New York, 9: 179-246, 1975.

5. Crissman, H. A., and Steinkamp, J. A. Rapid, Simultaneous Measurement of DNA, Protein and Cell Volume in Single Cells from Large Mammalian Cell Populations. J. Cell Biol., 59:766-771, 1973.

6. Schepartz, S. A. In: Summary Reports, Report of the Division of Cancer Treatment, National Institutes of Health. U. S. Department of Health, Education, and Welfare, Bethesda, Maryland, 1: 2.1-2.9.

7. Geran, R. I., Greenberg, N. H., MacDonald, M. M., Schumacher, A. M., and Abbott, B. J. Protocol for Screening Chemical Agents and Natural Products against Animal Tumors and Other Biological Systems. Cancer Chemotherapy Rep., 3:7-13, 1972.

8. Crissman, H. A., and Tobey, R. A. Cell Cycle Analysis in 20 Minutes. Science, 184:1297-1298, 1974.

9. Steinkamp, J. A., Fulwyler, M. J., Coulter, J. R., Hiebert, R. D., Horney, J. L., and Mullaney, P. F. A New Multiparameter Separator for Microscopic Particles and Biological Cells. Rev. Sci. Instr., 44:1301-1310, 1973.

10. Van Dilla, M. A., Trujillo, T. T., Mullaney, P. F., and Coulter, J. R. Cell Microfluorometry: A Method for Rapid Fluorescence Measurements. Science, 163:1213-1214, 1969.

11. Holm, D. M., and Cram, L. S. An Improved Flow Microfluorometer for Rapid Measurements of Cell Fluorescence. Exp. Cell Res., 80:105-110, 1973.

12. Mullaney, P. F., Steinkamp, J. A., Crissman, H. A., Cram, L. S., and Holm, D. M. Laser Flow Microphotometers for Rapid Analysis and Sorting of Individual Mammalian Cells. In: Laser Applications in Medicine and Biology. Ed.: M. L. Wolbarsht. Plenum Press, New York, 2: 151-204, 1974.

13. Horan, P. K., Romero, A., Steinkamp, J. A., and Petersen, D. F. Detection of Heteroploid Tumor Cells. J. Natl. Cancer Inst., 52:843-848, 1974.

14. Dean, P. N., and Jett, J. H. Mathematical Analysis of DNA Distributions Derived from Flow Microfluorometry. J. Cell Biol., 60:523-527, 1974.

15. Crissman, H. A., Kissane, R. J., Oka, M. S., Tobey, R. A., and Steinkamp, J. A. Flow Microfluorometric Approaches to Cell Kinetics. In: Growth Kinetics and Biochemical Regulation of Normal and Malignant Cells (Proceedings of the 29th Annual Symposium on Fundamental Cancer Research, Houston, Texas, March 10-21, 1976), 1976 (in press).

16. Simpson-Herren, L., Sanford, A. H., and Holmquist, J. P. Cell Population Kinetics of Transplanted and Metastatic Lewis Lung Carcinoma. Cell Tissue Kinet., 7:349-361, 1974.

ON THE NATURE OF CANCEROUS TRANSFORMATIONS AND CANCER THERAPY

Okan Gurel

IBM Corporation
1133 Westchester Avenue
White Plains, New York 10604

1. FORMALIZATION OF CANCER

The energy consideration for a cancerous cell in terms of its dynamics has been proposed in [3a,b (1970)] . This concept is based on the property that due to an energy increase in the cell, an additional biodynamic field is created, which is expressed as the energy principle [3b, p.570] . This principle can be stated in two parts, one on the existence of a biodynamic field, and the other on the complementarity, P1a and P1b :

P1a. *Energy Principle.* A *biodynamic field* is said to exist at a point, if a force of a biodynamic origin is exerted on a body placed at this point.

The concept of a biodynamic field points out two basic notions which can be restated for clarity as :

1. Cancer is a *dynamic state* of an *individual cell.*
2. The *elements* of the cell determine this state.

The second notion above can be formalized further by studying the entire set of biochemical macromolecules in a living system which can be denoted as the *set* of macro-molecules, B, [4b, p.378] . The important concept which is of a great significance in the living state of the set B is the *energy space* denoted by V ,[4b, p.380] . A function f on B with values in the space V, can be considered. The weak topologies on B is defined by the family of functions $[f]$, and denoted by $s(B,V)$. Referring to this topology on B, the complementarity principle is stated [4b, p.380] :

P1b. *Complementarity Principle.* The complementarity between the spaces B and V is defined by the weak topology $s(B,V)$.

These conclusions have been based on the acceptance that the cancerous state represents an *unstable dynamical field* [3a,b (1970)]   which manifests itself in an unstable behavior [1a,b(1969), 2(1969)]. This property is stated as the instability principle [3b, p. 576 and 5b, p.146]:

> P2. *Instability Principle.* If an unstable singular point at the center of the bio-dynamic field is expected, the acceleration of the particle lying in this field, $\ddot{x}$, should be positive. This implies that $\ddot{x}$ is proportional to the negative gradient of the potential energy, $\partial \Delta V/\partial x < 0$.

In addition, it was also observed [5a,b (1972)] that there is a *duality* between the two dynamic states of an individual cell, a cancerous state and the mitotic state. Denoting the negative gradient subspace of the energy space by H^- and the positive gradient subspace by H^+, similar to P2, a proposition for mitosis is given in [5b, p.146]:

> *Proposition of Mitosis.* A mitotic state corresponds to a variation belonging to the set H^+.

Based on P2 and the proposition of mitosis, the duality stemming from the stability properties of the two types of biodynamic fields is stated as the duality principle [5b, p.146]:

> P3. *Duality Principle.* Mitotic activities and cancerous activities are dual of each other.

These three items of formalization of observations characterize the cancer problem as follows:

> C1. Cancer is a dynamic phenomenon dual to mitosis, (P3).
> C2. Cancerous state is an unstable state, (P2).
> C3. The only 'measurable' quantity reflecting the 'phenomenon' of cancer is its increased energy state, (P1).

These three interrelated conclusions are significant, because they indicate the following results:

> R1. Any system (a cell) which goes through mitotic activity, i.e., all cells by definition, is *susceptible* to going through a cancerous transformation, (C1).
> R2. Cancerous state can exhibit many types of instabilities as well as bifurcations, thus cancerous alterations are *almost unlimited,* (C2).

Arguments leading to a third result will be developed in the next section, the statement of R3 is :

> R3. Based on the property P1, related to the energy state, cancerous state is an *irreversible state,* however it may be *repairable,* only if a reduction (absorption) of energy is induced, (C3).

The theory was also related to the *cause* of cancerous state in an earlier reference [4a,b (1971), p.385]. At the other end of the spectrum, the theory outlined above reveals additional information with *therapeutic implications.* In the light of the theory, the well known therapeutic modalities may be critically reevaluated. However, following arguments should be advanced which could easily be related to the cancer therapy.

2. THE NATURE OF THE ENERGY SPACE

In reference [3a,b] it was illustrated that the basic energy space V for interaction of one element interacting with another, thus entering the dynamics of the cell is represented by the function

$$f_1: R^1 \rightarrow V, \qquad\qquad V \subset R^1 \tag{1}$$

where R^1 is the one dimensional euclidean space, i.e. a line, Figure 1. The zero energy point is P_0, and at M the minimum energy is reached. On the other hand, if there are three elements contributing to the energy V, as two elements interacting with a third one, the energy function is,

$$f_2: R^1 \times R^1 \rightarrow V \tag{2}$$

It is noted that, for clarity in explanation, 1 and 2 are assumed to interact with 0, but not with each other. The interaction space is a product of two R^1's, a plane. On Fig.2, it is shown that L_{120} is the locus of zero energy points. Between the origin and L_{120} the energy is positive, beyond L_{120} the energy is negative reaching its minimum at M_{12}. The energy surface is also sketched on this figure. For the system of three elements, 1, 2, and 3 interacting with the fourth one, 0, the function is

$$f_3: R^1 \times R^1 \times R^1 \rightarrow V \tag{3}$$

or in short,

$$f_3: R^3 \rightarrow V.$$

The R^3 portion of this relation is depicted in Fig. 3. Since V forms the fourth dimension, the energy hypersurface can not be illustrated on this figure. The null surface S_{1230} is the locus of all those L_{ij0} line, thus that of all P_{i0}'s, and similarly S_{1230} devides the space into positive and negative energy portions.

In the section of R^n, $n=1,2,...,$ where the energy is negative, $f_n(R^n)<0$, there are various subregions which can be determined by referring to the gradient of f_n. Assuming that a coordinate system, $x_1, x_2,...$ is assigned to 1,2, ... and denoting the gradient of f with respect to x_i by $\partial f/\partial x_i$, $i=1,2, ...,$ it is noted that there can be various combinations of $\partial f/\partial x_i>0$ and $\partial f/\partial x_i<0$ for $i=1,2, ... $. For example, in the xase of x_1 only, Figure 1, since at M $\partial f/\partial x_1=0$,

in Region 1, where $x_1(P)<x_1<x_1(M)$, $\qquad \partial f/\partial x_1<0$,
in Region 2, where $x_1(M)<x_1$, $\qquad\qquad\qquad \partial f/\partial x_1>0$.

In short, r_1 and l_1, referring to the regions with positive gradient and that with negative gradient, respectively, can be used.

In the case of $n=2$, the following four regions exist:

$$r_1 r_2, \qquad r_1 l_2, \qquad l_1 r_2, \qquad l_1 l_2.$$

In the case of $n=3$, there are eigth different regions,

$$r_1 r_2 r_3, \qquad r_1 r_2 l_3, \qquad r_1 l_2 l_3, \qquad l_1 l_2 l_3,$$
$$r_1 l_2 r_3, \qquad l_1 r_2 l_3,$$
$$l_1 r_2 r_3, \qquad l_1 l_2 r_3.$$

These regions can easily be visualized in Fig.3. In general, for n, there are 2^n different regions.

In the most severe case, $l_1 l_2 l_3$, all the elements of overall gradient are negative. By the stability principle, P2, $l_1 l_2 l_3$ corresponds to the portion of the energy space where cancerous alterations take place. In addition, all the regions with r and l combinations are of a cancerous nature. In terms of the theory of dynamic stability, these regions correspond to saddle points of the system. That is to say, a cell with a dynamics representing these regions possess both stable and unstable characteristics (manifolds). On the other hand, according to the duality principle, P3, $r_1 r_2 r_3$ is the unique region of mitotic activity.

3.   IRREVERSIBILITY OF CANCEROUS STATE

The nature of the energy space as discussed above, points out another characteristics of the cancerous state, its irreversibility. This can be explained by the following observations.

As the instability principle, P2, and the duality principle , P3, reveal, the two dual dynamic activities, mitosis and cancerous state, are differentiated by the first derivative of the energy space,

Cancerous state: $\qquad V'=\partial V/\partial x_i < 0,$
Mitosis: $\qquad\qquad V' \qquad > 0.$

It was pointed out in [4] that V is a class of C^∞, i.e., possessing all the derivatives. Among these, the   first derivative, V', is instrumental in determining the duality between mitosis and cancerous state, see Fig. 4. In addition, the rate of V' is V'', the second derivative of the energy V. This is shown in Fig. 4 dividing x into two parts:

$V'' < 0$ corresponds to decreasing rate of V',
$V'' > 0$ corresponds to increasing rate of V'.

It is, therefore, clear that in the case of mitosis, once the dynamic activity starts, it diminishingly increases (slowing down) and when F is reached, the peak mitotic activity is reached. Then, the process is ready to return to M by a reverse process.

In the case of a cancerous state, however, V'' enhancingly increases, the dynamic activity never to reach a similar position of F of mitosis. This property of the energy space characterizes the irreversibility of cancerous transformations. There is never a natural slowing down similar to the mitotic activity. The two results discussed earlier, R1 and R2, may then be augmented by the third result:

R3. Based on the propert P1, related to the energy state, cancerous state is an *irreversible state*, however, it may be *repairable*, only if a reduction (absorption) of energy is induced, (C3).

4. SOME THEORETICAL MODELS OF MITOSIS

It should be mentioned that a mathematical model of the cell given in [6] is based on a globally stable biodynamic field corresponding to cell differentiation. This is an example of the duality principle, P3, thus the model proposed independently, agrees with the present energy view. This model represents the entire cell cycle, a part of which is the mitotic phase. In a similar fashion, a model oscillator for control of mitosis is described in [7]. Here again, the dynamic field possesses a stable limit cycle, which indicates that the biodynamic field of mitosis is bounded by a stable limit cycle.

Further examples of mitosis are discussed as a process of bifurcations in [8]. In this model, the field is bounded by a stable limit cycle. The singular point lying in the nucleus is a stable focus which goes through a bifurcation during prophase corresponding to that portion of the mitotic model presented in [5a,b].

Another study is based on the biochemistry of the cell division. The sensitivity to perturbation of various elements indicates that the equations based on mass equilibrium correspond to a stable synatic process [9]. Moreover, it is illustrated that in the case of cancerous transformations model points out the irreversibility of the process, thus the result R3 is independently reached. These findings are also experimentally verified, [9].

In addition to these four independent theoretical models agreeing with and supporting the energy view of cell dynamics, there are also purely experimental observations on the dynamics of cancerous alterations ina cell discussed in [1b, 2 and 3b] which stribgly support the remark R2 regarding variations of instabilities in cancerous states.

5. EVALUATION OF CURRENT THERAPEUTIC METHODS

Returning to the therapeutic modalities, various possibilities can be reevaluated in terms of the concepts discussed above.

a. *Surgeo-therapy*. This therapy, of course, may appear to be the most direct was of attacking the problem. That is, removing the cell community by excision. This 'treatment' neither guarantees nonoccurence of the cancerous state nor reveals any understanding of the nature of the cancerous state.

b.   *Radio-therapy.* This is a sophisticated surgery in the sense that by a physical technique the cancerous cell colony is 'removed' by ending their life. Here again, no knowledge about the cause or the nature of cancerous state is obtained. Moreover, radiotherapy has one additional characteristic which touches upon the present theory in a negative fashion. That is, it violates the characteristic C3 and the result R3 such that while a proable repair (treatment) method is by absorption of energy from the cell, the radio - therapy does just the opposite, additional energy is introduced into the system resulting in 'burning out' the region.

c.   *Chemo-therapy.* Another controversial treatment method is chemotherapy. However, if the characteristic C2 is considered, the concept of chemotherapy fails to be effective. The chemical agent administred must approach the cancerous cell while an unstable field dominates the cell, repelling incoming particles. There is, of course, the consideration as pointed out by the result R3 and the recent explanations on the classes of possible instabilities that a sufficient amount of a *proper* chemical may be able to enter the system (the cell). This is possible, if the *time* and *parameters* (other chemical and physical conditions) are such that chemicals are under the influence of stable manifolds of the unstable biodynamic field.

This characteristic of chemotherapy which distinguishes it from the two previous therapies is a delicate one. It can be discussed in two directions.

The first one is the answer to the question of how a particle, a chemical substance, can approach the cell?The only path is along the stable manifold. However, in a saddle point environment, to get on a stable manifold, and stay on it long enough to approach the singular point, and be effective during this short period is always 'distracted' by the existence of unstable manifold which will tend to take the particle away from the biodynamic field of the cell. Thus the effectiveness of the chemical substance is severely restricted to almost an impossibility.

The second approach can be explained in terms of the regions of negative and positive gradients discussed above. As an illustration of the idea, the role of adding a chemotherapeutic agent can be discussed by referring to the $n=2$ case, Fig.2. The four regions exist. These are shown in Fig. 5 a-d as l_1l_2, l_1r_2, r_1l_2, and r_1r_2.

Since the energy space is defined by x_1 and x_2, if x_2 is lost from the system, Case i results, Fig.6. If x_1 is lost, the second case takes place. Thus, replacing a chemical agent 'acting' as x_2 in Case i, or as x_1 in Case ii would 'pull' the system into a non-accelerated state, Fig. 5c, or Fig. 5d. If the time of 'action' is sufficient, and the stability manifold overpowers the role of the instability manifold, then it is possible to be effective in bringing the energy state back to its non-critical domain.

d.   *Immuno-therapy.* The most critical result, R3, in devising a therapeutic method already eliminates the surgeo-, radio- and to a lesser extent chemo-therapies as totally effective therapies. In a brief form, recapitulating these therapies, it can be stated that :

Surgeo-therapy is used to remove a colony of cells from the patient and does not reveal an understanding of the cancer phenomenon. Thus it can not be evaluated by referring to the theory presented here.

Radio-therapy, in addition to having similarities to surgeo-therapy, it introduces energy into the system rather than comsuming energy. Thus, theoretically it takes the system into even a more inbalanced energy state than the case of pre-therapy.

Chemo-therapy may be effective in cases exhibiting C3 of saddle points provided that R3 is also satisfied.

The general idea of immuno-therapy [10], on the other hand, appears to be attacking the property P1, however with an unrelated motivation. That is to say, the basic assumption in immuno-therapy of cancer is that the cell either originally has an immune system to all cancers or it can subsequently acquire one. Therefore, if a portion of the immune system is lost, it may be restrored or an immune system may be introduced by immuno-therapy. Evaluating this therapy by referring to the theory presented here, the assumption of immunity appears to be incorrect. Immunotherapists focus on immunology and ignore the conclusions C1 and C2 altogether. The result is that, after trial and error experiments, in vivo and clinical, a 'statistically' better success than that by chemotherapy is obtained, however, considering the energy theory, no more should be expected.

In terms of their effectiveness, however limited, the immuno-therapeutic 'techniques' give a partial answer to the result R3 by being effective in attacking the energy level of the cancerous cell. This success should not be interpreted as a result of the immunological property of the cell, because according to the duality principle P3, the cell is never immune, instead it is susceptible to a cancerous state (disease), R1. Therefore, the name immuno-therapy is perhaps misleading one in the treatment of cancer.

6.   CONCLUSIONS AND RECOMMENDATIONS : ENERGY THERAPY

Starting from the premise that in attacking a cancerous cell, the only open door for the therapists is the result R3, namely reduction of energy, concentration must be on the following points:

Diagnosis: 1.   Measurability of the energy state, C3.

               2.   The elements entering this measurement.

Therapy: 3.   Method of absorbing the excess energy.

It is theoretically conceivable, therefore, to administer a cancerous state with a chemical system which requires (absorbs) energy. A biological system, such as BCG, C. parvum, etc. may well be a suitable energy absorber. But it should be kept in mind that once a cancerous cell is forced into the normal state, by the definition of life (the energy property-dynamics) it is again dually susceptible to mitosis as well as cancerous transformations. Thus the system is never immune to cancerous state (disease).

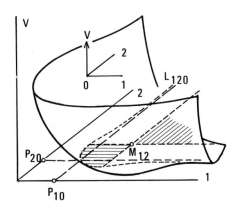

FIG. 1. (left) Energy space of one element interacting with another. Regions with positive and negative gradients are shown as r_1 and l_1, respectively.

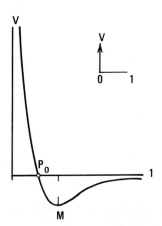

FIG. 2. (right) Energy space of two elements interacting with another. Regions with positive and negative gradients are shown as shaded areas, $r_1 r_2$ and $l_1 l_2$, respectively.

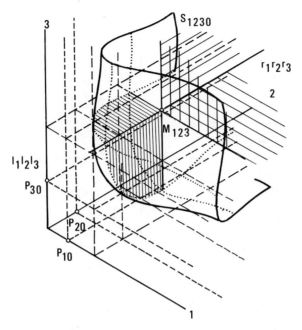

FIG. 3. Energy space of three elements interacting with another. Regions with positive and negative gradients are shown as shaded areas $r_1r_2r_3$ and $1_11_21_3$. respectively.

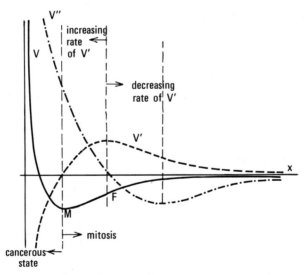

FIG. 4. Energy curve of two interacting elements, V, and its first and second derivatives. Various regions of significance determined by these curves are as marked.

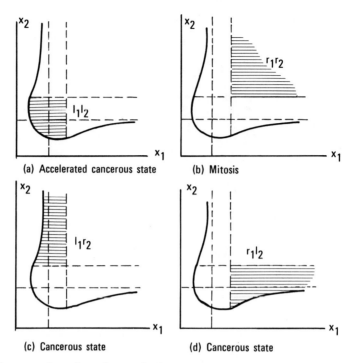

FIG. 5. An example of regions of the energy space with various combinations of negative and positive gradients. Corresponding biological states are also shown.

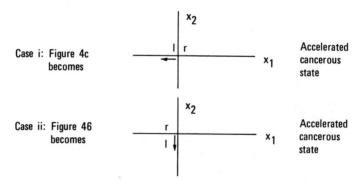

FIG. 6. Loss of an interacting element and its impact on the type of cancerous state.

REFERENCES

1. a. Gurel, O. The Dynamics of Cancerous Cells (Abstract), *Arch. Union Med. Balkan,* 7, p. 84, 1969.
   b. Gurel, O. Dynamics of Cancerous Cells, *Cancer, 23*:497-505, 1969.
2. Gurel, O. Qualitative Study of Unstable Behavior of Cancerous Cells, *Cancer, 24*: 945-947, 1969.
3. a. Gurel, O. Biodynamics of Cancerous Cells (Abstract), *10th Internl. Cancer Congress, Houston, Texas,* p.708, 1970.
   b. Gurel, O. Unstable Dynamic Field of an Individual Cancerous Cell, *Physiol. Chem. & Physics, 2*:570-580, 1970.
4. a. Gurel, O. Fundamental Weak Topologies in Living Systems (Abstract) *Biophysical Society Abstracts 10*:233a, 1970.
   b. Gurel, O. Biomolecular Topology and Cancer, *Physiol. Chem. & Physics, 3*:371-388, 1971.
5. a. Gurel, O. Dual Bifurcation Models of Cell Division, *Phys. Med. Biol. 17(5)*717,1972.
   b. Gurel, O. Bifurcation Models of Mitosis, *Physiol. Chem. & Physics, 4*:139-154,1972.
6. a. Sel'kov, E. E. Two Alternative Auto-Oscillatory Steady States in the Metabolism of the Thiols-Two Alternative Types of Cell Multiplication: Normal and Malignant, *Biophysica, 15*:1065-1073, 1970 [English Translation, *Biophysics,* 1104-1112,1970.
   b. Gilbert, D. A. The Nature of the Cell Cycle and the Control of Cell Proliferation, *BioSystems, 5*:197-206 , 1974.
7. Kauffman, S. Measuring a Mitotic Oscillator: The Arc Discontinuity, *Bulletin of Math. Biol. 36*:171-182, 1974.
8. Thom, R. Stabilite Structurelle et Morphogenese, W. A. Benjamin, Inc., Reading, Mass., p.267, 1972.
9. Davison, E. J. The Simulation of Cell Behavior: Normal and Abnormal Growth, *Bulletin of Math. Biol.* (To appear)
10. International Conference on Immunotherapy of Cancer, The New York Academy of Sciences, New York, New York, November 5-7,1975 (Annals to appear).

Chapter 2

GENETICS AND MUTAGENESIS

SEQUENTIAL CHROMOSOMAL SURVEYS IN THE MANAGEMENT OF CHRONIC GRANULOCYTIC LEUKEMIA

Kathryn E. Fuscaldo, Isadore Brodsky, James Conroy,
Barry J. Erlick, Anthony A. Fuscaldo, S. Benham Kahn,
Christie Lamping, and Ruthann Wieczoreck

Divisions of Genetics and Medical Oncology, Cancer
Institute and University Laboratories of Medicine (ULMI),
Hahnemann Medical College and Hospital, Philadelphia,
Pennsylvania.

Introduction

The use of chromosomal analysis to confirm the diagnosis of chronic granulocytic leukemia (CGL or CML) has been well documented (1-13). The presence of the Ph^1 chromosome in a variety of hematopoietic tissues has become a standard diagnostic criterion. Almost ninety percent of patients with the clinical signs of CGL are Ph^1 positive (14-15). Ezdinli (14) has suggested the term "sub-acute myelocytic leukemia" be applied to the Ph^1 negative disease since statistical differences have been found with respect to natural history of the disease, response to treatment, age at onset, sex prevalence, and possibly etiology.

Specific chromosomal markers have not as yet been confirmed for other myeloproliferative disorders although reports of non-random chromosome changes have appeared in the literature (16-20). Among the preneoplastic conditions leading to acute leukemia, CGL, polycythemia vera (PV), essential thrombocytosis (ET) and myelofibrosis and myeloid metaplasia (MM) are often characterized by abnormal karyotypes particularly as the disease progresses or enters the undifferentiated phase (20-40). CGL may in fact be a broad clinical entity encompassing several subgroups which may have different chromosomal anomalies, etiology and clinical courses (14,25,37). Substantial evidence is now available to suggest that CGL is a stem cell disorder (41,42), and that a viral agent may be involved in the etiology of the disease (43-47). The cause and effect relationship between (1) the genesis of Ph^1 in CGL (48-52); (2) stem cell evolution in CGL as well as other myeloproliferative disorders (52,53,41, 42); (3) the presence of oncornaviruses in CGL, ALL, AML and PV (43-47,55) and (4) the onset and progression of the leukemic process have not been elucidated.

Several investigators have observed that when CGL undergoes metamorphosis, it is often accompanied by the appearance of more bizarre chromosomal anomalies (55-60) and have suggested that serial chromosomal analysis might be useful in monitoring the disease and in prognosis (37,39-41,54,60-63). We elected to determine whether sequential karyotypic analysis of patients undergoing aggressive chemotherapy could be used to (1) monitor the efficacy of therapy (2) predict an impending metamorphosis in the nature of the disease and (3) correlate specific chromosomal anomalies other than Ph[1] with hematologically defined phases of the leukemic process, particularly in CGL. The ultimate aim of this study was to develop and evaluate a prognostic test that could aid in formulating more effective therapy.

Procedures and Materials Used

Twenty-five patients, whose diagnoses of CGL were established hematologically and chromosomally, were entered into the study along with 10 with a diagnosis of ET and 10 with PV.

Chronic Granulocytic Leukemia

Hematologic remission was induced in these patients with busulfan, $4mg/M^2$/day. After satisfactory remission was achieved, splenectomy was performed. Four to six weeks following removal of the spleen, intensive chemotherapy was instituted with cyclic active drugs including cytosine arabinoside 60 mg/M^2 and 6-Thioguanine 70 mg/M^2. These drugs were administered in divided doses every twelve hours for five days. The cycle was repeated every six weeks. The doses were excalated usually to 100 mg/M^2 in subsequent cycles. Intermittent maintenance therapy with busulfan was continued between cycles of intensive therapy.

Bone marrow aspirates were prepared for chromosomal analysis according to a modification of Tjio and Whang's method (65). Aspirates were taken at the time of initial diagnosis, prior to splenectomy and at regular intervals thereafter, usually three to six months.

With the appearance of significant aneuploidy, pseudodiploidy or other chromosomal anomalies, chemotherapy was both intensified and modified in an attempt to prevent hematologic deterioration and reverse the karyotypic abnormalities. Methotrexate, Hydroxyurea and Duanorubicin were added as indicated. Since each patient's response to therapy was highly variable, intensive therapy was individualized.

Polycythemia vera and Essential Thrombocythemia

Patients presenting with these preneoplastic conditions were karyotyped at the time of diagnosis and periodically thereafter. Patients whose platelet counts were in excess of 1,000,000/mm^3 at the time of diagnosis were phlebotomized. The platelets were analyzed biochemically for viral RNA directed DNA polymerase (RDDP) (reverse transcriptase) (46) and electron microscopically for the presence of type C oncornaviruses (47). Chemotherapy with Busulfan was usually instituted.

Interpretation of Cytogenetic Data

Suggested patterns of stem cell or clonal evolution are given for several index cases in the series. These are meant to show possible lines of evolution. At least three cells must exhibit the same abnormal karyotype in order to be classified as a clone. Cells to be studied were obtained from bone marrow aspirates and unstimulated peripheral blood cultures. A minimum of 25 metaphases were analyzed in each case.

The cytogenetic nomenclature used here is based on the recommendations made at the Paris conference (66).

Abbreviations used in the Text

Adr - Adriamycin	HU - Hydroxyurea
Asp - L Asparaginase	MTX - Methotrexate
Ara-C - Cytosine Arabinoside	32P - Radioactive Phosphorous
Bus - Busulfan	Pred - Prednisone
CTX - Cytoxan	6TG - 6 Thioguanine
DA - Daunorubicin	VCR - Vincristine

Results

CGL - Three index cases are presented.

Patient M.S. is a 44-year-old white male, initially diagnosed in July of 1973. Remission was induced with Bus and a splenectomy was performed in February, 1974. As can be seen in Table I, 100% of the dividing bone marrow cells were Philadelphia chromosome positive at the time of diagnosis. This was reduced to 80% post-splenectomy, but the reduction was transitory. The correlations between courses of therapy and percent aneuploidy are also shown in Table I. Figure 1 shows the clonal evolution of the karyotypic abnormalities. Several clones appear to persist regardless of the type of therapy. However, intensification and modification of therapy seems to have eliminated one of the more ominous clones shown in Figure 1 and 2.

Patient G.T. is a 48-year-old, white female whose diagnosis of CGL was established in February, 1970. An objective remission was achieved in less than six weeks with Bus. A splenectomy was performed in September of 1971. A sharp drop was noted in the percentage of dividing cells in the bone marrow that were Philadelphia chromosome positive post-splenectomy (Table II, Figure 3). As can be seen in Table II, the patient remained relatively stable chromosomally until late 1973. G.T. received 14 cycles of Ara-C and 6TG during this period. In June, 1974, hyperdiploidy involving C group chromosomes (probably C8 or C9) was noted. Ara-C, 6G and HU were discontinued and cyclic chemotherapy was instituted with Bus, 6TG and HU. On this regimen, the WBC and platelet counts were well controlled for about a year. The hyperdiploid clone noted in June of 1974 (Figure 4) was no longer detectible; the hypodiploid clone, -C, persisted. In October, 1975, the hypodiploid, -C, clone evolved into a -C and -E clone. At the same time a new clone appeared showing a small metacentric marker. These clones persisted to December, 1975. Therapy was again altered. DA, CTX and Ara-C were administered in December, 1975. Sequential chromosomal analysis was done in February, 1976. Clones with the marker disappeared. A low level of hypodiploidy, 10%, -C remains at this time, (Figure 3). The patient is in excellent clinical control.

Patient J.F. is a 27-year-old, white male diagnosed in August, 1972. 100% of the dividing cells in a bone marrow aspirate were Philadelphia chromosome positive. Busulfan therapy was initiated in March, 1973, and an objective hematologic remission was obtained within three months. A splenectomy was performed in June, 1973. The percentage of Philadelphia chromosomes dropped continuously from 100% pretreatment to 60% one year post-splenectomy. The only hypodiploidy noted during this period was a clone lacking the Y chromosome. Seven cycles of chemotherapy with Ara-C and 6TG were given during this time. The white count ranged from

5,000 to 30,000 and the platelet count from about 145,000 to 475,000. There appeared to be no correlation between the two hematologic parameters and the clinical or chromosomal pictures.

Five additional cycles were administered between July and December, 1974. However, in October, chromosomal analysis revealed evolution of two additional aneuploid clones, one with an additional C group and one with a deletion of a C group chromosome (Figure 5). Neither the white count, nor the platelet count were well controlled during this period. In April of 1975, Bus was substituted for Ara-C and in September, HU was added (Table III). Neither of these therapeutic regimens were effective as can be seen in Figure 5. Chromosomal analysis of a bone marrow aspirate in May and of a non-stimulated peripheral blood culture and bone marrow aspirate in December of 1975, revealed the presence of significant aneuploidy, including the evolution of clones with double Philadelphia chromosome (Figure 6). On the basis of these karyotypic findings, therapy was changed. DA and Ara-C were administered in December, 1975. Sequential chromosomal analyses were again performed in late December, January and March 1976. As can be seen in Figure 5, there was a significant reduction in aneuploidy and the elimination or reduction of some of the more ominous clones.

PV and ET

Nine patients presenting with platelet counts of one million or more and diagnosed as having ET or PV were studied cytogenetically and for the presence of viral particles in platelet homogenates. Table--IV summarizes the results of these studies. Four of the patients L.F., D.S., F.P., and E.F., had varying degrees of aneuploidy, from 20 to 50%. In all cases a C group chromosome was missing, most likely a C8 or C9. No spontaneous mitosis were found in unstimulated peripheral blood cultures.

Viral-like particles were detected electron microscopically and biochemically (Table IV). Repeated phlebotomies did not adequately reduce the platelet count, but each of the four patients in this group responded to busulfan therapy clinically and chromosomally.

Two of the nine patients, B.D. and R.G. were hypodiploid (-C) but evidence for viral particles was not found. Bone marrow aspirates from R.G. were studied sequentially for chromosomal anomalies. Clonal evolution could be followed in this case. The percentage of hypodiploid cells increased and a marker chromosome appeared. This patient died of acute leukemia shortly after the last karyotypes were done. Viral particles, as noted elsewhere in the report, have never been found in the platelets of acute leukemics. B.G., although presenting with a platelet count of one million may also be in the process of converting to a more aggressive disease.

Eight other patients are also being studied in this program. Four of the group show hypodiploidy while the remaining four do not. Their platelets have not been examined for the presence of virus as yet.

Discussion

Approaches to the therapy of chronic granulocytic leukemia have been modified over the last several years (31, 33,37,67-77) but with few exceptions, the survival rate has not been significantly changed. Gomez and his collegues at Roswell Park Memorial Institute have analyzed 172 patients who had diagnosis of CGL established between 1950 and 1972 and who were followed through 1974 (76). The median survival for the entire group was 31 months. More pertinent for the purposes of this study was the median survival for the group of patients who were Philadelphia chromosome positive. Ninety patients in this group had a median survival of 43 months (p<.001). This is similar to the median survival of an untreated group of patients reported by Minot in 1924 (79). The recommended therapy for CGL until very recently has been induction of remission with Bus and subsequent maintenance with continuous low dose administration of the same drug (80, 81). More aggressive approaches to therapy have included splenectomy, splenic irradiation (69), 32P, intensive cycle active chemotherapy (37,70,74,75) and immunotherapy (72). Splenectomy, as a therapeutic modality in the chronic phase of the disease has had varied success in the past primarily because of the apparent lack of efficacy and prohibitive operative mortality (82). Unfortunately, however, many of the patients subjected to splenectomy were not in adequate hematologic remission at the time of surgery, were not in the chronic phase of the disease, were not given platelet transfusions or their infections were not adequately controlled. Present studies indicate that splenectomy can be performed in the early phase of the disease with little or no mortality or morbidity if sufficient care is taken in the selection and preparation of patients (37,69). Following splenectomy, intensive chemotherapy with the cycle active drugs has been initiated. One of the arguments used to support the contention that removal of the spleen early in CGL may be beneficial is that the spleen may be a reservoir for Ph positive cells, may be of significance in initiating metamorphosis and may be the preferred site of viral replication and action (25,31, 33,36,37,43,44,70,83,84). However, splenectomy alone cannot be considered effective therapy for CGL. Metamorphosis can occur after splenectomy if chemotherapy is not administered. Clinical trials are currently being conducted in Great Britain by the Medical Research Council's Working Party of Leukemia (MRC) and in Italy by the European Organization for Research and Treatment of Cancer (EORTC) to evaluate the efficacy of splenectomy and are being considered by the Eastern Cooperative Oncology Group (ECOG) in the United States. A proposal for splenectomy and intensive chemotherapy will be considered by ECOG at its May meeting (85).

Considerable attention is also being given to the types, doses and combination of drugs to be used in the post-splenectomy phase of treatment. Since CGL appears to be a stem cell disorder (37,41,42,86) which results in altered megakaryocytopoiesis, erythropoiesis and granulopoiesis, chemotherapy should be aimed at attacking these cells. The cyclic active drugs Ara-C and 6TG were originally chosen for this reason. Significant reductions have been observed in the percentage of marrow dividing cells possessing Ph' (Tables II and III). Other cyclic active drugs have been added to the armentarium. These include HU, MTX, VCR, PRED. ASP, DA and ADR.

Regardless of the mode of therapy, most cases of CGL enter a transition phase (metamorphosis) (85) which if unchecked will terminate in a blast crisis or acute transformation. The term blast crisis is used here in the restricted sense as defined by Spiers (85). "Rapid onset of increasing leukocytosis, preponderance of blasts, rapidly developing neutropenia and thrombocytopenia, progressive course, death coming in 2-6 weeks." Five to ten percent of CGL patients fall in this category. Fifty percent of patients undergo an acute transformation which is characterized by a "picture superficially resembling AML: some gradual development of neutropenia and thrombocytopenia (unless aggravated by therapy) survival for 3-6 months not uncommon". The remaining 40-45% compose a "mixed group exhibiting a variety of clinical and hematologic pictures including: thrombocytosis, thrombocytopenia, refractory anemia, polycythemia, myelofibrosis, leukopenia, accelerated granulopoiesis without excessive left shift and erythropoietic aplasia cannot justifiably be termed either blastic or acute; may have a course of months or years. AML-type therapy is quite inappropriate".

The diagnosis of metamorphosis preferably before the clinical signs appear would be distinct advantage in the management of the disease. There is ample evidence in the literature to suggest that transformation is accompanied by the appearance of abnormal clones first in the spleen, then in the bone marrow and finally in the peripheral blood.

We have attempted to predict an impending transformation by sequentially analyzing dividing bone marrow cells for chromosomal anomalies.

A group of eight patients (Table V) were entered into an ECOG protocol (#6472, Chairman, I. Brodsky) to evaluate the efficacy of splenectomy and intensive chemotherapy in the treatment of CGL. The initial chromosomal studies to confirm the diagnosis were done by Dr. Peter Nowell of the University of Pennsylvania (Tables II and III). Follow-up studies in our laboratory suggested that the appearance of chromosomal anomalies in dividing bone marrow cells preceded clinical deterioration and transformation into a more aggressive form of the disease.

As can be seen in Table I, patient M/S. first developed hypodiploidy between March and September 1974. During this period the white blood cell and platelet counts remained within acceptable limits. Five courses of therapy with Ara-C and 6TG were administered. However, by November of 1974, the white count had increased to 92,000. The sixth course of Ara-C and 6TG were given in November. The patient did not appear to be responding to therapy. Chromosomal analysis in July of 1975 revealed the presence of additional clones; 46% of all cells hypodiploid and 100% of all Ph' positive.

The decision was made at this time to alter treatment in an attempt to reverse the chromosomal and clinical pictures. 6TG, Bus and HU were given in July 1975. Both the chromosomal and clinical condition of the patient continued to deteriorate. DA and Ara-C were substituted for the previous therapeutic regimen in March 1975 with the dramatic results seen in Figure 1 and Table 1. Hypodiploidy dropped from 90% to 60% after the first course and to 20% after the second course of DA and CTX in December. More significantly, the clone containing the iso-17 chromosome was no longer detectible. The patient remains in excellent clinical control at this time.

Similar results were obtained with patients G.T. and J.F. Patient E.M., not described in this report, has had the longest survival of the group and has not shown any significant chromosomal changes. Patient C.U., also not described in this report, has had a similar course until very recently. In July of 1975, chromosomal analysis revealed the presence of two abnormal clones, 45, XO and 44, XO, -C. These persisted into March of 1976. CTX, MTX, and HU were administered in March, 1976. The latest hematologic findings show a reduction in the white blood count. A bone marrow aspirate will be surveyed for chromosomal anomalies in May.

Two cases in which chemotherapy was not based on chromosomal analysis are instructive. The first, F.S. was entered into the protocol prior to the initiation of the present study. This patient was followed chromosomally but no attempt was made to alter therapy based on the findings. At the time of diagnosis 100% of the dividing cells in the bone marrow were Ph' positive. No other chromosomal abnormalities were found. Five years after diagnosis and three years after splenectomy hyperdiploidy (30%) and triploidy (50%) were noted. Thrombocytopenia and subsequently acute granulocytic leukemia developed with the major symptom being severe bone pain. A sharp rise in WBC did not occur. The patient became refractory to all chemotherapeutic agents including DA, VTX, PRED and ASP. She expired early in 1975, 68 months after CGL had been diagnosed. The second patient, M.A.B. has had a benign and somewhat unusual form of CGL since 1968. A splenectomy was performed in February, 1972. She has had over 25 courses of Ara-C and 6TG to date and has tolerated them well, the only side effects being minimal nausea and slight fever. However, her disease has been characterized from the beginning by persistent thrombocytosis and leukocytosis. The platelet count is frequently in excess of one million and rarely below 700,000. In spite of the thrombocytosis, thromboembolic phenomena have not occurred. In 1975, therapy with Melphalan was initiated in an attempt to control the elevated platelet count but without success. Attempts to monitor the course of this patient's disease with sequential chromosomal surveys have been equally unsuccessful because of our inability to aspirate due probably to a fibrotic bone marrow. Peripheral blood studies have been negative until recently. However, the appearance of chromosomal anomalies in the peripheral blood has been accompanied by clinical deterioration and the appearance of blasts in the circulating blood. None of the patients whose therapy has been based on chromosomal findings in bone marrow aspirates have undergone transformation in their disease to date. As can be seen in Table V, the median survival in the group of six patients, three of whom are in this study is 72 months. This is 31 months longer than reported by Gomez (78). Six other patients have been splenectomized and are being followed chromosomally. An additional 12 patients are in the induction of remission phase of the protocol and will be followed sequentially.

Another group of patients (Table IV) who have had the initial diagnosis of PV or ET established and who we feel to be at risk for conversion of their disease to a more aggressive form have also been studied. The polycythemia study group (40) has reported the results of a survey of a large group of patients. Cytogenetic analysis revealed that a significant percentage of these patients had chromosomal abnormalities. It has also been known for some time and confirmed by this study that long time survivors of polycythemia develop myeloid fibrosis and myeloid metaplasia and in some cases acute leukemia. However, no significant correlations have been made between the cytogenetic findings and ultimate progression of disease. The Wurster-Hill study has shown, however, that there is no correlation between treatment of PV and metamorphosis into a more aggressive disease.

Based on our preliminary results (Table IV) a correlation does appear to exist between chromosomal abnormalities and the presence of virus-like particles in platelets of patients with PV or ET. In all cases (4) where the karyotype was abnormal, virus-like products were detected. In those cases where the karyotype was normal (3) no viruses were detectable in platelet homogenates. Two exceptions were found. Patient R.G. had hypodiploidy and a marker chromosome but no viruses were found. This patient showed increasing aneuploidy and died of acute leukemia. It is of interest to note, that virus-like particles have never been found in the platelets of patients with acute or chronic granulocytic leukemia (46,47) but have been found in the spleens of such patients (43,44).

The second patient, B.G. who has exhibited hypodiploidy and whose platelets are negative in tests for virus particles has an unusual form of polycythemia and may in fact be in the process of transforming to an acute disease entity. The combination of cytogenetic and viral surveys of polycythemia patients may be useful in predicting progression of disease.

Summary

Several tentative conclusions may be drawn from both an analysis of the results of the present study and the work of other investigations (1a). Sequential chromosomal surveys are useful in predicting the metamorphosis of CGL (1 b) chemotherapeutic intervention based on chromosomal findings may delay or prevent the onset of metamorphosis (1c). Splenectomy and intensive chemotherapy appear to be effective in prolonging survival of patients with CGL.

Untreated patients with a diagnosis of polycythemia vera or essential thrombocythemia may develop chromosomal anomalies (2a). Such patients may also harbor a virus-like particle in their platelets (2b). There may be a correlation between the development of clones of cells exhibiting an altered karyotype, the presence of detectable virus-like particles and the onset of more aggressive disease (2c).

Obviously, many more patients will have to be entered into the experimental studies, adequate controls will have to be included and the data must be subjected to vigorous statistical analysis. However, the initial studies appear to show enough promise to merit continued attention. In our hands, chromosomal analysis of bone marrow aspirates has proven efficacious in the diagnosis, prognosis and therapeutic management of patients with CGL, PV and ET.

ACKNOWLEDGMENTS

This investigation was supported in part by Program Project -- Medical Oncology Grant CA17053-01 and Eastern Cooperative Oncology Group Grant CA13611-03 from the National Cancer Institute, National Institutes of Health.

TABLE I. Summary of Chromosomal Abnormalities and Dates of Therapy, Patient M.S.

Date	Hypodiploidy	Ph'	Therapy
7/10/73	0	100%	
2/20/74			Splenectomy
3/15/74	0	80%	
5/29/74		73%	ARC-C, 6TG
9/25/74	20%	84%	ARA-C, 6TG
7/19/75	49%	100%	ARA-C, 6TG
8/16/75	70%	100%	6TG, HU, BUS
9/18/75	31%	100%	DA, CYT
11/10/75	90%	100%	DA, CYT
12/8/75			DA, ARA-C
12/22/75	60%	100%	
1/14/76			HU, MTX, CYT, 6TG
2/11/76			HU, MTX, CYT
3/3/76	20%	100%	

TABLE II. Summary of Chromosomal Abnormalities and Therapeutic Regimens, Patient G.T.

Date of Study	Aneuploidy Hypodiploid	Quasidiploid Hyperdiploid	Total	Ph'	Therapy
6/72*	0	0	0	12%	
9/73					ARA-C, 6TG
1/73*	0	0	0	20%	
11/73					ARA-C, 6TG
11/1/73*	0	0	0	70%	
1/74					ARA-C, 6TG
2/12/74*	0	0	0	38%	
3/74					ARA-C, 6TG, HU
4/74					ARA-C, 6TG, HU
6/17/74	7	37	44	66%	ARA-C, 6TG, HU
9/11/74					ARA-C, 6TG, HU
11/13/74					BUS, 6TG, HU
12/12/74	8	0	8	75%	
6/75					BUS, 6TG, HU
6/17/75	9	0	9	80%	
8/6/75	5	0	5	96%	
10/29/75	10	10	20	100%	
12/10/75	10	20	30	100%	DA, CTX, ARA-C
2/25/75		5	5	100%	

*Done in Dr. Nowell's Laboratory at the University of Pennsylvania

TABLE III. Summary of Chromosomal Abnormalities and Dates of Therapy, Patient J.F.

Date of Study	Aneuploidy Hypodiploid	Quasidiploid Hyperdiploid	Total	Ph'	Ph'Ph'	Therapy
1/23/73	0	0	0	100%	–	
6/8/73						Splenectomy
7/17/73						ARA–C, 6TG
9/6/73						ARA–C, 6TG
9/27/73	0	0	0	90%	–	
10/7/73						ARA–C, 6TG
11/16/73						ARA–C, 6TG
1/5/74						ARA–C, 6TG
1/16/74	12%	0	12%	82%	–	
2/15/74						ARA–C, 6TG
5/22/74	10%	0	10%	60%	–	ARA–C, 6TG
7/1/74						ARA–C, 6TG
8/12/74						ARA–C, 6TG
9/22/74						ARA–C, 6TG
10/22/74	7%	2%	9%	64%	–	
11/3/74						ARA–C, 6TG
12/15–74						ARA–C, 6TG
4/2/75						BUS, 6TG, HU
4/9/75						BUS, 6TG, HU
5/23/75	38%	2%	40%	100%	7%	
9/24/75						BUS, 6TG, HU
12/5/75	25%	17%	42%	100%	50%	
12/16/75						DA, ARA–C
12/25/75	20%	2%	22%	100%	20%	
1/16/76	10%	0	10%	100%	20%	
3/3/76	12%	0	12%	100%	16%	

TABLE IV. Correlation Between Karyotype and Virus Particles in PV and ET

Patient	Age/Sex	Diagnosis	Karyotype	Virus*	Comment
LF	75 F	PV	Hypo	+	
DS	59 F	ET	Hypo	+	
FP	80 F	ET	Hypo	+	
SS	64 M	PV	N	–	
BG	64 F	PV	Hypo	–	Possible conversion
EF	67 F	PV	Hypo	+	
EB	70 F	ET	N	–	
RG	74 M	PV	Hypo, Mr	–	Acute Leukemia, died
IF	54 M	ET	N	–	

*Electron microscopic and biochemical (RDDP) surveys.

TABLE V. Survival CML

Patient	Age/Sex	Diagnosis	Splenectomy	Months Survival to 4/76
EM	41 F	3/68	4/72	98
MAB	35 F	11/68	2/72	90
FS	49 F	7/69	11/71 died 2/75	68
GT	48 F	2/70	9/71	74
CU	54 M	8/71	2/72	56
JF	27 M	8/72	6/73	44
MS	45 M	7/73	2/74	34
RF	52 M	1/74	9/75	28
JH	28 M	6/74	9/75	22
JL	50 F	10/74	3/75	18
FF	51 F	5/75	10/75	11
DS	33 M	6/75	11/75	10
CB	43 F	9/75	4/26	8

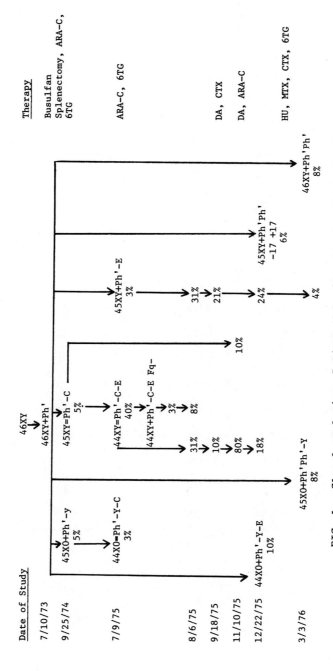

FIG. 1. Clonal evolution, Patient M.S. (Done in Dr. Peter Nowell's laboratory, University of Pennsylvania.)

118

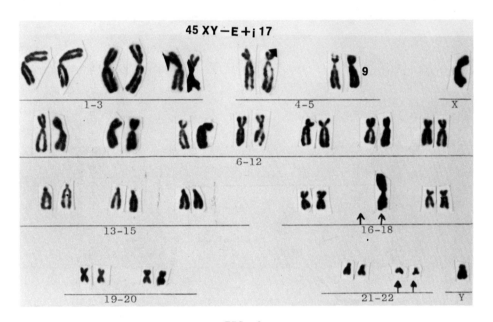

FIG. 2

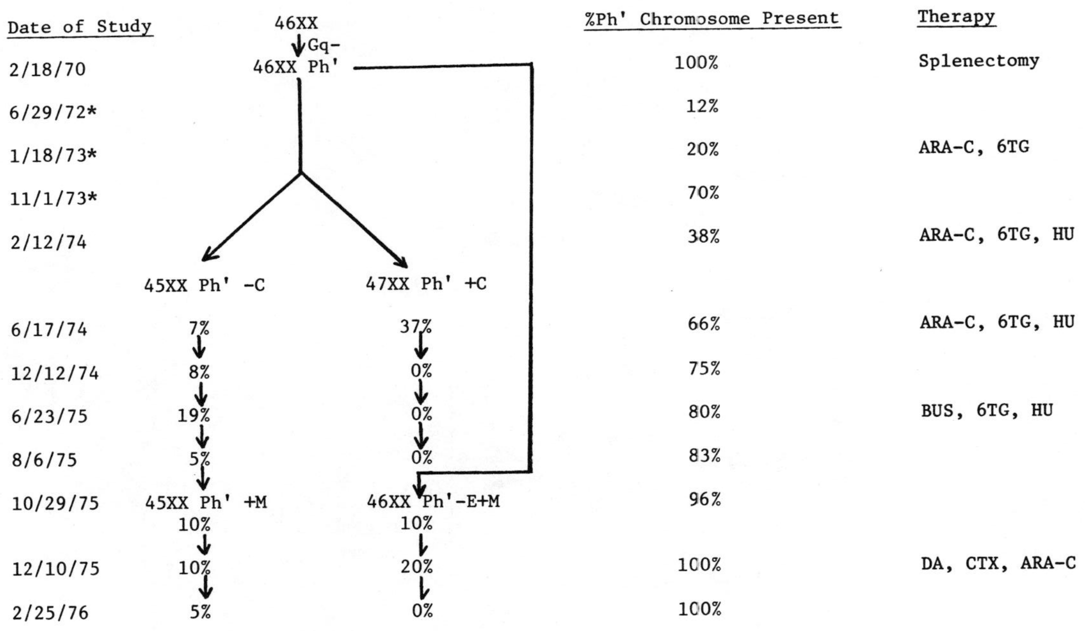

FIG. 3. Clonal evolution, Patient G.T. (*Done in Dr. Peter Nowall's laboratory, University of Pennsylvania.)

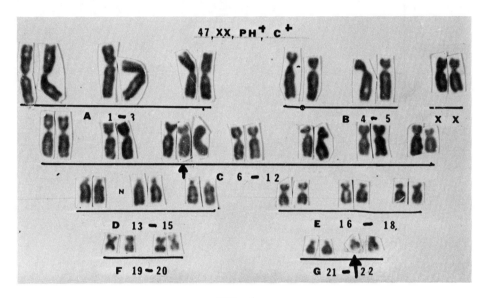

FIG. 4

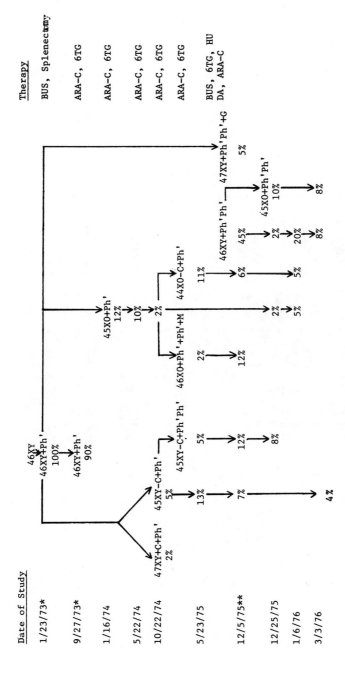

FIG. 5. Clonal evolution, Patient J.F. Data for 12/5/75 is for a non-stimulated blood culture. (*Done in Dr. Peter Nowell's laboratory, University of Pennsylvania.)

122

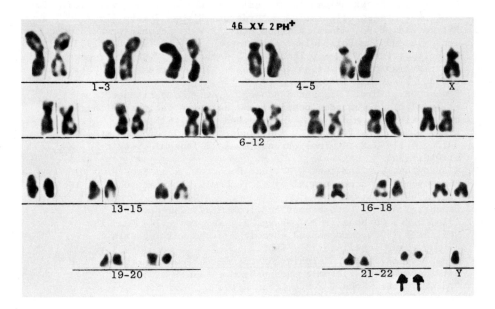

FIG. 6

REFERENCES

1. Baikie, A.G., Court-Brown, W.M., Buckton, K.E., Harriden, D.G., Jacobs,, P.A.,, and Tough, I.M.: A possible specific chromosome abnormality in human chronic myeloid leukemia, _Nature (London)_ 188: 1165.
2. Nowell, P.C. and Hungerford, D.A.: A minute chromosome in human chronic granulocytic leukemia. _Science_ 132:1497, 1960.
3. Nowell, P.C. and Hungerford, D.A.: Chromosome studies on normal and leukemic leucocytes. _J. Nat. Can. Inst.,_ 25:85, 1960.
4. Adams, A., Fitzgerald, P.H., and Gunz, F.W.: A new chromosomal abnormality in chronic granulocytic leukemia. _Brit. Med. J.,_ 2:1474, 1961.
5. Sandberg, A.A., Ishikara, T., Crosswhite, L., and Hauschka, T.S.: Comparison of chromosome constitution in chronic myelocytic leukemia and other myeloproliferative disorders. _Blood,_ 20:393, 1962.
6. Fitzgerald, P.H., Adams, A., and Gunz, F.W.: Chronic granulocytic leukemia and the Philadelphia chromosome. _Blood,_ 21:183, 1963.
7. Whang, J., Frei III, E., Tjio, J.H., Carbone, P.P., and Brecher, G.: Distribution of Philadelphia chromosome in a patient with CML. _Blood,_ 22(6):664, 1963.
8. Krauss, S., Sokol, J., and Sandberg, A.A.: Comparison of Philadelphia chromosome positive and negative patients with chronic myelocytic leukemia. _Ann. Intern. Med.,_ 6(4):625, 1964.
9. Kemp, N.S., Strafford, J.L, and Tanner, R.: Chromosome studies during early and terminal chronic myeloid leukemia. _Brit. J. Med.,_ 1:1010, 1964.
10. Kiossoglou, K.A., Mitus, W.J., and Dameshek, W.: Two Ph[1] chromosomes in acute granulocytic leukemia. _Lancet,_ Oct. 2, 1964: 665, 1965.
11. Sandberg, A.A.: Chromosomes and leukemia. _Cancer,_ 15:2, 1965.
12. Tjio, J.H., Carbone, P.P., Whang, J., and Frei III, E.: The Philadelphia chromosome and chronic myelogenous leukemia. _J. Nat. Can. Inst.,_ 36:567, 1966.
13. Stemple, R.M.: _Philadelphia chromosome in leukemia research,_ a bibliography, U.S. Atomic Energy Comm., ORNL:TM2103, 1968.
14. Ezdinli, E.Z., Sokal, J.E., Crosswhite, L., and Sandberg, A.A.: Philadelphia positive and Philadelphia negative chronic myelocytic leukemia. _Ann. Intern. Med.,_ 72:175, 1970.
15. Whang-Peng, J., Canellos, G.P., Carbone, P.P., et al, Clinical implications of cytogenetic variants in chronic myelocytic leukemias. _Blood,_ 32:755, 1968.
16. Rowley, J.: Abnormalities of chromosome 1 in myeloproliferative disorders. _Cancer,_ 36(5):1748, 1975.
17. Rowley, J.: Nonrandom chromosomal abnormalities in hematologic disorders in man. _Proc. Natl. Acad. Sci. (USA),_ 72:152, 1975.
18. Engel, E., McKee, L.C., Flexner, J.M., and McGee, B.J.: 17 long arm isochromosome: A common anomaly in malignant blood disorders. _An. Genet.,_ 18(1):56, 1975.
19. Ford, J.H., Pittman, S.M., Singh, S., Wass, E.J., Vincent, P.C., and Gunz, F.W.: Cytogenetic bases of acute myeloid leukemia. _J. Nat. Can. Inst.,_ 55(4):761, 1975.
20. Rowley, J.D.: Acquired trisomy 9, _Lancet,_ 2:390, 1973.
21. Khan, M.H., and Martin, H.: Presence of 2 Ph[1] chromosomes in cells with 49 clone from a patient in blast crisis of granulocytic leukemia. _Acta Haemat.,_ 42:357, 1969.

22. Meisner, L., Inhon, D.L, and Neilson, M.T.: Karyotypic evaluation of cells with Philadelphia chromosome. Acta Cytologica, 14(4):192, 1970.

23. Baikie, J.: Klonal evaluation in spalstadum der chronische myeloischen leukame. Detsh Med. Wschr, 98:195, 1973.

24. Whang-Peng, J., Knutsen, T.A., and Lee, E.O.: Dicentric Ph[1] chromosome, J. Nat. Cancer Inst., 51:2009, 1973.

25. Baccarani, M., Zaccanica, A., and Tura, S.: Splenic lymphocytes in CML. Lancet, Aug. 17, 1974:401, 1974.

26. Lawler, S.D., Lobb, D.S., and Wiltshaw, E.: Philadelphia-chromosome positive bone marrow cells showing loss of the Y in males with chronic myeloid leukemia. Br. J. Haematol., 27:247, 1974.

27. Rowley, J.D.: A new consistent chromosomal abnormality in chronic myelogenous leukemia identified by quinacrine fluorescence and giemsa staining. Nature, 243:290, 1973.

28. Rowley, J.D.: Missing sex chromosomes and translocations in acute leukemia. Lancet, 2:835, 1974.

29. Shiffman, N.J., Steiker, E., Conen, P.E., and Gardner, H.A.: Males with chronic myeloid leuekmia and the 45 xo Ph[1] chromosome pattern. Can. Med. Assoc. J., 110:1151, 1974.

30. Trujillo, J.M, Ahearn, M.J., and Cork, A.: General implication of chromosomal alterations in human leukemia. Human Pathology, 5(6):675, 1974.

31. Gomez, G., Hossfeld, D.K., and Sokal, J.E.: Removal of abnormal clone of leukemic cells by splenectomy. Brit. Med. J., 2:421, 1975.

32. Kohn, G., Noga, M., Eldar, Al., and Cohen, M.M.: De novo appearance of the Ph[1] chromosome in a previously monosomic bone marrow (45, XX, -6), conversion of a myeloproliferative disorder to AML. Blood, 45(5):653, 1975.

33. Mitelman, F., Nilsson, P.G., and Brandt, L.: Abnormal clones resembling those seen in the spleen in CML, J. Nat. Can. Inst. 54(6):1319, 1975.

34. Oberling, F., Stall, C., Lang, J.M., and Mayer, G.: Duplication of Philadelphia chromosome in acute transition of CGL. Ann. of Int. Med., 83(2)231, 1975.

35. Shaw, M.T., Bottomley, R.H., Grozea, P.N., and Nordquist, R.E., Herterogeniety of morphological, cytochemical and cytogenetic features in blastic phase of CGL. Cancer, 35(1), 199, 1975.

36. Spiers, A.S.D., Baikie, A.G., Dartnall, J.A., and Cox, J.E.: Cytogenetic studies of the spleen in chronic granulocytic leukemia. Aust. Nz J. Med., 5:295, 1975.

37. Brodsky, I., Fuscaldo, K.E., Kahn, S.B., and Lamping, C.G.: Chronic myelogenous leukemia: A clinical and experimental evaluation of splenectomy and intensive chemotherapy. Acta Hematol. (in press) 1976.

38. Nigam, R., and Dosik, H.: Chronic myelogenous leukemia presenting in blastic phase and its association with 45, XO, Ph[1] karyotype, Blood, 47(2):223, 1976.

39. Sukarai, M. and Sandberg, A.A.: Chromosomes and causation of human cancer XI, correlation of karyotypes with clinical features of acute myeloblastic leukemia. Cancer, 37(1):285, 1976.

40. Wurster-Hill, P., Whang-Peng, J., McIntyre, R., Hsu, L.F., Herschhorn, K., Nodan, B., Pisciotto, Aiv., Pierre, R., Balcerzak, S.P., Weinfeld, A., and Murphy, S.: Cytogenetic studies in polycythemia vera. Sem. Hemat., 13(1):13, 1976.

41. Fialkow, P.J.: The origin and development of human tumors studied with cell markers. N. Eng. J. Med., 291:26, 1974.

42. Faiklow P.J.: Clonal origins and stem cell evaluation, Natl. Found. of Birth Defects and Natl. Cancer Inst. Conference on Genetics of Human Cancer, Orlando, Fla., Dec., 1975 (in press) 1976.
43. Fuscaldo, K.E., Bacak, J., and Brodsky, I.: Electorn microscope studies of chronic myelogenous leukemia splenic tissue. Proc. Am. Soc. Clin. Onc., 15:180, 1974.
44. Witkin, S.S., Ohnu, T., Spiegelman, S.: Purification of RNA instructed DNA polymerase from human leukemia spleens. Proc. Nat. Acad. Sci. (USA), 72:4133, 1975.
45. Brodsky, I., and West, W.: Analysis of oncornaviruses in human and murine platelets. Proc. Am. Assoc. Can. Res., 17:508, 1976.
46. Brodsky, I., Fuscaldo, A.A., Erlick, B.J., Kingsbury, E.M., Schultz, G.M., and Fuscaldo, K.E.: Analysis of platelets from patients with thrombocythemia for reverse transcriptase and virus-like particles. J. Nat. Can. Inst., 55:1069, 1975.
47. Fuscaldo, A.A., Erlick, B.J., West, W., Fuscaldo, K.E., and Brodsky, I.: Use of critical point drying in electron microscopy as a screen for human oncornaviruses, submitted - Cancer Res., 1976.
48. Sandberg, A.A., Hossfeld, D.K., and Exdinli, E.Z.: Chromosomes and causation of human cancer and leukemia. VI. Blastic phase, cellular origin and the Ph^1 in CML, Cancer, 27:176, 1971.
49. Whang-Peng, J., Henderson, E.S., Knudzen, I., Freeneuk, E.J., and Cart, J.J.: Cytogenetic studies in acute myelogenous leukemia with special emphasis on the occurrence of Ph^1 chromosome. Blood, 36:448, 1970.
50. Gahrton, G., Lindsten, J., and Zech, L.: Clonal origin of the Philadelphia chromosome in either paternal or maternal chromosome #22 Blood, 43(3):837, 1974.
51. Mitelman, F.: Heterogeneity of Ph^1 in chronic myeloid leukemia, Hereditary, 76:315, 1974.
52. Whang-Peng, J., Lei, E.C., and Krietsen, T.A.: Genesis of the Ph^1 chromosome. J. Nat. Can. Inst., 52(4):1035, 1974.
53. Baike, J.: Clonal evolution in spalstadum der chronische myeloeschen leukame. Dtsh. Med. Wschr, 98:195, 1973.
54. Fuscaldo, K.E., Brodsky, I., Conroy, J.F., Kahn, S.B., and Wieczoreck, R.A.: Value of sequential chromosomal analysis for diagnosis, prognosis and monitoring of patients with CML. Am. Assoc. Can. Res., 17:506, 1976.
55. Gallagher, R.E., and Gallo, R.C.: Type C RNA virus isolated from cultured human acute myelogenous leukemic cells. Science, 187:350, 1975.
56. Gahrton, G., Zech, L., and Lindsten, J.: A new variant translocation (19q+, 228-) in CML, Exptl. Cell Res., 86:214, 1974.
57. Hsu, L.Y.F., Papenhausen, P., Greenberg, M.L., and Hirschron, K.: Trisomy D in bone marrow cells in a patient with CML. Aeta Hemat. 52:61, 1974.
58. Hayata, I., Kahati, S., and Sandberg, A.A.: Another translocation related to Ph^1 chromosome. Lancet, June 7, 1975:1300, 1975.
59. Engel, E., McGee, B.J., and Flexner, J.M., Russell, M.T., and Myer, B.J.: Philadelphia chromosome (Ph^1) translocation in an apparently Ph^1 negative, minus G22 case of CML. N. Engl. J. Med. July 18, 1975:154, 1974.
60. Carbone, P.P., Tjio, J.H., Whang, J., Brock, J.B., Kramer, W.B., and Frei III, E.: The effect of treatment in patients with chronic myelocytic leukemia. Ann. Intern. Med., 5:622, 1963.
61. Backie, A.G.: Chromosomes and leukemia, Acta Haemat., 36:157, 1966.
62. Amronin, G.D.: Pathology of leukemia. Harper Row, N.Y., 1968.

63. Sukurai, M., Hayata, I., and Sandberg, A.A.: Prognostic value of chromosomal findings in Ph[1] positive chronic myelocytic leukemia. Cancer Res, 36:313, 1976.

64. Mulvihill, J.J.: Cogenital and genetic diseases in persons at high risk of cancer. An approach to cancer etiology and control. J.R. Fraumeni, Jr. (Ed) Academic Press, Inc., New York, 1975.

65. Tjio, J.H. and Whang, J.: Chromosome preparations of bone marrow cells without prior in vitro culture and in vivo colchicine administration. Stain Technology 37:17, 1962.

66. Paris conference 1971. Standardization in human cytogenetics. Cytogenetics 11:313, 1972.

67. Sokal, V.E., Elias, E.G. and Mitelman, A.: Splenectomy in chronic myelocytic leukemia (CML) and related states. Proc. Am. Assoc. Can. Res., 12:37, 1971.

68. Canellos, G.P., Nordland, J. and Carbone, P.P.: Splenectomy for thrombocytopenia in chronic granulocytic leukemia. Cancer 29:660, 1972.

69. Kahn, S.B., and Brodsky, I.: Therapy of myeloproliferative disorders. In Cancer Chemotherapy II, Brodsky, I. and Kahn, S.B. (Eds), Grune and Stratton, New York, and London, pp. 347-359, 1972.

70. Sokal, V.E., Aungst, S.W., and Grace, J.J.: Immunotherapy in well controlled chronic myelocytic leukemia. New York State J. Med., 73:1180, 1973.

71. Dowling, M.D., Hopfan, S., Krapper, W.H., Vaqntage, T., Gee, I. Haghblin, M., and Clarkson, B.D.: Attempt to induce true remission in chronic myelogenous leukemia (CML). Proc. Am. Assoc. Can. Res., 189, 1974.

72. Goeggel, C., Kahn, S.B., and Brodsky, I.: Splenectomy in chronic myelogenous leukemia. Results of a pilot study. Proc. Am. Soc. Clin. Onc., 15:163, 1974.

73. Clarkson, B.D., personal communication, 1975.

74. Spiers, A.S.D., Baikie, A.G., Galton, D.A.G., Richards, H.G.H., Wiltshaw, E., Goldman, J.M., Catovsky, D., Spencer, J., and Peto, R.: Chronic granulocytic leukemia: effect of elective splenectomy on the course of disease. Brit. Med. J. 1:175, 1975.

75. Spiers, A.S.D., Galton, D.A.G., Kaier, J., and Goldman, J.M.: Thioguanine as primary treatment of chronic granulocytic leukaemia. Lancet, 1:829, 1975.

76. Spiers, A.S.D.: The treatment of chronic granulocytic leukemia. Brit. J. Haem. 32:291, 1976.

77. Tura, S.: Splenectomy and intensive chemotherapy in CML. International Society of Hematology, London, England, 1975. Acta Hemat. (in press) 1976.

78. Gomez, G.A., Sokal, J.E., Stutzman, L. and Reese, P.: Prognostic factors at the time of diagnosis (DX) in chronic myeloid leukemia (CML), Proc. Am. Assoc. Clin. Onc., C-177, 1976.

79. Minot, G.R., Buchman, J.E., Isaacs, R.: Chronic myelogenous leukemia: Age, incidence, duration and benefit derived. JAMA 82: 1486, 1924.

80. Galton, D.A.G.: Chemotherapy of chronic myelocytic leukemia. Sem. in Hemat. 6:323, 1969.

81. Strychkmans, P.A.: Current concepts in chronic myelogenous leukemia. Seminars in Hematology: P.A. Mieschker, and E.R. Jaffe (Eds) Grune and Stratton, New York and London, Vol. II, p. 101-127, 1974.

82. Strumia, M.M., Strumia, P.V., Bassert, D.: Splenectomy in leukemia: Hematologic and clinical effects on 34 patients and review of 299 unpublished cases. Cancer Res., 26:519, 1966.

83. Pegrum, G.D., Thompson, E., and Lewis, C.M.: Possible cell recruitment in human leukemia. <u>Lancet</u>, September 15:585, 1973.
84. Warner, R.F.C.S.: Cell recruitment in leukemia. <u>Lancet</u>, October 20:910, 1973.
85. Brodsky, I., Kahn, S.B., Spiers, A.S.D.: Effect of splenectomy and intensive chemotherapy on onset of metamorphosis, cytogenetics and survival in chronic granulocytic leukemia (CGL). Protocol submitted to ECOG, 1976.
86. Brodsky, I.: The role of the megakaryocyte in the leukemic process in mice and men. A review and hypothesis, <u>J. Natl. Cancer Inst.</u>, 51:329, 1973.

DETECTION OF ADENOVIRUS INTEGRATION SITES IN HOST CELL CHROMOSOMES

James K. McDougall, Ashley R. Dunn and Phillip H. Gallimore

Cold Spring Harbor Laboratory, New York 11724
and
Department of Cancer Studies, Medical School
University of Birmingham, England

INTRODUCTION

The ability of a number of DNA-containing viruses to induce tumors in experimental animals and to morphologically transform cultured cells in vitro has provided basic cancer research with an array of techniques for studying the pathways involved in the phenotypic changes from normal to malignant characteristics.

Adenoviruses, which are widespread in many species, including man, have been extensively utilized in such studies since the discovery by Trentin, Yabe and Taylor (1962) that this virus group can cause tumors in rodents. One of the most interesting facets of the tumor-inducing properties of this DNA virus group is that there are wide variations in oncogenic potential of the eighty or so different serotypes known. Some human adenoviruses are highly oncogenic, e.g. type 12 (Huebner, 1967) whereas at the other end of the spectrum the oncogenicity of type 2 genes is frequently only expressed in cells which, following in vitro transformation by the virus, are injected into immunosuppressed hosts (Gallimore, 1972).

During the past two years the use of restriction endonucleases to generate specific fragments of DNA molecules has resulted in very precise analyses of the integrated viral DNA sequences in many DNA virus-transformed and tumor cell lines (Sambrook et al., 1974). Among these the adenovirus type 2 lines, which never release virus (Dunn et al., 1973), have been shown to contain a consistent small fragment of the viral DNA molecule and to have only a portion of that fragment transcribed into messenger RNA (Sharp, Gallimore and Flint, 1974). The transcribed region is only sufficient to specify one or two proteins and these therefore might be considered to be the necessary factors involved in initiation and maintenance of the transformed and oncogenic phenotype.

The co-valently integrated viral sequences could exert their influence on the host genome either by the regulatory effect of the proteins translated from the known transcripts, for example the tumor antigen (T-ag) found in cells transformed by DNA viruses, or by a steric effect affecting host DNA transcription. In either case, an understanding of the specificity of viral gene integration may be the key to a final assessment of the role of viruses in oncogenicity.

This paper describes approaches we have made to determine the location and function of integrated adenovirus DNA sequences in rodent and human cells.

PROCEDURES AND MATERIALS USED

Adenovirus transformed cells

The development and properties of the cells used in this study have been described previously (Gallimore, 1974; McDougall et al., 1974; Graham et al., 1974).

T-antigen immunofluorescence

Detection of viral T-antigen was carried out as described by Gallimore (1974).

Chromosome identification

The Giemsa banding technique as described by Gallimore and Richardson (1973) was used to identify rat chromosomes. In situ hybridization of mouse satellite cRNA (Jones, 1970) was utilized for mouse centromere recognition.

Isozyme identification

Starch gel electrophoresis of cell extracts was carried out by the method of Nichols and Ruddle (1973).

In situ hybridization for viral sequences

i) Iodinated DNA

Cells were grown on sterile microscope slides in 9 cm petri dishes to sub-confluent monolayers fixed in 70% methanol and air dried.

The iodinated adenovirus DNA, prepared as described by Minson and Darby (1976), has an estimated specific activity of 5×10^7 dpm/ug and is 150-200 nucleotides in length.

Heat denatured iodinated DNA was 97% susceptible to digestion with S1 nuclease after incubation for 1 hour at $22^{\circ}C$ in the presence of calf thymus DNA.

A 5 micro-litre sample (12,000 cpm) of ^{125}I labelled DNA was denatured by boiling for 10 min in 0.1 x SSC, adjusted to 2 x SSC and applied to fixed preparations of cells. Hybridization was carried out for 5 hours at 65°C under a coverslip sealed with a gum solution after which slides were rinsed in Sl buffer (0.03M sodium acetate pH 4.5; 0.002M zinc sulphate and 0.01N NaCl). 5 micro-litres of the Sl enzyme made up in the same buffer was applied to each slide in the presence of 5 ug of denatured calf thymus DNA and digestion carried out at room temperature (22°C) for 1 hour. Slides were thoroughly washed in several changes of 2 x SSC at room temperature for 24 hours, run through a series of graded alcohols (70%, 90%, 95% and absolute) and air dried. Autoradiographs were established using Ilford K2 nuclear emulsion and after the appropriate exposure at 4°C, developed in Kodak D-19, rinsed, fixed in 30% sodium thiosulphate, washed for 15 minutes in running tap water and stained for 1 hour in 10% Giemsa pH 6.8.

ii) ^{3}H cRNA

The method used was that described by McDougall et al. (1972).

RESULTS

Somatic cell hybrids were derived by fusion of virus transformed rat cells and mouse cells deficient in thymidine kinase (LMTK⁻ Clone 1D). Fusion was mediated by β-propiolactone inactivated sendai virus which is known to increase the frequency of cell fusion.

A double selective system has been employed which favors the survival of hybrid cells over the parental cells. After fusion, cells were incubated in the presence of HAT, which selects against cells deficient in thymidine kinase (TK), and in growth medium containing calcium ions. Adenovirus transformed cells show a variable sensitivity to Ca^{++} (Freeman et al., 1967). The surviving hybrid cells must necessarily contain the rat gene coding for thymidine kinase.

14-21 days after seeding the mixed fused cell population at low density and incubation in the selective medium, morphologically distinct clones of cells were picked, plated out at low density and re-cloned. A total of 57 cloned hybrid lines was established.

In the hybrid lines examined, the only rat chromosomes positively identified are numbers 1, 2, 11, 12, 17 and 19; however, none of these chromosomes is consistently present in every hybrid cell line. In the majority of cloned cell lines, the content of rat chromosomes remains stable. As all the hybrid cell lines survive in HAT medium, they must by definition contain the rat thymidine kinase (TK) gene. The absence of a consistently identifiable rat autosome in every hybrid line suggests that this gene can be present as a part of a translocated chromosome. In support of this fact is the observation that 4 of the 6 clones seen in Table I derived from fusion of the Ad-2/F4 line contain the TK gene but not the galactokinase (GaK) gene. Since the structural genes for these two enzymes are known to be closely linked in a number of mammalian species (Elsevier et al., 1974; Orkwiszewski et al., 1974; Chen et al., 1976), it seems probable that the translocation has occurred at a point in the chromosome somewhere between the sequences coding for these enzymes.

In no hybrid cell line have we identified the marker chromosomes known to be present in the parental rat transformed cell lines and the rat chromosomes only appear as single copies in the hybrid lines, even though the parental cells are near triploid.

Using reassociation kinetics in solution the viral transcripts in a number of adenovirus 2 transformed cell lines, including the two cell lines (Ad-2/F4 and Ad-2/F17) used in this study, have been catalogued (Flint et al., 1975). Moar and Jones (1975) have shown that virus mRNA can be detected in a line of adenovirus transformed cells (line Ad-2/B1) by in situ hybridization using ^{3}H-thymidine labelled adenovirus DNA as probe. We have used a method for screening large numbers of mouse/rat hybrid lines for the presence of virus RNA transcripts. By using ^{125}I labelled adenovirus DNA in the in situ reaction, we have been able to achieve high specific activity probes (>10^7 cpm/ug) as well as reducing autoradiographic exposure time to 2 weeks. Following hybridization to fixed monolayers of cells and subsequent treatment with S1 nuclease, autoradiographs are examined for the presence of grains. In most autoradiographs grains are predominantly found in the nucleus with a lower level of cytoplasmic graining. This situation is true for lytically infected cells, the parental rat transformed cells, and in some mouse/rat hybrid lines. Uninfected human embryo kidney cells (HEK), rat embryo fibroblasts and a number of hybrid lines show low levels of grains only slightly higher than equivalent areas of non-cellular background. The predominantly nuclear graining probably represents hybridization to viral mRNA which forms part of a large HnRNA molecule comprising viral and cellular sequences, some of which never get transported to the cytoplasm in productive infections.

All of the hybrid lines established from both Ad-2/F4 and Ad-2/F17 which contain virus mRNA also contain T-antigen as determined by immuno-fluorescence. None of the hybrids which show a negative in situ hybridization show a positive reaction for T-antigen.

The results from an extensive study of a series of cloned cell lines are shown in Table I. None of the 6 rat chromosomes identified in hybrid lines was consistently present in T-antigen or viral mRNA positive lines and none of the 15 rat isozymes tested, apart from TK, was found to be always present in hybrid cells expressing viral functions.

The situation with an adenovirus transformed human cell line was similar, in that these cells were heterogeneous in chromosome constitution with an average count in the triploid range and with only a small amount of viral DNA per diploid quantity of human DNA (Sambrook, personal communication). Our preliminary experiments with this cell line hybridized to TK[-] mouse cells indicate a dilution of T-antigen and an association of this viral function with retention of human chromosome E17. This autosome carries the adenovirus inducible human TK gene (McDougall et al., 1973) and must be retained in the hybrid cell for survival in HAT medium. If in fact a viral integration site is not finally shown to be in this chromosome and associated with the virus induced uncoiler region, then the most probable explanation will be that there are presently undetectable trans-locations occurring during hybrid cell formation and chromosome segregation. One of the findings reported in this paper certainly supports this unwelcome prospect in that we have found separation of two enzymes known to be closely linked in mammalian cells, i.e. TK and GalK.

DISCUSSION

The finding that adenovirus or SV40 DNA molecules can persist as multiple copies of fragments occurring at different frequencies does not seem to be immediately compatible with the concept of integration at a single locus. It is nevertheless possible that one integration site could have more significance than others and the results with SV40 transformed human and primate cells (Croce and Koprowski, 1974; Croce et al., 1974; Khoury and Croce, 1975) would certainly be consistent with this hypothesis.

The significance of such a locus would be (i) that it allows transcription of the integrated viral genes by utilization of host promoters, resulting in a product controlling the transformed phenotype or (ii) that the integrated viral DNA effects a steric change in the host genome with consequent alteration in host transcription and regulation.

The present study is providing a series of hybrids some of which contain virus DNA sequences which serve as templates for virus RNA transcription. Although our data show that certain rat chromosomes appear with high frequency in hybrid cell lines, some of which contain virus mRNA and express T-antigen, the integration site(s) of adenovirus DNA sequences in this limited number of transformed cell lines does not appear to have segregated together with a single identifiable rat chromosome or isozyme.

Adenovirus transformed cell lines are karyotypically abnormal and the two parental rat cell lines used to produce these hybrids are no exception to the rule. Ad-2/F4 has a majority of cells (68%) which are triploid (63 chromosomes) and an average chromosome number of 66. There are 2-3 abnormal and stable marker chromosomes in every cell. The Ad-2/F17 C8 line is more heterogeneous than Ad-2/F4 with a higher average chromosome count (76) and with 4-5 large acrocentric markers.

The fact that none of the hybrid cell lines which are positive for viral mRNA and T-antigen contain any marker chromosome from the virus transformed cells indicates that the viral integration site is not associated with the markers. In a recent study of herpesvirus type 2 transformed hamster cells, no correlation has been found between marker chromosomes, viral sequences and oncogenicity (Copple and McDougall, 1976).

If identical autosomes have the same capability to integrate viral sequences, as might be expected, then the triploidy of these rat lines would tend to result in a dilution of viral gene dosage in hybrid lines when, as we have found, there is a tendency for only haploid copies of rat chromosomes to be retained in the hybrids. This is compatible with our observation that there is decreased T-antigen immunofluorescence in the positive hybrid cells, compared with the transformed rat cell.

The methods described in this paper are allowing selection of hybrid lines for a more critical quantitative analysis of viral sequences and the part these sequences play in determining the transformed and oncogenic

133

phenotypes. This approach, together with improved in situ hybridization techniques, should eventually provide a better understanding of the nature of integration of virus genes in transformed cells. The somatic cell hybrid approach is the optimum method for determining whether (i) the integration of specific viral genes, (ii) expression of T-antigen, (iii) the transformed phenotype in vitro and (iv) oncogenicity in vivo are all related phenomena which cannot be segregated. It is worth re-iterating that the first three characteristics do not inevitably lead to the fourth (McDougall, 1975).

SUMMARY

A series of hybrid cell lines resulting from the fusion of adenovirus transformed rat cells and mouse cells has been isolated using a double selective system. Identification of chromosomes in the hybrids bearing mouse centromeres has been made by using in situ hybridization with mouse satellite cRNA as the probe. The rat/mouse hybrid cells segregate rat chromosomes and established hybrid cell lines contain only a limited number of rat chromosomes, however none of these chromosomes is present in every cell line. All hybrids have been screened for virus mRNA by in situ hybridization using ^{125}I labelled adenovirus DNA. All lines containing virus transcripts are also positive for T-antigen by immunofluorescence.

Cytogenetic analysis and rat isozyme segregation data indicate that many of the hybrids contain new chromosome translocations which were not present in the parental cell lines and also that none of the marker chromosomes present in the transformed rat cells have appeared in the hybrid cell lines.

Although the results from these experiments indicate that integration of adenovirus DNA is into only a few chromosomes of the rat cells, it has not been possible to define a specific chromosome associated with the expression of adenovirus T-antigen.

ACKNOWLEDGMENTS

We thank Dr. K. W. Jones, Dr. A. Minson and Dr. G. Darby for help and valuable discussions. We are grateful to Delia Knox and Ann Maguire for excellent technical assistance and to the Cancer Research Campaign (CRC) and the National Institute of Health for supporting this work. J. K. McDougall is a Life Fellow of the CRC.

134

TABLE I. Analysis of Hybrid Cell Lines

Cell type	No. of rat chromosomes	Ad-2 T-antigen	Ad-2 mRNA	Rat enzymes[§]
Ad-2/ F17 C8	76*	+	+	+ (15 tested)
Ad-2/F17/LMTK⁻/A1	3	-	-	GaK,TK,IPO$_A$,RPPK
A3	3	-	-	GaK,TK,RPPK
B1	2	+	+	GaK,TK,RPPK
B2	3	+	+	GaK,TK,IPO$_A$
E1	1	-	-	GaK,TK
E3	1	-	-	GaK,TK
D1	1	-	-	GaK,TK,NP
Ad-2/F4	66*	+	+	+ (15 tested)
Ad-2/F4/LMTK⁻/ A1	3	-	-	GaK,TK,IPO$_A$,RPPK
A2	3	-	-	TK,NP,LDH-A,GPI,G6PD
A3	2	-	-	TK,NP,G6PD
B1	3	+	+	GaK,TK,NP
B2	3	-	-	TK,NP,Pep-A,MOD-1
B3	5	+	+	TK,NP,Pep-A,MOD-1
HEK infected with Ad-2(20 pfu/cell)[†]	-	+	+	-
HEK	-	-	-	-
Rat embryo fibroblasts	42	-	-	+ (15 tested)
LMTK⁻	-	-	-	-

+ = positive result.
*Average chromosome number.
[†]pfu = plaque forming units.
[§]TK - Thymidine kinase (E.C. no. 2.7.1.75), GaK - Galactokinase (E.C. no.
2.7.1.6), IPO$_A$ - Indophenoloxidase-A (E.C. no. 1.15.1.1), NP - Nucleoside
phosphorylase (E.C. no. 2.4.2.1), LDH-A - Lactate dehydrogenase-A (E.C. no.
1.1.1.27), GPI - Glucose phosphate isomerase (E.C. no. 5.3.1.9), G6PD -
Glucose-6-phosphate dehydrogenase (E.C. no. 1.1.1.49), Pep-A - Peptidase-A
(E.C. no. 3.4.11.), MOD-1 - Malic enzyme (soluble) (E.C. no. 1.1.1.40),
RPPK - Ribosephosphate pyrophosphokinase (E.C. no. 2.7.6.1), HGPRT -
Hypoxanthine phosphoribosyltransferase (E.C. no. 2.4.2.8), APRT - Adenine
phosphoribosyltransferase (E.C. no. 2.4.2.7), Pep-B - Peptidase-B (E.C. no.
3.4.11.), Pep-C - Peptidase-C (E.C. no. 3.4.11.), MPI - Mannose phosphate
isomerase (E.C. no. 5.3.1.8).

Enzyme nomenclature: Recommendations (1972) of the International Union of
Pure and Applied Chemistry and the International Union of Biochemistry.
Published in 1973 by Elsevier (Amsterdam) and American Elsevier (New York).

REFERENCES

Chen, S., McDougall, J.K., Creagan, R.P., Lewis, V., and Ruddle, F.H. Mapping of genes and adenovirus-12 induced gaps using chimpanzee-mouse somatic cell hybrids. Cytogen. Cell Genet., in press, 1976.

Copple, C.D., and McDougall, J.K. Clonal derivatives of a herpes type 2 transformed hamster cell line (333-8-9): Cytogenetic analysis, tumorigenicity and virus sequence detection. Int. J. Cancer, 17, in press, 1976.

Croce, C.M., and Koprowski, H. Concordant segregation of the expression of SV40 T-antigen and human chromosome 7 in mouse-human hybrid subclones. J. Exp. Med., 139: 1350-1353, 1974.

Croce, C.M., Huebner, K., Girardi, A.J., and Koprowski, H. Genetics of cell transformation by simian virus 40. Cold Spring Harbor Symp. Quant. Biol., 39: 335-343, 1974.

Dunn, A.R., Gallimore, P.H., Jones, K.W., and McDougall, J.K. In situ hybridization of adenovirus RNA and DNA. II. Detection of adenovirus specific DNA in transformed and tumor cells. Int. J. Cancer, 11: 628-636, 1973.

Elsevier, S.M., Kucherlapati, R., Nichols, E.A., Willecke, K., Creagan, R.P., Giles, R.E., Ruddle, F.H., and McDougall, J.K. Assignment of the gene for human galactokinase (EC 2.7.1.6) to chromosome E17 band q21-22. Nature, 251: 633-636, 1974.

Flint, S.J., Gallimore, P.H., and Sharp, P.A. Comparison of viral RNA sequences in adenovirus 2-transformed and lytically infected cells. J. Mol. Biol., 96: 47-68, 1975.

Freeman, A.E., Black, P.H., Vanderpool, E.A., Henry, P.H., Austin, J.B., and Huebner, R.J. Transformation of primary rat embryo cells by adenovirus type 2. Proc. Nat. Acad. Sci., 58: 1205-1212, 1967.

Gallimore, P.H. Tumor production in immunosuppressed rats with cells transformed in vitro by adenovirus type 2. J. gen. Virol., 16: 99-102, 1972.

Gallimore, P.H. Interactions of adenovirus type 2 with rat embryo cells. Permissiveness, transformation and in vitro characteristics of adenovirus transformed rat cells. J. gen. Virol., 25: 263-273, 1974.

Gallimore, P.H., and Richardson, C.R. An improved banding technique exemplified in the karyotype analysis of two strains of rat. Chromosoma, 41: 259-263, 1973.

Graham, F.L., Abrahams, P.J., Mulder, C., Heijneker, H.L., Waarnar, S.O., De Vries, F.A.J., Fiers, W., and Van der Eb, A.J. Studies on in vitro transformation by DNA and DNA fragments of human adenoviruses and simian virus 40. Cold Spring Harbor Symp. Quant. Biol., 39: 637-650, 1974.

Huebner, R.J. Adenovirus-directed tumor and T-antigens. In: Perspectives in Virology, V. Ed.: J. Pollard. Academic Press, New York, 1967.

Jones, K.W. Chromosomal and nuclear location of mouse satellite DNA in individual cells. Nature, 225: 912-915, 1970.

Khoury, G., and Croce, C.M. Quantitation of the viral DNA present in somatic cell hybrids between mouse and SV40-transformed human cells. Cell, 6: 535-542, 1976.

McDougall, J.K. Adenoviruses--Interaction with the host cell genome. Progr. med. Virol., 21: 118-132, 1975.

McDougall, J.K., Dunn, A.R., and Jones, K.W. In situ hybridization of adenovirus RNA and DNA. Nature, 236: 346-348, 1972.

McDougall, J.K., Kucherlapati, R.S., and Ruddle, F.H. Localization and induction of the human thymidine kinase gene by adenovirus 12. Nature New Biol., 245: 172-175, 1973.

McDougall, J.K., Dunn, A.R., and Gallimore, P.H. Recent studies on the characteristics of adenovirus-infected and transformed cells. Cold Spring Harbor Symp. Quant. Biol., 39: 591-600, 1974.

Minson, A.C., Thouless, M.E., Eglin, R.P., and Darby, G. The detection of virus DNA sequences in a herpes type 2 transformed hamster cell line (333-8-9). Int. J. Cancer, 17, in press, 1976.

Moar, M.H., and Jones, K.W. Detection of virus-specific RNA base sequences in individual cells transformed by adenovirus type 2. Int. J. Cancer, 16: 998-1007, 1975.

Nichols, E.A., and Ruddle, F.H. A review of enzyme polymorphism, linkage and electrophoretic conditions for mouse and somatic cell hybrids in starch gels. J. Histochem. and Cytochem., 21: 1066-1081, 1973.

Orkwiszewski, K.G., Tedesco, T.A., and Croce, C.M. Assignment of the human gene for galactokinase to chromosome 17. Nature, 252: 60-62, 1974.

Sambrook, J., Botchan, M., Gallimore, P., Ozanne, B., Pettersson, U., Williams, J., and Sharp, P.A. Viral DNA sequences in cells transformed by simian virus 40, adenovirus type 2 and adenovirus type 5. Cold Spring Harbor Symp. Quant. Biol., 39: 615-632, 1974.

Sharp, P.A., Gallimore, P.H., and Flint, S.J. Mapping of adenovirus 2 RNA sequences in lytically infected cells and transformed cell lines. Cold Spring Harbor Symp. Quant. Biol., 39: 457-474, 1974.

Trentin, J.J., Yabe, Y., and Taylor, G. The quest for human cancer viruses. Science, 137: 835-841, 1962.

EFFECTS OF CYTOCHROME P-448 AND P-450 INDUCERS ON MICROSOMAL
DIMETHYLNITROSAMINE DEMETHYLASE ACTIVITY AND THE CAPACITY
OF ISOLATED MICROSOMES TO ACTIVATE DIMETHYLNITROSAMINE TO A
MUTAGEN

J.B. Guttenplan
Department of Biochemistry
New York University College of Dentistry
New York, N.Y. 10010

A.J. Garro and F. Hutterer*
Department of Microbiology and Department of Pathology
Mount Sinai School of Medicine of the City
University of New York, New York, N.Y. 10029

INTRODUCTION

Dimethylnitrosamine, DMN, is a carcinogen which is not
mutagenic by itself but is metabolically activated to a
mutagen by enzymes present in hepatic microsomes [21]. It
has been suggested that DMN induced mutations result from
the alkylation of nucleic acid bases by the methyldiazonium
ion, $CH_3N_2^+$[16,18], which is produced from DMN by oxidative
demethylation to the unstable monomethylnitrosamine [24].
A microsomal DMN demethylase activity has been described
which appears to function as part of the cytochrome P-450
mixed function oxidase system as judged by its requirements
for molecular oxygen and NADPH, its inducibility and its
inhibition by CO which is reversible by light in the
vicinity of 450 nm [6,22,28].

We and others have previously demonstrated, using a
Salmonella auxotroph reversion test to assay DMN dependent
mutagenesis, that both the oxidative demethylation of DMN

*Presently: Department of Molecular Pathology
             University College of Medicine
             275 Martinel Drive
             Kent, Ohio   44240

and its activation to a mutagen followed typical Michaelis-Menton kinetics with respect to DMN concentration [6,8,10]. We also have shown, with microsomes from mice maintained on protein deficient diets [5] and with microsomes from human liver biopsy specimens [4], that there is a linear relationship between cytochrome P-450 levels and the capacity of isolated hepatic microsomes to convert DMN to a mutagen.

It has seemed reasonable to assume that activation of DMN to a carcinogen proceeds by the same pathways as its activation to a mutagen. There are, however, a number of observations derived primarily from carcinogenesis experiments which suggest that the activation scheme outlined above cannot fully account for either the mutagenic or carcinogenic activities of DMN. For example, the ethyl homologue of DMN, diethylnitrosamine, is also a potent carcinogen, however, it is only 0.01-0.03 as effective an alkylating agent of nucleic acid bases as DMN [12]. In another study in which different species and sexes of mice with widely different susceptibilities to DMN induced liver tumors were compared, it was observed that liver microsomes from the group with the lowest incidence of tumors had the highest DMN demethylase activity [7]. Furthermore, a number of laboratories have been unable to observe a significant correlation between the degree of alkylation of nucleic acid bases in different organs and the localization of tumors induced by exposure to various nitroso compounds [7,12,19,31,33]. However, there is evidence that the inability of certain tissues to eliminate one of the alkylation products, O^6-methylguanine, may increase suseptibility of these tissues towards DMN induced tumor formation [26]. DMN appears to be relatively efficient at O-alkylation of DNA [16]. In a study where several microsomal N-demethylase activities and cytochrome P-450 levels were monitored as a function of microsomal storage time, it was found that DMN demethylase activity decayed at a much slower rate than other N-demethylases or cytochrome P-450. From these and other data, the authors concluded that the rate limiting

140

step in DMN demethylation does not appear to involve cyto-chrome P-450 [15]. Alternative mechanisms to explain the mutagenic and carcinogenic activities of different nitro-samines have been proposed which postulate that reactions between DNA and the nitroso moieties of these compounds con-tribute to their biological activities [29,32].

In this study we have attempted to analyze the relation-ship between DMN demethylase and the activation of DMN mutagenicity through the use of different types of micro-somal enzyme inducers. One of these, phenobarbital, PB, increases cytochrome P-450 levels and enhances the activity of a wide variety of microsomal enzymes including those involved in N-demethylations of a number of drugs such as aminopyrine [3]. Another inducer 3-methylcholanrene, 3-MC, produces an effect typical of polycyclic hydrocarbons, in-creasing the level of a different cytochrome, P-448, and enhancing the activity of only a few enzymes one of which is aryl hydrocarbon hydroxylase [1,25]. This enzyme activity is not inducible by polycyclic hydrocarbons in one of the two strains of mice, DBA/2, used in this study [9]. Polychlorinated biphenyls such as Aroclor 1254 comprise a third type of inducer and enhance the metabolism of both P-450 and P-448 substrates [1].

PROCEDURES AND MATERIALS USED

Reagents
     Chemicals were obtained from the following sources: DMN and aminopyrine, Eastman Kodak Co., Rochester, N.Y.; PB, Merck Co., Rahway, N.J.; Aroclor 1254, Monsanto Chemical Corporation, St. Louis, MO; isocitrate dehydrogenase (20 milliunits/ul) and disodium $NADP^+$, Boehringer Mannheim Co., New York, NY; benzo(a)pyrene, BP, Aldrich Chemical Co., Milwaukee, WI; chenodeoxycholic acid, Calbiochem, San Diego, CA; SKF-525-A, was a gift from J.B. Schenkman, Yale Univer-sity School of Medicine.

141

Microsome preparations

Male C57 and DBA/2 mice were divided into groups of 10 animals and were fed a pelleted standard protein diet, Nutritional Biochemical Co., Cleveland, Ohio, ad libitum until 12 h before sacrifice. For induction of microsomal enzymes separate groups were given: PB, a single i.p. injection of 80 mg/kg and 0.1% in their drinking water for 7 days; Aroclor 1254 dissolved in corn oil and administered as a single i.p. injection of 500 mg/kg 4 days before sacrifice; 3MC, 80 mg/kg dissolved in corn oil and injected i.p. one day before sacrifice. The pooled livers from 10 animals were homogenized in 4 vol. of ice cold 0.1M phosphate buffer, 1 mM EDTA, pH 7.4 and the microsomal fraction was isolated by differential centrifugation as previously described [6]. The concentration of CO binding pigment in the microsomes was determined spectrophotometrically using the method of Omura and Sato [27] and protein concentrations were measured by the Biuret reaction [17] using human albumin as a standard.

Assay of mutagenic activity

Activation of DMN to a mutagen was assayed by a bacterial auxotroph reversion test using one of the His$^-$ Salmonella typhimurium tester strains, TA 1530, described by Ames et al. [2]. The bacteria, centrifuged from 1 ml of a culture growing exponentially (6-9 X 10^8 cfu/ml), in tryptone broth, were resuspended in 0.5 ml of 0.1 M phosphate buffer, pH 7.4 containing 3 mg of microsomal protein. This suspension was mixed with an equal volume of an NADPH generating system, consisting of 32 mM trisodium DL-isocitrate, 1.3 mM NADP$^+$, 10 mM MgCl$_2$ and 40 ul isocitrate dehydrogenase, all of which had been pre-incubated at 37°C for 15 min. DMN was then added to a final concentration of 100 mM and the whole system incubated with aeration at 37°C for 15 min before assaying for His$^-$ revertants. Under these conditions there is no significant decrease in cell viability and the DMN induced reversion frequency increases linearly for at least 30 min [5,8]. In a similar experimental system, Frantz and Malling have shown that DMN dependent

mutagenesis increases linearly with microsomal protein concentration at concentrations greater than 1.4 mg/ml [8].
No revertants were detected when formaldehyde (200 nmol) was
added directly to the reaction mixture instead of DMN or
when this concentration of formaldehyde was generated in situ
by substitution of aminopyrine for DMN in the reaction
mixture.   In all experiments the spontaneous reversion
frequency measured in the absence of added mutagen was less
than 10 per 10^8 cfu. The bacterial counts used in calculating the DMN induced reversion frequencies were taken from
plates containing between 10^2 and 10^3 cfu.

Enzyme assays
    DMN demethylase activity was determined by measuring
formaldehyde production colorimetrically as described by
Schenkman et al [30]. The reaction mixture used was the
same as that used for the mutagenesis assay with the
bacteria omitted.

    Aminopyrine demethylase activity also was determined by
measuring formaldehyde production. The reaction mixtures
consisted of 1.5 ml of a 2 mg/ml microsomal suspension, 0.5
ml of 36 mM aminopyrine in 0.1 M phosphate buffer, pH 7.4
and 1 ml of the NADPH generating system. Incubation was for
6 min at 37°C.

    Benzo(a)pyrene hydroxylase activity was determined in
reaction mixtures containing 0.5 mg microsomal protein in
0.5 ml 0.1 M Tris-HCl, 1 mM pH 7.4, 100 uM benzo(a)pyrene
added as 5 ul of a 2.0 X 10^{-2} M solution in dimethylsulfoxide, and 0.5 ml of the NADPH generating system. The mixture
was incubated for 5 min at 37°C and the reaction stopped
by the addition of 1.0 ml cold acetone. The product,
hydroxylated, benzopyrene(s) was measured fluorimetrically
by the method of Nebert and Gelboin [25], with one modification; 10^{-3}M cysteine was added to the alkali solution used
to extract hydroxylated benzopyrene(s). This concentration
of cysteine retarded the fluctuations in fluorescence
intensity occasionally encountered in this assay.

The inhibitors, SKF-525A and chenodeoxycholic acid were prepared at 10 X the concentrations to be used in inhibitor experiments and added, 0.1 ml/ml incubation mixture, to the microsomes before addition of substrate and NADPH generating system. SKF was dissolved in distilled water and chenodeoxylcholate acid in 2.5×10^{-2} M NaOH. The addition of the chenodeoxycholic acid solution to the microsomes raised the pH several tenths of a pH unit. This pH rise was necessary for detergent action. Control experiments were carried out in which an equal volume of NaOH solution was added, without chenodeoxycholic acid. The NaOH solution showed no effect on any of the enzyme or mutagenesis assays. Benzpyrene, when added as an inhibitor was prepared as a 2 mM solution in dimethylsulfoxide and 10 ul of this solution was added to the microsomal suspension.

All enzyme assays were performed in duplicate. Activities obtained from individual determinations were within 10% of each other.

RESULTS

The effects of the various inducers of DMN demethylase and DMN mutagenic activities in the two inbred strains of mice, C57 and DBA/2, are presented in Table I. Aminopyrine demethylase and benzo(a)pyrene hydroxylase activities were also monitored as representative of enzymes which are primarily cytochrome P-450 and P-448 dependent respectively. In the case of the C57 mice all three inducers produced significant increases in DMN demethylase and mutagenic activities. The capacity of microsomes from PB, 3-MC and Aroclor treated animals to convert DMN to a mutagen was increased to a greater extent than their capacity to demethylate DMN. This effect was particularly pronounced with the Aroclor induced microsomes which exhibited an 18.6-fold increase in their capacity to activate DMN to a mutagen and only a 2.6-fold increase in DMN methylase activity.

In the case of the DBA/2 mice, 3-MC, as expected, was ineffective as an inducer for any of the activities monitored This is the result of a genetic lesion which blocks induction by polycyclic hydrocarbons in these animals [9]. They do respond normally, however, to induction by phenobarbital. The reduced effectiveness of Aroclor as an inducer in this strain relative to its effect in C57 mice is particularly interesting. Its efficiency as an inducer of DMN activation and benzo(a)pyrene hydroxylase activity is reduced to a much greater extent than its effectiveness as an inducer of DMN or aminopyrine demethylase activities. Nevertheless, as was observed with the C57 mice, Aroclor, as well as PB produced a greater increase in the capacity of the microsomes to convert DMN to a mutagen than to demethylate the compound.

In addition to the above approach, which demonstrated that the enzymes responsible for DMN demethylation and DMN mutagenesis could be differentially induced, we sought to determine if these activities could be differentially inhibited. For this purpose we examined the effects of adding SKF 525-A and benzo(a)pyrene to the enzyme and mutagenesis reaction mixtures. The compound SKF 525-A has been shown to inhibit the metabolism of many substrates of cytochrome P-450 [23] as well as DMN induced mutagenesis [8,22]. Benzo(a) pyrene was chosen as a more selective inhibitor of P-448 dependent substrates since its metabolism would presumably complete with these substrates for the terminal oxygenase. Although benzo(a)pyrene is converted to a frame shift mutagen by the microsomes the test strain, Salmonella TA 1530, is not reverted by this mutagen since it is only sensitive to base substitution mutagens [2]. As seen in Table II, SKF was effective at inhibiting mutagenic activation and the enzyme activities of control and 3MC induced microsomes, but much more so with the control microsomes. On the other hand benzo(a)pyrene was more effective at inhibiting mutagenic activation and the enzyme activities of 3MC induced microsomes, than control microsomes. In all cases mutagenesis was inhibited to a greater extent than any of the enzyme activities.

Chenodeoxycholic acid, 0.6 mM, when added to microsomes and allowed to stand inhibits enzyme action by a noncompetitive inhibition [14], probably through detergent action, as the microsomal suspensions became noticeably clearer. With 3MC induced microsomes, chenodeoxycholic acid completely deactivated AP demethylase, DMN demethylase and mutagenesis, however, BP hydroxylase activity was still present at 70% of its initial value, and at lower BP concentrations than the 100 uM usually used in the assay i.e., < 20 uM, chenodeoxycholic acid increased BP hydroxylation activity.

We also considered the possibility that formaldehyde produced by demethylation of DMN or aminopyrine might be consumed by the microsomes, either by active metabolism by the NADPH dependent cytochrome P-450 or P-448 oxidase system, or by simple reaction with microsomal protein. To test this idea, 120 nmoles of formaldehyde were added to complete microsomal incubation mixtures, without added substrate. After a fifteen minute incubation, 91% of the formaldehyde was still present in tubes containing microsomes from untreated animals and 84% was still present in tubes containing microsomes from PCB animals. Omission of NADPH had no significant effect on formaldehyde consumption.

DISCUSSION

The results of the studies described here indicate that microsomal metabolism of DMN is more complex than a simple P-450 dependent demethylation, followed by spontaneous breakdown to methyldiazonium ion.

DMN demethylase as well as the microsomal factor(s) involved in DMN mutagenesis exhibit characteristics of P-448 dependent functions. Both activities are inhibited by the presence of benzo(a)pyrene and neither is inducible by 3-MC in DBA/2 mice. The fact that SKF 525-A also can inhibit DMN demethylation and especially DMN mutagenesis indicates that some fraction of these activities proceeds via cytochrome P-450. The extent of inhibition of benzo(a)pyrene hydroxy-

146

lase by SKF 525-A is consistent with a report that in microsomes from uninduced animals cytochrome P-450 contributes
significantly to the activity of enzymes normally considered
as being primarily P-448 dependent [11]. It seems particularly noteworthy, with respect to the presumed relationship
between DMN demethylation and mutagenesis, that DMN induced
mutagenesis is much more sensitive to inhibition by both
benzo(a)pyrene and SKF 525-A than is the demethylase. One
interpretation of these observations is that activation of
DMN to a mutagen requires both cytochromes P-448 and P-450.

The polychlorinated biphenyl, Aroclor 1254, is clearly
a very potent inducer of the factor(s) involved in DMN
activation. It is also a potent inducer for microsomal
enzyme activities dependent on cytochromes P-450 and P-448.
At the present time it is still not known whether Aroclor
induces a mixture of cytochromes or induces a cytochrome
P-448 that is catalytically different from the 3-MC induced
cytochrome P-448 [1].

The results of the induction and inhibitor studies
suggest that both cytochromes P-450 and P-448 contribute to
DMN demethylase and mutagenicity, and that high levels of
both cytochromes are necessary for efficient activation of
DMN to a mutagen. It may be relevant that microsomes
treated with chenodeoxycholic acid, at the described conditions, do not activate DMN to a mutagen. These microsomes
contain little P-450 dependent activity but retain substantial P-448 activity.

ACKNOWLEDGEMENTS
    The authors gratefully acknowledge the support and
encouragement of Dr. F. Schaffner. This investigation was
supported by a grant from the American Cancer Society,
BC 200 National Institute of Health Grants, Nos. AM 03846
and CA 19023-01.

Table I. Comparative inductive effects of phenobarbital, 3-methylcholanthrene, and Aroclor 1254 on aminopyrine demethylase, dimethylnitrosamine demethylase, benzo(a)pyrene hydroxylase, microsomal CO binding hemoprotein and dimethylnitrosamine mutagenic activities in C57 and DBA/2 mice.

Strain	Treatment	Aminopyrine[a] demethylase activity	dimethylnitrosamine[a] demethylase activity	benzo(a)pyrene[b] hydroxylase activity	Microsomal[c] CO binding hemoprotein	Revertants[d] per 10^8 survivors
C57	Controls	$10.2(1.0)^e$	4.4(1.0)	536(1.0)	0.83(1.0)	$1.9 \times 10^3(1.0)$
	PB	23.4(2.3)	9.8(2.2)	1078(2.0)	2.20(2.7)	$8.5 \times 10^3(4.5)$
	3-MC	15.8(1.6)	8.4(1.9)	3020(5.6)	1.42(1.7)	$6.9 \times 10^3(3.6)$
	Aroclor 1254	26.5(2.6)	11.5(2.6)	4658(8.7)	3.21(3.9)	$35.4 \times 10^3(18.6)$
DBA/2	Controls	10.3(1.0)	4.2(1.0)	541(1.0)	0.87(1.0)	$2.2 \times 10^3(1.0)$
	PB	25.1(2.4)	9.6(2.3)	1022(1.9)	2.30(2.6)	$9.4 \times 10^3(4.3)$
	3-MC	10.5(1.0)	4.6(1.1)	520(0.9)	0.83(0.9)	$1.8 \times 10^3(0.8)$
	Aroclor 1254	16.1(1.6)	5.9(1.4)	769(1.4)	1.32(1.5)	$5.2 \times 10^3(2.4)$

a) n moles HCHO/mg protein-min

b) p moles hydroxybenzpyrene/mg protein-min

c) n moles/mg protein

d) His[+] revertants of Salmonella TA1530

e) The numbers in brackets give the relative increases in the respective activities

Table II. Inhibitory effects of SKF 525-A and benzo(a)pyrene on microsomal enzyme activities and DMN mutagenesis

Treatment	Inhibitor	Aminopyrine[a] demethylase activity (n moles HCHO min-mg protein)	DMN[a] demethylase activity (n moles HCHO min-mg protein)	Benzo(a)pyrene[b] hydroxylase activity (p moles hydroxybenzpyrene min-mg protein)	His+ revertants per 10^8 survivors
Control	None	9.5(1.00)[b]	4.4(1.00)	437(1.00)	1.9×10^3(1.00)
	SKF 525-A(1mM)	3.2(0.34)	1.3(0.30)	264(0.60)	0.026×10^3(0.01)
	Benzo(a)pyrene(20uM)	9.2(0.96)	0.8(0.18)	--	0.86×10^3(0.05)
3MC	None	17.0(1.00)	10.6(1.00)	3948(1.00)	10.4(1.00)
	SKF 525-A(1mM)	7.4(0.44)	6.9(0.65)	3356(0.85)	3.2(0.31)
	Benzo(a)pyrene(20uM)	10.2(0.60)	2.8(0.26)	--	0.21(0.02)

a) n mol HCHO/mg protein/min   b) p mol hydroxybenzpyrene/mg protein/min

REFERENCES

1. Alvares, A.P., D.R. Bickers and A. Kappas, Polychlorinated biphenyls: a new type of inducer of cytochrome P-448 in the liver, Proc. Natl. Acad. Sci. U.S.A., 70 (1973) 1321-1325.
2. Ames, B.N., F.D. Lee and W.E. Durston, An improved bacteria test system for detection and classification of mutagens and carcinogens, Proc. Natl. Acad. Sci. U.S.A., 70(1973) 782-786.
3. Conney, A.H., Pharmacological implications of microsomal enzyme induction, Pharmacol. Rev., 19, (1967) 317-366.
4. Czygan, P., H. Greim, A.J. Garro, F. Hutterer, J. Rudick, F. Schaffner and H. Popper, Cytochrome P-450 content and the ability of liver microsomes from patients undergoing abdominal surgery to alter the mutagenicity of a primary and secondary one, J. Natl. Cancer Inst., 51(1973) 1761-1764.
5. Czygan, P., H. Greim, A. Garro, F. Schaffner and H. Popper, The effect of dietary protein deficiency on the ability of isolated hepatic microsomes to alter the mutagenicity of a primary and a secondary carcinogen, Cancer Res., 34(1974) 119-123.
6. Czygan, P., H. Greim, A.J. Garro, F. Hutterer, F. Schaffner, H. Popper, O. Rosenthal and D.Y. Cooper, Microsomal metabolism of dimethylnitrosamine and the cytochromes P-450 dependency of its activation to a mutagen, Cancer Res., 33(1973) 2983-2986.
7. Den Engelse, L., The formation of methylated bases in DNA by dimethylnitrosamine and its relation to differences in the formation of tumors in the livers of GR and C3Hf mice, Chem.-Biol. Interactions, 8(1974) 329-338.
8. Frantz, C.N., and H.V. Malling, Factors affecting metabolism and mutagenicity of dimethylnitrosamine and diethylnitrosamine, Cancer Res., 35(1975) 2307-2314.

9. Gielen, J.E., F.M. Goujon and D.W. Nebert, Genetic regulation of aryl hydrocarbon hydroxylase induction II. Simple Mendelian expression in mouse tissues in vivo, J. Biol. Chem. 247(1972) 1125-1137.

10. Gletten, E., U. Weekes and D. Brusick, In vitro metabolic activation of chemical mutagens.I. Development of an in vitro mutagenicity assay using liver microsomal enzymes for the activation of dimethylnitrosamine to a mutagen, Mutation Res., 28(1975)113-122.

11. Gnosspelius, Y., H. Thor and S. Orrenius, A comparative study on the effects of phenobarbital and 3,4-benzopyrene on the hydroxylating enzyme system of rat-liver microsomes, Chem. Biol. Interactions, 1(1969) 125-135.

12. Goth, R., and M.F. Rajewski, Ethylation of nucleic acids by ethylnitrosourea-1-^{14}C in the fetal and adult rat, Cancer Res., 32(1972) 1501-1505.

13. Hoch-ligeti, C., M.F. Argus and J.C. Arcos, Combined carcinogenic effects of dimethylnitrosamine and 3-methylcholanthrene in the rat, J. Natl. Cancer Inst., 40(1968) 535-540.

14. Hutterer, F., H. Denk, P.G. Bacchin, J.B. Schenckman, F. Schaffner and H. Popper, 1. Effect of bile acids on microsomal P-450 dependent biotransformation in vitro, Life Sci. 9(1970) 877, Part II.

15. Lake, B.J., C.E. Heading, J.C. Phillips, S.D. Gangolli and Alun G. Lloyd, Some studies on the metabolism in vitro of dimethylnitrosamine by rat liver, Biochem. Soc. Trans. 2(1974) 610-612.

16. Lawley, P.D., Some chemical aspects of dose-response relationships in alkylation mutagenesis, Mutation Res., 23(1974) 283-295.

17. Layne, E., Spectrophotometric and turbidimetric methods for measuring proteins, Methods Enzymol., 3(1957) 447-454.

18. Lijinsky, W., J. Loo and A.E. Ross, Mechanism of alkylation of nucleic acids by DMN, Nature, 218(1968) 1174-1175.

19. Lijinsky, W., H. Garcia, L. Keefer, J. Loo and A.E. Ross Carcinogenesis and alkylation of rat liver nucleic acids by nitrosomethylurea and nitrosoethylurea administered by intraperitoneal injection, Cancer Res., 32(1972) 893-897.

20. Lu, A.Y.H., R. Kuntzman, S. West, M. Jacobson and A.H. Conney, Reconstituted liver microsomal enzyme system that hydroxylates drugs, other foreign compounds, and endogenous substrates, J. Biol. Chem., 247(1972) 1727-1734.

21. Malling, H.V., Dimethylnitrosamines: formation of mutagenic compounds by interaction with mouse liver microsomes, Mutation Res., 13(1971) 425-429.

22. Malling, H.V. and C.N. Frantz, Metabolic activation of dimethylnitrosamine and diethylnitrosamine to mutagens, Mutation Res., 25(1974) 179-186.

23. Mannering, G.J., Properties of cytochrome P-450 as affected by environmental factors: qualitative changes due to administration of polycyclic hydrocarbons, Metabolism, 20(1971) 228-245.

24. Miller, J.A., and E.C. Miller, Metabolism of drugs in relation to carcinogenicity, Ann. N.Y. Acad. Sci. 123 (1965) 125-140.

25. Nebert, D.W. and H.V. Gelboin, Substrate-inducible microsomal aryl hydroxylase in mammalian cell culture, J. Biol. Chem., 243(1968) 6242-6249.

26. Nicoll, J.W., P.F. Swann and A.E. Pegg, Effect of di-methylnitrosamine on persistence of methylated guanines in rat liver and kidney DNA, Nature 254(1975) 261-262.

27. Omura, T. and R. Sato, The carbon monoxide-binding pigment of liver microsomes. II. Solubilization, purification and properties, J. Biol. Chem., 239(1964) 2379-2385.

28. Popper, H., P. Czygan, H. Greim, F. Schaffner and A.J. Garro, Mutagenicity of primary and secondary carcino-gens altered by normal and induced hepatic microsomes, Proc. Soc. Exp. Biol. Med., 142(1973) 727-729.

29. Rosenkranz, H.S., S. Rosenkranz and R.M. Schmidt,
    Effects of nitrosomethylurea and nitrosomethylurethan
    on the physical properties of DNA, Biochem. Biophys.
    Acta, 195(1969) 262-265.

30. Schenkman, J.B., H. Remmer and R.W. Estabrook,
    Spectral studies of drug interaction with hepatic
    microsomal cytochrome, Mol. Pharmacol., 3(1967)
    113-123.

31. Schoental, R., Lack of correlation between the pre-
    sence of 7-methylguanine in DNA and RNA of organs
    and localization of tumors after a single carcinogene-
    tic dose of N-methyl-N-nitrosourethane, Biochem. J.,
    114(1969) 55P.

32. Schoental, R., The mechanism of action of the carcino-
    genic nitroso and related compounds, Br. J. Cancer,
    28(1973) 436-439.

33. Swann, P.F. and P.N. Magee, Nitrosamine induced
    carcinogenesis. The alkylation of N-7 of guanine of
    nucleic acids of the rat by diethylnitrosamine, N-
    ethyl-N-nitrosourea and ethyl methanesulphonate,
    Biochem. J., 125(1971) 841-847.

STUDIES ON THE MUTAGENICITY OF VINYL CHLORIDE METABOLITES AND RELATED CHEMICALS

A. D. Laumbach, S. Lee, J. Wong, and U. N. Streips

Department of Microbiology and Immunology
University of Louisville School of Medicine
Department of Chemistry
Louisville, Kentucky 40201

I. INTRODUCTION

The studies by Viola et al (26) and Maltoni et al (15) established the carcinogenic potential of vinyl chloride monomer. The detection of angiosarcoma in industrial workers exposed to polyvinyl chloride suggested a causal relationship between this chemical and the development of hepatic abnormalities (4,12). Hefner et al (7) have delineated the metabolic fate of inhaled vinyl chloride in rats and proposed that the epoxide, chlorooxirane, and chloroacetaldehyde were the carcinogenic intermediates. Their hypothesis has been supported by the work of several laboratories (3,14,16,19, Elmore, Wong, Laumbach and Streips, submitted for publication) using bacterial strains as mutagenic indicators.

In this communication we present additional data concerning the mutagenicity and the potential mechanisms of action of several vinyl chloride metabolites, including the previously unreported chloroacet-adehyde monomer hydrate, chloroacetaldehyde dimer hydrate, and chloroacetaldehyde trimer. Epichlorohydrin, a mutagenic/carcinogenic (21,25) methylene homolog of chlorooxirane was also examined.

II. PROCEDURES AND MATERIALS USED

A. Bacterial Strains

The bacterial strains utilized in these studies are presented in Table I. The Bacillus subtilis strains were all maintained on AK agar (BBL). Salmonella typhimurium cultures were obtained from B. N. Ames (1) and were stored on Nutrient Agar (Difco) plus 5g NaCl per liter.

B. Mutagenicity Assays

The indirect assay utilized repair deficient strains of B. subtilis. The procedure was a modification of the "rec-assay" described by Kada et al (9). Cells were grown overnight in Nutrient Broth (Difco) at 37C in a rotary incubator shaker, then diluted tenfold in phosphate buffer (pH 7.0). The suspended cultures were streaked onto Nutrient Agar plates (Difco). Filter paper discs (6 mm) were saturated with the chemical solutions to be examined, then were placed onto the agar plates next to the streaked bacterial cultures. Following incubation at 37C overnight the plates were examined and the lethality and mutagenic potential of the test chemicals were assessed by comparing inhibition zones between the B. subtilis 168 wild type, a repair-capable strain and the various DNA repair-deficient strains. In all these studies 4-nitroquinoline-1-oxide (4NQO) was used as the positive mutagenic control.

Direct mutagenicity assays utilized the S. typhimurium tester strains described by Ames (1). The chemicals were examined by the methods of McCann et al (16). The cultures were grown in Nutrient Broth plus 0.5% NaCl overnight in a rotary incubator shaker at 37C. A mixture of the test chemical (0.1 ml) in dimethyl sulfoxide (DMSO) and 2 ml of soft agar (0.6% agar, 0.6% NaCl, 0.5 mM biotin, and 0.5 mM histidine) was added to 0.1 ml of the bacterial culture. The solutions were mixed thoroughly and overlaid onto minimal plates [Vogel-Bonner E medium (27), 1.5% agar, and 2% glucose]. Control samples were prepared by omitting the test chemicals. For the positive mutagenesis control, 4NQO was added to the mixtures in place of the test chemicals. All plates were incubated for 48 hr at 37C prior to the enumeration of revertant colonies.

C. Chemical Compounds

The chemical compounds utilized in these studies were prepared, purified, and analyzed by previously reported techniques (Elmore, Wong, Laumbach, and Streips, submitted for publication).

D. Preparation of DNA

Transforming DNA was isolated from B. subtilis cultures by the method described by Young and Wilson (29). In some of the experiments the cultures were pretreated for 15 min either with chloroacetaldehyde (16 mM) or epichlorohydrin (16 mM) prior to the extraction procedure. In alternate experiments S-9 liver homogenate mix was added to the compounds prior to addition to bacteria. The S-9 liver homogenate contains per ml, 0.3 ml of the S-9 fraction, 8 mM $MgCl_2$, 33 mM KCl, 5 mM glucose-6-P, 4 mM NADP, and 100 mM sodium phosphate (pH 7.4). The DNA concentration in all lysates were assayed by the method of Richards (20).

E. Treatment of DNA In vitro with Chemicals

A sample of B. subtilis transforming DNA (0.9 ml) in standard saline citrate (SSC) (0.15 M NaCl-0.015 M trisodium citrate, pH 7.0) was combined with 0.1 ml chloroacetaldehyde (1.0 M in DMSO) or 0.1 ml epichlorohydrin (1.0 M in DMSO). The mixture was allowed to react for 1 hr with occasional shaking. Following this treatment the treated DNA was dialyzed at OC against three 500 ml changes of SSC for 24 hrs. In alternate experiments the DNA-chemical mixtures were placed in a dialysis bag and immersed in the S-9 liver homogenate mix. These samples were dialyzed in SSC as above.

F. Competent Cultures for Transformation Assays

The procedures for the development of competence were similar to those described (23). B. subtilis cells were grown in a modified Spizizen's minimal medium (GMI) (29) for 90 min at 37C after cessation of logarithmic growth in a rotary incubator shaker. The cells were then diluted tenfold into GMII medium (29) and incubated for an additional 60 min at 37C in the shaker. At this time the culture has attained maximum competence.

G. Transformation Procedures

A sample (0.1 ml) of extracted, treated or untreated DNA was added to 0.8 ml of the competent cultures and incubated at 37C for 30 min in the shaker. The reaction was terminated by the addition of 0.1 ml of deoxyribonuclease (500 µg/ml, Worthington Biochem. Corp.) for 15 min at 37C. The cells were plated on appropriate selective minimal media and incubated at 37C for 48 hrs.

III. RESULTS

A summary of preliminary mutagenesis screening experiments with potential vinyl chloride monomer metabolites and related compounds is presented in Table II. It is evident that chlorooxirane and chloro-acetaldehyde are the ultimate mutagens in this system. These results agree with the published data (3,16). In addition, this table describes the mutagenicity of the other chemical forms of chloroacetaldehyde, not-ably a monomer hydrate, a dimer hydrate, and a trimer. The hydrate and dimer hydrate forms have been shown to form an equilibrium mixture by the spontaneous rearrangement of chloroacetaldehyde under physiological conditions (Elmore, Wong, Laumbach, and Streips, submitted for publication),and these hydrate forms must be regarded as potential metabolites of consequence. Purified dimer hydrate and trimer were synthesized under laboratory conditions. Neither acetaldehyde, chloro-acetic acid, nor chloroethanol showed a significant level of mutagenicity in these assays. Other investigators have reported the mutagenicity of chloroethanol, however, either high concentrations or activation with microsomal enzymes was required for activity (3,16). Our results agree with those of McCann et al (16). These experiments suggest a molecular relationship involving the proximity of the chloride group to the aldehyde moiety for mutagenic activity. In this regard we are currently examining structurally analogous ketones, substituted with various halogens. Epichlorohydrin (1-chloro-2,3 epoxypropane) was also mutagenic in screens using the Salmonella tester strain TA100.

157

Further experiments examined the effect of proposed metabolites on several different DNA repair deficient strains of B. subtilis. Chlorooxirane and the different forms of chloroacetaldehyde were all found to specifically inhibit the growth of strain MC-1, which lacks recombination repair (17) (Table III). Epichlorohydrin was capable of moderate reactivity only in the presence of the S-9 fraction.

Quantitative mutagenesis assays with Salmonella strain TA100, an indicator for base-pair substitution mutations, revealed that chloroacetaldehyde monomer had the highest mutagenic capacity of all the reactive metabolites (Table IV). The monomer-dimer hydrates, dimer hydrate, and trimer show progressively decreasing mutagenic efficiency as evidenced by the higher chemical concentration required for eliciting maximum reversion. All forms of chloroacetaldehyde were very toxic, thus the mutagenic response of each compound was limited to a narrow range of concentrations. However, epichlorohydrin, a weak mutagen by comparison, has a broad mutagenic spectrum and a corresponding low toxicity.

Since the mutagenic activity of the compounds constituted strong evidence that DNA was a primary target of attack, we examined the interaction of chloroacetaldehyde and epichlorohydrin with transforming DNA. It is known that the biological activity of transforming DNA can be altered by exposure to physical and chemical agents (8,22). Previous studies have shown that chloroacetaldehyde can bind to DNA in vitro (11). Accordingly, transforming DNA isolated from B. subtilis 168WT was treated with either chloroacetaldehyde or epichlorohydrin as described in Materials and Methods. The treated DNA was examined in transformation assays utilizing several different auxotrophic strains of B. subtilis as the recipients. Data presented in Table V reveals that in vitro treatment of DNA with either compound has little or no apparent effect on the biological activity of this DNA in transformation.

Since both chloroacetaldehyde and epichlorohydrin demonstrated mutagenic activity in the Salmonella TA100 strain, we examined the effect of these two compounds on B. subtilis DNA in vivo. Transforming DNA was isolated from B. subtilis following a 15 min exposure to the mutagenic chemicals. The DNA concentration was calculated from these samples, and levels equivalent to those used in the in vitro assays were added to competent cultures. The results of these transformation assays are shown in Table VI. Two major effects are evident with chloroacetaldehyde in vivo treated DNA. First, there was a major depression of the biological activity in the transforming DNA. Secondly, the depression showed genetic marker specificity. Moreover, the DNA segments containing genetic markers which have previously been shown to be associated to macromolecular structures such as the cell membrane (6,24,28) or the cell wall (Streips, Doyle, Sueoka, Brown, and Fan, submitted for publication) were selectively protected from attack by chloroacetaldehyde and epichlorohydrin. The activity of epichlorohydrin was less in these experiments, however, the patterns of specific marker inactivation are quite similar. The addition of the S-9 mix to the chemicals prior to addition to the cells, did not cause significant alteration in transformation efficiency (results not shown). In some samples there was an effect on the transforming DNA by DMSO, therefore all transformation values were corrected to account for this parameter.

IV. DISCUSSION

The major findings reported in this manuscript can be summarized:
1) We have confirmed the mutagenicity of chloroacetaldehyde and chloro-oxirane, and extended it to include the additional potential metabolites, chloroacetaldehyde monomer hydrate, dimer hydrate and trimer, as well as the previously unreported chlorooxirane homolog, epichlorohydrin. 2) We have shown that recombination repair appears to be the mechanism for the correction of vinyl chloride metabolite elicited damage. 3) Chloro-acetaldehyde causes a decrease in the biological activity of transforming DNA only if the cells are treated with the mutagen prior to the extraction of the DNA. In vitro studies showed no effect. 4) Epichlorohydrin apparently differs markedly from the vinyl chloride metabolites in mutagenic activity.

To understand the mutagenic potential of an environmental carcinogen, such as vinyl chloride and related chemicals, it is necessary to determine both its metabolic fate and probable mechanism of action for alteration of cellular processes. This report, as well as others, (3,14,16) has identified the potential active metabolites in vinyl chloride monomer mediated carcinogenesis. Furthermore, on the basis of a series of studies in microbial systems, we can postulate probable mechanisms of action of the vinyl chloride monomer metabolites and related chemicals. Under-standing of these mechanisms is necessary for the development of possible blocking agents to the carcinogenic activity.

Recombination repair appears to be induced to correct DNA lesions caused by vinyl chloride monomer metabolites and epichlorohydrin. Salmonella strain TA100 which lacks excision repair (uvr⁻), yet retains the capacity for recombination repair is capable of recovery and can express mutation following exposure. Furthermore, experiments with several repair-deficient B. subtilis mutants demonstrate that only the recombination repair mutant is specifically sensitive to the active metabolites, whereas the excision repair mutants and the wild type strain are relatively unaffected. The nature of the lesions may specifically evoke the recombination repair mechanism (10), or, alternatively, the chemical reactivity of the metabolites may directly suppress other repair. It is known that recombination repair is inducible, while other types of repair are mostly constitutive (5). Since chloroacetaldehyde has been shown to specifically interact with proteins containing -SH groups (J. Hoffman, personal communication), it is possible that the chemical could inactivate the constitutive repair enzymes leaving the repair to an inducible system.

The requirement for recombination repair of damage induced by these chemicals suggests the potential route of mutagenesis in bacteria. Recombination repair has been shown to be error prone (16). In this sense it resembles postreplication repair in mammalian cells (13). Thus, we can postulate that the analogous error prone repair pathway, post-replication repair, may function in mammalian cells in response to vinyl chloride metabolite elicited damage. A relationship between post-replication repair caused errors and somatic mutation and carcinogenesis has been suggested in patients with the skin disease, xeroderma pig-mentosum (13).

The increased inhibitory activity of the chloroacetaldehyde dimer and trimer forms for the other repair-deficient B. subtilis strains (Table III) may have been nonspecific killing of the cells, since all the strains other than MC-1 showed identical levels of inhibition. The necessity for metabolic activation of epichlorohydrin could reflect either a lack of permeability of the nonactivated compound or the requirement of a metabolite of this compound as the true mutagenic species.

Neither chloroacetaldehyde nor epichlorohydrin seemed to affect transforming DNA in vitro (Table V). Although several investigators have reported that CAA specifically modifies bases and causes mismatched base pairs (2,11), this reaction in vitro does not seem to affect the biological activity of the DNA. In contrast, DNA which was isolated from cells treated with either chloroacetaldehyde or epichlorohydrin (in vivo, Table VI) was severely affected. The overall biological activity of the transforming DNA is depressed, and it appears that the regions of the genome which are not protected by either the cell membrane or cell wall are most susceptible to attack and inactivation. It has also been postulated both in Escherichia coli and B. subtilis that the replication origin, terminus, and replication fork are all outer surface bound (18,24). Thus, these would be protected regions from chloroacetaldehyde attack and the nonreplicating DNA in the cytoplasm would be most susceptible. In this connection, recent experiments in our laboratory (Laumbach, Lee, Wong, and Streips, manuscript in preparation) have shown that chloroacetaldehyde causes enhanced mutation levels in cultures with nonreplicating genomes. This may imply that chloroacetaldehyde could be active in mammalian cells during growth stages where little DNA synthesis occurs.

The mode of action of epichlorohydrin, a known carcinogen (25), differs from that of the vinyl chloride monomer metabolites. Although epichlorohydrin causes similar base substitution mutations in Salmonella tester strain TA 100, it is a comparatively weaker alkylating agent based on quantitative assay. Epichlorohydrin also exhibits a lower toxicity level than vinyl chloride monomer metabolites, thus epichloro- hydrin can demonstrate mutagenic activity through a wider range of concentrations. In addition, our laboratory has preliminary evidence that epichlorohydrin produces higher levels of mutation in Salmonella cultures which are actively replicating DNA than in cultures which have been arrested in DNA replication (Laumbach, Lee, Wong, and Streips, manuscript in preparation). The different activity spectra between chlorooxirane and its homolog epichlorohydrin points out the necessity for a multifaceted study of carcinogens.

V. SUMMARY

Our laboratories have utilized strains of B. subtilis and Salmonella typhimurium to investigate the mutagenicity of vinyl chloride metabolites and related compounds. The major findings reported in this manuscript are: 1) Confirmation of mutagenicity of chloroacetaldehyde and chlorooxirane. 2) Description of mutagenicity of additional potential metabolites of vinyl chloride, chloroacetaldehyde monomer hydrate, dimer hydrate, and trimer, as well as the mutagenic carcinogenic chlorooxirane homolog, epichlorohydrin. 3) Recombination repair is postulated to be the mechanism for correcting vinyl chloride metabolite elicited damage. 4) Chloroacetaldehyde affects the transformation activity of DNA only if cells are treated with the mutagen prior to the extraction of the DNA. In vitro the chemical had no effect. 5) Epichlorohydrin differs from vinyl chloride metabolites in mode of action.

VI.   ACKNOWLEDGEMENTS

We wish to thank Mary A. Kinnaman for her extremely able technical assistance. We are grateful to Dr. Jerald Hoffman for making available preliminary results and to Dr. B. N. Ames for providing the Salmonella tester strains. This work was supported by a grant from the B. F. Goodrich Company to the Cancer Center at the University of Louisville, School of Medicine.

Table I

Bacterial Strains

Bacillus subtilis	Genotype	Origin and Comments
RUB 783	purB6, leu-8, hisA1, metB10	U. Streips
BR 151	trpC2, lys-3, metB10	B. Reilly
BUL 709	ura-1, hisA1, leu-8, metB10	This laboratory
BUL 714	cysA, hisA1, leu-8, metB10	This laboratory
Hcr-9 (JB01-200)	trpC2	S. Okubo and W. Romig, hcr⁻
MC-1	trpC2, recB2	S. Okubo and W. Romig, rec⁻
FB-13	trpC2	C. Hadden, uvr⁻
168WT	prototroph	A. Laumbach and I. Felkner

Salmonella typhimurium	Mutations in Strains				
	His⁻	LPS	DNA Repair	R Factor	Mutation Detected
TA1535	hisB46	rfa	uvrB	–	base-pair substitution
TA100	hisB46	rfa	uvrB	pKM101	base-pair substitution
TA1537	hisC3076	rfa	uvrB	–	frameshift
TA1538	hisD3052	rfa	uvrB	–	frameshift
TA98	hisD3052	rfa	uvrB	pKM101	frameshift

Table II

Mutagenic Activity Assayed by Bacterial Test Systems

Compounds	Indirect Screen B. subtilis "Repair-Assay"	Direct Test[a] S. typhimurium Strain TA100
Acetaldehyde	NR[b]	NR
Chloroacetic Acid	NR	NR
Chloroethanol	NR	NR
Vinylidene Chloride	NR	NR
Vinyl Chloride	NR	NR
Chlorooxirane	+[c]	++[d]
Chloroacetaldehyde (monomer)	+++[e]	+++
Chloroacetaldehyde (monomer-dimer hydrates)	++	++
Chloroacetaldehyde (dimer hydrate)	+	+
Chloroacetaldehyde (trimer)	+	+
Epichlorohydrin	NR	+

[a]Experiments performed in absence of liver homogenate-mediated activation.

[b]NR no reaction detected

[c] + Reactive

[d]++ Moderately reactive

[e]+++ Very reactive

Table III

"Repair-Assay" with Bacillus subtilis Strains

Compounds	Molar Concentration	Growth Inhibition in Millimeters[a]			
		168WT (hcr+, rec+)	MC-1 (hcr+, rec-)	Hcr-9 (hcr-, rec+)	FB-13 (uvr+, rec+)
Chloroacetaldehyde (monomer)	0.10	2.0	28.0	4.0	3.0
Chloroacetaldehyde (monomer-dimer hydrate)	0.115	NI[b]	23.0	NI	NI
Chloroacetaldehyde (dimer hydrate)	0.097	2.0	10.0	2.0	2.0
Chloroacetaldehyde (trimer)	0.096	7.0	15.0	6.0	7.0
Chlorooxirane	0.26	NI	10.0	NI	NI
Epichlorohydrin	0.997	NI	NI	NI	NI
Epichlorohydrin (plus liver homogenate)[c]	0.997	NI	3.0	NI	NI

[a] Average inhibition calculated from multiple experiments.
[b] No inhibition detected.
[c] 9,000 x g supernatant (S-9) + NADPH generating system.

Table IV

Quantitative Mutagenicity Assay by <u>Salmonella</u> TA100 Reversion

Compound	Concentration in Soft Agar Layer mM/Plate[a]	Average Number Revertants/Plate[b]
Chloroacetaldehyde (monomer)	0.0004	265
Chloroacetaldehyde (monomer-dimer hydrate)	0.054	977
Chloroacetaldehyde (dimer hydrate)	0.490	311
Chloroacetaldehyde (trimer)	0.240	159
Epichlorohydrin	4.746	2856

[a]Highest effective non-toxic concentration for reversion.
[b]Spontaneous background revertants subtracted.

Table V

Effect of Chloroacetaldehyde and Epichlorohydrin of Transforming DNA _In vitro_

Recipient Strains [c]	Relative Transformation Efficiency[a]							
	metB10	leu-8	cysA	hisA1	ura-1	trpC2	lys-8	purB6
Epichlorohydrin treated DNA								
BUL 714	.92	.97	.97	1.16				
RUB 783	.91	.60		.98				.77
BUL 709	.99	.95		1.02	.85			
BR 151	1.48					1.07	.62	
Chloroacetaldehyde treated DNA								
BUL 714	1.43	.92	.55	.91				
RUB 783	.93	1.45		.75				.89
BUL 709	.86	1.33		.90	.75			
BR 151						ND[b]	.77	

[a]Relative transformation efficiency calculated: $\dfrac{\text{number of transformants with treated DNA}}{\text{number of transformants with untreated DNA}}$

[b]Not determined.

[c]Conditions for competence and transformation as described in Materials and Methods.

Table VI

EFFECT OF CHLOROACETALDEHYDE AND EPICHLOROHYDRIN ON TRANSFORMING DNA IN VIVO

Recipient Strains[b]	Relative Transformation Efficiency[a]							
	metB10	leu-8	cysA	hisA1	ura-1	trpC2	lys-3	purB16
Chloroacetaldehyde in vivo treated DNA								
BUL 714	.54	.09	.08	.36				
RUB 783	.33	.10		.35				.10
BUL 709	.53	.07		.32	.34			
BR 151	.37					.13	.11	
Epichlorohydrin in vivo treated DNA								
BUL 714	.55	.17	.25	.46				
RUB 783	.52	.15		.38				ND[c]
BUL 709	.59	.15		.50	.36			
BR 151	.37					.11	.19	

[a]Relative transformation efficiency calculated: number transformants with treated DNA / number transformants with untreated DNA

[b]Conditions for competence and transformation as described in Materials and Methods.

[c]Not determined.

167

LITERATURE CITED

1. Ames, B. N., Lee, F. D., and Durston, W. E. An Improved Bacterial Test System For Detection And Classification Of Mutagens And Carcinogens. Proc. Nat. Acad. Sci., U.S.A., 70: 782-786, 1973.

2. Barrio, J. R., Secrist, J. A., and Leonard, N. J. Fluorescent Adenosine And Cytidine Derivatives. Biochem. Biophys. Res. Comm., 46: 597-604, 1972.

3. Bartsch, H., Malaveille, C., and Montesano, R. M. Human, Rat, And Mouse Liver-Mediated Mutagenicity Of Vinyl Chloride In S. typhimurium Strains. Int. J. Cancer, 15: 429-437, 1975.

4. Creech, J. L., and Johnson, M. N. Angiosarcoma Of The Liver In The Manufacture Of Polyvinyl Chloride. J. Occup. Med., 16: 150-151, 1974.

5. Ganesan, A. K., and Smith, K. C. Recovery Of Recombination Deficient Mutants Of Escherichia coli K-12 From Ultraviolet Irradiation. Cold Spring Harbor Symp. Quant. Biol., 33: 235-242, 1968.

6. Ganesan, A. T., and Lederberg, J. A Cell-Membrane Bound Fraction Of Bacterial DNA. Biochem. Biophys. Res. Comm., 18: 824-835, 1965.

7. Hefner, R. E., Watanabe, P. G., and Gehring, P. G. Preliminary Studies Of The Fate Of Inhaled Vinyl Chloride Monomer (VCM) In Rats. Ann. N. Y. Acad. Sci., 246: 135-148, 1975.

8. Jensen, R. A., and Haass, F. L. Analysis Of Ultraviolet Light-Induced Mutagenesis By DNA Transformation In Bacillus subtilis. Proc. Nat. Acad. Sci., U.S.A., 50: 1109-1116, 1963.

9. Kada, T., Tutikawa, K., and Sadaie, Y. In vitro And Host-Mediated "Rec-Assay" Procedures For Screening Chemical Mutagens; And Phloxine, A Mutagenic Red Dye Detected. Mutation Res., 16: 165-174, 1972.

10. Laumbach, A. D., and Felkner, I. C. Formation Of A 4-Nitro-quinoline-1-Oxide Complex With DNA In Normal And Repair-Deficient Strains Of Bacillus subtilis. Mutation Res., 15: 233-245, 1972.

11. Lee, C. H., and Wetmur, J. G. Physical Studies Of Chloro-acetaldehyde Labeled Fluorescent DNA. Biochem. Biophys. Res. Commun., 50: 879-885, 1973.

12. Lee, F. I., and Harry, D. S. Angiosarcoma Of The Liver In A Vinyl Chloride Worker. Lancet, 1: 1316-1318, 1974.

13. Lehmann, A. R. Postreplication Repair Of DNA In Mammalian Cells. Life Sci., 15: 2005-2016, 1974.

168

14. Malaveille, C. H., Bartsch, H., Montesano, R., Barbin, A., Camus, A. M., Croizy, A., and Jacquignon, P. Mutagenicity Of Vinyl Chloride, Chloroethylene Oxide, Chloroacetaldehyde And Chloroethanol. Biochem. Biophys. Res. Commun., 63: 363-370, 1975.

15. Maltoni, C., and Lefemine, G. Carcinogenicity Bioassays Of Vinyl Chloride. Environm. Res., 7: 387-405, 1974.

16. McCann, J., Simmon, V., Streitwieser, D., and Ames, B. N. Mutagenicity Of Chloroacetaldehyde, A Possible Metabolic Product Of 1,2-Dichloroethane (Ethylene Dichloride), Chloroethanol (Ethylene Chlorohydrin), Vinyl Chloride, And Cyclophosphamide. Proc. Nat. Acad. Sci., U.S.A., 72: 3190-3193, 1975.

17. Okubo, S., and Romig, W. R. Impaired Transformability Of Bacillus subtilis Mutant Sensitive To Mitomycin C And Ultraviolet Radiation. J. Mol. Biol., 15: 440-454, 1966.

18. Olsen, W. L., Heidrich, H. G., Hannig, K., and Hofshneider, P. H. Deoxyribonucleic Acid-Envelope Complexes Isolated From Escherichia coli By Free-Flow Electrophoresis: Biochemical And Electron Microscope Characterization. J. Bacteriol., 118: 646-653, 1974.

19. Rannug, U., Johansson, A., Ramel, C., and Wachtmeister, C. A. The Mutagenicity Of Vinyl Chloride After Metabolic Activation. AMBIO, 3: 194-197, 1974.

20. Richards, G. Modifications Of The Diphenylamine Reaction Giving Increased Sensitivity And Simplicity In The Estimation Of DNA. Anal. Biochem., 57: 369-376, 1974.

21. Strauss, B., and Okubo, S. Protein Synthesis And The Induction Of Mutations In Escherichia coli By Alkylating Agents. J. Bacteriol., 79: 464-473, 1960.

22. Strauss, B., Reiter, H., and Searashi, T. Recovery From Ultra-violet And Alkylating Agent-Induced Damage In Bacillus subtilis. Rad. Res. Supp., 6: 201-211, 1966.

23. Streips, U. N., and Young, F. E. Transformation In Bacillus subtilis Using Excreted DNA. Molec. Gen. Genetics, 133: 47-55, 1974.

24. Sueoka, N., and Quinn, W. Membrane Attachment Of The Chromosome Replication Origin In Bacillus subtilis. Cold Spring Harbor Symp. Quant. Biol., 33: 695-705, 1968.

25. Van Duuren, B. L. On The Possible Mechanism Of Carcinogenic Action Of Vinyl Chloride. Ann. N. Y. Acad. Sci., 246: 258-267, 1975.

26. Viola, P. L., Bigotti, A., and Caputo, A. Oncogenic Response Of Rat Skin, Lungs And Bones To Vinyl Chloride. Cancer Res., 31: 516-522, 1971.

27. Vogel, H. J., and Bonner, D. M. Acetylornithinase Of _Escherichia coli_: Partial Purification And Some Properties. J. Biol. Chem., _218_: 97-106, 1956.

28. Yamagudin, K., and Yoshikawa, H. Association Of The Replication Terminus Of The _Bacillus subtilis_ Chromosome To The Cell Membrane. J. Bacteriol., _124_: 1030-1033, 1975.

29. Young, F. E., and Wilson, G. A. _Bacillus subtilis_. In: Handbook Of Genetics. _Ed._: Robert C. King, Plenum Press, New York, _1_: 69-114, 1974.

Chapter 3

VIROLOGY AND ONCOGENESIS

GENETIC AND IMMUNOLOGICAL CONTROLS OF MURINE LEUKEMIA
VIRUSES IN AKR MICE

Robert C. Nowinski* and Joyce M. Baron**

*Fred Hutchinson Cancer Research Center
1124 Columbia Street
Seattle, Washington 98104
McArdle Laboratory for Cancer Research
University of Wisconsin
Madison, Wisconsin 53703

The intimate relationship between host genetic factors and oncogenesis was established in the 1930's with the development of mouse strains that differed significantly in their incidence of spontaneous leukemia (1,2). These early studies of inbred mice from high leukemic strains (AKR, C58) and low leukemic strains (C3Hf/Bi, C57BR) revealed that heritable factors played an essential role in leukemogenesis.

Transmission of leukemia by virus isolated from mouse embryos as well as by virus isolated from leukemia cells, suggested that murine leukemia virus (MuLV) was vertically transmitted from parent to offspring (3-6). The concept of vertical transmission was further supported by the findings that *(a)* foster-nursing of mice of high leukemic strains on mothers of low leukemic strains (and vice versa) had no effect on leukemia incidence (2,7) and *(b)* transplantation of ova of AKR mice into mothers of low leukemic strains did not affect the incidence of spontaneous leukemia in these mice (8). Subsequently, it was proposed (9,10) that mice of all strains carried latent tumor viruses that were inducible by X-irradiation and chemical carcinogens.

Formal proof of these postulates was accumulated during the next decade: these lines of evidence included the findings that *(a)* viral particles and antigens were identified in mice of divergent genetic backgrounds during different stages of development (11-14); *(b)* virus-specified antigens could be expressed in the normal tissues of mice in the absence of infectious virus or leukemia (13,15-17); *(c)* chemically-induced tumors of mice of low leukemic strains contained MuLV antigens, although the normal tissues of those mice did not show overt signs of virus infections (13,14,18-20); *(d)* cells from mice of low leukemic strains could be induced to release MuLV after treatment with halogenated pyrimidines (21-23) or inhibitors of protein synthesis (24); *(e)* the production of infectious MuLV was transmitted as a dominant Mendelian trait in genetic crosses between mice of high leukemic strains and mice of sensitive low leukemic strains; and *(f)* virus-specific DNA has been identified by molecular hybridization in the chromosomal DNA of mice of all strains examined (26-28).

Recent biological analysis indicates that the murine leukemia viruses actually constitute a family of closely related agents (29,30). Thus, MuLV can be separated into ecotropic or xenotropic groups on the basis of growth in selected target cells in culture (31,32). Ecotropic MuLV infect mouse cells *in vivo* or *in vitro* with high efficiency; these viruses can be further separated into N- or B-tropism on the basis of relative plating efficiencies on NIH Swiss or BALB/c embryo fibroblasts (31). Xenotropic MuLV, although derived from mouse cells, can only infect cells of other species (32, 33). Distinctions between various MuLV isolates also can be demonstrated by immunological analysis (33,65); furthermore, in some cases the genetic divergence between MuLV isolates is sufficiently great to enable detection of these differences by molecular hybridization (66).

Host genetic factors have been demonstrated to play a significant role in controlling the overt production of MuLV at the level of *(i)* the expression of viral proteins, *(ii)* the production of infectious virions, *(iii)* the spread of infectious virus, and *(iv)* the development of immune response to virus or viral-associated antigens.

Mice from high leukemic strains chronically produce infectious MuLV and contain high levels of viral proteins p30 and gp70 in their tissues; however, expression of these proteins also has been observed in the absence of infectious MuLV in the tissues of mice from low leukemic strains (34,35). In mice of the 129 strain the gp70 envelope protein (previously referred to as G_{IX} antigen) (17) was detected on thymocytes in the absence of infectious virus. The G_{IX} phenotype of thymocytes was controlled by independent dominant *(Gv-1)* and semidominant *(Gv-2)* genes; the presence of both genes was required for the G_{IX} phenotype. Similarly, the expression

174

of p30 antigen in the absence of infectious MuLV has been observed in the lymphoid tissues of mice of the C57L and DBA/2 strains (35,37). From genetic studies, it has been demonstrated that a single recessive gene *(Mlv-1)* controls the expression of MuLV p30 in DBA/2 mice (37). In AKR mice, at least two, and possibly three independent dominant genes, control the expression of MuLV p30 (36,38,39,40).

The production of infectious ecotropic MuLV appears to be subject to different host gene controls in various inbred mouse strains. Production of N-ecotropic MuLV in AKR mice is controlled by two independent dominant loci *(Akv-1, Akv-2)* (25). *In vitro* studies have shown that both virus inducibility and persistence of the virus phenotype are coordinately inherited (25,41). One of the viral production genes *(Akv-1)* has been mapped on the Ist linkage group, in close proximity to the enzyme marker glucose phosphate isomerase *(Gpi-1)* (23,25). In BALB/c mice two independent loci control the production of two biologically distinguishable endogenous viruses (an N-ecotropic and a xenotropic agent) (29,42). In C58 mice, three or more independent dominant loci have been demonstrated to control production of N-ecotropic MuLV (43,44), whereas a semidominant locus influences expression of an endogenous xenotropic virus in cells of NZB mice (43).

Resistance or susceptibility of mice to infection with naturally occurring MuLV of different host ranges is controlled by the Fv-1 locus (31,45-47). *Fv-1* maps in the VIII linkage group (48), in close proximity to the enzyme marker glucose phosphate dehydrogenase *(Gpd-1)*. Two alleles, $Fv-1^n$ and $Fv-1^b$, determine susceptibility of mouse cells to N-tropic or B-tropic MuLV, respectively. Resistance to MuLV, as conferred by *Fv-1*, is dominant to susceptibility. Since a strong correlation exists between the expression of MuLV and leukemogenesis, the Fv-1 genotype plays a major role in host susceptibility to leukemogenesis (49).

Although it was originally thought that the mouse was immunologically tolerant to endogenous MuLV (53), it has been recently shown that mice of a variety of inbred strains are immunologically responsive to MuLV antigens. For example, antibodies have been detected in mice for the MuLV envelope antigens gp70 and p15 (54-56), as well as for the viral core protein p30 (57), and the viral RNA-dependent DNA polymerase (58). Resistance or susceptibility of mice to induction of leukemia by MuLV has been found to be associated with the H-2 locus in the IXth linkage group (49-51). The *Rgv-1* locus, which governs resistance to Gross virus, is closely linked to *H-2K* (45,42); furthermore, certain haplotypes of *H-2*

($e.g.$, H-2^k) are associated with the susceptibility allele of $Rgv-1$, while other haplotypes of $H-2$ ($e.g.$, H-2^b) are associated with the resistance allele of $Rgv-1$.

Thus, a variety of host genetic factors are instrumental in the control of the overt expression of MuLV and/or leukemia in mice. In the following studies we specifically describe the role of host genetic and immunological factors in the control of expression of MuLV in mice of the high leukemic strain AKR. In these studies we have examined AKR mice (genetically characterized as: MuLV$^+$, Fv-1^n, H-2^k) and mice of the low leukemic C57L strain (genetically characterized as: MuLV$^-$, Fv-1^n, H-2^b), as well as genetic crosses of these strains, for the production of the MuLV antigen p30, the production of infectious N-ecotropic MuLV, and the development of immunity against various proteins of the endogenous virion.

METHODS AND MATERIALS

Mice. AKR and C57L mice were obtained from the Jackson Laboratories (Bar Harbor, Maine). (AKR x C57L)F$_1$ hybrid and C57L x (AKR x C57L)F$_1$ backcross mice were bred in our laboratory. Mice were caged according to sex and age, with no consideration given to viral status.

XC Assay for Ecotropic MuLV. Tail biopsies were performed on individual mice that were under ether anesthesia (25). Tail segments (2 cm in length) were ground in 6 ml of tissue culture medium in a mortar and pestle. The extract was clarified by centrifugation at 500 g for 10 minutes and then used for infection in the XC assay.

Infectious ecotropic MuLV were assayed by the XC plaque assay (59) with the feral SC-1 mouse cell line (60) as the target cell. Sixty millimeter petri dishes were seeded with 10^5 SC-1 cells; 24 hours later each dish was infected with 0.2 ml of virus extract (containing 20 µg/ml polybrene) for two hours at 37°C. Infected SC-1 cells were maintained in MEM containing 5% fetal calf serum for five days; the cell monolayer was then lethally irradiated with UV and overlaid with 10^6 XC cells. Two or three days later, depending upon the appearance of the plaques, the dishes were fixed and stained.

176

Radioimmunoassay (RIA) for MuLV p30 Protein. RIA for p30 protein was performed by the double antibody competition procedure of Scolnick *et al* (61).

Purified Rauscher (R)-MuLV p30 protein was a gift of Dr. John Stephenson, National Cancer Institute, Bethesda, Maryland. The p30 protein had been isolated from detergent-disrupted R-MuLV by G-100 Sephadex chromatography and isoelectric focusing. This preparation was >95% pure when analyzed by polyacrylamide gel electrophoresis (PAGE).

R-MuLV p30 was iodinated by the method of Greenwood *et al* (62). The reaction mixture contained: 2-5 µg p30 protein, 25 µl buffer (0.4 M Tris-HCl, 0.004 M EDTA, pH 7.4), 1 mCi ^{125}I, 10 µl Chloramine T (2.5 µg/ml). The reaction was quenched after 60 seconds by the addition of 25 µl $Na_2S_2O_5$ (2.5 mg/ml). Residual free iodine was separated from the iodinated protein by gel filtration in Biogel P-10 (100-200 mesh). Iodinated p30 had a specific activity of between 2×10^7 and 1×10^8 cpm/µg.

Goat anti-R-MuLV p30 was obtained from Dr. Jack Gruber, (National Cancer Institute). Rabbit anti-goat IgG antiserum was purchased from Cappel Laboratories (Downington, Pennsylvania).

Spleens from individual mice were teased apart in 0.5 ml cold buffer (0.01 M Tris-HCl, 0.01 M NaCl, pH 7.8) and sonicated to disrupt the cells. Triton X-100 was added to a final concentration of 0.5%; the extracts were incubated for 15 minutes at 37°C, followed by three cycles of freezing and thawing in a dry ice/methanol bath. Extracts were clarified by centrifugation at 1,000 g for 15 minutes and the supernatants were frozen at -70°C. The protein content of each extract was determined by the procedure of Lowry (63).

Radioimmune Precipitation (RIP) Assays for the Detection of Anti-MuLV Antibodies. RIP assays were performed according to Ihle *et al* (55). Fifty microliters of radiolabeled virus preparation (6000 dpm) was initially incubated with 200 µl of diluted mouse serum for 1 hour at 37°C. Mouse immunoglobulins were then precipitated by the addition of 200 µl of undiluted antiglobulin (Goat anti-mouse 7 S gamma globulins; purchased from Hyland Laboratories, California) for 1 hour at 37°C, and then for 2 hours at 4°C. Precipitates were collected by centrifugation at 1000 g for 10 minutes; residual radioactivity was measured in 350 µl of supernatant.

Radiolabeled MuLV antigen was prepared from a continuously-producing AKR embryo cell line that was radiolabeled *in vitro* by the addition of ^{3}H-labeled leucine to the tissue culture medium. In order to increase specific labeling of viral proteins the cell line was first depleted of leucine by growth for one hour in leucine-free MEM: cells were then radiolabeled in leucine-free MEM containing ^{3}H-leucine (50 µC/ml) and 1% fetal calf serum (FCS). Culture fluids were harvested 16 hours after labeling and the viruses purified by density-gradient centrifugation. The virus band (in sucrose) was then divided into small samples and stored frozen at -70°C.

PAGE of viral proteins or antibody:virus complexes was performed overnight at 1.5 mA in cylindrical gels (12 cm in length; 12.5% polyacrylamide) according to the method of Laemmli (64). Samples were dissolved in SDS-sample buffer (3% SDS, 5% β-mercaptoethanol, 10% glycerol, in 0.06 M Tris-HCl, pH 6.8) by heating at 100° for 2 minutes.

RESULTS

Infectious Ecotropic MuLV in the Tissues of AKR, C57L, and (AKR x C57L)F$_1$ Hybrid Mice. AKR, C57L, and (ARK x C57L)F$_1$ hybrid mice were typed for infectious ecotropic MuLV by the XC plaque assay with tail biopsies. The results of these tests are shown in Figures 1A and 1B. AKR mice were uniformly positive for infectious MuLV at a titer ranging from $10^{4.7}$-$10^{5.7}$ PFU/ml. The production of high titered infectious MuLV in the F$_1$ hybrids demonstrated that the AKR viral phenotype was inherited as a dominant trait, in accord with the findings of Rowe *et al* (25).

Infectious Ecotropic MuLV in the Tissues of C57L x (AKR x C57L)F$_1$ Backcross Mice. Production of infectious ecotropic MuLV in mice of the C57L x (AKR x C57L)F$_1$ backcross exhibited Mendelian segregation; thus, the two parental phenotypes were observed in the majority of backcross mice. As shown in Figure 1C, 68% (79/117 mice tested) were positive for virus production. Although the majority of virus-positive mice of the backcross were of the AKR phenotype, there were some mice that displayed a considerable range of virus titers ($10^{1.7}$-$10^{5.7}$ PFU/ml). By statistical analysis, this data is most compatible with a two gene model for the control of virus production. The lower titer of virus in certain mice, as well as the occurrence of a slightly lower number of virus-positive mice (as predicted by a two gene model) may be explained by modifying (suppressive) gene(s) contributed by the C57L genome.

Detection of p30 Antigens in the Spleens of AKR, C57L, and (AKR x C57L)F$_1$ Hybrid Mice. RIA with splenic extracts from mice of the C57L and AKR strains are shown in Figures 2 and 4A. AKR mice uniformly had high levels of MuLV p30 (163±19 ng/mg tissue protein); female AKR mice expressed higher levels of p30 than did the males (females 180±21 ng/mg; males 111±21 ng/mg). Mice of the C57L strain expressed lower levels of MuLV p30 (12±3 ng/mg) than AKR mice; in the C57L strain the levels of p30 were the same in males and females. Although the upper limit of values for p30 protein in the spleens of C57L mice and the lower limit of values of p30 protein in the spleens of AKR mice were contiguous, most of the animals could be separated into two distinct classes; these two classes could be distinguished by a one log difference in mean values of MuLV p30 levels ($P<0.01$).

The (AKR x C57L)F_1 hybrid mice showed levels of MuLV p30 (191±20 ng/mg) comparable to those of the AKR strain (Figure 4B), indicating the inheritance of the expression of p30 protein as a dominant trait.

Detection of p30 Antigen in the Spleens of Mice of the C57L x (AKR x C57L)F_1 Backcross. RIA with splenic extracts from mice of the C57L x (AKR x C57L)F_1 backcross are shown in Figures 3 and 4B. The quantitative distribution of MuLV p30 in mice of this backcross showed a continuum (range: 3 ng/mg to 631 ng/mg), rather than a discrete grouping of values. This suggested the possibility of complex polygenic control of the inheritance of the expression of MuLV p30. However, when these same mice were analyzed for the coordinate expression of infectious ecotropic MuLV and MuLV p30, a more interpretable pattern emerged.

Coordinate Analysis of Infectious Ecotropic MuLV and MuLV p30 Antigen in the Tissues of C57L x (AKR x C57L)F_1 Backcross Mice. Sixty-eight percent of mice of the C57L x (AKR x C57L)F_1 backcross produced infectious ecotropic MuLV (Figure 5); of these mice, the majority expressed high levels of MuLV p30 (157±16 ng/mg). Although the majority of virus-producing backcross mice appeared similar to the AKR parent, there was significant variation in both the levels of infectious MuLV and MuLV p30 protein expressed in the backcross mice that was not seen in either the AKR or (AKR x C57L)F_1 hybrids. In several instances the virus-producing mice of the backcross had a lower titer of infectious MuLV, or a lower level of MuLV p30 protein, than mice of the AKR strain. Since this decreased expression of viral functions was not observed in the (AKR x C57L)F_1 hybrid, it was concluded that this effect was the result of recessive resistance gene(s) contributed by the C57L genome.

Thirty-two percent of mice of the C57L x (AKR x C57L)F_1 backcross did not produce infectious ecotropic MuLV; of these mice, the majority (28/38 tested) coordinately expressed low levels of MuLV p30 protein (9±2 ng/mg), comparable to mice of the C57L strain (Figure 5C). However, a proportion (10/38) of mice with virus-negative phenotypes expressed levels of p30 protein that were significantly higher (87±12 ng/mg) than that of mice of the C57L strain. Mice of this latter phenotype were distinguished on the basis that the level of p30 protein in their spleens was greater than two standard deviations above the mean level of p30 protein in the spleens of C57L mice. The MuLV⁻ p30+ phenotype of these mice could conceivably be related to (a) a suppressive effect of recessive C57L gene(s) on the expression of infectious MuLV, (b) the production of an AKR MuLV in these mice that was defective in the induction of XC plaques or (c) incomplete expression of genes from an endogenous MuLV of AKR mice that resulted in the production of p30 antigen in the absence of infectious virions. Continued genetic analysis through the second backcross should clarify these possibilities.

Antibodies Against MuLV in the Sera of AKR, C57L, and (AKR x C57L)F_1 Hybrid Mice. Results of RIP assays with the sera of AKR, C57L, and (AKR x C57L)F_1 hybrids, are presented in Figure 6. Mice of the AKR strain contained low titers of antibody against MuLV. In most instances, sera of these mice failed to show detectable reactions at a dilution of 1/20. Mice of the C57L strain also contained low titers (<1/20) of antibody against MuLV, although some mice of this strain also showed intermediate titers (1/20-1/40) of antibody. Sera of (AKR x C57L)F_1 hybrid mice generally contained titers of antibody that was higher (1/40-1/320) than either of the parental strains. It was inferred from these findings that the AKR genome contributed the immunogenic virus *(Akv-1 and Akv-2)* to the F_1 hybrid, while the C57L genome contributed a dominant immune response *(Ir)* gene(s). In order to test this hypothesis, mice of the C57L x (AKR x C57L)F_1 backcross were examined for the production of antibody against MuLV; these animals would be expected to be uniformly positive for dominant C57L *Ir* genes, but to segregate for genes that control the production of endogenous MuLV.

Antibodies Against MuLV in the Sera of Mice of the C57L x (AKR x C57L)F_1 Backcross. RIP assays were performed with the sera of 103 mice of the C57L x (AKR x C57L)F_1 backcross. Antibody titers varied considerably from one animal to another, although three major quantitative classes could be distinguished: *(1)* mice of the low responder class had antibody titers of

<1/20, *(2)* mice of the intermediate responder class had antibody titers of 1/40-1/120, and *(3)* mice of the high responder class had antibody titers of 1/320-1/1280. Data from RIP assays of five of these experiments (representing 59 mice) are presented in Figure 7.

Concordance of Antibody Production and Virus Production in Mice of the C57L x (AKR x C57L)F$_1$ Backcross. One hundred and three mice of the C57L x (AKR x C57L)F$_1$ backcross were concordantly typed for infectious MuLV by the XC test and for antibody against AKR MuLV in the RIP assay (Figures 7 and 8). All virus-producing mice produced antibody against MuLV; quantitatively, these mice were of the intermediate or strong responder types. In contrast, a significant proportion (44%) of mice of the virus-negative class produced extrememly low or non-detectable levels of antibodies against MuLV. Due to the multi-modal distribution of antibody titers this data was statistically examined by the Mann-Whitney test; the differences between the virus-free and virus-producing mice was significant to $P<.03$. In fact, all eleven mice of this backcross that *did not* produce detectable antibodies against MuLV were of the virus-negative class. This was a particularly striking observation, especially when considering that the virus-negative class constituted only a third of the total backcross population. The remainder of virus-negative mice (56%) produced antibody against MuLV with titers comparable to that of mice in the virus-producing class.

The degree of concordance between the production of infectious MuLV and the production of anti-MuLV antibody in backcross mice was influenced by the age of the host. When the data presented in Figure 8 was examined for age-related effects, it was found that the degree of concordance between these two parameters was most striking in younger mice (9-17 weeks old). Thus, only 36% (5/14) of young virus-free mice produced detectable anti-MuLV antibody, whereas 100% (42/42) of young virus-producing mice produced anti-MuLV antibody. This difference between the virus-free and virus-producing mice was highly significant ($P<.001$) when examined by the Mann-Whitney test.

Identification of MuLV Proteins that were Immunogenic in Mice of the C57L x (AKR x C57L)F$_1$ Backcross. In order to identify MuLV proteins that were immunogenic in mice of the C57L x (AKR x C57L)F$_1$ backcross, RIP reactions were performed with detergent-disrupted (0.5% NP40) AKR MuLV and the immune complexes were then separated by PAGE.

Several representative PAGE patterns of virus:antibody immune complexes are shown in Figure 9. Control preparations of AKR MuLV contained seven virion polypeptides (gp70, gp45, p30, p17, p15, p12, and p10). Mouse antibodies reacted primarily with the viral proteins p15 and gp70. Minor reactions also were observed with the viral proteins gp45 and p12, although these appeared to represent non-specific reactions. In subsequent studies the minor reactions with gp45 and p12 were eliminated when the NP40-disrupted AKR MuLV was centrifuged at high speed (10,000 g for 5 minutes) immediately before use.

Precipitation of p15 and gp70 from detergent-disrupted MuLV was observed with sera from mice that had high-titers of antibody against intact MuLV in the RIP assay (Figure 9). Sera from mice with low-titers of antibody in the RIP assay did not react with detergent-disrupted MuLV (Figure 9). A qualitatively similar immune response to proteins p15 and gp70 was observed in mice of both MuLV[+] and MuLV[-] phenotypes.

DISCUSSION

Although the DNA sequences of endogenous MuLV exist in the genome of mice of all inbred strains, genetic studies demonstrate that the expression of these endogenous proviral sequences are under strain-specific genetic control. In the high leukemic AKR strain, two independent dominant loci *(Akv-1 and Akv-2)* control the production of N-ecotropic MuLV (25), whereas in the C58 strain, the production of N-ecotropic virus is regulated by three or more dominant independent loci (44). Furthermore, in some strains of mice, viral proteins can be expressed in the absence of overt virus production (13,15,17). Expression of MuLV p30 antigen is a common occurrence in mice of different genetic backgrounds (13,15); yet, mice of some of these strains do not coordinately express infectious MuLV.

Genetic regulation of the expression of p30 protein varies in mice of different strains. Taylor *et al* (37) demonstrated that the expression of p30 protein in the B10.D2(58N)Sn congenic line was controlled by a single recessive locus. The regulation of p30 expression in AKR mice is controlled by multiple dominant loci, although there is some ambiguity as to the exact number of genes involved. Taylor *et al* (67), using a complement fixation assay for the detection of the gs antigen of MuLV, reported that two independent dominant genes controlled the expression of p30 protein in mice of the AKR strain; these results were somewhat unclear, however,

182

since an analysis by the same authors of recombinant inbred lines between C57L and AKR suggested a single gene effect. Hilgers *et al* (38), using a quantitative immunofluoresence absorption technique, reported that two dominant genes controlled the expression of p30 protein in various genetic crosses, but these results were obscured by the effect of the Fv-1 gene. With similar methodology, Ikeda *et al* (68) demonstrated that p30 protein of AKR MuLV was controlled by three independent dominant loci; two of these loci were linked to *Akv-1* and *Akv-2*, while the third locus (designated *Akvp*) was not associated with the production of infectious virus. These studies were supported by the preliminary findings of Strand *et al* (36) with RIA, who showed that multiple genes (most likely three) were responsible for the expression of p30 protein in AKR mice.

In the study reported here, mice of the high leukemic AKR strain, mice of the low leukemic C57L strain, and mice of genetic crosses between these strains, were examined for the expression of infectious ecotropic MuLV (by the XC plaque assay) and for the expression of MuLV p30 protein (by RIA) in the spleen. These strains were utilized since the AKR mice express high titers of infectious MuLV throughout life, while the C57L does not express infectious MuLV; furthermore, there is Fv-1 compatibility between these strains, such that extracellular spread of the AKR MuLV is not restricted.

AKR mice uniformly expressed high titers of infectious MuLV (mean: $10^{5.1}$ PFU/ml) whereas C57L mice were uniformly negative for the expression of infectious MuLV ($<10^{0.7}$ PFU/ml); thus, a five log difference in infectious MuLV distinguished these two strains. F_1 hybrid mice uniformly expressed high titers of infectious MuLV (mean: $10^{5.2}$ PFU/ml) comparable to that of the AKR parent. In the backcross C57L x (AKR x C57L)F_1 68% of the mice were positive for infectious MuLV (mean: $10^{4.4}$ PFU/ml) whereas 32% of these mice were negative for infectious MuLV ($<10^{0.7}$ PFU/ml). These results were compatible with the two gene model of Rowe *et al* (67).

In RIA it was observed that AKR mice uniformly expressed high levels of MuLV p30 (mean: 163±19 ng/mg) while C57L mice expressed lower, but appreciable levels of MuLV p30 (mean: 12±3 ng/mg); thus, a one log difference in p30 levels distinguished these two strains. F_1 hybrid mice expressed levels of MuLV p30 (mean: 191±20 ng/mg) comparable to that of the AKR parent. In the backcross C57L x (AKR x C57L)F_1 76% of the mice expressed high levels of MuLV p30 protein. Analysis of these backcross mice for the coordinate expression of infectious MuLV and MuLV p30 protein revealed three distinct classes of segregants. *Class I* mice (24%) resembled the C57L parent; they did not express infectious MuLV ($<10^{0.7}$ PFU/ml) and they expressed low levels of MuLV p30 (mean: 9 ± 2 ng/mg). *Class II* mice (68%) resembled the AKR parent; they expressed high titers of infectious MuLV (mean: $10^{4.4}$ PFU/ml) and high levels of MuLV p30 (mean: 157 ± 16 ng/ml). *Class III* mice (8%) did not resemble either parental class; they did not express infectious MuLV ($<10^{0.7}$ PFU/ml), although they did express levels of MuLV p30 (mean: 87 ± 12 ng/mg) that were intermediate between the AKR and C57L levels.

It is interesting to note the apparent dichotomy between the levels of MuLV p30 protein and the titer of infectious MuLV observed in mice of the AKR and C57L strain. Although mice of these two strains differ by greater than five logs of infectious virus activity, there is only a one log difference in the levels of MuLV p30 protein expressed in the spleen. Possible explanations for this seemingly paradoxical situation could include: *(1)* C57L mice express an MuLV that is not detectable by the XC plaque assay (32, 69); *(2)* C57L mice may not produce the entire complement of MuLV proteins that are required for virus assembly, hence, there would only be partial expression of the viral genome; or *(3)* C57L mice may express the precursor protein of the p30 antigen that is not processed correctly for virion assembly (70).

Data presented here also demonstrates that the production of endogenous MuLV provides a major antigenic stimulus in the mouse for the synthesis of anti-MuLV antibody. Effective repression of the viral genome by the host removes this immunogenic stimulus, such that virus-free mice may not produce antibody against MuLV. Since virus-free and virus-producing mice in these studies often are reared by the same mother, and housed together in the same cage, it can be concluded that the horizontal infection with MuLV is not the primary antigenic stimulus for the anti-MuLV immune response.

The findings reported here also point to the fact that continued virus production does not render the host immunologically tolerant to MuLV. Persistent viremia in mice of backcrosses to AKR can be demonstrated as early as two weeks of age (25). Furthermore, the presence of high levels of circulating MuLV in the mouse does not prevent (*e.g.*, by absorption of antibody) the demonstration of humoral immunity. In fact, our results indicate that antibody is produced *in excess* of virus in mice of this genetic cross--a direct implication of these findings is that infectious ecotropic MuLV of these mice exists as a virus:antibody complex. Studies by Hanna *et al* (71) indicate that natural antibodies bind to ecotropic MuLV, but do not neutralize viral infectivity; more recently, we have demonstrated (72) that these natural anti-viral antibodies are cytotoxic for virus-producing cells.

The occurrence in the C57L x (AKR x C57L)F_1 backcross of mice that are virus-free, but which are producing anti-MuLV antibody, may be explained by *(a)* a sporadic activation (with concommitant repression by unknown mechanisms) of infectious MuLV in these mice, *(b)* the presence of inefficiently-replicating XC-defective MuLV (69) in these mice, *(c)* the production of viral antigens (23) in these mice in the absence of intact virions, or *(d)* horizontal infection of these mice with low levels of MuLV (73). In this regard, we have found that mice of the virus-free antibody-nonproducing class uniformly (10/10 tested) contained low levels of p30 antigen (2-14 ng/mg total protein) in their spleens, analogous to that of the C57L parent. On the other hand, some mice (7/27) of the virus-free antibody-producing class contained high levels (30-60 ng/mg total protein) of p30 antigen in their spleens, suggesting that possibilities "*b*" and/or "*c*" were correct for these mice. Lastly, the presence of anti-viral antibody in some (11/27) virus-free mice that had low levels of p30 protein (2-18 ng/mg total protein) could be the consequence of possibilities "*a*" or "*d*". Possibility "*d*" can be entertained since it has been shown (73) that continued contact (common caging) between mice of high and low leukemic strains leads to immunization of the low leukemic strains against the Gross virus soluble antigen (GSA). In our studies we have found that the production of antibody in virus-free backcross mice increased with age--this may be the result of horizontal infection and immunization that occurs upon common caging of virus-producing and virus-free mice.

SUMMARY

Mice of the low leukemic C57L strain do not produce infectious ecotropic MuLV ($<10^{0.7}$ PFU/ml of tail extract); the expression of MuLV p30 protein in the spleen of C57L mice also is characteristically low (12 ng/mg tissue protein). In contrast, mice of the high leukemic AKR strain produce high titers of infectious ecotropic MuLV ($10^{5.1}$ PFU/ml); the expression of MuLV p30 protein in the spleens of AKR mice also is high (163 ng/mg). Virus production and expression of MuLV p30 protein are dominant characteristics in the F_1 hybrid. F_1 hybrid mice produce high titers ($10^{5.2}$ PFU/ml) of infectious ecotropic MuLV and express high levels (191 ng/mg) of p30 protein in their spleens.

Mice of the backcross C57L x (AKR x C57L)F_1 genetically segregate for the expression of infectious MuLV and MuLV p30 protein. Sixty-eight per-cent of the backcross mice produce infectious MuLV, whereas thirty-two percent of these mice did not contain detectable infectious virus. These segregation ratios are statistically compatible with a two gene model for the control of infectious MuLV. Virus-producing backcross mice express high levels of MuLV p30 protein; in contrast, virus non-producing back-cross mice can be separated into two classes--the majority of virus non-producers express low levels of p30 protein, while a minor population of virus non-producers express high levels of p30 protein. This latter class of mice represents a phenotype distinct from that of the AKR and C57L parents.

Mice of the AKR and C57L strains produced low titers of natural antibody against ecotropic murine leukemia viruses (MuLV). The F_1 hybrid of these strains produced anti-MuLV antibody in higher titer than mice of either of the parental strains. Progeny of the genetic backcross C57L x (AKR x C57L)F_1 were examined for the production of antibody against MuLV. All mice of this backcross that contained infectious MuLV produced anti-MuLV antibodies. Thus, the persistent production of high-titered MuLV in these mice did not result in immunological tolerance towards viral antigens. In contrast, mice that did not contain infectious MuLV could be separated into antibody-producing and antibody-nonproducing classes. The absence of detectable antibody to MuLV in an individual mouse was invariably associated with a virus-free phenotype. Antibody against MuLV reacted primarily with p15 and gp70 proteins of the viral envelope. It was concluded that overt production of endogenous ecotropic MuLV served as a major immunogenic stimulus for the production of anti-MuLV antibody in these mice.

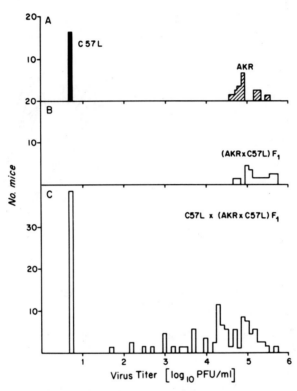

FIG. 1. Infectious ecotropic MuLV in mice of the AKR, C57L, (AKR x C57L) F_1, and C57L x (AKR x C57L)F_1 genotypes. Tail extracts from individual mice (age 2-7 mos.) were tested in the XC plaque assay (SC-1 target cells) for the presence of infectious ecotropic MuLV. (A) Tests with tail extracts from AKR and C57L mice; (B) Tests with tail extracts from (AKR x C57L)F_1 hybrid mice; (C) Tests with tail extracts from C57L x (AKR x C57L)F_1 backcross mice.

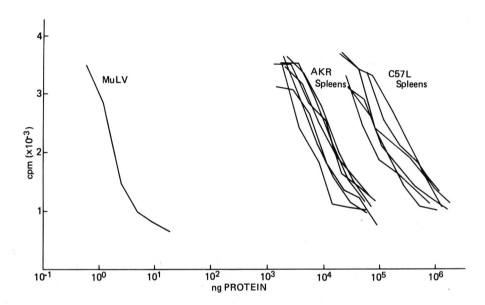

FIG. 2. Radioimmunoassay of p30 antigen in the spleens of AKR and C57L
mice. Each curve represents an RIA competition assay with a splenic
lysate (0.04% Triton X-100) from an individual mouse (age 2-7 mos.) AKR
MuLV (disrupted with Triton X-100) was used as the standard p30 source;
p30 represented 15% of the total viral protein. The standard curve of AKR
MuLV is graphed on the basis of p30 content. Antibody in this essay was
goat anti-Rauscher MuLV p30 (1/15,000 dilution); the ^{125}I-labeled antigen
was purified Rauscher MuLV p30 protein (input: 7400 cpm). Immune complexes were precipitated by rabbit anti-goat IgG. In this assay 3600 cpm
of ^{125}I-labeled p30 was precipitated in the absence of competing antigen.

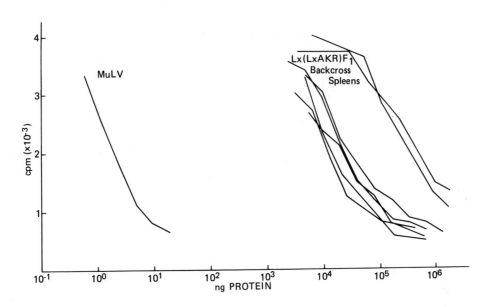

FIG. 3. Radioimmunoassay of p30 antigen in the spleens of C57L x (AKR x C57L)F_1 backcross mice. Conditions for this assay were the same as in Fig. 2, with the exception that the input of ^{125}I-labeled p30 was 7200 cpm, and 3600 cpm of ^{125}I-p30 was precipitated in the absence of competing antigen.

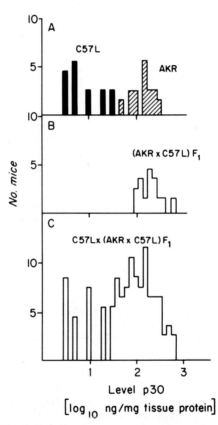

FIG. 4. MuLV p30 antigen in mice of the AKR, C57L, (AKR x C57L)F_1 and C57L x (AKR x C57L)F_1 genotypes. Splenic extracts from individual mice (age 2-7 mos.) were tested in RIA for the levels of MuLV p30. (A) Tests with splenic extracts from AKR and C57L mice; (B) tests with splenic extracts from (ARK x C57L)F_1 hybrid mice; (C) tests with splenic extracts from C57L x (AKR x C57L)F_1 backcross mice.

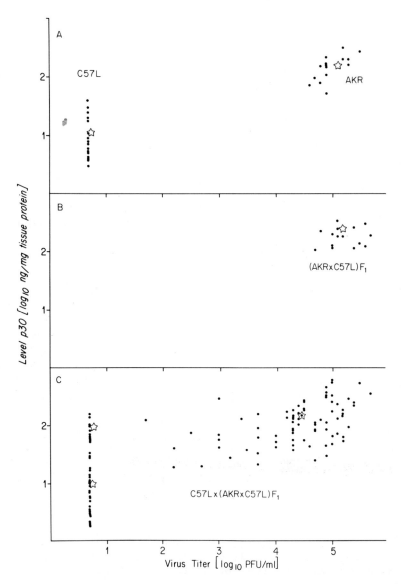

FIG. 5. Coordinate analysis of infectious ecotropic MuLV and MuLV p30 antigen in the tissues of mice of the AKR, C57L, (AKR x C57L)F_1 and C57 x (AKR x C57L)F_1 genotypes. (A) AKR mice (15 tested) and C57L mice (16 tested). AKR and C57L mice were distinguished by a five log difference in infectious virus; the same strains were distinguished by a one long difference in the level of MuLV p30 protein. (B) (AKR x C57L)F_1 hybrid mice (15 tested). The F_1 hybrid mice coordinately expressed high titers of infectious MuLV and high levels of MuLV p30 protein. (C) C57L x (AKR x C57L)F_1 backcross mice (117 tested). Three classes of backcross mice were observed: Class I mice (28/117) were of the C57L parental type; mice of this class expressed low levels of MuLV p30 and did not produce infectious virus. Class II mice (79/117) were of the AKR parental type; mice of this class expressed high levels of MuLV p30 and produced high titers of infectious MuLV. Class III mice (10/117) were a nonparental class; these mice expressed high levels of MuLV p30 but did not produce infectious MuLV. The star indicates the mean levels of infectious MuLV and of MuLV p30 antigen.

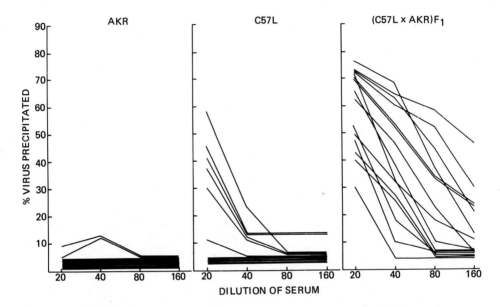

FIG. 6. RIP assays with sera from AKR, C57L, and F_1 hybrid mice. Sera from individual mice were examined for antibody against AKR MuLV by the RIP assay. Sera from AKR and C57L mice contained low-titered anti-MuLV antibodies; sera from the F_1 hybrids contained anti-MuLV antibodies in higher titer than mice of either of the parental strains.

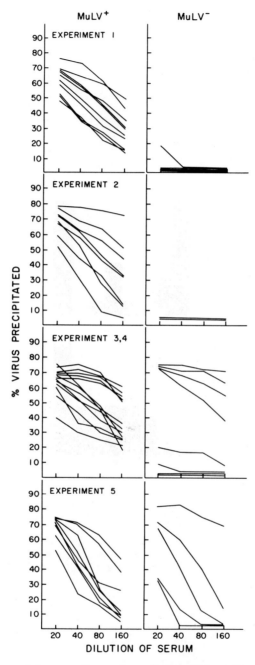

FIG. 7. RIP assays with sera from mice of the C57L x (AKR x C57L)F_1 back-cross. Sera from 59 individual mice were examined for antibody against AKR MuLV by the RIP assay. A tail biopsy from each mouse also was examined in the XC plaque assay for infectious econtropic MuLV. All mice that con-tained infectious MuLV produced antibody against MuLV. Mice that did not contain infectious MuLV could be separated into antibody-producer and antibody-nonproducer classes.

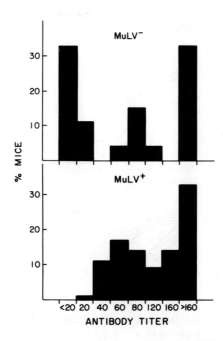

FIG. 8. Concordance between the production of infectious MuLV and the production of anti-MuLV antibodies. This figure represents the results of RIP assays and XC plaque assays that were performed concurrently on 103 mice of the C57L x (AKR x C57L)F$_1$ backcross. The presence of infectious MuLV in mice of this cross was associated with the production of antibody against MuLV. Mice that did not produce anti-MuLV antibody were of the virus-free phenotype.

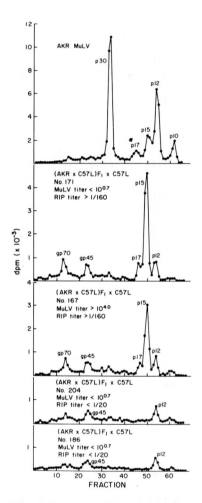

FIG. 9. PAGE of immune precipitates that were formed between IgG₂ antibodies in mouse sera and NP40-disrupted AKR MuLV. The control preparation
of AKR MuLV contained seven polypeptides (gp70, gp45, p30, p17, p15, p12,
and p10); the AKR virus shown in this figure does not demonstrate the gp70
and gp45 peaks, since these proteins contain a relatively low percentage
of the ^{3}H-leucine in the virion. Sera from mice that had high-titered
anti-MuLV antibody in the RIP assay reacted with the viral proteins p15
and gp70. In contrast, sera from mice that had low-titered anti-MuLV
antibody in the RIP did not react with the NP40-disrupted AKR MuLV.

REFERENCES

1. Furth, J., H.R. Seibold, and R.R. Rathbone. Amer. J. Cancer 19: 521-590, 1933.
2. MacDowell, E.C., and M.N. Richter. Archiv. Pathol. 20: 709-724, 1935.
3. Gross, L. Proc. Soc. Exptl. Biol. Med. 76: 27-32, 1951.
4. Gross. L. Proc. Soc. Exptl. Biol. Med. 78: 342-348, 1951.
5. Gross, L. Cancer 9: 778-791, 1956.
6. Gross, L. Proc. Soc. Exptl. Med. Biol. 107: 90-93, 1961.
7. Barnes, W.A., and R.K. Cole. Cancer Res. 6: 99-101, 1941.
8. Fekete, E., and H.K. Otis. Cancer Res. 14: 445-447, 1954.
9. Gross, L. Acta Haemat. 19: 353-361, 1958.
10. Lieberman, M., and H.S. Kaplan. Science 130: 387-388, 1959.
11. Abelev, G.I., and D.A. Elgort. Int. J. Cancer 6: 145-152, 1970.
12. Carnes, W.H. Fed. Proc. 26: 748, 1967.
13. Huebner, R.J., G.J. Kelloff, P.S. Sarma, W.T. Lane, H.C. Turner, R.V. Gilden, S. Oroszlan, H. Meier, D.D. Myers, and R.L. Peters. Proc. Natl. Acad. Sci., U.S.A. 67: 366-376, 1970.
14. Kajima, M., and M. Pollard. Nature 218: 188-189, 1968.
15. Nowinski, R.C., L.J. Old, E.A. Boyse, E. deHarven, and G. Geering. Virology 34: 617-627, 1968.
16. Parks, W.P., D.M. Livingston, G.J. Todaro, R.E. Benveniste, and E.M. Scolnick. J. Exptl. Med. 137: 622-635, 1973.
17. Stockert, E., L.J. Old, and E.A. Boyse. J. Exptl. Med. 133: 1334-1355, 1971.
18. deHarven, E. Proc. 6th Int. Congr. Elec. Micro., Kyoto. 221-222, 1966.
19. Geering, G., L.J. Old, and E.A. Boyse. J. Exptl. Med. 124: 754-772, 1966.
20. Whitmire, E.C., R.A. Salerno, L.S. Rabstein, et al. J. Natl. Can. Inst. 47: 1255-1265, 1971.
21. Aaronson, S.A., G.J. Todaro, and E.M. Scolnick. Science 174: 157-159, 1971.
22. Lowy, D.R., W.P. Rowe, N. Teich, and J.W. Hartley. Science 174: 155-156, 1971.
23. Rowe, W.P., J.W. Hartley, and T. Bremmer. Science 178: 860-862, 1972.
24. Aaronson, S.A., and C.Y. Dunn. Science 183: 422-424, 1974.
25. Rowe, W.P. J. Exptl. Med. 136: 1272-1285, 1972.
26. Chattopadhyay, S.K., P.R. Lowy, N.M. Teich, A.S. Levine, and W.P. Rowe. Proc. Natl. Acad. Sci., U.S.A. 71: 167-171, 1974.
27. Chattopadhyay, S.K. Cold Spring Harb. Symp. Quant. Biol. 39: 1085-1101, 1975.
28. Lowy, D.R., S.K. Chattopdhyay, N.M. Teich, W.P. Rowe and A.S. Levine. Proc. Natl. Acad. Sci., U.S.A. 1971: 3555-3559, 1974.
29. Aaronson, S.A., and J.R. Stephenson. Proc. Natl. Acad. Sci. U.S.A. 70: 2055-2058, 1973.
30. Stephenson, J.R., J.C. Crow, and S.A. Aaronson. Virology 61: 411-419, 1974.
31. Hartley, J.W., W.P. Rowe, and R.J. Huebner. J. Virol. 5: 221-225, 1970.
32. Levy, J.A. Science 182: 1151-1153, 1973.
33. Stephenson, J.R. et al. Virology 61: 56-63, 1974.
34. Bilello, J.A., M. Strand, and J.T. August. Proc. Natl. Acad. Sci. U.S.A. 71: 3234-3238, 1974.
35. Strand, M., F. Lilly, and J.T. August. Proc. Natl. Acad. Sci., U.S.A. 71: 3682-3686, 1974.

36. Strand, M., F. Lilly, and J.T. August. Cold Spring Harb. Symp. Quant. Biol. 39: 1117-1122, 1975.
37. Taylor, B.A., H. Meier, and R.J. Huebner. Nature 241: 184, 1973.
38. Hilgers, J., and J. Galesloot. Int. J. Cancer 11: 780-793, 1973.
39. Meier, H., B.A. Taylor, M. Cherry, and R.J. Huebner. Proc. Natl. Acad. Sci., U.S.A. 70: 1450-1455, 1973.
40. Ikeda, H., W.P. Rowe, E.A. Boyse, E. Stockert, H. Sato, and S. Jacobs. J. Exp. Med. 143: 32-46, 1976.
41. Stephenson, J.R., and S.A. Aaronson. J. Exptl. Med. 136: 175-184, 1972.
42. Stephenson, J.R. and S.A. Aaronson. Proc. Natl. Acad. Sci., U.S.A. 69: 2798-2801, 1972.
43. Aaronson, S.A., and J.R. Stephenson. Cold Spring Har. Symp. Quant. Biol. 39: 1129-1137, 1975.
44. Stephenson, J.R., and S.A. Aaronson. Science 180: 865-866, 1973.
45. Lilly, F., and T. Pincus. Advan. Cancer Res. 17: 231-277, 1973.
46. Pincus, T., J.W. Hartley, and W.P. Rowe. J. Expt. Med. 133: 1219-1233, 1971.
47. Pincus, T., W.P. Rowe, and F. Lilly. J. Exptl. Med. 133: 1234-1241, 1971.
48. Rowe, W.P., J.B. Humphrey, and F. Lilly. J. Exptl. Med. 137: 850-853, 1973.
49. Lilly, F., M.L. Duran-Reynals, and W.P. Rowe. J. Explt. Med. 141: 882-889, 1975.
50. Aoki, T., E.A. Boyse, and L.J. Old. J. Natl. Cancer Inst. 41: 97-101, 1968.
51. Lilly, F. Bibl. Haemot. 36: 213-220, 1970.
52. Sato, H., E.A. Boyse, T. Aoki, C. Iritani, and L.J. Old. J. Expt. Med. 138: 593-606, 1973.
53. Huebner, R.J., P.S. Sarma, G.J. Kelloff, R.V. Gilden, H. Meier, D.D. Myers, and R.L. Peters. Annals. N.Y. Acad. Sci. 181: 246-271, 1971.
54. Aoki, T., E.A. Boyse, and L.J. Old. Cancer Res. 26: 1415-1419, 1966.
55. Ihle, J.M., M.G. Hanna, L.E. Roberson, and F.T. Kenney. J. Exp. Med. 139: 1568-1581, 1974.
56. Nowinski, R.C., and S.L. Kaehler. Science 185: 869-871, 1974.
57. Nowinski, R.C. and A. Watson. J. Immunol., in press.
58. Aaronson, S.A., W.P. Parks, E.M. Scolnick, and G.J. Todaro. Proc. Natl. Acad. Sci. U.S.A. 68: 920-924, 1971.
59. Rowe, W.P., W.F. Pugh, and J.W. Hartley. Virology 42: 1136-1139, 1970.
60. Hartley, J.W., and W.P. Rowe. Virology 65: 128-134, 1975.
61. Scolnick, E.M., W.P. Parks, and D.M. Livingston. J. Immunol. 109: 570-577, 1972.
62. Greenwood, F.C., W.M. Hunter, and J.S. Glover. Biochem. J. 89: 114-123, 1963.
63. Lowry, O.H., N.J. Rosenbrough, A.L. Farr, and R.J. Randall. J. Biol. Chem. 193: 265, 1951.
64. Laemmli, U.K. Nature 277: 680, 1970.
65. Old, L.J., Boyse, E.A. Fed. Proc. 24: 1009-1017, 1965.
66. Callahan, R., M.M. Lieber, G.J. Todaro. J. Virology 15: 1378-1384, 1975.
67. Taylor, B.A., H. Meier, and D.D. Myers. Proc. Natl. Acad. Sci 68: 3190, 1971.
68. Ikeda, H., W.P. Rowe, E.A. Boyse, E. Stockert, H. Sato, and S. Jacobs. J. Exp. Med. 143: 32-46, 1976.
69. Rapp, U.R. and R.C. Nowinski. J. Virol., in press.

70. Eisenman, R. and V.M. Vogt. In, Tumor Virus-Host Cell Interactions. Ed.: A. Kolber. Plenum Press, 303-310, 1975.
71. Hanna, M.G., J.M. Ihle, B.L. Batzing, R.W. Tennant and C.K. Schenley. Cancer Res. 35: 164-171, 1975.
72. Nowinski, R.C., and P.A. Klein. J. Immunol. 115: 1261-1268, 1975.
73. Aoki, T., E.A. Boyse, and L.J. Old. J. Natl. Canc. Inst. 41: 103-110, 1968.

PRELIMINARY STUDIES OF A NON-VIRIONIC ANTIGEN ASSOCIATED WITH HERPES SIMPLEX VIRUS 1 AND 2 (HSV_1- HSV_2)

R.Accinni[1], R.Ferrara[1], G.Tarro[4], E.Sisillo[3], L.Privitera[3], C.Biancardi[1], and A.Bartorelli[1,2]

1 Clinica Medica II dell'Università di Milano- Direttore: C.Bartorelli
2 II Cattedra Radiologia dell'Università di Milano- Direttore: G. Dragoni
3 Clinica del Lavoro "L.Devoto" dell'Università di Milano- Direttore: E. Vigliani
4 Oncologia Virale, Ospedale D. Cotugno, Università di Napoli - Direttore: G. Tarro

INTRODUCTION

It is important to increase our knowledge of the tumor-specific non-virion herpes antigens (1,2) in order to differentiate them from the thermostable structural antigens to which antibodies are found distributed generally throughout the population. The results of such a differentation would be to eliminate the necessity for absorbing the sera and make possible to test them directly for the presence of antibodies specific for tumoral antigens.

By means of polyacrilamide Gel electrophoresis (P.A.G.E.) Hollinshead et al. (3,4) were able to separate soluble HSV-induced antigens from membranes of cells which had undergone lytic infection with the virus and also from living cells grown from squamous cells carcinomas of the head, mouth, pharynx, larinx (5).

It would be especially desirable to be able to replace the complement-fixation test with a more sensitive procedure. A radioimmunological procedure would make it possible to study the distribution of specific antibodies in tumor patients as compared with a control population by determining the presence of the non-virion antigens induced by HSV_1 and HSV_2 .

Ansai et al. (6) have reported that sera from patients with cancer of the uterine cervix show a high degree of reactivity against the early non-structural proteins of HSV_2 , whereas sera from patients with breast tumor or from equiparous control women do not, and that this reactivity of the serum is independent of the neutralizing antibodies for HSV_2 . The method they used was an indirect test, with radioimmunological precipitation followed by analysis of the immune precipitate by P.A.G.E.

PROCEDURES AND MATERIALS USED

A. Virus and antigens

The non-virion antigens of herpes virus (HSV$_1$, Schooler strain) was prepared in vitro in guinea pig kidney cells by the technique described by Tarro and Sabin (7).
Table 1 summarizes the process for preparation of the 50% (w/v) cell sediment suspension from which the virion and non-virion antigens were extracted.

B. Sera

Five sera taken from patients with neoplasias (K sera) and three sera obtained from healthy control donors (C sera) were adsorbed with the virus (Herpes virus types 1 Schooler and 2 Justin) (Tables 2 and 3).
The K sera were all positive in the complement fixation test in respect of non-virion Antigen and all the C sera were negative.
Complement fixation tests were carried out elsewhere by the method described by Lennette, adapted by Tarro and Sabin (7).

C. Radioimmunological Study

Each serum was tested at various dilutions (1:100, 1:200, 1:800). The volume of each dilution used was 0.1 ml. All determinations were done in triplicate.

D. Gel Filtration on Sephadex

Glass columns (1x100 cm) were packed with Sephadex G-200 (height 90cm Pharmacia-Uppsala Sweden) and eluted with PBS (Na/Na$_2$ 0;075 M + 0,075 M NaCl) pH 7,2 at a hydrostatic pressure of 6 cm. The void volume was approximately 30 ml., measured with Blue Dextran 2000. For every preparation, fresh solution, fresh gel and clean glassware were used, in order to avoid any possibility of contamination.

E. Electrophoresis on Polyacrylamide Gel (P.A.G.E.)

The method of Hollinshead (8) was used. Every glass column (0.6x12cm) was filled with four different concentrations of acrylamide and N,N,N',-methylene bis-acrylamide (Bis) (10%, 7%, 4.75%, 3.5%) to a total height of 10 cm (2). The intensity of the current was 4 mA/column. The buffer was Tris-Glycine 0.5M, pH 8.3. Bromophenol Blue was used as tracking dye.

F. Extraction of soluble fractions from suspension of non-infected normal control and infected cells

Three ml aliquots of the 50% (w/v) cells suspension (Table 1) from infected and non-infected cells were centrifuged at 100,000 x g x Ih. between sonication.
The five soluble fractions in the supernatant after sonication and centrifugation from normal cells, SN, or infected cells, SI, were pooled

and concentrated by ultrafiltration with PSAC membrane, (nominal molecular weight limit: 1.000 daltons) (Millipore Ultrafiltration Equipment)
(Table 4).

The two final pellets, normal and infected were treated with 3 M KCl in
phosphate buffer (Na/Na$_2$) 0.05 M, pH 7.2, and stirred for 24 hours at
+4°C. The solutions obtained in this way were centrifuged at 30,000 x g
for 30'. The pellets were discarded and the supernatants (ISP and NSP)
were dyalized exhaustively against distilled water to remove the chloride
and then against PBS and finally concentrated to the initial volume of 3ml.

G. Labelling

To 0.1 ml of the solution to be labelled were added:
1 mCi ^{125}NaI (10 µl) (Amersham)
50 µl   Chloramine T (16 mg/10 ml PBS) (Merck)
50 µl   Na Metabisolfite (48 mg/10 ml PBS) (Merck)
Labelling time: 35" at room temperature
The labelled material was gel-filtrated on Sephadex G 200

H. Radioimmunological Study

0.1 ml of each central fraction of every Gel-filtration peak of the labelled material diluted to 15,000 cpm/0.1 ml in PBS + 3% bovine serum
albumin (BSA) was incubated with K and C sera for 24 hours at 37°C.
Rabbit anti-human- γ -globulin serum at a final dilution of 1:8 in PBS
was added to separate bound from free radioactivity with incubation of
1 hr at 37°C and 20' at 4°C and centrifuged at 7,000 x g for 15'. The
supernatant was discarded by aspiration, the tubes were washed twice and
then counted in a gamma counter (Packard 5130 Autogamma Scintillation
Counter, efficiency 70%).

RESULTS

1 ml aliquots of the pooled soluble fractions of the pellet extracts, obtained by sonication and centrifugation of normal or infected cells were
loaded on 4 columns of Sephadex G-200. Elution resolved three groups
of different molecular size from each column, as determined by the
absorption at 280 mm (fig. 1). The central fractions of each peak (fig.1)
were concentrated by ultrafiltration, labelled by the method described,
and an aliquot of 210 µl loaded again on Sephadex G-200. 60 ml/fractions
were collected from each column.

The results of the second gel filtration after labelling are summarized in
fig. 1 that show that every group of different molecular size (as dected
at 280 mm) could be separated into several peaks. The first gel filtration on Sephadex G-200 (unlabelled material, 1 ml load) did not permit
resolution of the several materials present. After labelling of the central pooled fractions (fig. 1) for every group of different molecular size,
the smaller column load (210 µl) permitted a very much degree of resolution. Such small amounts of material can be evaluated after gel filtration elution only when they are labelled.

The Gel-filtration of labelled supernatant and labelled "soluble pellet" (NSP, ISP) from the control and infected cells (fig. 1) showed that there was no qualitative differences between normal and infected cell with regard to the labelled supernatants. However, in the soluble labelled pellet some materials were present in extracts from infected cells that were absent in the soluble labelled pellet of control cells.

The results obtained after the second Gel filtration on Sephadex G-200 of the labelled material yelded information on the range of molecular weights of the materials present. The electrophoretic mobilities of these substances have been studied on polyacrylamide gel.

All the first peaks of the gel filtration after labelling of the supernatant from control and infected cells, were combined and concentrated by ultrafiltration. 50 μl aliquots were loaded on polyacrylamide gel columns, as described above. After electrophoresis, the gels were cut into 100 slices of about 1 mm each and each slice was counted in the gamma counter. The first peaks were found to have similar molecular weight materials (as shown on Sephadex G-200 after labelling) and analogous electrophoretic mobilities (all the labelled material remained in the cathodic zone).

The same procedure was applied to all the second peaks after labelling. The migration of the labelled material, in this case, showed the presence of materials with similar molecular weights but differing electrophoretic mobilities on polyacrylamide gel (fig. 2). In the second peak obtained with supernatants from extraction of infected cells, there were some radioactive bands which were not present in the second peaks from supernatants of normal cells.

All the first peaks from supernatant were dyalized to remove the free iodine, and when placed on polyacrylamide gel contained insufficient radioactivity to give any useful information.

A. Results of Radioimmunological Study

Blanks: a series of blanks was run with each determination. In the presence of PBS alone, 44% of the labelled material of the first peaks (infected and normal) remained adherent to the walls of the tubes. This phenomenon increased with the time and the centrifugation. Different substances were added to the buffer to overcome inconvenience. The best results were obtained with 3% BSA (blank values below 20%).

All the other peaks showed negligible blank values.

The rabbit anti-human immunoglobulin serum used as second antibody, when incubated alone with the labelled material from each peak did not change the blank value.

For the radioimmunological study six pooled fractions were made, consisting of each of the three peaks from control and infected cells. These six pool were then incubated as described in "Procedures and Materials used" with the five sera from cancer patients (K sera) and the three normal sera (C sera) diluted 1:100 (fig. 1).

The incubations of the three labelled peaks from control cell soluble extracts (NS) and of the second and third labelled peaks from infected cell soluble extract (SI) demonstrated no appreciable binding with either K or C sera. However, incubation of the K sera with the pooled labelled first peaks from soluble extracts of infected cells (SI) gave a radioactive precipitate which was 14-30% greater than that of the blanks when the same pooled material was incubated with C sera no such effect was seen.

Graduated dilution of the K sera from 1/200 to 1:1800 produced a descending curve of the percentage of the radioactivity in the precipitate (fig. 3). When the serum dilution (K sera) was maintained constant and the concentration of the second antibody varied the binding capacity was modified as shown in fig. 4.

When K and C sera were incubated with the peaks derived from the pellet extracts of either normal or infected cells (NSP and ISP), no noticeable binding was seen.

The specific labelled peaks seen only on material extracted from the pellets of infected cells could not be tested by R.I.A. because the amount of label available was insufficient for running the necessary blanks and serum controls.

DISCUSSION

With radioimmunological study, soluble extracts of normal or infected cells incubated with pathological sera, were found to possess different immunological properties.

Gel Filtration on Sephadex (G-200). High resolution of gel filtration of labelled materials obtained from pellet extracts from infected cells demonstrated the presence of two peaks which were absent in analogous extracts from normal cell pellets.

P.A.G.E. Soluble extracts from suspensions of infected cells contained three radioactive bands which were absent in soluble extracts from normal cells (fig. 2).

We can't rule out the idea that any labelled residue of viral material might have been present in the preparations from infected cells on the basis of the results obtained in the gel filtration and P.A.G.E. studies. The results of the R.I.A. studies indicate that it will be worthwhile to undertake a preparative-scale extraction, not just an analytical one.

In order to demonstrate any possible existing biochemical or immunological difference in this work we used labelled crude extracts immediately after extraction. We would have preferred to apply this technique only after having demonstrated by classical immunological methods that there is an immunological affinity between sera of patients with malignant epithelial tumors and materials extracted from infected cells. Unfortunately, in our laboratory we have a very limited capacity for growing infected and control cells and we felt it would be unwise to store the preparations of antigen for a long time since we could not check them for denaturation of the infective material (7). For these reasons, we were forced to work with very small amounts of material for each extraction. For such small amounts of protein, the only possible detection method is the use of labelled materials, since the differences would not be detectable by U.V. absorption of fractions obtained from Gel filtration or by traditional methods of P.A.G.E. Moreover, R.I.A. was possible only with labelled material, and this was needed to determine the interaction of the extracted fractions with sera from patients. The very low concentrations of material in each peak obtained from Gel filtration ruled out complement fixation and immunoelectrophoretic techniques.

TABLE I   Preparation of the antigen

1. Hep_2 cells collected when shown 100% cytopathic effect (ECP) for virion antigen preparation
   Guinea-pig kidney cells, collected 3 hours after infection for non virion antigen (NVA) preparation

2. Cells washed and centrifuged at 1500 x g for 10'.
   Sedimented cells resuspended in Eagle's essential medium.
   Recentrifugation.
   Cell sediment resuspended: 50% (w/v) in bidistilled water for antigen preparation, 10% (w/v) in bidistilled water for storage of virus stock.

3. Cell suspension quickly frozen and thawed, then sonicated for 30".

4. Virion antigen suspension stored at 4°C for 2-3 weeks before use.
   Non virion antigen stored at -80°C, used within 2 days of preparation

TABLE II   Pathological sera (K) and control sera (C), with their identifying symbols in the R.I.A.

TYPE OF PATHOLOGY OR CONTROL	SYMBOLS
Clear cell carcinoma of the kidney	K_1
Spinocellular carcinoma of the uterine cervix	K_2
Squamous cell carcinoma of the nasopharynx	K_3
Clear cell carcinoma of the kidney	K_4
Adenocarcinoma of the prostate	K_5
Healthy donor	C_1, C_2, C_3

TABLE III   Preparation of the absorbed antisera

A. Guinea-pig antisera

    1. Obtained from guinea-pig immunized with guinea-pig renal cells grown in a culture medium containing guinea-pig serum and collected 3 hours after infection with herpes virus (HSV).

    2. Adsorbed with virion antigen to remove antibodies to HSV_1 and HSV_2.

    3. Centrifuged at 100.000 x g for 2 hours at 4°C Supernatant inactivated at 60°C for 20'.

B. Human sera

    1. Obtained from normal subjects and from cancer patient.

    2. Diluted 1:4 and adsorbed 3 x with virion antigen.

    3. Prepared as in A-3 and used as HSV-antibody-free sera.

TABLE IV Extraction scheme

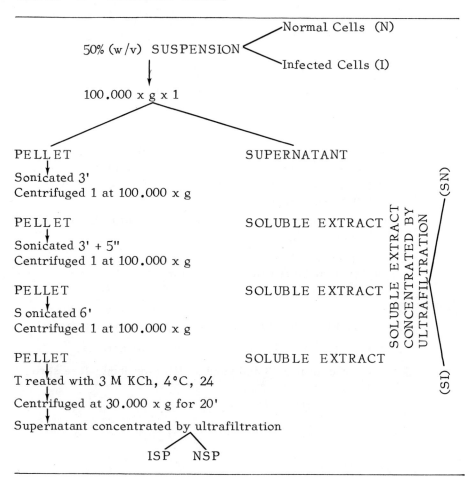

ISP   NSP

SOLUBLE EXTRACT

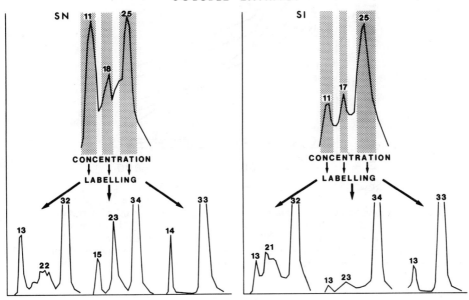

SOLUBLE PELLET EXTRACT

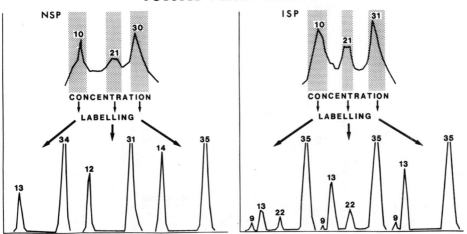

FIG. 1. See text for details.

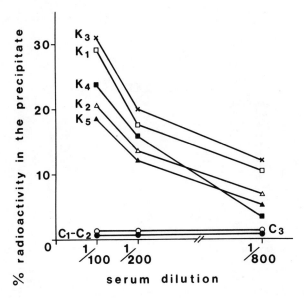

FIG. 2. Polyacrylamide gel electrophoresis (P.A.G.E.) of the material from the second peaks obtained by Sephadex G-200 gel filtration of soluble extracts from infected cells (SI). The positions of the radioactive bands were different from those obtained on P.A.G.E. of the second peak material from control cells (SN). Material labelled with [125]I.

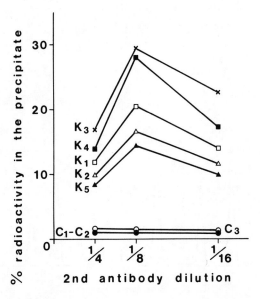

FIG. 3. Percent of total radioactivity of the precipitate, corrected for the blank value, obtained on incubation of pathological sera and control sera with the first peaks obtained from Sephadex G-200 gel filtration of soluble extracts from infected cells (SI). The abscissa shows the varying dilutions of serum.

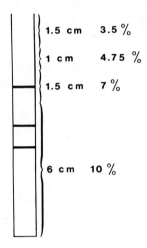

FIG. 4. Variation of the percent radioactivity in the precipitates (with sera K and C) when the serum concentration was maintained constant at 1:100 and the dilution of the second antibody was varied.

REFERENCES

1. Tarro, G., Sabin, A.B. Nonvirion Antigens Produced by Herpes Simplex Viruses 1 and 2. Proc. Nat. Acad. Sci. 70, 1032, 1973.

2. Sabin, A.B., Tarro, G. Appearance in Trypsinized Normal Cells of Reactivity with Antibody Presumably Specific for Malignant Cells. Proc. Nat. Acad. Sci. 70, 3225, 1973.

3. Hollinshead, A.B., Chretien, P.B. et al. Antibodies to Herpesvirus Nonvirion Antigens in Squamous Carcinomas. Science 182, 713-715, 1973.

4. Hollinshead, A.B., Tarro, G. Soluble Membrane Antigens of Lip and Cervical Carcinomas: Reactivity with Antibody for Herpesvirus Non-virion Antigens. Science 179, 698, 1973.

5. Hollinshead, A.B., Tarro, G., Rawls, W., Chretien, P. Caracterization of Herpesvirus Nonvirion Antigens: Relation to Squamous Cell Carcinoma. Viral Immunodiagnosis 301, 1974, Academic Press, New York.

6. Ansai, T., Dreesman, G.T., Courtney, R.J., Adam, E., Melnick, J.L. Antibody to Early Nonstructural Proteins of Herpes Virus Type 2 in Women with Cervical Cancer and in Control Groups. J.N.C.I. May 1975.

7. Tarro, G., Sabin, A.B. Virus-specific, Labile, Nonvirion Antigen in Herpes Virus-Infected Cells. Proc. Nat. Acad. Sci. 65, 753, 1970.

GENITAL HERPESVIRUS IN THE ETIOLOGY OF HUMAN CERVIX UTERI CANCER

Irving I. Kessler, M.D.

Department of Epidemiology
The Johns Hopkins University
Baltimore, Maryland 21205

INTRODUCTION

Herpesviruses are large, enveloped virions with icosahedral capsids consisting of 162 capsomeres and arranged around cores of deoxyribonucleic acid (19). The group includes varicella-zoster, cytomegalovirus and herpes simplex, among others. The latter in turn, consist of two principal types differing from one another in physical, biological and immunological properties (13,22). Herpesvirus Type 1 (HSV-1) is associated with herpes labialis, gingivostomatitis, keratoconjunctivitis, meningoencephalitis, and a variety of vesicular skin eruptions above the waist (7). Herpesvirus Type 2 (HSV-2) has a predilection for the genitalia and is probably transmitted venereally (14,18).

The observed relationships of cervical cancer to coital practice, circumcision, syphilis, prostitution, and socioeconomic class suggested to a number of investigators (4,16,20) that it might have a venereally transmitted viral etiology.

Naib and his colleagues (15) observed cervical carcinoma or squamous atypia in 23.7 percent of 245 biopsied cervices which gave cytologic evidence of active herpetic infection. Out of 44 biopsies taken after the herpetic infection had been diagnosed, 26 (or 59%) revealed anaplasia. By way of contrast, among 245 control biopsies without cytologically detectable herpetic infection only 4 (or 1.6%) were anaplastic. Among 56,418 women screened over an eight year period in the same hospital, only 2.7 percent were diagnosed as having invasive cancer, carcinoma in situ or squamous atypia of the cervix.

Such findings can be explained on the basis of a secondary association between herpetic infection and cervical neoplasia resulting from the relationship of each to sexual promiscuity. Alternatively, the data are consistent with a primary etiologic role for HSV-2 in cervical cancer. In support of the latter hypothesis is the observation that the modal age of the women with genital herpetic infections was ten or more years younger than that of those with cervical neoplasia.

A more systematic approach to testing the herpesvirus hypothesis came in the form of a series of seroepidemiological studies in which neutralizing antibodies to HSV-2 were measured in groups of women with and without cervical neoplasia (8). Despite a lack of uniformity in the types of patients studied, in the specific serologic techniques employed and in the degree to which the cases and controls were epidemiologically comparable, a positive association between cervical cancer and HSV-2 antibodies is clearly evident.

Despite the concordant results of these studies with respect to the association of cervical cancer with HSV-2, sizeable differences are apparent in the levels of HSV-2 antibodies in different population groups. Aurelian (1) suggested that these variations might be due to antigenic differences between the herpesvirus strain indigenous to each population under study and the viral prototypes used in the serologic assays. In order to inquire into this question, we attempted to isolate strains of herpesvirus from various groups of women in Yugoslavia during the course of an epidemiological study to be described below. Fifty-seven Yugoslav women were investigated, 17 from Zagreb, 10 from Skopje, and 30 from Rijeka. Included were infertile middle class women, patients attending an abortion clinic and prostitutes seen at a local venereal disease center. None of the women studied gave evidence of active herpetic lesions on pelvic examination when the cervical swab specimens were collected.

A recurrent lesion from the thigh of a professional woman yielded herpesviruses which were very similar to HSV-2 prototypes from the United States (2). On the other hand, an isolate from the cervix of a 29 year old prostitute induced the formation of large polykaryocytes in HEp-2 cells.

Another source of variation in the results of the seroepidemiological studies lies in the serological tests themselves. We previously reported on a double blind analysis of sera tested by plaque reduction (PR) (1), microneutralization (MN) (17) and indirect hemagglutination (IHA) (6). Out of a total of 108 sera antibody-positive by PR, 38.0% were positive by MN and 26.9% by IHA. Of the 22 antibody-negative sera by PR, 81.8% and 77.3% were also negative by MN and by IHA respectively. On the other hand, out of 48 specimens tested positive by MN, 85.4% were also positive by PR but only 41.7% by IHA. Of 95 sera negative by MN, 18.9% were also negative by PR and 77.9% by IHA. Among 35 sera antibody-positive by IHA, 82.9% were also positive by PR but only 48.8% by MN. Of 102 sera negative by IHA, 16.7% were also negative by PR and 72.5% by MN.

These results suggest that Aurelian's adaptation of the plaque reduction technique is substantially more sensitive than the microneutralization or indirect hemagglutination methods employed. This may be deduced not only from the higher positivity rates obtained but also from the observation that the method tested positive in over 80 percent (90%, including borderline values) of sera found to be positive by either of the other two methods, whereas the latter agreed in only 40 or 50 percent of the cases when the one or the other was positive. It is not possible to draw any conclusions at this time on the relative specificities of the three techniques because of the absence of an absolute standard for antibody titer.

Recently, Aurelian (3) summarized the evidence that cervical cancer cells possess at least a fragment of the HSV-2 viral genome, messenger RNA and some viral proteins. She also demonstrated the presence of a tumor specific antigen, AG-4, in all cervical cancer specimens studied to date, and showed that this is a virion structural polypeptide located on the surface of 2 to 5 percent of the infected cells. All of these observations provide further evidence for the role of HSV-2 in active cervical cancer growth and suggest a possible mechanism for its role in cervical oncogenesis.

However, in view of the fact that the large majority of women with antibodies against HSV-2 never develop cervical cancer it is apparent that this virus, while necessary, is probably not a sufficient cause of the neoplasm. The possible roles of environmental, hormonal, and constitutional factors must not be ignored.

PROCEDURES AND MATERIALS

Two investigations on the possible role of herpesviruses in cervical cancer were undertaken. The first was a retrospective, case-control study of 350 women with histologically confirmed squamous carcinoma of the uterine cervix and a similar number of control women randomly selected from among all currently hospitalized patients without cervical cancer, dysplasia, syphilis or gonorrhea who resembled a case in age (± 5 years), marital status (ever/never married), religion (Moslem/Non-Moslem), and residence (urban/rural). All patients were interviewed and their medical records abstracted. Complete gynecologic examinations including colposcopy and (for the controls) cervical cytology were performed. Cervical smears of the controls and biopsy specimens of the cases were reviewed by a single group of pathologists.

Aliquots of blood were collected for serologic analysis. A microneutralization technique, employing constant amounts of virus and varying dilution of serum, was employed to ascertain the presence of HSV-2 antibodies (9). The $\log_{10}$ HSV-2 antibody titer of each patient was divided by $\log_{10}$ HSV-1 antibody titer to form a "log titer ratio" which was then multiplied by 100 to form a "II/I index" of prior infection with HSV-2. II/I indexes $\geq$ 85 have been shown to discriminate between patients with and without a previous HSV-2 infection (17). In addition to the seroepidemiological measurements, a number of epidemiologic factors of possible significance were assessed on the basis of the patients' interview responses, their medical records and the findings on physical examination (10).

The second study, still in progress, involves direct observation on two large groups of women: one group married to men who, at some other time, had wives who developed cervical cancer and a second group married to men without such histories. An answer is sought to the following question: "Is the risk of developing cervical cancer increased among the wives of men who, at some other time in their lives, were married to other women who developed cervical cancer?"

We begin by identifying a large cohort of women diagnosed over the past 20 years as having squamous carcinoma of the uterine cervix. The husbands of these women are investigated to the extent of identifying their previous and subsequent wives ("case" wives). A random sample of "control" wives, similar to the "case" wives in demographic and marital characteristics, is then selected. The cohorts of "case" and "control" wives are being traced prospectively forward through time to death or survival. A flow chart indicating the manner in which the "case" and "control" wives are assembled and followed is illustrated in Table I. The cumulative risk of cervical neoplasia among the two cohorts of women is ascertained by means of personal interview, medical record review, and exfoliative cytological screening by self-administered irrigation pipette. Cervical scrapings on direct visualization are obtained from all women with non-normal irrigation findings. This approach affords us an epidemiologic test of the role of any venereally transmitted male factor in cervical cancer, herpesvirus genitalis among others.

RESULTS

Seroepidemiological Findings

Among both Moslem and non-Moslem cases in each age category, as well as for all ages combined, HSV-2 antibody titers were higher than among controls, though statistical significance was not attained with the present sample sizes. Among both Moslems and non-Moslems, the II/I index was significantly higher in cases as compared with controls. The same was true for 7 out of 8 specific age groups, except that the differences failed to reach statistical significance (9). Only the Moslem cases below 35 years of age demonstrated a lower antibody prevalence than their controls. Excluding the latter, the risks of cervical cancer in the herpesvirus-positive Moslem patients ranged from 1.71 to 2.28 (overall: 1.83) times that in the herpesvirus-negatives. Among non-Moslems the risk increases ranged from 1.57 to 2.70 (overall: 2.00). There was no apparent relationship between relative risk and age [Table II].

The antibody prevalence data were also analyzed in terms of matched pairs of cases and controls. Few differences from the unmatched results were obtained. With one exception, matched pairs of each age and religious category showed increased relative risks among patients with HSV-2 antibodies. The relative risks ranged from 0.60 to 2.33 among Moslems (overall: 1.86) and from 1.38 to 4.00 among non-Moslems (overall: 1.94). With the exception of Moslems aged 20-34 years, the magnitude of the relative risk in patients of each religion was inversely related to their age.

Epidemiologic Findings

The epidemiologic characteristics of the Yugoslavian cases and controls were examined in great detail. It was noted that women who developed cervical cancer were more likely to manifest behavioral characteristics such as smoking, drinking of alcohol, and diminished religiosity. They tended to be significantly shorter, lighter and less endomorphic than controls similar to them in age, marital status, religion and urban/rural residence. The cases also had somewhat higher systolic and diastolic blood pressures measured at two different times. Their parents tended to be older, especially over 40, than the control parents at the time of the patients' birth. Multiple marriages and early initiation of coitus were more common among the cases. However, coital frequency was consistently lower among Moslem and non-Moslem cases than controls, both at the onset of coital practice and later. Cases tended to have more "normal" menstrual histories than controls, with relatively fewer long, heavy, painful, or irregular cycles [Table III]. Absences from home and extramarital sexual experiences were significantly more common among the first husbands of the cases.

An unexpected finding was the two-or threefold greater mortality, especially at young ages, of the first husbands of cases as compared with those of the controls. The cases tended to experience more frequent and longer widowhoods, beginning at earlier ages, than did the controls. For most of the variables studied, case-control differences among the Moslem women closely resembled those among the non-Moslems.

In order to further investigate the role of HSV-2 in cervical carcinogenesis, a multiple regression model was employed to control for case-control variation due to 34 other factors found to be significantly or substantially different among the Yugoslavian cases and controls. The independent variables so controlled are listed in Table IV. A multiple logistic function suggested by Cornfield, Walker and Duncan (5,23) was employed. Utilizing this approach, an odds ratio adjusted for the 34 independent variables was calculated as an estimate of the relative risk associated with HSV-2 in cervical cancer. The adjusted odds ratio, R, was calculated to be 1.68, a value significantly increased above unity $(p < 0.05)$.

In the previously described male role study, a total of 1,436 wives have been completely traced, to date. Non-normal pap tests were observed in 13.6 percent of the "case" wives as compared with 7.2 percent in the "control" wives, a statistically significant difference $(p < 0.05)$. Cervical cancer or carcinoma in situ were diagnosed in 3.5% of the "case" wives and 1.2% of the "control" wives $(p < 0.05)$. The latter percentage may be compared with an expected incidence of approximately 1.0 percent calculated from population statistics for Baltimore women of similar ages over the same time span.

These results may also be analyzed in terms of the numbers of observed and expected "marital clusters", i.e. the number of multiply-married men, each of whose wives developed cervical cancer during or subsequent to the given marriage. A total of 30 such marital clusters have been observed so far, against an expectation of 10.6. Selected details on these marital clusters are given in Table V.

DISCUSSION

HSV-2 is a venereally transmitted virus. Cervical cancer behaves as a venereal disease (11). Therefore, is cervical cancer transmitted by HSV-2? Validation of this syllogism must await evaluation of a number of ongoing investigations as well as studies still to be undertaken. Completed work in a multiplicity of disciplines -- virology, immunology, epidemiology, cytopathology, etc. -- is highly consistent with such a conclusion, however.

The findings reported here are supportive of the hypothesized role of HSV-2 in cervical pathogenesis. Utilizing a serological method which is not especially sensitive, no distinctive pattern in the distribution of HSV-1 titers between women with and without cervical cancer could be discerned. However, among both Moslems and non-Moslems, HSV-2 titers were clearly higher among cases than controls. The consistent direction of these findings among the various ethnic and age groups, rather than their absolute numerical value, are especially impressive. They lend further credence to the herpesvirus hypothesis in cervical cancer.

The epidemiological findings in the Yugoslavian study are also highly consistent. Particularly compelling is the fact that the relationship with HSV-2 persists at a statistically significant level even after controlling for the effect of 34 other variables which distinguish in one degree or another between cervical cancer cases and controls. This suggests that, while other factors may be operative in the disease process, prior infection with HSV-2 is a necessary condition, at least in some women, for the ultimate development of the neoplasm.

The epidemiological data suggest that hormonal factors may be involved as well. Women with cervical cancer, both Moslem and non-Moslem, revealed small but impressively consistent differences in their menstrual patterns as compared with control patients. Though the direction of the differences might be considered anomalous (i.e. more normal menses among women destined to develop cervical cancer) there is no logical reason why this should not be so, especially in view of the evidence that estrogens

217

and cervical atypia may be associated (21) and that HSV-2 and steroidal hormones may interact in the development of cervical cancer in certain laboratory animals (12).

The results of our ongoing investigation of the male role in cervical cancer are consistent with an effect of HSV-2 but do not exclude the operation of a number of other venereally transmitted factors, though it seems to us that none of these are as consistent with the biological and clinical characteristics of the disease as genital herpesvirus. The study protocol suffers from at least one theoretical weakness, viz. that we are following only marital partners rather than all sexual contacts of the suspect males. This is, of course, unavoidable and, in our opinion, is preferable to following selected sexual contacts of the males. That is to say, it is methodologically advantageous to identify all wives of subject males and to follow them to the development of cervical cancer, rather than to follow only those sexual contacts whom we are able to identify. The selective biases in the latter approach could not be controlled and the analysis would suffer accordingly.

If the final results of this investigation suggest that women marrying men whose previous wives had cervical cancer experience a significantly increased risk of this disease themselves, two alternative inferences might then be drawn. First, the increased cancer risk might be attributed to an extrinsic characteristic of the spouses, such as a venereally transmitted carcinogen or procarcinogen (HSV-2?); or second, the clustering might be due to an intrinsic factor, such as the tendency for certain men to marry women destined to develop cervical cancer. The second of these possibilities cannot be summarily dismissed because cervical neoplasia is associated with certain social and sexual characteristics which conceivably could influence particular men to repeatedly choose certain classes of women for their marital or coital partners. To some extent, we have controlled for this possibility by matching the controls to the "case" wives on age, race, place of marriage and prior marital status. In addition, detailed information on each woman's sexual practices as well as other known and suspected risk factors is obtained at interview and will be taken account of in the analysis.

Assuming that bias and confounding factors cannot explain the observed marital clustering in cervical cancer, it would seem reasonable on the basis of all of the accumulated epidemiological, serological, virological and immunological evidence to implicate the genital herpesvirus as the likeliest agent in the pathogenesis of this disease. Should our present findings be confirmed, we would proceed to a detailed characterization of the case and control spouses, with special emphasis on their HSV-2 infections.

More definitive conclusions on the association between HSV-2 and cervical neoplasia must also await the design and execution of appropriate prospective studies. We have previously suggested one possible approach (27). A large cohort of women free of both cervical neoplasia and HSV-2 antibodies would be selected for study in a given geographic area. All would be examined for cervical lesions, active herpetic infections, and initial HSV-2 antibody status. A brief interview designed to secure basic demographic information as well as marital, coital and social data would also be conducted. Thereafter, the live/dead status, marital status, cervical cytology and HSV-2 serology of each woman would be determined on an annual or, perhaps, biennial basis. Whenever cervical neoplasms were diagnosed, the patients would be serologically tested for HSV-2 antibodies. Conversely, whenever sero-positivity developed in a woman, her cervix would be cytologically screened for neoplasia.

From such an effort could be derived estimates of the true risk of cervical neoplasia among women with and without prior histories of HSV-2 infection. The findings, together with those of the retrospective and laboratory-based studies should, within a reasonable time, enable definitive conclusions to be drawn about the herpesvirus hypothesis. These, in turn, could lead to the initiation of the appropriate preventive measures.

SUMMARY

Two investigations on the possible role of herpesviruses in human cervix uteri cancer were undertaken. The first was a retrospective case-control study of 350 Yugoslavian women with histologically confirmed squamous carcinoma of the uterine cervix and a similar number of controls randomly selected from among all currently hospitalized patients who resembled the cases in age, marital status, religion and area of residence. All were interviewed and complete gynecologic examinations performed. Exfoliative smears and biopsy specimens were reviewed by a single group of pathologists. In addition, blood was collected for analysis of neutralizing antibodies to herpesvirus genitalis (HSV-2).

HSV-2 antibody titers were higher among both Moslem and non-Moslem cases of each age category as compared with controls. The relative risk of cervical neoplasia in women positive for HSV-2 was significantly increased even after adjusting for the effects of 34 epidemiologic factors associated with cervical cancer. A number of epidemiologic observations were also made. Women who developed cervical cancer were more likely to smoke and to drink alcoholic beverages. They had somewhat higher systolic and diastolic blood pressures. Their parents tended to be older at the time of their birth than control parents. Multiple marriage and early initiation of coitus were more common among them. However, their coital frequency was consistently reduced, both at the onset of coital practice and later. Cases were more likely than controls to have normal menstrual histories, free of long, heavy, painful or irregular cycles. Absences from home and extramarital sexual experiences were significantly more common among the first husbands of the cases. An unexpected finding was the two-or threefold greater mortality, especially at younger ages, of the first husbands of the cases as compared with those of the controls.

In a second study, still in progress, direct observations are being made on two large groups of women: one married to men who, at some other time, had wives who developed cervical cancer and a second married to men without such histories. An answer is being sought to the following question: "Is the risk of cervical cancer increased among the wives of men who, at some other time in their lives, were married to other women who developed cervical cancer?" To date, non-normal pap tests have been observed in 13.6% of the "case" wives as compared with 7.2% of the control wives (p < 0.05). Cervical cancer or carcinoma in situ have been diagnosed in 3.5% of "case" wives and 1.2% of control wives (p < 0.05).

These findings are supportive of an etiological role for HSV-2 in cervical oncogenesis. In addition, the epidemiological data suggest that hormonal factors may be involved in the process as well. In any event, further characterization of the suspect males, with special reference to HSV-2 antibody status, should be undertaken. Prospective studies designed to estimate the true risk of cervical neoplasia among women with and without prior herpetic infections are also needed. The results of such investigations could open the door to the initiation of appropriate preventive measures.

ACKNOWLEDGEMENTS

These studies were supported by P.H.S. research grant no. CA 11489; N.C.I. grant no. CA 16605, Regional Medical Programs Service (H.S.M.H.A.) project no. 02-802 and Faculty Research Award no. PRA-112 from the American Cancer Society.

I am most grateful to Dr. James A. Tonascia for the multiple regression analysis and to Mmes. Lucy Hare and Page Clark and their staffs for technical assistance. The Yugoslavia study was conducted in collaboration with Drs. Zivko Kulcar and Marija Strnad and their colleagues, in whose debt I remain.

TABLE I. Male Role Study Flowchart

PROBANDS

```
┌─────────────────────────────┐
│   All cervix cancer*        │
│   cases in Baltimore        │
│        1950-69              │
└─────────────────────────────┘
```

HUSBANDS

```
┌─────────────────────────────┐
│   All husbands of           │
│   probands, prior to        │
│   cancer diagnosis          │
└─────────────────────────────┘
```

OTHER WIVES

```
┌─────────────────────────────┐
│   All other wives of        │
│   proband husbands,         │
│   previous and subsequent   │
└─────────────────────────────┘
```

CONTROLS

```
┌─────────────────────────────┐
│ Random women, similar in    │
│ age, race, yr. marriage and │
│ prior marital status to     │
│ other wives, selected from  │
│ marriage records            │
└─────────────────────────────┘
```

PROSPECTIVE FOLLOW UP

```
┌─────────────────────────────┐
│ To death, ascertain causes  │
│            or               │
│ To survival, interview and  │
│         pap test            │
└─────────────────────────────┘
```

*Invasive and in situ.

TABLE II. Prevalence of HSV-2 Antibodies Among Cases and Controls by Age and Religion*

| Age (yr) | Moslems | | | | | Non-Moslems | | | | |
| | Cases | | Controls | | Rela-tive Risk† | Cases | | Controls | | Rela-tive Risk† |
	Num-ber	Per-cent	Num-ber	Per-cent		Num-ber	Per-cent	Num-ber	Per-cent	
20 to 34	13	23.1	14	28.6	0.75	12	33.3	12	16.7	2.49
35 to 44	50	38.0	52	21.2	2.28	61	45.9	70	23.9†	2.70
45 to 54	54	35.2	58	24.1	1.71	89	36.0	91	26.4	1.57
55 to 64	33	33.3	26	19.2	2.10	38	42.1	26	26.9	1.98
ALL AGES	150	34.9	150	22.7	1.83‡	200	40.0	200	25.0	2.00 ‡

*Figures give total number of patients in each category and the percent with HSV-2 antibodies.

†Extimated from odds ratio.

‡P < 0.05 for given case-control difference.

TABLE III. Menstrual Characteristics of Study Patients*

Characteristic	Moslems		Non-Moslems	
	Cases	Controls†	Cases	Controls†
I. Age at menarche:				
A. % < 14 yr.	23.8	30.0 (29.8)	34.5	38.0 (36.3)
B. Mean age, yr.	14.4	14.4 (14.4)	14.4	14.2 (14.3)
II. Menstrual regularity:				
A. % "regular"	92.6	88.7 (87.9)	92.0	84.0‡(85.4)‡
III. Menstrual interval:				
A. % < 27 days	8.7	14.7 (14.0)	10.1	20.0‡(20.8)‡
B. Mean interval, days	28.6	28.2 (28.3)	28.5	28.0 (27.9)
IV. Menstrual duration:				
A. % > 6 days	14.7	18.7 (17.7)	14.6	30.8‡(33.7)‡
B. Mean duration, days	4.9	4.8 (4.7)	4.8	4.4‡(5.6)‡
V. Menstrual flow:				
A. % heavy	18.1	23.3 (25.0)	25.6	35.0‡(38.0)‡
B. % painful	11.7	23.2‡(23.5)‡	17.9	31.2‡(32.1)‡
VI. Menstrual hygiene:				
A. % douching	86.6	86.7 (84.7)	71.9	75.9 (74.7)

*Excluding a few patients with characteristic of interest unknown.
 For only the proportions with painful menstrual flow were there >5%
 of patients with characteristic unknown.

†Values excluding controls hospitalized for menstrual problems are in
 parentheses.

‡P < 0.05 for observed case-control difference.

‡P < 0.01 for observed case-control difference.

TABLE IV. Independent Variables Used in the Multiple Regression Analysis

1. Cervical cancer case/control
2. Diastolic blood pressure > 100 mm Hg
3. Education < 5 years
4. Born in urban area
5. Ponderal index ≤ 12
6. Cigarettes smoked
7. Alcohol drunk
8. Menarche ≤ 13 years of age
9. Menses regular
10. Menses heavy
11. Menses duration < 7 days
12. Menses interval > 26 days
13. Menses painful
14. 1st married ≤ 18 years of age
15. Married ≥ 2 times
16. Pregnancies > 4
17. Abortions 1+

18. 1st abortion < 20 years of age
19. No. coital partners > 1
20. 1st coitus ≤ 16 years of age
21. Coital frequency at 1st < 30 times per month
22. Coital frequency later < 15 times per month
23. Coitus during menses
24. Coitus during final 6 weeks of pregnancy
25. Coitus during pregnancy
26. Coital satisfaction frequent
27. Patient's father at her birth ≥ 40 years of age
28. Patient's mother at her birth ≥ 40 years of age
29. Husband married ≤ 20 years of age
30. Husband educated < 5 years
31. Husband absent from home
32. Husband had other coital partners
33. Husband had extramarital partners during this marriage
34. Husband died < 40 years of age

225

TABLE V. Selected Details on Marital Clusters

Cluster	Wife	Age at Marriage Husband	Age at Marriage Wife	Wife's Age at Cervical Cancer		Yrs. Marriage Prior to Cervical Cancer Married to This Husband	Married to Another	Other[a]
I	1st	19	18	39	In situ carcinoma	10	3	8
	2nd	32	32	38	In situ carcinoma	6	-	-
II	1st	19	19	34	Squamous cell carcinoma	4	9	1
	2nd	24	22	--	- - - - - - - -	-	-	-
	3rd	29	24	29	Micro-invasive carcinoma	5	5	1 1/2
III	1st	20	20	34	Squamous cell carcinoma	14	-	-
	2nd	42	25	27	In situ carcinoma	2	-	-
IV	1st	22	18	47	Transitional cell carcinoma	28	1	-
	2nd	56	41	43	Squamous cell carcinoma	3	-	-
V	1st	18	15	35	In situ carcinoma	2	18	1
	2nd	32	26	34	In situ carcinoma	9	-	-
VI	1st	25	26	38	Micro-invasive carcinoma	12	-	-
	2nd	40	41	44	In situ carcinoma	3	-	-
VII	1st	DK[b]	15	41	Papillary adenocarcinoma	15	-	11
	2nd	DK	39	40	Squamous cell carcinoma	1	DK	DK
VIII	1st	18	19	35	In situ carcinoma	3	11	1
	2nd	21	36	40	Adenocarcinoma	4	-	-
	3rd	32	45	--	- - - - - - - -	-	-	-
IX	1st	DK	DK	48	Micro-invasive carcinoma	DK	24	5
	2nd	34	31	33	In situ carcinoma	1	-	-
X	1st	21	16	25	In situ carcinoma	6	3	-
	2nd	27	19	25	Micro-invasive carcinoma	6	-	-
XI	1st	17	16	26	Micro-invasive carcinoma	10	-	-
	2nd	29	35	36	In situ carcinoma	1	-	-

226

XII	1st	24	19	In situ carcinoma	4	18	5
	2nd	29	30	In situ carcinoma	13	-	-
XIII	1st	DK	DK	In situ carcinoma	DK	DK	DK
	2nd	60	59	In situ carcinoma	9	23	13
XIV	1st	DK	DK	- - - - -	--	--	--
	2nd	30	32	In situ carcinoma	4	--	--
	3rd	50	50	In situ carcinoma	9	--	--
XV	1st	20	18	- - - - -	--	--	--
	2nd	DK	DK	Squamous cell carcinoma	DK	DK	DK
	3rd	47	37	Squamous cell carcinoma	4	DK	DK
XVI	1st	18	18	- - - - -	--	--	--
	2nd	DK	DK	In situ carcinoma	DK	DK	DK
	3rd	30	21	In situ carcinoma	12	2	1
XVII	1st	23	18	In situ carcinoma	1 1/2	21	0
	2nd	28	21	In situ adenocarcinoma	24	0	0
XVIII	1st	DK	DK	Adenocarcinoma	DK	DK	DK
	2nd	24	24	In situ carcinoma	26	DK	DK
XIX	1st	25	19	Invasive cervical cancer, Type?	23	0	0
	2nd	59	51	Squamous cell carcinoma	8	DK	7.5
XX	1st	22	15	In situ carcinoma	4	0	0
	2nd	34	35	Squamous cell carcinoma	0	18	1
XXI	1st	21	19	In situ carcinoma	5	11	1
	2nd	27	26	In situ carcinoma	12	DK	DK
XXII	1st	DK	DK	Squamous cell carcinoma	DK	1	DK
	2nd	DK	DK	Squamous cell carcinoma	DK	DK	DK
XXIII	1st	22	20	Squamous cell carcinoma	9	0	0
	2nd	DK	DK	In situ carcinoma	DK	DK	DK

a – Years lived while unmarried, divorced or widowed, between the 1st marriage indicated and diagnosis of cervical cancer.
b – DK denoted data unavailable at the time of this report.

REFERENCES

1. Aurelian, L. The Possible Role of Herpesvirus Hominis, Type II in Human Cervical Cancer. Fed. Proc. 31: 1651-1659, 1972.

2. Aurelian, L., Smerdel, S., Kessler, I.I., and Kulcar, Z. Three Yugoslav Herpes Simplex Viruses: Biologic and Antigenic Properties and Formation of Giant Cells in Vitro by a Cervical Isolate. J. Infect. Dis. 129: 465-469, 1974.

3. Aurelian, L. Sexually Transmitted Cancers? The Case for Genital Herpes. J. Am. Vener. Dis. Assoc. 2: 10-20, 1976.

4. Ayre, J.E. Role of the Halo Cell in Cervical Cancerigenesis. A Virus Manifestation in Premalignancy? Obstet. Gynecol. 15: 481-491, 1960.

5. Cornfield, J. Joint Dependence of Risk of Coronary Heart Disease on Serum Cholesterol and Systolic Blood Pressure: A Discriminant Function Analysis. Fed. Proc. Suppl. No. 11, pp. 58-61, 1962.

6. Fuccillo, D.A., Moder, F.L., Catalano, L.W., Jr., Vincent, M.M., and Sever, J.L. Herpesvirus Hominis Types I and II: A Specific Micro-indirect Hemagglutination Test. Proc. Soc. Exp. Biol. Med. 133: 735-739, 1970.

7. Kaplan, A.S. Herpes Simplex and Pseudorabies Viruses. Virology Monograph No. 5. New York, Springer-Verlag, 1969.

8. Kessler, I.I. Perspectives on the Epidemiology of Cervical Cancer with Special Reference to the Herpesvirus Hypothesis. Cancer Res. 34: 1091-1110, 1974.

9. Kessler, I.I., Kulcar, Z., Rawls, W.E., Smerdel, S., Strnad, M., and Lilienfeld, A.M. Cervical Cancer in Yugoslavia. I. Antibodies to Genital Herpesvirus in Cases and Controls. J. Natl. Cancer Inst. 52: 369-376, 1974.

10. Kessler, I.I., Kulcar, Z., Zimolo, A., Grgurević, M., Strnad, M., and Goodwin, B.J. Cervical Cancer in Yugoslavia. II. Epidemiologic Factors of Possible Etiologic Significance. J. Natl. Cancer Inst. 53: 51-60, 1974.

11. Kessler, I.I. Human Cervical Cancer as a Venereal Disease. Cancer Res. 36: 783-791, 1976.

12. Muñoz, N. Effect of Hormonal Imbalance and Herpesvirus Type 2 on the Uterine Cervix of the Mouse. In: Oncogenesis and Herpesviruses. Ed.: Biggs, P.M., de-Thé, G. and Payne, L.N. International Agency for Research on Cancer, Lyon, pp. 443-447, 1972.

13. Nahmias, A.G. and Dowdle, W.R. Antigenic and Biologic Differences in Herpesvirus Hominis. Prog. Med. Virol. 10: 110-159, 1968.

14. Nahmias, A.J., Dowdle, W.R., Naib, Z.M., Josey, W.E., McLone, D., and Domescik, G. Genital Infection with Type 2 Herpes Virus Hominis. A Commonly Occurring Venereal Disease. Br. J. Vener. Dis. 45: 294-298, 1969.

228

15. Naib, Z.M., Nahmias, A.J., Josey, W.E., and Kramer, J.H. Genital Herpetic Infection: Association with Cervical Dysplasia and Carcinoma. Cancer 23: 940-945, 1969.

16. Pereyra, A.J. The Relationship of Sexual Activity to Cervical Cancer. Obstet. Gynecol. 17: 154-159, 1961.

17. Rawls, W.E., Iwamoto, K., Adam, E., and Melnick, J.L. Measurement of Antibodies to Herpesvirus Type 1 and 2 in Human Sera. J. Immunol. 104: 599-606, 1970.

18. Rawls, W.E., Gardner, H.L., Flanders, R.W., Lowry, S.P., Kaufman, R.H., and Melnick, J.L. Genital Herpes in Two Social Groups. Am. J. Obstet. Gynecol. 110: 682-689, 1971.

19. Roizman, B. The Herpesviruses - A Biochemical Definition of the Group. Curr. Top. Microbiol. Immunol. 49: 1-79, 1969.

20. Rotkin, I.D. Adolescent Coitus and Cervical Cancer: Associations of Related Events with Increased Risk. Cancer Res. 27: 603-617, 1967.

21. Rubio, C.A. Estrogenic Effect in Vaginal Smears in Cases of Carcinoma in Situ and Micro-Invasive Carcinoma of the Uterine Cervix. Acta. Cytol. 17:361-365, 1973.

22. Terni, M., and Roizman, B. Variability of Herpes Simplex Virus: Isolation of Two Variants from Simultaneous Eruptions at Different Sites. J. Infect. Dis. 121: 212-216, 1970.

23. Walker, S.H. and Duncan, D.B. Estimation of the Probability of an Event as a Function of Several Independent Variables. Biometrika 54: 167-179, 1967.

COMPARED HUMORAL AND CELLULAR IMMUNE RESPONSE TO HERPES
SIMPLEX (HSV-2) ANTIGENS IN WOMEN WITH CERVICAL
CARCINOMA.

Lise THIRY, S. SPRECHER-GOLDBERGER, E. HANNECART-POKORNI,
I. GOULD and M. BOSSENS.
Institut Pasteur du Brabant, Institut Bordet
and Université libre de Bruxelles.

Introduction.

The presence of herpes simplex virus (HSV) antigens in necrotic
cells exfoliated from cervical carcinoma has been demonstrated (1), as
well as that of a specific HSV polypeptide, named Ag4, in living cells
from biopsies of the same tumors (2). These antigens elicit immune
responses, such as antibodies which fix complement in the presence of
Ag4 (3). These antibodies are only present in patients with precancerous
and cancerous lesions, while antibodies which neutralise the virions
persist in any patient who has experienced a previous herpes genitalis
infection. However, the HSV proteins expressed in exfoliated cells from
the cervical carcinoma probably act as booster antigens, since **neutralising**
antibody activity increases in patients with prolonged dysplasia or
carcinoma, and decreases after treatment (4); on the other hand, some HSV
antigens of the cancer cells probably adsorb complement dependent
cytotoxic antibodies, since these antibodies decrease with time in
patients with prolonged dysplasia or carcinoma (5). Decreasing antibody
titers to membrane antigens of herpes simplex virus infected cells also
ran parallel to the severity of the lesions (6).

We have tried to further characterize the specific immune status of
these patients, with a study of cell-mediated response of their lymphocytes to stimulation by killed HSV virions and cells transformed with
these viruses. Also, we have investigated whether, in the cancer and in

231

the control groups, neutralising antibodies to HSV are of IgG nature only, or whether IgM and/or IgA are also present. For this purpose, sera from the patients were absorbed with suspensions of staphylococcus aureus Cowan I, a procedure which removes IgG_1, IgG_2 and IgG_4 (7).

Materials and methods.

Patients. Women attending a center for screening of cancer were entered into the study when dysplasia or carcinoma in situ was diagnosed; controls with normal cervical smear were matched for age ($\pm$ 5 years). All the women belonged to a broadly similar middle class socio-economic group. Diagnosis of dysplasia corresponded to the presence in smears of squamous cells showing abnormally large, hyperchromatic nuclei and premature keratinization of cytoplasm. Another group of women was studied; they were entering two university hospitals with the diagnosis of squamous cell cervical carcinoma of various documented stages. These women were not matched with controls but their immune response to HSV antigens was followed at 2–6 months intervals before and after treatment with irradiation or surgery.

Absorption of sera with staphylococcus Cowan A. The bacterial strain was kept lyophilized and grown on solid tryptose soja agar for the first passage. It was then passed once in liquid medium CCY (8) for 18 h. with agitation. The final suspension was grown in the same medium in a fermentor with constant pH7 and killed by formaldehyde and heat, as described (8), except that heating was performed for 10 min. at 80°C in sealed vials of 150 ml. A 15% suspension was kept at +4°C for 1–2 months.

Sera were adsorbed with freshly washed staphylococci; one volume of 10% staphylococci suspension was mixed with one volume of serum diluted 1:10 and left for 30 min. at room temperature, before centrifugation. This procedure was repeated once.

Assay for neutralising antibodies. HSV-2 was mixed with the patient's sera and assayed for residual infectivity after 2 minutes contact at 37°C, and the constant K of inactivation was calculated as previously described (4).

For the assay of non IgG antibodies, 50 ul of serum adsorbed with staphylococcus Cowan A were mixed with 50 ul of tissue culture medium containing 2500 plaque forming units of HSV-2, and similar mixtures were made with non adsorbed serum. After 20 min. contact at 37°C, residual infectivity of HSV-2 was assayed by plating the mixtures at dilutions 1:40, 1:60 and 1:120 on primary cultures of chick embryofibroblasts in

232

Sterilin 306V plastic dishes. The plaques were read after 3 days at 37°C.
With most of the sera from normal individuals, and with hyperimmune
rabbit antisera to HSV-2, all neutralising activity was removed after a
double adsorption with the staphylococci; these sera were considered to
possess only IgG neutralising antibodies to HSV-2. With other sera,
neutralising activity remained after staphylococcus absorption, and
amounted to 50-100% of the activity of the non adsorbed sera; these were
counted as non IgG containing sera. Only a few per cent of the sera
showed intermediate results; they were not entered into the statistics.
Lymphocyte transformation test. As previously described (9), cells from
heparinized blood were washed and grown in the presence of heated HSV
virions or mitomycin-C treated cells, and ^{3}H-thymidine incorporation into
acid-insoluble material was studied after 6 days at 37°C. Indices of
stimulation were expressed as ratios of cpm with and without virions;
specific stimulation by the HSV-2 transformed hamster cell line (333-8-9)
was evaluated by comparison with results obtained with two hamster cell
lines (Nil and BHK-21) not transformed by viruses or chemicals. Some
blood samples were also assayed for specific stimulation by SV40
transformed hamster cells, as compared to the same non transformed cells.

Results.

Specific humoral and cell-mediated responses in five groups of
patients are shown in table I. We shall first analyse the differences
between women with normal cervical smears and those with precancerous
and cancerous lesions. Antibodies to HSV-2, as measured by kinetics of
neutralisation, were found in 20% of the women with normal cervical
smears and in 45% and 56% of those with dysplasia or cervical carcinoma,
respectively ($P < 0.001$). The constant K evaluated neutralising activities
of the sera to HSV-2 after a 2 minutes contact with the virus. This short
contact period ensures a fairly good specificity to the test, since sera
from children with primary herpes simplex type 1 infection only reacted
with HSV-1 by this procedure. However, the situation may be different in
adults with viral reactivations and possibly even reinfections. This
means that most but possibly not all of the positive tests were indicative of a previous herpes genitalis infection.

The sera were then absorbed with staphylococcus Cowan A; no
neutralising activities were left in the supernatants when sera were
assayed after 2 minutes contact with HSV-2. Since IgM antibodies react
more slowly than IgG, the tests were repeated using a 20 minutes contact

period with preadsorbed and adsorbed sera. The latter sera were then able to neutralise HSV-2 in 66% of the 32 cases of carcinoma, as compared to 56% with the kinetics of neutralisation test; thus, 3 of these patients had non IgG antibodies to HSV, in the absence of detectable IgG in the non adsorbed sera. Such examples were not found in the other study groups. The dysplasic cases, however, also differed from the control group since non IgG antibodies were found in 42% of the women with dysplasia and in only 6% of the women with norma smears $(P < 0.001)$. A striking difference between the patients groups and the controls was also found when the lymphocytes from heparinised blood were stimulated by mitomycin C treated HSV-2 transformed cells. No positive responses were observed in women with normal cervical smears while there were responses in 24% and 36% of the women with dysplasia or carcinoma, respectively. On the other hand, the difference between these groups was poorly significant $(0.01 < P < 0.05)$ when HSV-1 and HSV-2 virions were used as antigens in the stimulation tests. This was due to the fact that 20% and 24% of the control women sera were positive in these tests.

Let us now turn to the differences between cancer patients before and after treatment. Eleven women were treated with irradiation and 24 with surgery. During irradiation, the number of women whose lymphocytes responded to HSV-2 transformed cells, increased highly, since 82% now responded in this test, as compared to 36% in the group of non treated cases of carcinoma. In contrast, many of these women lost their non IgG antibodies to HSV-2, during irradiation, while this treatment did not modify the proportion of women with IgG antibodies to the same virus. Later on, six months after treatment with irradiation or surgery, the immune status of these women was similar to that of the control group with no cervical lesion. Actually, only 10% of the treated women had lymphocytes which responded to HSV-2 virions, as compared to 24% in the control group; the cell mediated response to HSV-2 was then statistically lower in the treated group than in the cancer group. This does not necessarily indicate that the removed cancer cells did contain HSV antigens, since one may argue that removal of the cervix decreased the chances for herpes simplex genital reactivation or reinfection. In order to assess the specificity of the lymphocyte responses to HSV-2 transformed cells, 37 samples of heparinised blood, chosen at random in the five patient groups, were assayed for lymphocyte transformation in the presence of SV40 transformed hamster cells. Only one index of

234

stimulation was positive, in a patient who did not respond to HSV-2 transformed cells.

Figure 1 illustrates that two tests discriminated more clearly than the others between diseased and non diseased patients : these were the assay for non IgG antibodies and the lymphocyte stimulations by HSV-2 transformed cells.

We then calculated how often these two tests were simultaneously positive in a given blood sample : it was striking that this only occurred exceptionally. The calculations were made for two major groups of blood samples (fig.2) : the normal group comprised 47 samples from healthy or treated women and the cancer group was composed of 30 samples obtained from women with a current diagnosis of squamous cells carcinoma of the cervix or dysplasia. Only one of these 77 samples possessed non IgG antibodies to HSV-2 in the serum together with lymphocytes responding to HSV-2 transformed cells. In the cancer group, a majority of the samples (72%) were positive in one of the two tests, while most samples of the normal group (78%) were negative in both tests. The differences were less clearcut when coexistence of non Ig antibodies with lymphocytes responses to the virions was studied. The latter responses were however also significantly rarely associated with non IgG antibodies, since they were found in 7-8% of blood samples of the normal and cancer groups.

A negative correlation between humoral and cell-mediated responses is also demonstrated in figure 3, where only the cancer patients with combined positive lymphocyte response to HSV-2 and positive constant of neutralising antibodies to this virus were taken into account. High constants of neutralisation were associated with the lowest positive indices of lymphocyte stimulation ($r = -0.6$ with a confidence limit of 95%). When results were similarly plotted for the other groups of patients without current cervical carcinoma, the points were scattered, with no positive or negative correlations (results not shown).

Discussion.

For the sake of brevity we have named "non IgG" those antibodies which remained in the sera after absorption with staphylococcus Cowan A; protein A of this staphylococcus, however, does not bind IgG_3 and antibodies of this class may have remained in the serum supernatant, but they represent only 5% of the total IgG content of human serum and could probably not account for the high neutralising activities to HSV-2 which were found in the adsorbed sera of some of the women with cervical carcinoma. The presence of specific IgM in these adsorbed sera was verified in a few cases by ultracentrifugation in sucrose gradients, which showed neutralising activity in the 19S region, but the presence of IgA was not assayed.

Thus, IgG3 and IgA may have played some part in the positive reactions which we observed, but the role of IgM was probably predominant. It is now progressively recognized that IgM production is not restricted to primary infections, since IgM antibodies to varicella virus were found in cases of herpes zoster, caused by reactivation of a latent varicella virus (11). Also, the continued presence of an endogenous oncornavirus in mice induces 19S but not 7S neutralising antibodies (12). Our findings that IgM neutralising antibodies to HSV-2 are present almost exclusively in cases of dysplasia and cervical carcinoma, as compared to the healthy and treated groups, fits with other indications that these precancerous and cancerous lesions bear herpesvirus antigens which continuously stimulate immune responses. Complement fixing antibodies to Ag4, which are also restricted to cases with simular lesions of the cervix, were also shown to be of IgM nature (10).

Cell-mediated response, as assayed by lymphocyte transformation in the presence of HSV virions, was more frequent, but not very significantly, in cases of dysplasia or cervical carcinoma than in the control groups; actually, one fifth of the healthy women had lymphocytes sensitized to some HSV antigens which were common to HSV-1 and HSV-2, since the reactions were most often simultaneously positive with both serotypes. This indicates that latent herpetic infection, or unsuspected reactivations, may be sufficient to maintain lymphocyte responsiveness. It was thus striking that none of the healthy or cured women showed in vitro lymphocyte response to HSV-2 transformed cells, in contrast to 24-36% responses in the dysplasia and carcinoma groups. The responses were not due to non specific antigens present on any type of tumor cells, since the responses were not paralleled by similar results if SV40 transformed cells were used as stimulating antigens. There is no proof, however, that the lymphocytes from the cancer patients responded to some herpesvirus antigens present in the transformed cells. These cells were not in early passages and they had ceased demonstrating herpesvirus antigens with current immunofluorescent or radioimmunoassay techniques; however, hamsters bearing tumors caused by these cells had serum

antibodies which were specifically cytotoxic to herpes simplex virus
infected cells, in the presence of complement, indicating that the
tumors developed in vivo expressed some herpesvirus antigens.

It is clear from our results that some mechanism must exist in
vivo which modulates the immune reactions in such a way that the
simultaneous presence of non IgG antibodies to HSV-2 and lymphocyte
responsiveness to this virus is excluded. In one case of prolonged
dysplasia who was followed, non IgG antibodies were detected two times at
2 months interval; they had disappeared 6 months later, at a moment when
lymphocyte response to HSV-2 had become positive. Two other cases of
prolonged dysplasia also showed that non IgG antibodies preceded
lymphocyte response, indicating that cell-mediated reactions may switch
off the synthesis of these antibodies. T helper cells have indeed been
shown to be needed for efficient conversion of 19S to 7S immune response
in mice (13) and in vitro studies showed that supraotpimal numbers of T
helper cells decreased the number of antibody forming cells (14).

It would be very interesting to know whether regressions of the
dysplasic lesions to atypia which were not rarely observed in this study
were due to the action of non IgG antibodies or to the appearance of
cell-mediated response. On the one hand, IgM may help to reject a tumor
as indicated by the fact that mice inoculated with Moloney sarcoma virus
and undergoing regression of the tumor possessed IgM antibodies, and
these could induce specific cytotoxicity against the sarcoma cells by
normal thymocytes (15); on the other hand, the cytotoxicity of IgM
antibodies in the presence of complement may be efficient only on target
cells with high antigen density : in the situation of renal allografts in
rats, IgM antibodies were cytotoxic to the donor's lymphocytes, but they
enhanced the graft (16).

One of the reasons why tumors are not rejected resides in their
low antigen density.

Summary.

Neutralising antibodies to herpes simplex type 2 virus (HSV-2)
were studied by kinetics of neutralisation, before and after adsorption
of 141 sera with staphylococcus Cowan A. Antibodies remaining in the
supernatant were non IgG antibodies. These antibodies were found in 5% of
women with normal cervical smears, in 42 and 66% of women with dysplasia
or cervical carcinoma, respectively, and in 6% of treated cases.
Heparinized blood was obtained from most of these patients. Thymidine

incorporation into washed non purified lymphocytes was studied in the presence of killed HSV-2 and HSV-1, as well as in the presence of mitomycin C treated hamster cells transformed by HSV-2, or by SV40, or not transformed. Specific stimulation by the HSV-2 transformed cells was obtained in 0%, 24% and 36% of women with normal cervical smears, dysplasia or carcinoma of the cervix, respectively, as well as in 82% of 11 cases studied during irradiation treatment, and 11% of 29 treated cases.

Differences between the various groups were less clearcut when virions instead of transformed cells were used as antigens to stimulate the lymphocytes, since 24% of the control women had lymphocytes responding to HSV virions. Non IgG antibodies to HSV-2 were not present at the same time as cell response to HSV-2 transformed cells. There was also a negative correlation between neutralising activities of the sera and the indices of lymphocyte stimulation, indicating a regulation between humoral and cell-mediated responses.

Table I. Neutralising antibodies to HSV - 2 and lymphocyte response to HSV virions and HSV - 2 transformed cells, in various groups of patients.

| | Humoral response | | | Lymphocyte response | | | |
	N° tested	% positive K*	% positive non Ig**	N° tested	% positive with Transf. cells	HSV - 2	HSV - 1
Normal Cervix	30	20	6	30	0	24	20
Dysplasia	33	45	42	32	24	37	28
Cervical carci-noma	32	56	66	22	36	45	32
During irra-diation	11	60	27	11	82	40	50
After treatment	35	31	6	29	11	10	21

* Constant of the kinetics of neutralisation

** Presence of neutralising antibodies in sera adsorbed with Staphyloccus Cowan I

*** Index of stimulation determined by (^3H) thymidine incorporation into acid insoluble material.

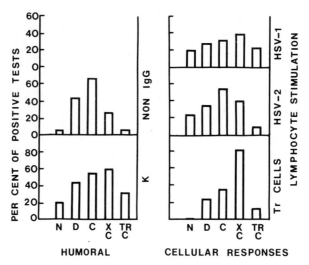

FIG. 1. Illustration of the results shown in Table I, for the following groups of women: N = normal cervical smears; D = dysplasia; C = cervical carcinoma; XC = irradiated carcinoma; Tr C = treated carcinoma, 6-12 months after irradiation or surgery.

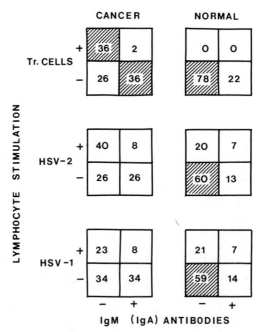

FIG. 2. Percentage of patients showing combined presence (+) or absence (-) of IgM and/or IgA antibodies with or without lymphocyte response to HSV virions or HSV-2 transformed cells. The hatched boxes show the most frequent combinations of immune responses in the cancer group (cervical carcinoma and dysplasia) and the normal group (normal cervical smear and treated carcinoma).

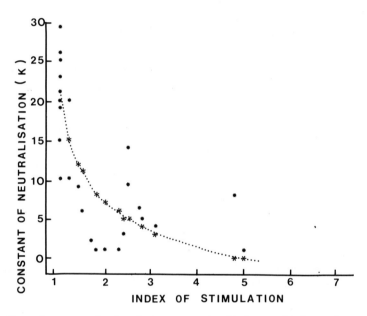

FIG. 3. Negative correlation between neutralising activity of sera to HSV-2 and index of lymphocyte stimulation by HSV-2, in cancer patients who showed positive results in both tests; (*) experimental results for each patient; (*) calculated results.

References.

1.- Royston, I., and Aurelian, L. Immunofluorescent detection of herpesvirus antigens in exfoliated cells from human cervical carcinoma. Proc. Nat. Acad. Sci., 67, 204–212, 1974.

2.- Aurelian, L., Davis, H., and Julian, C. Herpesvirus type 2 induced, tumor-specific antigen in cervical carcinoma. Al. J. Epidem., 98, 1–9, 1973.

3.- Aurelian, L., Schumann, B., Marcus, R., and Davis, H. Antibody to HSV-2 induced tumor specific antigens in serums from patients with cervical carcinoma. Science, 181, 161–163, 1973.

4.- Sprecher-Goldberger, S., Thiry, L., Gould, I., Fassin, Y., and Gompel, C. Increasing antibody titers to herpes simplex virus type 2 during follow-up of women with cervical dysplasia. Am. J. Epidem., 97, 103–110, 1973.

5.- Thiry, L., Sprecher-Goldberger, S., Fassin, Y., Gould, I., Gompel, C., Pestiau, J., and de Halleux, F. Variations of cytotoxic antibodies to cells with herpes simplex virus antigens in women with progressing or regressing lesions of the cervix. Am. J. Epidem., 100, 251–261, 1974.

6.- Christenson, B., and Espmark, A., Long-term follow-up studies on herpes simplex antibodies in the course of cervical cancer. II. Antibodies to surface antigen of herpes simplex virus infected cells. Int. J. Cancer, 17, 318–325, 1976.

7.- Ankerst, J., Christensen, P., Kjellen, L., and Kronvall, G. A routine diagnostic test for IgA and IgM rubella antibodies by absorption of IgG antibodies with staphylococcus aureus. J. Infect. Dis., 130, 268–273, 1974.

8.- Arvidson, S., Holme, T., Wadström, T. Influence of cultivation conditions on the production of extracellular proteins by staphylococcus aureus. Acta Pathol. Microbiol. Scand. (B), 79, 399–405, 1971.

9.- Sprecher-Goldberger, S., Thiry, L., de Halleux, F., Bossens, M., Gould, I. Cell mediated response to herpes simplex virion and non-virion antigens in patients with cervical carcinoma with a depressed response to phytohemagglutinin. Biomedicine Express, 23, 399–401, 1975.

10.- Aurelian, L., and Strnad, B.C. Herpesvirus type 2-related antigens and their relevance to humoral and cell-mediated immunity in patients with cervical cancer. Cancer Res., 36, 810–820, 1976.

242

11.- Ross, C.A., and Mc Daid, R. Specific IgM antibody in serum of patients with Herpes Zoster infections. Brit. Med., $\underline{4}$, 522-523, 1972.

12. Lee, J.C., Hanna, M.G., Ihle, J.N., and Aaronson, S.A. Autogenous immunity to endogenous RNA tumor virus : differential reactivities of immunoglobulins M and G to virus envelope antigens. J. Virology, $\underline{14}$, 773-781, 1974.

13.- Romano, T.J., and Thorbecke, G.J. Thymus influence on the conversion of 19S to 7S antibody formation in the response to TNP-Brucella. J. Imm., $\underline{115}$, 332-334, 1975.

14.- Feldmann, M. T cell suppression in vitro. I.Role in regulation of antibody responses. Eur. J. Imm., $\underline{4}$, 660-666, 1974.

15.- Lamon, E.W., Whitten, H.D., Skwizak, H.M., Andersson, B., and Lidin, B. IgM antibody-dependent cell-mediated cytotoxicity in the Moloney sarcoma virus system : the involvement of T and B lymphocytes as effector cells. J. Imm., $\underline{115}$, 1288-1294, 1975.

16.- van Breda Vriesman, P.J.C., Swanen-Sierag, L., and Vlek, L.F.M. Cytotoxic and enhancing properties of early γ M allo-antibodies elicited by first set renal allografts. Transplantation, $\underline{20}$, 385-392, 1975.

EVALUATION OF THE EFFECTS OF PHOSPHONOACETIC ACID AND 2-DEOXY-D-GLUCOSE ON HERPESVIRUS SAIMIRI AND EPSTEIN-BARR VIRUS

by

Dharam Ablashi[2,5], Gary Armstrong[2], Charles Fellows[3],

John Easton[2], Gary Pearson[4], and Daniel Twardzik[2]

INTRODUCTION

Phosphonoacetic acid (PAA) has been shown to be effective in significantly reducing mortality in mice experimentally infected with herpes simplex virus (28). PAA was also shown to be able to reduce herpesvirus lesions on the corneas of infected rabbits (28). PAA is apparently much less toxic than compounds such as cytosine arabinoside, which is also an inhibitor of herpesvirus replication.

The multiplication of both herpes simplex virus and human cytomegalovirus is reversibly inhibited in vitro by PAA (11, 19). The compound inhibited viral DNA synthesis, and acted on virus-induced DNA polymerases (11, 16, 19).

[1] This work was supported in part by the National Cancer Institute under Contract No. NCI-CO-25423 with Litton Bionetics, Inc.

[2] National Cancer Institute, Bethesda, Maryland 20014.

[3] Frederick Cancer Research Center, Fort Detrick, Frederick, Md. 21701

[4] Mayo Clinic, Rochester, Minnesota 55901.

[5] Presenter. To whom requests for reprints should be addressed at: NCI-Frederick Cancer Research Center, Fort Detrick, Frederick, Maryland 21701.

In this paper, we present in vitro experiments in which we studied the effect of PAA on Herpesvirus saimiri (HVS) (2, 17) and on Epstein-Barr virus (EBV) (5). The former virus is oncogenic in nonhuman primates, and the latter, in addition, causes heterophile-positive infectious mononucleosis in man, and is associated with Burkitt's lymphoma and nasopharyngeal carcinoma. We also present data on the effect of 2-deoxy-D-glucose (2-DG) on HVS (13, 15, 23). HVS provides a good model system for possible herpesvirus-induced neoplasia in man. These experiments were performed in anticipation of assaying the effects of these compounds on HVS and EBV tumors in nonhuman primates and nude mice (7, 21).

PROCEDURES AND MATERIALS USED

HVS. HVS, originally supplied by Dr. L. V. Meléndez, was plaque-purified three times and repeatedly passaged in our laboratory. A virus pool, having a titer of $10^{6.8}$ 50% tissue culture infective doses ($TCID_{50}$) per ml, was prepared in owl monkey kidney cells and used in these experiments. One ml of this virus pool induced malignant lymphoma and lymphocytic leukemia in an adult owl monkey.

EBV. A pool of nontransforming EBV was prepared from the supernatant fluid of P3HR-1 cells (9), an EBV producer lymphoblastoid line, by Dr. L. J. Charamella, Frederick Cancer Research Center. The virus was concentrated by a factor of 100. One ml of a 10^{-5} dilution of this concentrate induced early antigen (EA) in Raji cells, but failed to transform human umbilical cord blood lymphocytes.

Cell Cultures. Vero cells, a continuous line derived from African green monkey kidney (26), were grown in Eagle's Minimal Essential Medium (MEM) containing 10% heat treated (56°C for 0.5 hr.) fetal calf serum (ΔFCS) and maintained in MEM with 2% ΔFCS. Raji cells, a nonproducer lymphoblastoid line derived from a case of Burkitt's lymphoma (22), were allowed to replicate in medium RPMI 1640 containing 10% ΔFCS. All media contained penicillin (100 units/ml) and streptomycin (100 µg/ml). Media and serum were purchased from Grand Island Biological Company, Grand Island, New York. Cultures were incubated at 37°C. Owl monkey kidney cells were originally supplied by Dr. L. Meléndez. These cells were later cloned.

Compounds. Phosphonoacetic acid (PAA) was purchased from Richmond Organics. 2-deoxy-D-glucose (2-DG) was purchased from Sigma Chemical

Company, St. Louis, Missouri. Stock solutions (1 mg/ml) were prepared
in buffered saline (pH 7.2), filtered through 0.45µ Millipore membranes,
and stored at -20°C.

Determination of Drug Toxicity and Effect on Virus. In determinations with Vero cells, confluent tube cultures were employed. Medium
was changed two times weekly. In toxicity studies, four cultures were
incubated with a given concentration of compound, and observed for
14 days. Assays of the effect of a compound on HVS replication were
performed with Vero cell cultures inoculated with 0.2 ml of ten-fold
dilutions of the virus pool. Compound was added to all cultures,
under the conditions specified for each experiment. Four cultures
were used for each dilution of virus, and $TCID_{50}$ were calculated by
the method of Reed and Muench (24). In most experiments the final
reading for HVS cytopathic effect (CPE) was made 14 days after virus
inoculation. Experiments with Raji cells were performed in 75 cm^2
plastic Falcon flasks containing 35 ml of medium.

Antisera. Serum from an owl monkey with an HVS-induced tumor was
used for the determination of HVS EA and late antigen (LA). The serum
was known to contain antibodies to both antigens (anti-EA titer 1:40;
anti-LA titer 1:128). Serum from a patient with nasopharyngeal
carcinoma was used for the determination of EBV early antigen (EA)
and nuclear antigen (EBNA). It was known to contain antibodies to
both antigens, and was supplied by Dr. G. B. de-Thé (anti-EA: 1:40,
anti-EBNA: 1:40).

Induction of Early Antigen in Raji Cells. EBV EA was induced in
Raji cells using either 5-iododeoxyuridine (IUdR) (6) or nontrans-
forming EBV derived from P3HR-1 cells (8). The IUdR was supplied by
Dr. R. Adamson, National Cancer Institute, Bethesda, Maryland.

Assays for HVS and EBV Antigens. Methods for the determination
of HVS EA and LA, and EBV EA, EBNA, viral capsid antigen (VCA), and
membrane antigen (MA), have been previously described (6, 8, 12, 25).
HVS MA assay has been described (20).

DNA Polymerase Assay. Vero cell DNA-dependent DNA polymerases
were purified from isolated nuclei and cytoplasmic extracts by DEAE-
cellulose and phosphocellulose column chromatography and glycerol
gradient centrifugation as previously described (29, 30). In this
study the cytoplasmic DNA polymerase (160,000 daltons) is designated
(α) and the nuclear enzyme (30,000 daltons) as (β). The DNA polymerase

assay measured the incorporation of [^{3}H] thymidine triphosphate (^{3}H-TTP) into trichloracetic acid precipitable material. Reaction mixtures contained in a volume of 0.1 ml: 50 mM TRIS-Cl pH8.2, 5mM MgCl$_2$, 1 mM dithiothreitol, 5 mM each dATP, dCTP, dGTP, 2.5 μCi ^{3}H-TTP (specific activity 30 Ci/mM), dA oligo dT$_{10}$ 5 μg or denatured calf thymus DNA 25 μg, and 100 μg of BSA.

RESULTS

Toxicity of PAA for Vero and Raji Cells. Table I shows that PAA in a concentration of 50 μg/ml was not toxic for Vero cells over a 14-day period. However, at higher concentrations, PAA was toxic. The cells became granular and there was an increase in giant cell formation. When PAA was present in a concentration of 300 μg/ml, 75 to 100 percent of the cell sheet was affected.

A concentration of 100 μg/ml of PAA was found to be only slightly toxic for Raji cells in the experiments reported in this paper. However, over longer periods of time, PAA did cause increased cell death.

Reversible Inhibition of HVS Replication by PAA. Table II shows that PAA at a concentration of 50 μg/ml significantly inhibited the replication of HVS in Vero cells. The compound was added to the cell cultures at the end of the 2-hour absorption period, and was maintained for 14 days. Additional preincubation of the Vero cells with PAA for 24 or 48 hours did not significantly affect the results. However, removal of PAA after 14 days enabled the HVS to reach a titer not significantly different from that of the untreated control. This occurred over a 10-day period.

Effect of PAA on the HVS Replicative Cycle. PAA, in a concentration of 50 μg/ml, inhibited HVS LA production and cytopathic effect, but not EA induction, when HVS was added to cells in the doses indicated in Table III. PAA was added to cells at the end of viral absorption. These results suggest that PAA does not inhibit early events in the viral cycle, but does inhibit viral DNA synthesis and the events which occur thereafter.

In experiments in owl monkey kidney cells, we found that PAA, in a concentration of 40 μg/ml, did not significantly inhibit the induction of HVS EA, but did inhibit LA and MA production (Table IV) almost completely.

Effect of PAA on EBV Antigens. Table V shows that PAA, in a concentration of 100 µg/ml, did not inhibit the induction of EBV EA in Raji cells. Induction of EA was brought about either by super-infection with nontransforming EBV or by IUdR treatment. These results are thus similar to those with HVS. Table V shows that PAA, in concentrations of 50 or 100 µg/ml, did not inhibit the persistence or expression of EBNA in actively dividing Raji cells. The existence of this antigen is not dependent on virus production, because it is present in almost all of the cells of EBV-genome carrying nonproducer lines. However, it is regularly associated with detectable EBV genomes, and the results of this experiment thus suggest that the replication of EBV DNA, along with that of the Raji cells, is not inhibited by PAA.

Other experiments with nontransforming EBV showed that PAA, in a concentration of 100 µg/ml, prevented the formation of EBV MA (Table IV) and VCA in Raji cells. PAA, in a concentration of 50 µg/ml, failed to do this. It caused only a slight reduction in VCA and MA (Table IV) under these conditions.

Absence of Direct Effect of PAA on HVS and on Its Absorption. Table VI shows that PAA, in a concentration of 50 µg/ml, had no significant effect on HVS replication when the virus was allowed to remain in the presence of the compound for 24 or 48 hours at 4°C, before addition to cell cultures. In this experiment, PAA was also present, in a concentration of 50 µg/ml, during the 2-hour absorption period of the virus. Thus, PAA had no significant effect on HVS itself, or on its absorption or penetration.

Absence of Effect of Preincubation of Vero Cells with PAA. Table VII shows that preincubation of Vero cells with PAA for 24 or 48 hours had no significant effect on the subsequent replication of HVS in them. The concentration of PAA was 50 µg/ml. Similar results are presented in Table II, and were discussed previously.

Absence of Effect of Subsequent Addition of PAA. Table VIII shows that addition of PAA to infected Vero cultures, at various time intervals after the end of HVS absorption, had no significant effect of HVS replication. The concentration of PAA used was 50 µg/ml. The time intervals before the application of PAA ranged from 2 hr to 9 days. These results should be contrasted with the data presented in Table II, in which PAA, added immediately after the 2 hr absorption period, had a marked effect on subsequent HVS replication.

Inhibition of Vero Cell DNA-Dependent DNA Polymerases by PAA. The incorporation of ^{3}H-TTP into trichloracetic acid precipitable material was markedly inhibited by small concentrations of PAA. A 50% inhibition of the $\propto$ and β DNA polymerases was seen at PAA concentrations of 15 and 150 μg/ml, respectively, when dA·dT$_{12}$ was used as template-primer; reaction mixtures containing denatured DNA as template exhibited a 50% inhibition at 25 μg for the $\propto$ enzyme and 200 μg for the β enzyme (Fig. 1). A preincubation of the enzymes with PAA was not necessary to achieve the inhibition and the addition of more template to inhibited reaction mixtures failed to reverse the inhibition. This suggests that PAA interacts directly with the enzymes.

Effect of 2-DG on Vero Cells and on HVS. 2-DG was found to be nontoxic for Vero cells in concentrations of 5 to 200 μg/ml. At a concentration of 200 μg/ml, 2-DG failed to inhibit the replication of HVS. Experiments were performed in a manner similar to those with PAA.

DISCUSSION

The results presented in this paper show that PAA reversibly inhibits the replication of HVS under certain specific conditions. HVS was markedly inhibited when PAA was added to infected cells immediately after absorption, but was not significantly inhibited when PAA was added 2 hours after the end of absorption, or later. Preincubation of Vero cells with PAA, preincubation of HVS with PAA, or the presence of PAA during HVS absorption also had no significant effect. In addition, PAA did not inhibit the induction of HVS EA when HVS LA production and CPE were inhibited. The induction of EA is an early function which does not require viral DNA synthesis (6, 8).

Results published previously, in which cytosine arabinoside was used to inhibit HVS replication, suggested that, at low virus input, significant amounts of HVS DNA synthesis may not occur until several days after infection (1). Thus, the block induced by PAA probably occurs before viral DNA synthesis, during the early part of an eclipse phase in which virus does not replicate. A short time later, however, input virus is refractory to the effects of PAA. This is also before viral DNA synthesis has begun. The failure of more template to reverse the inhibition of Vero cell DNA polymerases by PAA suggests that PAA

250

does not interact with the uncoated DNA of input HVS in Vero cells. Rather, PAA may block a cellular process essential for HVS replication.

The results with EBV suggest that PAA does not block either exogenously or endogenously induced EA, and, more significantly, does not block the appearance of EBNA in replicating lymphoblastoid cells. EBNA is widely believed to indicate the presence of the EBV genome (14); thus, PAA may not have stopped the replication of EBV DNA in Raji cells. This DNA may be present both as a free circular form and in a form integrated with the cell genome (3, 4, 18). However, PAA was found to block the expression of EBV MA and VCA under certain conditions.

If the resistance of HVS to PAA, beginning two hours after the end of absorption, is similar to that of EBV DNA in Raji cells, infecting HVS DNA may assume a relatively stable and resistant form within the infected cell. We do not know if this would involve integration of input HVS DNA with the cellular genome. Integration has been shown to occur in another lytic system; during the infection of bacteria with bacteriophase Mu, half of the infecting phage DNA has been found covalently linked to host DNA (10, 27).

Other investigators have found that PAA reversibly inhibits the replication of the DNA of herpes simplex virus and of human cytomegalovirus (11, 19). The inhibition was felt to involve the specific recognition of herpesvirus-induced DNA polymerases (11, 16, 19). HVS is unusual in that it has not been found to induce its own polymerase (30); in fact, HVS replication may progressively inactivate the nuclear DNA polymerase of cells in which it replicates (30). The experiments presented in this paper suggest that PAA, in the case of HVS, exerts its effect long before DNA replication begins. The inhibition of Vero cell DNA polymerases, although it occurs, may therefore not be the primary effect of PAA in this system.

The failure of 2-DG to inhibit the replication of HVS may have been due either to an inadequate dose or to competition with other sugars in the culture medium (13, 15).

SUMMARY

Phosphonoacetic acid significantly and reversibly inhibited the replication of Herpesvirus saimiri in Vero cells when the compound was added immediately after a 2-hour absorption period, but not later. The compound had no effect on the virus itself, on viral absorption, or on the induction of early antigen, but did inhibit production of

251

late antigen and membrane antigen almost completely. The failure of
more template to reverse the inhibition of Vero cell DNA polymerases
by the compound suggests that phosphonoacetic acid may block a cellular
process, early in the viral eclipse phase, essential for viral
replication. Phosphonoacetic acid had no effect on the induction of
endogenous or exogenous early antigen of Epstein-Barr virus, and did not
inhibit the appearance of Epstein-Barr virus nuclear antigen in actively
replicating Raji cells. The compound may thus have had no effect on
the replication of Epstein-Barr virus DNA in Raji cells. This DNA is
either integrated with the cell genome or in a free circular form.
However, under certain conditions, phosphonoacetic acid did inhibit
the expression of the membrane antigen and viral capsid antigen of
Epstein-Barr virus. We do not know if phosphonoacetic acid is unable
to act on Herpesvirus saimiri, beginning 2 hours after the end of
absorption, because viral DNA is integrated with that of the host cell.
We found 2-deoxy-D-glucose to be without effect on Herpesvirus saimiri.

ACKNOWLEDGMENTS

We thank Ms. Karen Cannon and Mrs. Linda Lyons for their able
secretarial assistance.

TABLE I. Toxicity of PAA for Vero Cells

PAA Conc. µg/ml	Toxicity[1]
50	None
100	1+
150	2+
200	2+
250	3+
300	4+

[1]Toxicity consisted of increased giant cell formation and increased granularity of cells. 1+ = 5-25% of cell sheet involved; 2+ = 25-50%; 3+ = 50-75%; 4+ = 75-100%. Cultures were incubated with PAA for 14 days, with medium changed two times weekly.

TABLE II. Reversible Inhibition of HVS Replication by PAA

Group[1]	HVS Titer (log $TCID_{50}$/ml)
1. Untreated Controls	6.4
2. Post-treatment with PAA	2.8
3. Pretreatment (24 or 48 hr) and post-treatment with PAA	1.8
4. Post-treatment and removal of PAA	6.1

[1]In group 2, cultures of Vero cells were incubated with 50 µg/ml PAA for 14 days, beginning immediately after the 2-hr. period for HVS absorption. In group 3, the Vero cells, in addition, were treated with 50 µg/ml PAA for 24 or 48 hours before addition of virus. In group 4, treated Vero cells were washed three times after 14 days, and medium was added without PAA. The final reading for CPE was made 24 days after the inoculation of HVS. These experiments were performed twice. Controls maintained the same titer between day 14 and day 24.

TABLE III. Effect of PAA on the HVS Replicative Cycle[1]

	CPE	EA	LA
Infected Vero cells without PAA	3+	-	2+
Infected Vero cells with PAA	None	2+	None

[1]Vero cells in both groups were infected with $10^{4.5}$ $TCID_{50}$ of HVS. Doses of $10^{3.5}$ $TCID_{50}$ and $10^{2.5}$ $TCID_{50}$ gave similar results. PAA (50 μg/ml) was added immediately after the 2-hour viral absorption period and maintained until cells were harvested for antigen assay. Cells showing EA had trabecular and punctate nuclear staining; cells showing LA had bright diffuse staining of the whole cell (12). LA masked EA in untreated cells. Antiserum was used in a dilution of 1:20 for EA and 1:100 for LA. 2+ = 25-50% of cells involved; 3+ = 50-75%. This experiment was performed twice.

TABLE IV. Effect of PAA on EBV and HVS Membrane Antigens

PAA Concentration (μg/ml)	MA	
	HVS	EBV
40	Almost completely inhibited	Not done
50	Not done	Slightly inhibited
100	Not done	Completely inhibited

Experiments with HVS were performed by infecting owl monkey kidney cells with HVS and then incubating the cells for 3 or 4 days in the presence of PAA. Experimental and control cells were then harvested by trypsinization and stained. Experiments with EBV were performed by superinfecting Raji cells with 10^4 infectious doses of EBV derived from P3HR-1 cells. The presence of membrane antigen in experimental and control cells was determined 3 or more days after superinfection.

TABLE V. Lack of Effect of PAA on EBV EA or EBNA

	Percent cells producing EA
Raji cells superinfected with nontransforming EBV[1] (PAA present or absent)[4]	50%
Raji cells induced with IUdR[2] (PAA present or absent)[4]	5-7%

	Percent cells producing EBNA
Raji cells[3] (PAA present or absent)[4]	98%

[1] Raji cells were superinfected with 10^4 infectious doses (1:10 dilution) of EBV derived from P3HR-1 cells. The presence of EA was determined 2 days after superinfection. PAA, in a concentration of 100 µg/ml beginning 1 hour after EBV superinfection, had no effect on EA induction.

[2] Raji cells were treated with 50 µg/ml IUdR for 2 days. The cells were then washed and PAA, in a concentration of 100 µg/ml was added for 5 days. This had no effect on EA induction.

[3] Raji cells were seeded at low density and allowed to replicate. Cells were examined for EBNA 3, 5, and 7 days after subpassage. PAA, in concentrations of 50 or 100 µg/ml, had no effect on the presence of EBNA.

[4] These experiments were performed twice.

TABLE VI. Absence of Direct Effect of PAA on HVS and on its Absorption

Group	HVS Titer (log TCID$_{50}$/ml)
Untreated controls	6.0
Pretreatment of virus with PAA (24 or 48 hr.). PAA present during 2-hr. absorption period[1]	5.5

[1] Virus was diluted in medium containing 50 µg/ml PAA, kept at 4°C for 24 or 48 hours, and then inoculated into Vero cultures. After the 2-hour absorption period, cells were washed three times. Fresh medium, not containing PAA, was then added. Controls were treated in a like manner, only in the absence of PAA. Final reading for CPE was made 14 days after inoculation. This experiment was performed twice.

TABLE VII. Absence of Effect of Preincubation of Vero Cells with PAA

Group	HVS Titer (log TCID$_{50}$/ml)
Untreated controls	6.6
Pretreatment (24 hr.)[1]	6.5
Pretreatment (48 hr.)[1]	5.8

[1] Cultures of Vero cells were treated with 50 µg/ml PAA for 24 or 48 hours, washed three times, and inoculated with serial dilutions of HVS. Final reading for CPE was made 14 days after inoculation. This experiment was performed twice.

TABLE VIII. Absence of Effect of Subsequent Addition of PAA

Time of PAA Addition[1]	HVS Titer (log $TCID_{50}$/ml)
Untreated control	6.8
2 hr	5.8
1 day	5.8
2 days	5.1
3 days	5.8
4 days	6.8
7 days	6.5
8 days	6.8
9 days	6.8

[1] PAA, in a concentration of 50 μg/ml, was added to Vero cultures at various time intervals after the end of absorption of serial dilutions of HVS. Final reading for CPE was made 14 days after HVS inoculation. This experiment was performed twice.

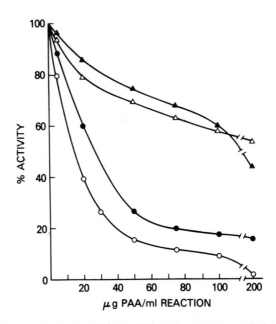

FIG. 1. Inhabition of DNA-dependent DNA polymerase activity by PAA.
Reaction mixtures containing varying amounts of PAA (0-200 µg/ml reaction)
were incubated for 30 minutes at 37°C. In the absence of added compound
"∝" DNA polymerase incorporated 15.8 and 8.2 p moles of ^{3}H-TMP per 5.0 µg
protein using dA·dT$_{12}$ and denatured DNA, respectively, as templates (100%
control value); the β enzyme incorporated 12.6 and 10.2 p moles per 2.8 µg/
protein per reaction. [(0 - 0)dA·dT$_{12}$; ● - ● denatured DNA; ∝ DNA poly-
merase]. [(▲ - ▲) dA·dT$_{12}$, (Δ - Δ) denatured DNA; β DNA polymerase.]

REFERENCES

1. Ablashi, D.V., Armstrong, G.R., Easton, J.M., Chopra, H.C., and Adamson, R.H. Evaluation of Effects of Cytosine Arabinoside on Herpesvirus Saimiri Replication in Owl Monkey Kidney Cells. Biomed. Express, 21: 57-60, 1974.

2. Ablashi, D.V., Loeb, W.F., Valerio, M.G., Adamson, R.H., Armstrong, G.R., Bennett, D.V., and Heine, U. Malignant lymphoma with lymphocytic leukemia induced in owl monkeys by Herpesvirus saimiri. J. Nat. Cancer Inst., 47: 837-855, 1971.

3. Adams, A., and Lindahl, T. Epstein-Barr Virus genomes with properties of circular DNA molecules in carrier cells. Proc. Nat. Acad. Sci. USA, 72: 1477-1481, 1975.

4. Adams, A., Lindahl, T., and Klein, G. Linear association between cellular DNA and Epstein-Barr virus DNA in a human lymphoblastoid cell line. Proc. Nat. Acad. Sci. USA, 70: 2888-2892, 1973.

5. Epstein, M.A., Achong, B.G., and Barr, Y.M. Virus particles in cultured lymphoblasts from Burkitt's lymphoma. Lancet, 1: 702-703, 1964.

6. Gerber, P. Activation of Epstein-Barr virus by 5-Bromodeoxyuridine in "Virus Free" human cells. Proc. Nat. Acad. Sci. USA, 69: 83-85, 1972.

7. Glaser, R., Ablashi, D.V., Nonoyama, M., Henle, W., Easton, J., Armstrong, G., and Fellows, C. Characteristics of transformation associated with the Epstein-Barr virus in non-lymphoblastoid cells. Manuscript in preparation.

8. Henle, W., Henle, G., Zajac, B.A., Pearson, G., Waubke, R., and Scriba, M. Differential reactivity of human serum with early antigen induced by Epstein-Barr virus. Science, 169: 188-190, 1970.

9. Hinuma, Y., Konn, M., Yamaguchi, J., Wudarski, D.J., Blakeslee, J.R., Jr., and Grace, J.T., Jr. Immunofluorescence and herpes-type virus particles in the P3HR-1 Burkitt lymphoma cell line. J. Virol., 1: 1045-1051, 1967.

10. Howe, M.M., and Bade, E.G. Molecular Biology of Bacteriophage Mu. Science, 190: 624-632, 1975.

11. Huang, E.-S. Human Cytomegalovirus IV. Specific Inhibition of virus-induced DNA polymerase activity and viral DNA replication by phosphonoacetic acid. J. Virol., 16: 1560-1565, 1975.

12. Klein, G., Pearson, G., Rabson, A., Ablashi, D.V., Falk, L., Wolfe, L., Deinhardt, F., and Rabin, H. Antibody reactions to Herpesvirus saimiri (HVS) induced early and late antigens (EA and LA) in HVS infected squirrel, marmoset, and owl monkeys. Int. J. Cancer, 12: 270-289, 1973.

13. Klenk, H.-D., Scholtissek, C., and Rott, R. Inhibition of glycoprotein biosynthesis of influenza virus by D-glucosamine and 2-Deoxy-D-Glucose. _Virology_, _49_: 723-734, 1972.

14. Lindahl, T., Klein, G., Reedman, B.M., Johansson, B., and Singh, S. Relationship between Epstein-Barr virus (EBV) DNA and the EBV determined nuclear antigen (EBNA) in Burkitt's lymphoma biopsies and other lymphoproliferative malignancies. _Int. J. Cancer_, _13_: 764-772, 1974.

15. Ludwig, H., Becht, H., and Rott, R. Inhibition of herpes virus-induced cell fusion by Concanavalin A, antisera and 2-Deoxy-D-Glucose. _J. Virol._, _14_: 307-314, 1974.

16. Mao, J.C.-H., Robishaw, E.E., and Overby, L.R. Inhibition of DNA polymerase from herpes simplex virus-infected Wi-38 cells by phosphonoacetic acid. _J. Virol._, _15_: 1281-1283, 1975.

17. Meléndez, L.V., Hunt, R.D., Daniel, M.D., Garcia, F.G., and Fraser, C.E.O. _Herpesvirus saimiri_ II. An experimentally induced malignant lymphoma in primates. _Lab. Animal Care._, _19_: 378-386, 1969.

18. Nonoyama, M., and Pagano, J.S. Separation of Epstein-Barr virus DNA from large chromosomal DNA in non-virus-producing cells. _Nature New Biol._, _238_: 169-171, 1972.

19. Overby, L.R., Robishaw, E.E., Schleicher, J.B., Rueter, A., Shipkowitz, N.L., and Mao, J.C.-H. Inhibition of herpes simplex virus replication by phosphonoacetic acid. _Antimicrob. Agents and Chemother._, _6_: 360-365, 1974.

20. Pearson, G.R., Ablashi, D.V., Orr, T., Rabin, H., and Armstrong, G.R. Intracellular and membrane immunofluorescence investigations on cells infected with _Herpesvirus saimiri_. _J. Nat. Cancer Inst._, _49_: 1417-1424, 1972.

21. Povlsen, C.O., Jacobsen, G.K., and Rygaard, J. The mouse mutant nude as a model for testing of anticancer agents. _In_: The Laboratory Animal in Drug Testing. 5th Symposium of the International Committee on Laboratory Animals. A. Spiegel, Ed., pp.63-72, Gustav Fischer Verlag, Stuttgart, 1973.

22. Pulvertaft, R.J.V. Cytology of Burkitt's Tumour (African Lymphoma). _Lancet_, _i_: 238-240, 1964.

23. Ray, E.K., Levitan, D.B.; Halpern, B.L., and Blough, H.A. A new approach to viral chemotherapy; inhibitors of glycoprotein synthesis. _Lancet_, _ii_: 680683, 1974.

24. Reed, L.J., and Muench, H. A simple method of estimating fifty percent end points. _Amer. J. Hyg._, _27_: 467-476, 1938.

25. Reedman, B.M., and Klein, G. Cellular localization of an Epstein-Barr virus (EBV)-associated complement-fixing antigen in producer and nonproducer lymphoblastoid cell lines. Int. J. Cancer, 11: 499-520, 1973.

26. Rhim, J.S., and Schell, K. Cytopathic and Plaque Assay of rubella virus in A line of African green monkey kidney cells (Vero). Proc. Soc. Exp. Biol. Med., 125: 602-606, 1967.

27. Schroeder, W. Mol. Gen. Genet., In Press.

28. Shipkowitz, N.L., Bower, R.R., Appell, R.N., Nordeen, C.W., Overby, L.R., Roderick, W.R., Schleicher, J.B., and Von Esch, A.M. Suppression of herpes simplex virus infection by phosphonoacetic acid. Applied Microbiol., 26: 264-267, 1973.

29. Twardzik, D.R., Papas, T.S., and Portugal, F.H. DNA polymerase in virions of a reptilian type C virus. J. Virol., 13: 166-170, 1974.

30. Twardzik, D.R., Simonds, J., Armstrong, G.R., and Ablashi, D.V. DNA polymerase activities in vero cells infected with Herpesvirus saimiri. Biomed. Express, 21: 1-5, 1974.

THE HERPESVIRUS OF MAREK'S

DISEASE AND HUMAN CANCER

Jack G. Makari
Makari Research Laboratories
Englewood, New Jersey U.S.A.
07631

INTRODUCTION

In earlier studies, using a modified Schultz-Dale technique, common antigenicity was demonstrated between glycoprotein antigens extracted from human cancers and those extracted from chicken tumors infected with Marek's Disease
Herpesvirus (MDHV) [1]. Common antigenicity was also demonstrated between TPS glycoprotein antigens from human cancers
and similarly prepared glycoprotein antigens from MDHV grown
in tissue culture.[2] It was believed that the basis for this
common antigenicity resided in the viral component rather
than the host's neoplastic response to the oncogenic virus.
The purpose of this study is to explore further this relationship between MDHV and human cancer.

METHODS

Antigens - A number of glycoprotein antigens both of tumor
and viral origin were prepared in accordance with methods
described earlier [1]. Those extracted from tumors of birds inoculated with MDHV and referred to as Tumor Polysaccharide
Substances (TPS) include: CR-64 (extracted from gonadal
tumors from animals infected with the CR-64 strain) kindly
supplied by Dr. H.G. Purchase, Regional Poultry Research
Laboratory, U.S. Department of Agriculture; GA-2 (extracted
from liver tumors of birds inoculated with the GA strain)
kindly supplied by Dr. J. Wetzel of Ayerst Research Laboratories; JM (extracted from the blood pellets of birds infected with the JM strain) kindly supplied by Dr. F. Melchior,
Jr. of Sterwin Laboratories. Those extracted from viral
tissue cultures referred to as Viral Polysaccharide Substances
(VPS) include: GA (extracted from a GA virus grown in tissue
culture on chick embryo cells, referred to earlier [2] as TPS-
GAV) kindly supplied by Dr. J. Wetzel; HSV-1 (extracted from
Herpesvirus hominis type 1, MacIntyre strain grown on human
foreskin fibroblasts); HSV-2 (extracted from Herpesvirus

hominis type 2 grown on human foreskin fibroblasts); Epstein-Barr Virus (EBV) or Burkitt's lymphoma agent (grown on human lymphoblast-oid cells; Mouse hepatitis virus or MHV, MHV 1 (Parkes) strain grown in mouse liver. These cultures were obtained from the American Type Culture Collection, Rockville, Maryland numbers: 539(HSV-2), 602(EBV), 261(MHV). VPS was also prepared from a bivalent vaccine purchased from Lederle Laboratories containing influenza strain A_2 (Japan 170/62), A_2 (Taiwan 1/64)and B(Mass 3/66).

Control normal polysaccharide antigens (NPS) were also prepared by the same method from normal chicken liver and normal chicken kidney, as well as from four human tissues, namely, liver(cirrhosis), colon(diverticulitis), lung(normal) and uterus(fibroid).

Desoxyribose-purine fragments (DPF) antigens were pre-pared from various cancerous tissues (carcinoma or ca ovary, ca stomach, ca lung, ca breast, ca colon, ca pancreas, ca liver, lymphoma and sarcoma.) This material gives a positive Dische reaction using diphenylamine, one of the most specific reactions for desoxyribose linked to purine. DPF is believed to represent a fragment of desoxyribonucleic acid (DNA). In addition, DPF was also prepared from normal lung and from fibroid uterus. The method for the extraction of DPF based on repeated freon extraction is detailed in an earlier publication.[5]

Human Sera, used as the source of antibodies, were kind-ly supplied by Dr. R. Herberman of the National Cancer Institute, and by Dr. E. Holyoke of the Rosewell Park Memorial Institute.

Immunization - Virgin female guinea pigs were immunized intra-peritoneally with .5 ml. of 1/1000 dilution of the DPF or the VPS to be tested. The animals were sacrificed from 2 to 5 days after immunization. Passive immunization was accomplished by coating uterine segments from unimmunized pigs with human serum at 27°C for 30 minutes.

In vitro Anaphylaxis - Uterine segments from animals immunized with DPF or with VPS, or passively coated with serum antibodies, were used in a modified Schultz-Dale technique [1]. The anaphylactic reaction was released by the addition of .25 ml. of NPS, TPS or VPS starting with higher dilutions and proceeding to lower dilutions until a positive re-action is obtained with a deflection of 20 mm or more on the Gould recorder. The maximum deflection obtainable is 40 mm. The titer is expressed as 10^{12} dilution of the releasing antigen. A titer below 1×10^{12} is regarded as a negative test while a titer of 1×10^{12} or above is considered positive. It has been estimated that the modification of this technique as used in this study is about a million times more sensitive than RIA testing.[4]

RESULTS

Serum Antibodies to MDHV in Subjects with and without Clinical Cancer - In these studies serum antibodies were passively coated on uterine segments from unimmunized pigs. The reaction was released by the addition of VPS, TPS and NPS antigens. The distribution of serum antibodies to MDHV

264

and to other herpesviruses for 141 subjects with and without clinical cancer is shown in Table I.

In the 141 subjects tested 96 or 68% had serum antibodies to MDHV as compared to 6% of the 111 subjects in whom serum antibodies to HSV-1, HSV-2 and EBV were found. P is < .001. Of the 65 subjects in the non-malignant group, 63% were positive reactors to MDHV as compared to 74% in the 69 subjects with carcinoma. The difference between the two groups is   found to be significant at the .05 level. In the 37 subjects with melanoma and sarcoma 57% were positive reactors. The difference between the malanoma, sarcoma group and the non-malignant disease category is not significant at the .05 level.

In Table II the incidence of antibodies to Marek's Herpesvirus in 26 subjects with early or late cancer of the colon and of the breast is compared with reference to the commonest associated strain of MDHV namely GA for ca colon and CR-64 for ca breast. All of the 8 subjects with early cancer reacted positively with the Marek's strains tested as compared to only 56% of the 18 subjects with late cancer. A similar pattern was observed when the titers, expressed in 10^{12} dilutions of VPS, were evaluated. The titer for VPS antigens tested was found to be 8.3 for the early cancer sera as compared to 3.3 for the late cancer sera. This 2.5 times difference is found to be significant. P < .05.

The distribution of serum antibodies to the 4 strains of MDHV tested in 76 subjects with cancer is shown in Table III. It is apparent from this table, that certain types of cancer are found to be more intimately associated with certain special strains of MDHV. Although, this association will be more clearly shown in the DPF studies to be described later, it is still apparent in these studies with serum antibodies. An association will be noted between ca colon and GA, between ca breast and CR-64 and between ca stomach and ca lung and GA-2.

Presence of MDHV Antigens in DPF obtained from Normal and Cancerous Tissues - In these studies, DPF was used as the immunizing antigen and the various VPS, TPS & NPS antigens used as releasing antigens. When normal DPF or DPF from a fibroid tumor was used as the immunizing antigens, no cross-reacting antigen with a titer above 1.0×10^{12} were dis-covered in either the control NPS, TPS and VPS antigens in-cluding VPS prepared from the various strains of MDHV and the other herpes strains tested. With DPF from cancerous tissues however, cross-reacting antigens were discovered in all of the 4 strains of Marek's disease tested (mean titer from 2.6 to 5×10^{12}) and to a much lesser extent with EBV virus (mean titer 1.3×10^{12}) No cross-reacting antigens with a titer of 1.0×10^{12} or more were found with HSV-1 and HSV-2, nor with the 6 NPS or 2 VPS control antigens.

The presence of MDHV antigens in the DPF from cancerous tissues was further explored in an effort to uncover any possible association between certain strains of these viruses and certain types of human cancer. The results of this in-vestigation are shown in Table V. Ca colon was found to be in association with the GA strain of MDHV, while ca breast, ca ovary and ca lung seem to be associated with the CR-64 strain. Ca liver and lymphoma were found to be associated with the GA-2 strain. In ca stomach and in sarcoma, two strains, CR-64 and JM were found to have equally high titers (4 x 10^{12} and 3 x 10^{12} respectively) suggesting the possibility of a hybrid strain between CR-64 and JM associated with these two types of cancer. Similarly, in ca pancreas (a hybrid strain between CR-64, JM and GA-2) may be associated with this disease.

Antigenic Relationship between MDHV and EBV - In this part of the investigation VPS antigens from the GA strain of MDHV and EBV were used as the immunizing antigens. The Schultz-Dale reactions were released with VPS antigens from the various MDHV strains, EBV, HSV-1 and MHV. The results are shown in Table VI and Fig. 1. When GA was used as the immunizing antigen, the highest titer (32 x 10^{12}) was obtained with the GA strain, followed by GA-2 (28 x 10^{12}), CR-64 (21 x 10^{12}). EBV (6 x 10^{12}), JM (1.3 x 10^{12}), HSV-1 (1.1 x 10^{12}), HSV-2 (1.0 x 10^{12}), and MHV (.2 x 10^{12}). When EBV was used as the immunizing antigen, the highest titer (4.4 x 10^{12}) was observed with EBV as expected, followed by GA (3.6 x 10^{12}0, GA-2 (3.2 x 10^{12}), JM (2.0 x 10^{12}), CR-64 (1.7 x 10^{12}), HSV-2 (.9 x 10^{12}) and HSV-1 (.6 x 10^{12}).

DISCUSSION

In studies reported earlier,[1] common antigenicity was demonstrated between glycoprotein antigens from human cancers and those from cancers of chickens with Marek's disease. Common antigenicity was also demonstrated between glyco-protein antigens from human cancers and those from MDHV grown in tissue culture.[2] This apparent association between MDHV and cancer was further explored in the present studies along two main avenues, namely the search for serum antibodies to MDHV in subjects with and without cancer, and the search for MDHV antigens in the DPF of normal and cancerous tissues.

MDHV is known to be present in more than 90% of chickens from commercial flocks.[5] It has been shown that the virus on feather follicles is very stable and can remain infectious at room temperature for a period of eight months.[6] It can travel in dust particles for long distances. As a result, this virus could be inhaled, it could pollute water lines through cross contamination from poultry houses, it could end up in sewerage infecting sea food, and it could be passed to adults and children through contamination kitchens and kitchen utensils during the preparation of the infected chickens. Opportunities for contact with this virus can therefore be presumed to be great indeed. It is not sur-prising therefore to find that in 63% of the 65 adult subjects with non-malignant diseases tested, serum antibodies to MDHV were found.

If a casual relationship between this virus and cancer did exist, one would expect that those at risk of developing

266

cancer would be individuals who had intimate and prolonged contact with this virus as revealed by serum antibodies to MDHV. This would require a longitudinal study and can not be answered at this time. However, the finding of approximately one-half of those tested to have no serum antibodies to any of the types of MDVH strains studied is in conformity with the finding by Lynch et al[7] in a thorough study of more than 4,000 consecutive persons that "approximately one-half of all families studied showed an absence of cancer (all sites) in first degree relatives." Furthermore, if MDHV is responsible for some forms of cancer in man, a high percentage of those developing cancer would be expected to have serum antibodies against MDHV especially in the early stages of the disease. The finding of 74% positive reactors in 69 subjects with carcinoma lends support to this concept.

Since such cases comprise, both early and late cancer cases, and since immunocompetence is impaired in the late stages of cancer, and antiviral antibodies may not be found, further analysis was made to obtain the incidence of serum antibodies to early , as contrasted with late cancer. In a small number of cases (shown in Table II), it was found that of the 8 early cases, 100% had serum antibodies to MDHV as compared with 56% of the 18 subjects with late cancer. The finding of serum antibodies to   MDHV in all the early cancer subjects with ca breast and ca colon is believed to strengthen this association between MDHV and human cancer. Furthermore, evidence for an association between certain strains of this virus and certain types of human cancer makes such an association more meaningful. In Table III for example, an association which is indicated by the highest titer of VPS has been found between ca breast and the CR-64 strain, ca colon and the GA strain.

If a viral agent is to be a candidate for a human cancer virus, it should be possible to discover some traces of this agent in the nucleus of certain types of human cancer. Glyco-protein VPS antigens of MDHV have been found to cross-react with DNA from various human cancer tissues but not from normal lung or from fibroid uterus. See Table IV. VPS antigens from the human herpesviruses studied (with the exception of EBV); VPS antigens prepared from two unrelated viruses (MHV, and influenza strains A_2 and B) as well as the six control TPS antigens prepared from various human and chicken tissues, all showed no cross-reactivity with DPF prepared from normal or cancerous tissues. EBV in this study behaved less like human herpesvirus and more like Marek's herpesvirus.

A further analysis of the pattern of cross-reactivity observed for each of the DPF prepared from cancerous tissues and the various strains of MDHV is detailed in Table V. It should be noted that in this Table, all of the 9 DPF preparations from cancerous tissues were positive reactors (1.0 x 10^{12} or more) with glycoprotein antigens of one or more of the four strains of MDHV tested. Furthermore, a pattern of cross-reactivity with these antigens similar to that observed in serum antibodies from subjects with cancer, has also been found. Ca colon has been found to be associated with the GA

strain (with a titer of 28 x 10^{12}); ca breast and ca ovary and
ca lung were found to be associated with the CR-64 strain
(with titers of 20 x 10^{12} and 4.5 x 10^{12} and 3.4 x 10^{12} respectively); ca stomach with both CR-64 and JM (with titers
of 3.8 x 10^{12} and 4.2 x 10^{12} respectively); and ca liver and
lymphoma with GA-2 strain (with titers of 4.0 x 10^{12} and
6.0 x 10^{12} respectively). In ca pancreas, three strains,
CR-64, JM and GA-2 had a weak association (with titers of 2.0
x 10^{12} and 2.1 x 10^{12} respectively); and in sarcoma, two
strains, CR-64 and JM, revealed a weak association (with
titers of 3.2 x 10^{12} and 3.0 x 10^{12} respectively). It is
possible that in both ca pancreas and sarcoma, some other
strain of MDHV not tested in this study may be found to be
more intimately associated.

It is interesting to compare the patterns of cross-reactivity observed in serum antibodies and in DPF preparations
with the various MDHV strains tested. In both systems, the
association of ca colon and the GA strain, and ca breast and
the CR-64 strain was established. In ca stomach and in ca
lung the patterns of cross-reactivity in the serum and in the
DPF preparations were different. Since detection of antigens
in DPF preparations is a direct measure of the presence of
virus while the detection of antibodies in serum represents
only an indirect measure, one may regard the association observed with the DPF preparations as the more meaningful one
since the host response is circumvented.

Whatever the strain specificity may be, the fundamental
issue is the presence of some form of MDHV antigens in the nuclear
fraction DPF of the 9 types of human cancer studied but not
in the two control DPF preparations tested.

Herpes viruses have been implicated in various neoplastic
and proliferative diseases of man. Of these EBV is the only
virus of man that is consistently associated with human tumors.
This association has been recently strengthened by the use of
molecular hybridization techniques for Burkitt's lymphoma[8]
and nasopharyngeal carcinoma[9], but not for American lymphoma,
Hodgkin's lymphoma and malignant melanoma.[10] Yet, evidence
is mounting that a transmissable agent may be important in
Hodgkin's disease.[11] Could this agent be MDHV? An association with lymphoma and GA strain of MDVH has been found in
our earlier studies [1,2] and has been confirmed in this study.
If EBV, a related herpesvirus, is implicated, why not MDHV?
This emphasized the need for a study of the antigenic relationship of EBV and MDHV.

It is important to find out if EBV is a human herpesvirus more related to HSV-1 and HSV-2, or of non-human origin
more related to the animal herpesviruses such as MDHV. The
cross-antigenicity studies reported in Table VI and Fig.1 indicate that EBV is more related to the chicken MDHV than it
is to the human (HSV-1 and HSV-2) viruses. Furthermore, in
other studies reported in Tables IV and V the behavior of EBV
has been found to be in conformity with this view, being more
like MDHV and less like the human herpesviruses tested.

Two other points need to be emphasized. Firstly, in
permissive cells of a natural host productive infection

usually occurs and resembles the lytic action of various animal viruses. In non-permissive cells of a foreign host, cell transformation results, whereby DNA is inserted in the host cell genome without lysis of the cell.[12] Since man is a foreign host to the herpesvirus of Marek's disease, transformation, rather than cell lysis, is expected to result. Secondly, glycoproteins in cells infected with HSV-1 have been shown to be specified by the virus and not by the host.[13] Glycoproteins specified by different strains of Herpes simplex virus differ in quantitative and qualitative characteristics.[14] The immunologically distinct properties exhibited by the various strains of Marek's disease as shown earlier [1] and as confirmed in this study, are consistent with these findings.

If a viral agent is to be a candidate for a human cancer virus, supporting epidemiologic evidence should be found. But if practically everyone is exposed to this virus, no clean cut results are expected from epidemiological investigations. The difference between those individuals who are over exposed to this virus and the majority who are simply exposed may not be perceivable. Other factors may have to be taken into consideration such as the route of entry, exposure to other carcinogenic agents, the presence of a helper virus and a variety of host factors which may determine whether such a viral agent is to be permitted by the host defenses to induce cell transformation and whether such transformed cells would escape the host defenses thereby resulting in neoplastic proliferation. This is especially pertinent in a country such as the U.S. where with the exception of few rural areas, every community is in contact with other communities and where, with the exception of certain religious and ethnic groups, contact with MDHV infected chickens has become universal. However, in a country such as China, where rural conditions still predominate and where links between population groups in various areas are still less developed, epidemiological studies can be more meaningful.

This may explain some inconclusive results from epidemiological investigations in the U.S. as compared to more conclusive results from China. Thus, California farm workers, presumably with greater exposure to poultry than nonfarm workers, had a slight excess mortality due to leukemia and a deficiency in mortality due to lymphoma and all cancers combined.[15] In Washington State and Oregon, there was a statistically significant association between farming occupations and mortality due to leukemia and myeloma; poultry farmers had the greatest proportionate excess leukemia mortality.[16]

The possible relationship between human cancer deaths and exposure to poultry was studied for ten Southeastern States for 1950 - 1969.[17] It was found in this study that deaths from uterine cervical and ovarian cancers and from multiple myeloma were excessive in high poultry population areas as compared with low poultry population areas. For ovarian cancer and myeloma, the significance disappeared when data from the high poultry population areas were compared with data from the total U.S. For myeloma, the difference between high versus intermediate units was not found significant. The study did not detect any excess risk of lymphoma, Hodgkins disease and leukemia in people occupationally exposed to poultry. If we assume that the population of the U.S. as a whole is exposed to this virus (comparable to the intermediate units studied), no significant difference from the over-exposed high poultry population areas or those occupationally exposed to poultry will be expected as explained earlier. A statistically significant difference may be anticipated however, between the over-exposed high poultry population areas and the under-exposed low areas. This was in fact observed in this study.

Other studies have also established that certain population groups which do not consume chickens have lower cancer rates than the general population. The risk of death from colon-rectal cancer in Seventh-day Adventists is two thirds that of the general population.[18] The recommended diet of the Seventh-day Adventists (which is followed by almost 50% of them) is a vegetarian diet to the exclusion of meat and chickens.

A markedly lower cancer rate among the Indians of the Southwest U.S. have been reported. [19,20, 21] The historical Indian diet consists of fried bread, coffee, mutton stew (well cooked) and corn which they raise. Poultry was conspiciously absent from their diet[21]. Of interest is the observation that the one case of prostatic cancer of an Indian encountered was one who raised a large flock of chickens.[21]

A very significant report which shows a casual relationship between cancer in chickens and cancer in man has recently been made by the Coordinating Group for Research on Etiology of Oesaphageal Cancer in North China.[22] This study included the provinces around the Taihang Mountains in North China and has been summarized in a recent issue of The Lancet. [23] In Linhsien County, the prevalence was 379 per 100,000 with mortality rates fairly steady over the years at 100 - 150 per 100,000 per annum (the corresponding figure for England and Wales is 6): and oesophageal cancer was the most common cause of death. One hundred and eighty one counties were studied, and some showed the same pattern of Linhsien, while others were not unusual. This study was initiated because of an epedemic of dysphagia. The diagnosis of oesaphgeal cancer was confirmed in three quarters of the cases.

Of special interest is the epedemiologic data obtained by Lynch and coworkers from studies with "cancer families". Familial association of such cancer types as ca breast, ovary, colon, stomach, prostate, endometrium have been documented by these workers. There is now general agreement, for example, that first degree relatives of probands with ca breast have two to fourfold increased risk of having similar lesions develop. If the cancer is both premenopausal and bilateral, the familial risk is increased to an even greater extent.[24] The familial occurences of a variety of premalignant disease and uncommon malignant neoplasms have prompted Lynch et al[25] to postulate an oncogenic virus operating in concert with a genotypically transmitted cancer diathesis. The familial association of ca breast and ca ovary [26], ca breast and sarcomas and ca breast and cancer of the gastrointestinal tract [27] have been described. It is of great interest to note that ca breast, ca ovary, ca gastrointestinal tract (other than ca colon and ca stomach) and to a lesser extent sarcoma, all show an association with the CR-64 strain of MDHV. A family exposed to this special viral stain, may therefore be expected to develop one or more of these cancer types.

SUMMARY

The association between Marek's disease herepesvirus and human cancer reported earlier, has been further investigated with a highly sensitive modified Schultz-Dale technique.

Serum antibodies to glycoprotein antigens prepared from MDHV were studied in 141 subjects with and without cancer. These were found in 63% of 65 subjects with non-malignant diseases, in 74% of 69 subjects with carcinoma and in 4 out of 7 subjects with melanoma and sarcoma. Serum antibodies to glycoprotein antigens prepared from other herpesviruses, HSV-1, HSV-2 and the Epstein-Barr viruses, were found in only 4% of the 52 subjects with non-malignant diseases, in 9% of the 54 subjects with carcinoma and in none of the 5 subjects with melanoma and sarcoma.

All of the 8 subjects with early carcinoma of colon and breast were found to have serum antibodies against MDHV as compared to 56% of 18 subjects with late disease.

Search for MDHV antigens in DPF of human cancer revealed the presence of these antigens in all of the 9 types of cancer tested but not in normal lung DPF or in DPF from fibroid uterus. No such antigens were detected with comparable glycoprotein antigens extracted from two other viruses, mouse hepatitis virus and influenza virus, or from 6 control tissue antigens prepared from human and chicken tissues.

An association was found between certain types of cancer and antigens prepared from various strains of MDHV. This association was found in both the serum antibody studies and in the studies with the DPF preparations. This was not the case with the glycoprotein antigens from the other herpesviruses studied.

The findings of serum antibodies to MDHV in subjects with non-malignant disease and more so in subjects with cancer especially early cancer, as well as the discovery of MDHV glycoprotein antigens in the DPF preparation of the 9 types of cancerous tissues studied, further implicates MDHV as a possible agent of human cancer. Although the Dische positive DPF preparations obtained by repeated freon extractions have not been subjected to enzyme action and cannot be considered as purified DNA preparations, yet the mere presence of such foreign viral antigens in the nuclear fraction of human cancer tissues is enough to arouse suspicion. Studies in this area are urgently needed.

Acknowledgement

I wish to thank Mr. William Pere for technical assistance and Ormont Drug and Chemical Co., Inc. for its interest

TABLE I. Serum Antibodies to Marek's and Other Herpesviruses
in 141 Subjects with and without Cancer

	MDHV		HSV-1,2, EBV.	
	Total	+ %	Total	+ %
Non-neoplastic	29	62	18	0
Peptic Ulcer	11	72	9	11
Bronchitis	11	72	11	9
Fibrocystic Disease Breast	14	50	14	0
	65	63	52	4
Ca Breast	18	72	15	0
Ca Lung	20	70	16	19
Ca Stomach	6	83	3	0
Ca Colon	21	76	17	12
Ca GI (other)	4	75	3	0
	69	74	54	9
Melanoma	4	50	4	0
Sarcoma	3	67	1	0
	7	57	5	0
Total	141	68	111	6

TABLE II. Incidence of Antibodies to Marek's Herpesvirus in 26 Subjects with Early and Late Cancer

Cancer Type	Stage	No.	Associated Type	Marek's Strain % +	Mean Titer*
Ca Colon	early	4	GA	(4/4)	8.9
Ca Breast	early	4	CR-64	(4/4)	7.8
		8		100	8.3
Ca Colon	late	11	GA	54	2.9
Ca Breast	late	7	CR-64	57	3.8
		18		56	3.3

*Mean titer is expressed in 10^{12} dilution of VPS.

TABLE III. Distribution of Serum Antibodies in 76 Subjects with Cancer in Relation to Strain of Marek's Herpesvirus

Cancer Type	No. Subjects	No. Tests	Mean Titer in 10^{12} dilution of VPS GA	CR-64	JM	GA-2
Ca Breast	18	32	0.8	3.6	3.5	3.5
Ca Colon	21	36	3.8	0.4	.7	3.0
Ca Lung	20	52	5.6	6.3	7.1	8.5
Ca Stomach	6	9	2.0	3.0	2.0	5.3
Ca-Other GI	4	12	1.2	4.0	0.9	0
Melanoma	4	7	1.1	0	1.6	
Sarcoma	3	3	1.3	0	1.6	

TABLE IV. Presence of Marek's Herpesvirus Antigens in DPF of Normal and Cancerous Tissues

Releasing Antigens	Normal Lung DPF		Uterine Fibroid DPF		Cancerous Tissues DPF	
	No Test	Mean* Titer	No. Test	Mean* Titer	No. Test	Mean* Titer
Controls#	32	0	29	0.1	249	0.4
Marek's						
GA	6	0	7	0.6	87	4.9
CR-64	8	0	4	0	90	4.5
JM	8	0	4	0	66	2.6
GA-2	4	0	5	0.4	46	3.3
Other Herpesvirus						
HSV-1	4	0	7	0.2	42	0.8
HSV-2	4	0	4	0	41	0.7
EBV	4	0	4	0	46	1.3

*Mean Titer is expressed as 10^{12} dilution of VPS

#Control antigens used include 6 normal (NPS) tissue antigens and 2 viral (VPS) antigens from MHV and Influenza A_2 and B strains.

TABLE V. Presence of Marek's Herpesvirus Antigens in DPF of Cancerous Tissues Titer Expressed as 10^{12} Dilution of VPS

	No. Tests	GA	CR-64	JM	GA-2	HSV-1	HSV-2	EBV
Ca Ovary	36	2.5	4.5	2.5	2.7	1.7	1.7	1.9
Ca Stomach	45	0.3	3.8	4.2	1.0	0.1	0.6	0.5
Ca Lung	46	1.9	3.4	1.6	0.7	0.8	0.1	1.6
Ca Breast	38	4.2	20.0	5.6	2.7	1.7	2.2	2.4
Ca Colon	80	28.0	0	1.9	8.0	0.3	0	0.1
Ca Pancreas	28	1.0	2.0	2.0	2.1	0.5	0.1	0.4
Ca Liver	29	0.9	2.5	0.7	4.0	0	0.1	1.2
Lymphoma	44	3.2	1.6	2.2	6.0	0.3	0.6	2.8
Sarcoma	34	2.2	3.2	3.0	2.4	1.5	0.4	1.2

TABLE VI. Antigens Relationship Between Marek's Disease
Herpesvirus (MDVH) and Epstein-Barr virus (EBV)

Releasing VPS Antigens	- Immunizing VPS Antigen			
	MHV - GA		EBV	
	No. Tests	Mean Titer	No. Tests	Mean Titer*
GA	7	32.0	8	3.6
CR-64	8	21.2	4	1.7
JM	4	5.2	4	2.0
GA-2	5	28.0	4	3.2
EBV	4	5.8	8	4.4
HSV-1	4	4.3	4	0.6
HSV-2	4	3.9	4	0.9
MHV	4	0.2	1	0.7

* Mean titer is expressed as 10^{12} dilution of VPS.

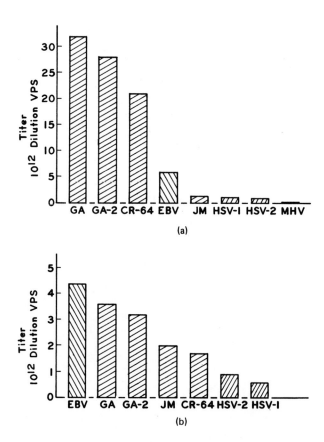

FIG. 1. (a) Cross-reactivity between GA strain of Marek's disease and other herpesviruses. GA is the immunizing antigen. (b) Cross-reactivity between EBV and other herpesviruses. EBV is the immunizing antigen.

REFERENCES

1. Makari, J.G. Association between Marek's Herpesvirus and Human Cancer. I. Detection of Cross-Reacting Antigens between Chicken Tumors and Human Tumors. Oncology, 28: 164, 1973.

2. Makari, J.G. Association between Marek's Herpesvirus and Human Cancer. II. Detection of Structural Viral Antigens in Chicken Tumors and Human Tumors. Oncology 28: 177, 1973.

3. Makari, J.G. Activity of a Tumour Polysaccharide Substance on Mice Transplanted with Sarcoma 180. Nature (Lond.), 205: 1178, 1965.

4. Makari, J.G. Unpublished Results.

5. Sevoian, M. University of Massachusetts, Amherst. Personal Communication.

6. Calnek, B.W. and Hitchner, S.B. Survival and Disinfection of Marek's Disease Virus and the Effectiveness of Filters in Preventing Airborne Dissemination. Science, 52: 35, 1973.

7. Lynch, H.T. Guirgis, H., Albert, S. and Brennan, M. Familial Breast Cancer in a Normal Population. Cancer, 34: 2080, 1974.

8. zur Hansen, H. and Schulte-Holthausen, H. Presence of EB Virus Nucleic Acid Homology in a "Virus-free" Line of Burkitt Tumor Cells. Nature (Lond.), 227: 245, 1970.

9. zur Hansen, H., Schulte-Holthansen, H., Klein, G. et al EBV DNA in Biopsies of Burkitt Tumours and anaplastic Carcinomas of the Nasopharynx. Nature (Lond.),228: 1056, 1970.

10. Pagano, J.S., Huang, C.H. and Levine, P. Absence of Epstein-Barr Viral DNA in American Burkitt Lymphoma. N.Engl. J. Med., 289: 1395, 1973.

11. Vianna, N.J., and Polan, A.K. Epidemiologic Evidence for Transmission pf Hodgkin's Disease. N.Engl. J. Med., 289: 499, 1973.

12. Allen, D.W. and Cole, P. Viruses and Human Cancer N.Engl. J. Med., 286: 70, 1972.

13. Roizman, B. and Spear, P.G. Herpesviruses: Current Information on the Composition and Structure; in Maramorosch and Kurstak Comparative Virology, Academic Press, Inc. New York, p. 135, 1971.

14. Spear, P.G., Keller, J.M. and Roizman, B. Proteins Specified by Herpes simplex virus 2. Viral Glycoproteins Associated with Cellular Membranes. J. Virol., 5: 123, 1970.

15. Fasal, E., Jackson, E.W. and Klauber, M.R. Leukemia and Lymphoma Mortality and Farm Residence. Am. J. Epidemiol. 87: 267, 1968.

16. Milham, S. Leukemia and Multiple Myeloma in Farmers. Am. J. Epidemiol. 94: 307, 1971.

17. Priester, W.A. and Mason, J. Human Cancer Mortality in Relation to Poultry Population, by County in 10 Southeastern States. J. Natl. Cancer Inst., 53: 45, 1974.

18. Phillips, R.L., Kuzma, J.W., Lemon, F.R. and Walden, R.T. Mortality from Colon-Rectal Cancer in California Seventh-Day Adventists. Presented at Annual Meeting of the Amer. Public Health Assoc., San Francisco, Nov. 8, 1973.

19. Muggia, A Diseases among the Navajo Indians. Rocky Mountain Med. J. 68: 39, 1971.

20. Creegan, E.T., Franmeni, J.F. Jr., Cancer Mortality Among American Indians 1950-67. J. Natl. Cancer Inst., 49:959, 1972.

21. Gibbons, D.L., in the press; Personal Communication. August 13, 1974.

22. Coordinating Group for Research on Etiology of Oesophogeal Cancer in North China. Paper Read at the 11th International Cancer Congress held in Florence, October, 1974; Chin. Med. J. 1: 167,1975.

23. Lancet, Editorial. Oesophageal Cancer in China. 1: 1413, 1975.

24. Lynch, H.T., Krush, A.J., Lemon, H.M. et al. Tumor Variations in Families with Breast Cancer. J. A. M. A. 222: 1631, 1972.

25. Lynch, H.T., Krush, A.J., Mulcahy, G.M. and Reed, W.B. Familial Occurrences of a Variety of Premalignant Diseases and Uncommon Malignant Neoplasms. Cancer. 33: 1474, 1974.

26. Lynch, H.T. Guirgis, H., Albert S., Brennan, M. et al. Familial Association of Carcinoma of the Breast and Ovary. Surg. Gynecol. Obste. 133: 644, 1971.

27. Lynch, H.T. Krush, A.J. and Guirgis, H. Genetic Factors in Families with Combined Gastrointestinal and Breast Cancer. Am. J. Gastroenterol. 59: 31,1973.

ACTIVATION OF RNA PARTICLES FROM HUMAN TUMORS BY HUMAN ADENOVIRUS

Wendell D. Winters*

Anthony Neri

John A. Sykes**

and

Carol O'Toole

UCLA School of Medicine, Los Angeles, CA

*The University of Texas Health Science Center, San Antonio, TX

**Southern California Cancer Center, Los Angeles, CA, U.S.A.

I.   INTRODUCTION

Activation of type C viruses from murine cells in vitro has been reported using physical means (1) and chemical agents (2,3). RNA virus particles have been biologically induced from animal tumor cells in vitro in mixed lymphocyte reactions (4) and by exposure to DNA viruses (5,6,7). RNA-containing virus-like particles were successfully activated by human adenovirus type 5 in primary cultures of guinea pig sarcomas of different histologic types (5) and in cultures of murine lymphoid cells (6), while more recently, type C virus has been activated from mouse cells using ultraviolet irradiated herpes simplex virus types 1 and 2 (7).

We present evidence in this communication that RNA-containing particles with DNA polymerase activities were detected and purified from cell-free fluids of cultures of different types of human tumor cells after biological activation with human adenovirus type 5 (Ad-5).

II.   PROCEDURES AND MATERIALS USED

A.   Cells and Medium

All early passage cell lines of different histologic types of normal and tumor cells used in this study were derived from explant cultures of surgical specimens under biocontainment conditions. Continuous cell

279

lines studied were derived from our original explant cultures, were generously donated by other investigators, or were obtained from Naval Biological Laboratories, Oakland, CA. Plating efficiencies and growth characteristics of many of the normal and neoplastic human cells used in this study have been previously described (8). All cells were subcultured at least twice in our growth medium (GM) before use in experiments. Growth medium (GM) consisted of Dulbecco's Minimum Essential Medium (DMEM; Microbiological Associates, Inc., Bethesda, MD), supplemented with 20% heat inactivated and sterile filtered fetal bovine serum (PBS). Maintenance medium used during the virus infection experiments consisted of DMEM supplemented with 0.5% FBS.

B. Adenovirus Propagation and Titrations

Human adenovirus type 5 (Ad-5; strain Ad-75), originally obtained from the Division of Virology, National Institute for Medical Research, Mill Hill, London, England, was grown in human embryonic kidney cells and in human sarcoma cells (9). Standard stocks of Ad-5 had an average titer of 2×10^{12} PFU/cc after serial purification on cesium chloride (CsCl) density gradients as previously described (10).

Samples of stock adenovirus preparations and fractions of cell-free fluids and soluble cell extracts from uninfected and adenovirus-infected cultures were assayed for infectious adenovirus according to previously described methods (11,12). Human newborn foreskin and human embryonic kidney fibroblast cells were routinely used as target cells for plaque titrations in 21 day assays.

C. Adenovirus Inactivation

Aliquots of Ad-5 suspensions at the different virus concentrations used for cell inoculation were heat inactivated at $100^{\circ}C$ for 1-3 minutes or were neutralized with human convalescent antiserum to Ad-5 for 2 hrs at $4^{\circ}C$ prior to inoculation.

D. Electron Microscopy

Normal and neoplastic cell cultures, both uninfected and after adenovirus inoculation, were scraped from the flasks and cell pellets were fixed, stained, processed and examined according to previously described methods (13).

E. Radioisotope Labeling and Profiles

^{3}H-uridine (28 Ci/mmol) and ^{3}H-thymidine (25 Ci/mmol) were purchased from Schwarz/Mann, Orangeburg, NY. Replicate cultures of untreated cells and of cells after adenovirus inoculation were labeled with ^{3}H-thymidine or ^{3}H-uridine for 16-24 hrs at 37°C at different intervals after virus inoculation. Samples of cells and culture fluids were harvested at different intervals and these materials were assayed for evidence of radiolabeled adenovirions by isopycnic centrifugation into cesium chloride density gradients (12). Cell-free fluids from uninoculated and adenovirus-inoculated cultures were also clarified by serial differential centrifugations, layered on 15-60% sucrose gradients and centrifuged in a Beckman SW-40 Rotor at 35,000 rpm for 16 hrs at 4°C. After bottom puncture, 200 μl fractions were collected and 50 μl of each fraction in the 1.12-1.20 gm/cc density range of the sucrose gradients was assayed for DNA polymerase activities. Fractions with highest radioactivity and DNA polymerase activity were pooled and further purified and concentrated on new 15-60% sucrose gradients. Cell-free fluids from corresponding cultures which did not receive radio-isotopes were treated in the same way. Fractions with highest DNA polymerase activities were pooled, diluted and pelleted by ultracentrifugation.

F. DNA Polymerase Assays

Following sequential sucrose density gradient purifications and pelleting cell-free fluids were assayed for DNA polymerase activities to detect RNA-dependent DNA polymerase. Synthetic templates, poly (rC)·oligo (dG) and oligo (dG), were used to increase detection of enzyme activity. Assays were performed according to methods originally described by Sarngadharan et al. (14), Gallagher et al. (5) and Winters et al. (5) with these modifications: ^{32}P-dGTP was used alternatively to confirm that material in the ^{3}H-uridine-labeled peak also had polymerase activity. Reactions proceeded for 60 minutes at 37°C in a shaker water bath and were stopped by the addition of cold 10% TCA containing 0.02 M sodium pyrophosphate. After 30 minutes in ice, TCA precipitable radio-activity was collected on cellulose acetate filters, washed twice with cold 5% TCA and the wet filters were placed into vials containing 10 ml Filter-Solv solution (Beckman). Counts were performed in a LS-250 scintillation counter (Beckman) after the vials were left at room temperature (22°C) for 16-24 hrs and then chilled to 4°C. After the filters were dissolved, total counts were enhanced 10 times or more over duplicate samples counted in standard toluene-based scintillation fluids. Control assay mixtures without template, without enzyme, and without template or enzyme were counted for levels of endogenous RNA-dependent DNA polymerase activity.

G. Experimental Plan

Replicate cultures of various histologic types of normal human cells grown in the same type of medium (GM) were inoculated with the same stock of Ad-5 at doses from 5 to 500 PFU/cell. Similarly, cell cultures of human tumors with the same and different histopathologic properties were grown in standard medium (GM) and then inoculated with various doses of stock Ad-5. Untreated and adenovirus-inoculated cultures were observed daily for the development of cytopathic effects (CPE). Cell-

free fluids were monitored at designated time periods for evidence of
productive adenovirus infection and for the production of other particles
released from the cell cultures. When the presence of adenovirus
particles or other particles was detected in cell-free fluids, replicate
cultures of the positive cells were then labeled with ^{3}H-thymidine or
^{3}H-uridine and the cell-free fluids from these cultures were then studied
as previously described.

III. RESULTS

A. Human Adenovirus Replication In Human Cell Cultures

Characteristics of the different types of human cells, both normal
and tumor, are presented in Tables 1 and 2. Replication of Ad-5 was not
observed to be influenced by the growth rate, the cell type, or the
subpassage level of any of the human cells examined in these studies.

Cells derived from 15 of 20 human sarcomas of different histologic
types, as well as those of all breast, cervical and squamous cell
carcinomas examined, readily supported Ad-5 replication (Table 1).
Different histologic types of human normal embryonic, fetal, newborn and
adult cells likewise supported the complete replication of Ad-5. Ad-5
also replicated in 9 of 10 cell cultures obtained from human melanomas
(Table 2).

In studies of the influence of the virus input multiplicity on the
time course of development of adenovirus effects, early cell detachment
was observed when replicate cultures of the different permissive cell
types were inoculated with Ad-5 input multiplicities of 300, 400 or 500
PFU/cell. Therefore, although all cell types were initially tested using
Ad-5 doses ranging from 5-500 PFU/cell, subsequent experiments were
performed in replicate cultures inoculated with Ad-5 at doses from 5
to 200 PFU/cell. CsCL density gradient profile analysis of radioisotope-
labeled viral DNA demonstrated that the earliest production of progeny
adenovirus occurred between 48 and 72 hrs after inoculation at doses of
5-50 PFU/cell in sarcoma line ONSA-8 and in both cervical carcinoma lines.
When the remaining human tumor cell types were assayed, sarcomas, breast
carcinomas and cervical carcinomas all displayed evidence of new virus
production earlier than melanomas, bladder carcinomas and normal cell
cultures. This same order was observed when cells of these different
tumor types were assayed for production of infectious adenovirus.
Although progeny adenovirus particles produced in most permissive tumor
cell types and normal cells remained cell-bound, it was found that two
human sarcoma cultures and two melanoma cultures released the majority of
new progeny virions into the supernatants. In cells where abortive (no
adenovirus antigens detected) or incomplete (early or capsid adenovirus
antigens produced) replication occurred, no infectious particles were
detected by infectivity assay, electron microscopy, and radioactivity
gradient profile analysis (Table 1 and Table 2). Electron micrographic
evaluations confirmed the presence of complete adenovirus particles in
permissive human normal and tumor cells.

282

B. Biological Activation of New Particles In Cell-Free Fluids

Human tumor cell cultures in which incomplete or abortive adenovirus replication had been confirmed were reexamined after Ad-5 inoculations ranging from 5 to 200 PFU/cell. In these experiments, replicate cultures of control and Ad-5-inoculated cells provided specimens of cell-free fluids. Cell-free fluids taken from these cultures at different time periods after adenovirus inoculation were assayed for infectious adenovirus and for DNA polymerase activities after purification and concentration.

C. RNA Directed DNA Polymerase Activities

Representative responses of permissive and non-permissive human tumor cells to different doses of human Ad-5 are presented in Table 3. Cell-free fluids of untreated or adenovirus-inoculated permissive human tumor and normal cell cultures had no DNA polymerase activities. Cell-free fluids of non-permissive human tumor cells were found to contain DNA polymerase activities from 3-9 days following Ad-5 inoculation. The activation of detectable DNA polymerase-containing particles was found to be both dose-and time-dependent. As represented in Table 3, all five activated human sarcoma cell types and the melanoma cell culture were induced with approximately 100 PFU/cell. Both 50 and 100 PFU/cell of Ad-5 were found to activate significant DNA polymerase activities in materials from cell-free fluids of the bladder carcinoma cells.

Additional studies designed to label specifically the DNA and RNA in replicate cultures revealed that cell free supernatants contained ^{3}H-uridine labeled particles with densities of 1.14-1.18 gm/cc in equilibrium sucrose density gradients. DNA polymerase activities were detected within this range of density in fractions taken from these gradients. Peak activities were observed in fractions from 1.15-1.16 gm/cc.

D. Electron Microscopic Observations

Membrane-bound particles of unique morphology were observed by electron microscopy in extracellular fluids and at plasma membrane sites of cells in the activated cultures (Fig. Ia), but not in cells from untreated cultures. These particles were observed to be contiguous with the outer plasma membrane of some activated cells and were found, in most cases, to be composed of multilayered laminar structures (Fig. lb). Electron microscopic examinations of cells over a time course suggested that the particles observed initially at the plasma membrane later lost a number of the membrane coats so that the free particles found in extra-cellular fluids contained 2-3 membrane layers.

E. Biologic and Immunologic Studies

The infectivity of suspensions of adenovirus at the different virus concentrations used for cell inoculations was completely abolished when these virus specimens were heat inactivated for 1-3 minutes or were neutralized with antiserum specific for Ad-5. Moreover, after inactivation by these methods, virus stocks were not capable of biologically activating RNA-containing particles from any of the cell types which had previously been found to   yield RNA-containing particles.

Concentrated, highly purified RNA-containing particles inoculated in monolayer and in suspension cultures have not been observed to consistently produce any significant changes in normal human cells. Likewise, these RNA particulates did not react immunologically with antisera prepared against human DNA viruses with known oncogenic potential (herpes virus types 1 and 2 and adenovirus types 12 and 18) or against RNA tumor viruses from murine, feline, simian or avian species.

IV. DISCUSSION

Our results indicate that human tumor cells derived originally from a number of different histologic types of human tumor tissues can readily support the complete replication of human adenovirus type 5. Although three continuous human carcinoma cell lines have historically been used as "standard" cells for studies of human adenovirus replication and propagation, i.e., cells derived from adenocarcinomas of the cervix (HeLa), nasopharyngeal carcinoma (Hep-2) and epidermoid carcinoma of the larynx (KB) (16,17,18), few other types of human tumor cells have been considered for similar studies (19). Our present findings confirm results of previous studies in some human tumor cell lines showing permissive infections with Ad-5 (16-18). More recently, remarkable differences in the replication of human Ad-5 in different types of human tumor cells were suggested by reports of Ad-5 replication in human Burkitt's lymphoma cells (20) and in human chondrosarcoma cells (9). Faucon and co-workers observed limited production of Ad-5 and differences of expression of EB viral antigen production in Ad-5-infected EB-virus positive and EB-virus negative human Burkitt's lymphoma cells. In addition, they suggested that human adenovirus might have the potential to derepress some functions of the original infecting EB virus in these human tumor cells (20).

In accord with the general possibility that super-infecting adeno-virus may function in some role to derepress latent viral functions, our present results indicate that RNA-containing particles with DNA polymerase (reverse transcriptase) activities were detected in cell-free fluids from cultures of different types of human tumor cells following biological activation with human adenovirus type 5. Our biological activation method, using a DNA virus of human origin (Ad-5), was similar to what has been described previously in the successful activations of murine RNA virus particles from murine lymphoma cells (6) and of RNA virus particles from different guinea pig sarcoma cells (5) with this human adenovirus type.

Classical viral approaches of attempting to grow viruses from human tumor cells and to visualize viruses in human tumors by electron microscopy have met with rare success. More recently, indirect approaches using biochemical, immunological, biological and biophysical methods have provided evidence that strongly suggests that viruses are associated with certain human tumors. However, the general lack of success using biophysical and biochemical methods to activate virus particles from human tumor cells suggested that alternative, less harsh treatments for viral activation might be of particular importance for examining human tumor cells. Thus, our method of biological activation may be of use in studying human tumor cells.

The present work implies that infectious viruses with which we normally have contact and with which we may be infected, could under the proper host conditions, play a role in activating latent viruses associated with human tumors.

The RNA-containing particles detected in cell-free fluids and at the surface of the activated cells may be "mimic" virus particles and as such they may have only a chance relationship as agents associated with cells of these human tumors. In this case, it is important to note that "mimic" virus particles can be activated from human tumor cells. Moreover, the particles that we observed to be budding and released from the human tumor cells after adenovirus activation may have significance in a relationship between the ability of these tumors to produce these particles and the ability of these tumors to metastasize rapidly. Since these human tumor cellular particles contained RNA, had unique biochemical activities, and demonstrated no immunologic relationships with any known viruses of other species, they may be important in the dissemination of tumor cells or tumor materials from the primary site in humans to sites of metastasis.

Finally, our results may be of considerable importance in virology and oncology. Type C virus particles have been observed in cells of lymphomas that developed late in hamsters which were originally inoculated with different types of human adenoviruses (21,22). Therefore the possibility exists that other adenoviruses, as well as other types of human DNA viruses, can assist in activation of oncornaviruses from different animal tumor cells in vivo.

We found no evidence of adenovirus replication in the two cell lines derived from human meningiomas nor was there any evidence of production of RNA-containing particulates. In view of the nature of multiple tumor-associated antigens known to be contained in these cells (23), one interesting possibility is that these completely non-permissive meningioma cell cultures might have been originally induced by a virus. Therefore, resistance of meningiomas to Ad-5 replication could be due to viral interference or inhibition. In addition, cells from meningiomas containing known tumor associated antigens could interfere with or block replication of any new virus introduced into the system.

V. SUMMARY

A human DNA virus, adenovirus type 5, has been shown to be capable of activating, on a dose and time-dependent basis, human tumor cells in culture. These cells contained observable membrane-enclosed particles and the culture supernatants contained RNA particles with specific DNA polymerase activities. Cell-free fluids from cultures of 5 of 20 sarcomas, 3 of 5 bladder carcinomas and 1 of 10 melanomas yielded ^{3}H-uridine-labeled particles with densities of 1.14-1.18 gm/cc in isopycnic sucrose density gradients. Reverse transcriptase (RT) enzyme activity was detected in both ^{3}H-uridine-labeled and unlabeled purified particles using ^{32}P-dGTP and ^{3}H-dGTP, respectively, in assays containing poly (rC)·oligo (dG) as the template primer. Replicate cultures of Ad-5-treated normal cells and most human tumor cells were permissive for complete Ad-5 replication. Cell-free fluids from untreated cultures of 18 various normal tissues (including adult, newborn, fetal and embryonic), as well as fluids from most ad-5-infected human normal and tumor cells, were negative for RNA particles and RT enzyme activities. Heat-inactivated and antiserum-neutralized Ad-5 did not infect or activate human tumor cells. Time course studies of tumor cells inoculated with 5-500 PFU/cell of Ad-5 showed that RNA-containing particles with maximum RT activities were released into culture fluids at 3 days in sarcoma and at 6 days in melanoma and bladder carcinoma cell cultures.

The method of biological activation (using one virus to activate another virus) successfully employed in cultured animal tumor cell systems, has now been found to be capable of activating RNA-containing particles from some cultured human tumor cells.

TABLE I

CHARACTERISTICS OF HUMAN SARCOMA AND CARCINOMA CELLS IN CULTURE

Histopathologic Type	Designation or Source[a]	Morpho-logy[b]	Passages Tested	Growth Rate[c]	Adenovirus Replication[d]
TUMOR CELLS:					
Osteogenic sarcoma	HT 1080	E	24-37	M	Incomplete
	AO 693	E	17-21	M	Complete
	2T	E	98-112	R	Complete
	SS-S	E	8-12	S	Complete
	SS-F	E	5-8	R	Complete
	SS-G	E	4-8	M	Complete
Chondrosarcoma	ONSA-8	E	12-79	R	Complete
	SS-T	E	11-13	M	Complete
	SS-V	E	12-19	M	Complete
Fibrosarcoma	MB 8387	E	144-180	S	Abortive
	AO 793	E	11-15	M	Incomplete
	LASA-05	E	88-98	R	Complete
Rhabdomyosarcoma	AO 867	E	63-66	R	Incomplete
	AO 812	E	31-35	R	Complete
	TE-32	E	46-52	M	Incomplete
	SS-M	E	4-9	R	Complete
	SS-O	E	3-11	M	Complete
Liposarcoma	SS-V	E	9-10	S	Complete
Leiomyosarcoma	SS-B	E	1-19	S	Complete
Giant Cell sarcoma	SS-K	E	4-6	S	Complete
Carcinoma, breast	MDA-MB-157	E	93-98	M	Complete
	MDA-MB-231	E	60-78	M	Complete
	ALAB	E	75-78	R	Complete
Carcinoma, cervix	HUCA	E	100+	R	Complete
	HeLa-S3	E	100+	R	Complete
Carcinoma, bladder	T-24	E	100+	R	Incomplete
	J-92	E	48-63	R	Complete
	SS-SU	E	2-5	M	Complete
	SS-R	E	2-5	M	Abortive
	J-257	E	2-8	M	Incomplete
Carcinoma, squamous cell	Colo-16	E	29-33	M	Complete

a, SS=surgical specimen
b, E=epitheloid, F=fibroblast
c, cell doubling times were used to calculate the growth rates for the cells, and the growth rates were designated as rapid for doubling in 14-24 hours, medium for doubling in 24-48 hours, and slow for doubling in 4- hours or longer from time of re-seeding into new cultures.
d, Replication as determined by EM, virus titrations and radioactivity gradient profiles after ^{3}H thymidine labeling

TABLE II

CHARACTERISTICS OF HUMAN MENINGIOMA, MELANOMA AND NORMAL CELLS IN CULTURE

Histopathologic Type	Designation or source[a]	Morphology[b]	Passages Tested	Growth Rate[c]	Adenovirus Replication[d]
TUMOR CELLS:					
Meningioma	SS-CH	E	3-5	S	Abortive
	SS-MF	E	2-4	S	Abortive
Melanomas	SS-M	E	16-18	F	Abortive
	Mel-1	E	52-57	M	Complete
	SS-AL	E	10-14	M	Complete
	SS-KO	E	24-26	M	Complete
	SS-W	E	31-35	M	Complete
	SS-E	E	15-19	R	Complete
	SS-D	E	31-33	R	Complete
	SS-R	E	17-19	M	Complete
	SS-Ro	E	11-13	M	Complete
	SS-CL	E	27-31	M	Complete
NORMAL CELLS:					
Bladder	HCV-29	F	92-110	R	Complete
Bladder	Embryonic-SS	F	2-4	S	Complete
Bladder	Embryonic-SS	F	2-4	S	Complete
Bladder	Fetal-SS	F	3-5	S	Complete
Bladder	Fetal-SS	F	3-4	S	Complete
Bladder	Adult[e]-SS	F	6-10	S	Complete
Bladder	Adult[f]-SS	F	5-12	S	Complete
Skin	Adult, SS-TA	F	8-21	S	Complete
Skin	Adult, SS-CL	F	15-17	S	Complete
Skin	Adult, SS-SE	F	9-12	S	Complete
Skin	Newborn-SS-A	F	10-14	S	Complete
Skin	Embryonic-SS	F	5-7	S	Complete
Skin	Fetal-SS	F	3-4	S	Complete
Kidney	Fetal-SS	F	12-17	S	Complete
Kidney	Adult-SS	F	6-9	S	Complete
Muscle	Fetal-SS	F	3-4	S	Complete
Muscle	Adult-SS	F	13-15	S	Complete
Lung	Fetal-SS	F	3-4	S*	Complete

a,b,c,d same as legend of Table 1
e, cells obtained from inflammatory bladder tissue specimen
f, bladder connective tissue specimen

TABLE III

RESPONSES OF HUMAN TUMOR CELLS TO DIFFERENT DOSES OF ADENOVIRUS

Tumor Cell Type	Inoculum Ad5(PFU/cell)	CPE[a]	DNA Polymerase Activities	
			Enzyme Positive[b]	Time of Enzyme Detection[c]
Rhabdomyosarcoma	5	0	0	0
	25		0	0
	50		0	0
	100		+	3-6
	200		0	0
	None	0	0	0
Osteogenic Sarcoma	5-200	+	0	0
	None	0	0	0
Carcinoma, bladder	50-100	0	+	5-7
	None	0	0	0
Melanoma	100	0	+	6-9
	None	0	0	0
Normal skin Muscle, and bladder	5-200	+	0	0
	None	+	0	0

a, CPE - cytopathologic effects observed in Ad5 inoculated cultures
b, Polymerase activity established by 3 times or greater increase over internal
      control in artificially templated reactions
c, Time (days) after Ad5 inoculation

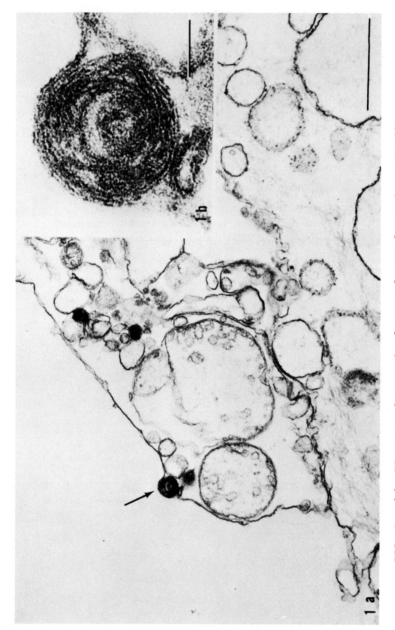

FIG. 1. (a) Electron micrograph of part of cell from a human bladder
carcinoma culture after inoculation with 15 PFU per cell of human adenovirus
type 5. Cell is necrotic and shows (arrow) typical large "mimic" particle
of 270 nm diameter budding from plasma membrane. The bar represents 1 um.
Magnification X 22,500. (b) High magnification of particle indicated by
arrow in Figure 1a. Particle is seen to be composed of multiple, concentric
double membranes. Bar represents 0.1 um. Magnification X 150,000.

VI. REFERENCES

1. Rowe, W.P., Hartley, J.W., Lander, M.R., Pugh, W.E., and Teich, N. Noninfectious AKR Mouse Embryo Cell Lines In Which Each Cell Has The Capacity To Be Activated To Produce Infectious Murine Leukemia Virus. Virology, 46:866-876, 1971.

2. Igel, H.S., Huebner, R.J., Turner, H.C., Kotin, P., and Falk, H.L. Mouse Leukemia Virus Activation By Chemical Carcinogens. Science, 166:1624-1626, 1969.

3. Lowy, D.R., Rowe, W.P., Teich, N., and Hartley, J.W. Murine Leukemia Virus: High-Frequency Activation In Vitro By 5-Iododeoxyuridine And 5-Bromodeoxyuridine. Science, 174:155-156, 1971.

4. Hirsch, M.S., Phillips, S.M., Solnik, C., Black, P.H., Schwartz, R. S., and Carpenter, C.B. Activation Of Leukemia Viruses By Graft-Versus-Host And Mixed Lymphocyte Reactions In Vitro. Proc. Nat. Acad. Sci. USA, 69:1069-1072, 1972.

5. Winters, W.D., Boddie, A.W., and Roth, J.A. Biological Activation Of Viruses-Like Particles From Chemically Induced Guinea Pig Sarcomas. Proc. Soc. Expt. Biol. Med., 149:714-722, 1975.

6. Winters, W.D., Hays, E.F., and Sykes, J.A. Biologic Activation Of Viruses From Murine Lymphomas. Abstr. Proc. Am. Assoc. for Cancer Res., 17:5, 1976.

7. Hampar, B., Aaronson, S.A., Derge, J.G., Chakrabarty, M., Showalter, S.D. and Dunn, C.Y. Activation Of An Endogenous Mouse Type C Virus By Ultraviolet-Irradiated Herpes Simplex Virus Types 1 and 2. Proc. Nat. Acad. Sci. USA, 73:646-650, 1976.

3. Winters, W.D., Tuan, A.L., and Morton, D.L. Differential Effects Of Rifampicin On Cultured Human Tumor Cells. Cancer Res., 34:3173-3179, 1974.

9. Winters, W.D., Neri, A., and Morton, D.L. New Cell Line Derived From A Human Chondrosarcoma. In Vitro, 10:70-76, 1974.

10. Russell, W.C., Valentine, R.C., and Pereira, H.G. The Effect Of Heat On The Anatomy Of The Adenovirus. J. Gen. Virol., 1:509-522, 1967.

11. Winters, W.D., and Khoobyarian, N. Fate Of Adenovirus Types 2 and 12 In Infected Serial Cultures Of Non-Primate Origin. J. Gen. Virol., 8:95-104, 1970.

12. Winters, W.D., and Russell, W.C. Studies On The Assembly of Adenovirus In Vitro. J. Gen. Virol., 10:181-194, 1971.

13. Sykes, J.A., Whitescarver, J. and Briggs, L. Observations On A Cell Line Producing Mammary Tumor Virus. J. Natl. Cancer Inst., 41:1315-1327, 1968.

14. Sarngadharan, M.G., Sarin, P.S., and Gallo, R.C. Reverse Transcriptase Activity Of Human Acute Leukaemic Cells: Purification Of The Enzyme, Response To AMV 70S RNA, And Characterization Of The DNA Product. Nature New Biol., 240:67-72, 1972.

15. Gallagher, R.E., Todaro, G.J., Smith, R.G., Livingston, D.M., and Gallo, R.C. Relationship Between RNA-Directed DNA Polymerase (Reverse Transcriptase) From Human Acute Leukemic Blood Cells And Primate Type C Viruses. Proc. Nat. Acad. Sci. USA, 71:1309-1313, 1974.

16. Herrmann, E.C. Experiences In Laboratory Diagnosis Of Adenovirus Infections In Routine Medical Practice. Mayo Clin. Proc., 43:635-644, 1968.

17. Evans, A.S. Establishment Of Human Adult Tonsil Cells In Continuous Culture And Their Virus Susceptibilities. Proc. Soc. Exp. Biol. Med., 96:752-757, 1957.

18. Pal, S.R., McQuillin, J., and Gardner, P.S. Comparative Study Of Susceptibility Of Primary Monkey Kidney Cells, Hep-2 Cells And HeLa Cells To A Variety Of Faecal Viruses. J. Hyg., 61:493-498, 1963.

19. Winters, W.D., Watson, D.A., and Sykes, J.A. Adenovirus Infections Of Cultured Human Solid Tumor Cells. Submitted for Publication, 1976.

20. Faucon, N., Chardonnet, Y., Perrinet, M.D., and Sohier, R. Superinfection With Adenovirus To Burkitt's Lymphoma Cell Lines. J. Natl. Cancer Inst., 53:305-308, 1974.

21. Stenback, W.A., Van Hoosier, G.L., and Trentin, J.J. Virus Particles In Hamster Tumors As Revealed By Electron Microscopy. Proc. Soc. Expt. Biol. Med., 122:1219-1223, 1966.

22. Trentin, J.J., Van Hoosier, G.L., and Samper, L. The Oncogenicity Of Human Adenoviruses In Hamsters. Proc. Soc. Expt. Biol. Med., 127:683-689, 1968.

23. Winters, W.D., and Rich, J.R. Human Meningioma Antigens. Int. S. Cancer, 15:815-822, 1975.

BIOSYNTHESIS OF RAUSCHER LEUKEMIA VIRAL PROTEINS

R. B. Arlinghaus, G. A. Jamjoom, L. J. Arcement, R. B. Naso and
W. L. Karshin

Biology Department, The University of Texas System Cancer Center
M.D. Anderson Hospital and Tumor Institute, Houston, Texas 77030

INTRODUCTION

Rauscher murine leukemia virus (RLV) has been reported to contain
four major nonglycosylated polypeptides (p30, p15, p12, and p10), and two
size classes of glycoproteins {gp69/71 and gp45 (1-4)}*. Recent studies
by Ikeda et al. (5) and Ihle et al. (6) have identified an additional
polypeptide (17,000 daltons), termed "envelope p15" or p15E, in murine
leukemia viruses. Work from this laboratory (7) has established that RLV
produced in several cell lines also contains a nonglycosylated precursor
polypeptide (≈65,000 daltons) that has p30 peptide sequences. This precursor migrates faster in polyacrylamide gels than gp69/71 and in some
analytical systems is not resolved from this viral glycoprotein.

RLV genomic RNA probably consists of two strands of RNA (8) which
is extracted from the virion as a RNA complex that sediments between 60-
70S (9). When denatured by heat or denaturing chemicals, a 35S subunit
RNA is obtained (9). This subunit RNA is thought to act as messenger RNA
since viral specific RNA of that size is found associated with polyribo-
somes in infected cells (10,11). The size of the subunit RNA indicates
that it is a polycistronic RNA and all polycistronic RNAs in mammalian
cells thus far investigated are translated into protein, at least in part,
by way of large precursor proteins (12-17).

Our studies on the translation of RLV genomic RNA in whole cells
(4,7,18-20) and cell-free systems (21,22) support the conclusion that
high molecular weight precursor polypeptides, which are in fact viral specific polyproteins, are the primary gene products produced during translation of the viral genomic RNA. These polyproteins are then cleaved in
vivo in stages to produce the mature viral proteins. These studies were
made possible by the development of sophisticated techniques that permit
the translation of genomic RNA in cell-free extracts, and allow specific
isolation of intracellular viral specific proteins which represent only
1-3% of the total proteins.

Studies with avian RNA tumor viruses have supported the idea that
such viral proteins are made by way of synthesis and cleavage of polyproteins. In cells infected with avian myeloblastosis virus (AMV), a 76,000
dalton precursor polypeptide, which contained peptide sequences of four
of the major nonglycosylated viral structural proteins was detected (23-
25). Translation of Rous sarcoma virus (RSV) 35S subunit RNA in a cell-
free system gave similar results in that the major product was the above-
mentioned 76,000 dalton precursor (26).

The overall objectives of our studies are to identify and charac-

---

*We have used the nomenclature for oncornaviruses as set forth in August
et al. (1).

terize the factor or factors involved in the conversion of normal cells to
tumor cells by RNA tumor viruses. Our initial approach has been to investigate the mechanism by which murine leukemia viral proteins are synthesized. It is this phase of our research that is presented here. In
the future, these findings will then be applied and extended to murine
sarcoma virus systems, since sarcoma viruses can transform fibroblasts
into tumor cells in tissue culture.

PROCEDURES AND MATERIAL USED

The materials and methods have been described previously (18-20,
27).

RESULTS

Analysis of RLV-infected Cell Cultures by Immune Precipitation of
^{35}S-Methionine Pulse-Labeled and Chased Cultures. Our studies with cell-
free systems primed with high molecular weight RLV RNA strongly suggest
that the viral structural proteins are made by way of high molecular
weight precursor polypeptides (21,22). RLV-specific precursor polypeptides should be unstable polypeptides that are rapidly labeled in infected
cells. To identify such precursor candidates, replicate cultures of RLV-
infected JLS-V16 cells were pulse-labeled with ^{35}S-methionine for 15 min.
One culture was lysed and the cytoplasmic extract was prepared. The other
cultures were incubated in complete growth medium containing excess unlabeled methionine for 15, 30, 60 min and 4 hr, respectively, and cytoplasmic extracts were prepared. Each cytoplasmic extract was treated
with anti-RLV serum, and the immune precipitates were analyzed by SDS-PAGE
(Fig. 1). There was no significant change in the total radioactivity of
the immune precipitates of the 15 min pulse and the 15-, 30-, or 60-min
pulse-chases. There was, however, a 10-20% reduction in radioactivity
following a 4 hr chase. The decrease in radioactivity in the immune precipitates of 4 hr pulse-chase samples probably reflects export of newly
made virus into the culture fluid.

The 15 min pulse-labeled immune precipitate (Fig. 1A) did not contain detectable amounts of p30 but did contain several large polypeptides
with molecular weights larger than 40,000. The predominant polypeptides
are identified as Pr4 ($\approx$65,000 daltons), Pr3 ($\approx$80,000 daltons), two
closely migrating polypeptides termed Pr2a+b ($\approx$90,000 daltons), and two
closely migrating polypeptides termed Pr1a+b ($\approx$200,000 daltons). After a
15 min chase, two changes were evident (Fig. 1B). First, p30 was detected,
and secondly Pr3 began to disappear. After a 30-min chase (Fig. 1C), Pr3
had almost completely disappeared and p30 became a prominently labeled
polypeptide. After a 60-min chase (Fig. 1D) Pr4 began to disappear and
p30 increased further. Two of the three polypeptide bands in the Pr1
region (Pr1a+b) began to disappear after a 30-min chase whereas a slower
migrating polypeptide near those two did not disappear. After a 4-hr
chase (Fig. 1E) only the above-mentioned slowly migrating polypeptide was
discernible. In recent experiments using anti-RLV serum absorbed with uninfected cell proteins, either two or three bands were detected in the Pr1
region when samples were analyzed in 6-12% or 6-20% gradient gels (Fig. 4).
The third band is termed Pr1c because it is related to Pr1a+b as shown by
tryptic digestion and mapping experiments. With respect to Pr2a+b, it
usually did not decrease following chases up to 2 hr. However, Pr2a+b
did finally begin to decrease in amount after a 4 hr chase period (Fig. 1D).

The results of these pulse-chase experiments indicate that Pr1a+b, Pr2a+b, Pr3, and Pr4 are unstable polypeptides and thus are possible precursors to mature viral polypeptides (both structural and functional).

RLV-Specific Glycoproteins. As mentioned above, Pr2a+b have the properties of glycoproteins. The evidence for this conclusion is as follows. RLV-infected JLS-V16 cells were labeled for 5½ hr with ^{14}C-glucosamine to detect viral glycoproteins. The cytoplasmic extract was divided into two portions, one portion was treated with anti-RLV serum and the second was treated with anti-gp69/71 serum. The immune precipitates were analyzed by SDS-PAGE. The anti-RLV serum precipitated two major bands corresponding to gp69/71 and Pr2a+b (Fig. 2C). Other minor ^{14}C-glucosamine-labeled bands were also observed. The anti-gp69/71 serum precipitated both gp69/71 and a wide band migrating with Pr2a+b; very few other ^{14}C-glucosamine-labeled bands were observed (Fig. 2D). The Pr2a+b band can usually be resolved into two bands, particularly when low amounts of protein are applied to 8% or 10% SDS polyacrylamide gels (see Fig. 1).

In order to compare the viral specific glycoproteins to amino acid labeled viral specific proteins, RLV-infected JLS-V16 cells were pulse-labeled with a ^{14}C-amino acid mixture for 10 min. ^{35}S-methionine labeling was not done because p15, p10 and (as seen below) gp69/71 are deficient in methionine. The viral specific proteins were isolated by specific immune precipitation with anti-RLV serum and the analyzed by SDS-PAGE (Fig. 2B). Polypeptides Pr2a+b, Pr3, and Pr4 as well as minor amounts of Pr1a+b were formed in the 10 min pulse-labeling. None of the mature structural proteins were detected. A 90 min chase incubation (Fig. 2E) with cold excess amino acids showed that Pr3 disappeared, as expected, and Pr4 decreased in amount, while bands corresponding to gp69/71, p30, p15E and p15 were formed. It should be pointed out here that p12 and p10 are difficult to detect in cells after a pulse-chase with a ^{14}C-amino acid mixture; but that polypeptides p15E and p12E are readily observed in ^{35}S-methionine pulse-chase experiments and p10 is readily detected by labeling with radioactive arginine and lysine.

Since anti-gp69/71 serum specifically precipitated two glucosamine labeled polypeptides corresponding to polypeptides Pr2a+b and gp69/71, it was of interest to determine whether anti-gp69/71 serum would in fact precipitate the amino acid-labeled gp69/71 and Pr2a+b. Infected JLS-V16 cells were labeled for 5½ hr with either ^{14}C-amino acids or ^{35}S-methionine. The cytoplasmic extracts were either treated with anti-RLV serum or anti-gp69/71 serum. The results with ^{14}C-amino acid-labeled extracts revealed that anti-gp69/71 serum did indeed precipitate mainly Pr2a+b and gp69/71. Labeling RLV-infected cells with ^{35}S-methionine showed that gp69/71 did not appear to be strongly labeled with ^{35}S-methionine, indicating that gp69/71 is deficient in methionine (see ref. 19 for details).

To determine whether Pr2a+b and gp69/71 are in fact viral specific polypeptides, we labeled uninfected and RLV-infected JLS-V16 cells with ^{14}C-glucosamine and analyzed the anti-RLV immune precipitates by SDS-PAGE. The results of this experiment showed that both these glycoproteins are present in RLV-infected cells (Fig. 3B) but not in uninfected cells (Fig. 3A). We note that uninfected JLS-V16 cells do not contain any of the major viral specific proteins, and do not produce detectable amounts of virus particles (7).

Fucose Content of RLV-Specific Glycoproteins. RLV-infected JLS-V16 cells were pulse-labeled for 5½ hr with ^{3}H-fucose or ^{14}C-glucosamine (Fig. 3C-F). The cytoplasmic extracts were immune precipitated and the precipitates were analyzed by SDS-PAGE. The results revealed that both Pr2a+b and gp69/71 contained glucosamine and that Pr2a+b is deficient in fucose whereas the gp69/71 component contained fucose.

295

The glycoproteins of purified RLV were also examined (Fig. 3G and H). Virion gp69/71 was labeled when RLV-infected JLS-V16 cells were incubated with either ^{3}H-fucose or ^{14}C-glucosamine. No labeled Pr2a+b was detected in purified virus preparation.

We conclude from these results that Pr2a+b is a methionine-containing glycoprotein deficient in fucose; it is viral specific but not present in virions. By comparison, viral glycoprotein gp69/71 is deficient in methionine and contains both fucose and glucosamine and is seen in both infected cells and virus but not in uninfected cells.

A Summary of the Analysis of Tryptic Maps of RLV Precursors and Mature Structural Proteins. To determine whether Pr1a+b, Pr2a+b, Pr3 and Pr4 contained mature structural viral protein sequences, we analyzed tryptic digests of these polypeptides by ion exchange chromatography on Chromo Bead Type P columns (see ref. 18 for details). Initially, we chose to label the proteins with either ^{3}H-methionine or ^{35}S-methionine in order to first simplify the complexity of the peptide patterns of high molecular weight polypeptides, and second, to allow simultaneous analysis of the precursor labeled with ^{35}S-methionine and mature proteins labeled with ^{3}H-methionine. The main drawback of such an approach is that gp69/71, p15 and p10 are deficient and possibly lack methionine, and therefore, these proteins could not be considered. Precursors were isolated from RLV-infected JLS-V16 cells whereas mature viral proteins were purified from virus produced in JLS-V5 cells. The results of these studies (18) showed that p30 sequences are present in Pr1a+b, Pr3 and Pr4. More recent experiments (unpublished results) have shown that this same p30 methionine-containing tryptic peptide fraction is found in two minor intracellular precursors termed Pr5 ($\approx$55,000 daltons) and Pr6 ($\approx$45,000). Viral p12E and the polypeptide termed p15E {$\approx$17,000 dalton (5,18)} have the same methionine-containing tryptic peptide fraction which is also found in Pr2a+b (18,19). Recently, a tryptic digest of ^{3}H-arginine and ^{3}H-lysine-labeled p15E was fractionated on ion exchange column along with a ^{14}C-arginine and ^{14}C-lysine-labeled tryptic digest p12E. The result showed that p15E was indeed a precursor to p12E, since all tryptic peptides of p12E were also present in p15E.

We should emphasize that the p12 region of polyacrylamide gels contains two proteins. These two proteins can be separated by chromatography on guanidine-HCl agarose columns in which p12E remains aggregated with p15E, gp69/71 and other components and thus elutes in the void volume (19). The other p12 elutes between p15 and p10 in such an analysis. P12E and p12 contain different methionine-containing tryptic peptides, the latter being acidic. In addition the total map of p12E compared to p12 as well as the tyrosine-labeled maps are very different. In addition p12 is phosphorylated whereas p12E appears not to be (28; Karshin, unpublished results).

In order to determine which precursors contained gp69/71, p15, p12 and p10, the proteins were labeled with a mixture of amino acids labeled with either ^{3}H- or ^{14}C. The results showed that gp69/71 peptide sequences are present in Pr2a+b (19) and p15, p12 and p10 sequences are present in Pr3 and Pr4 (Arcement, Karshin, Naso, and Arlinghaus, unpublished results). Pr5 (55,000-57,000 daltons) lacked tryptic peptides characteristic of p10. Thus, Pr5 contained p12, p15 and p30. Pr6 contained tryptic peptides characteristic of p30 and p12 but not p15 or p10. In summary: Pr2a+b is a precursor to gp69/71, p15E and p12E (19) while Pr1a+b, Pr3 and Pr4 are precursors to p30, p15, p12 and p10.

Effect of Protease Inhibitors on the Formation and Cleavage of RLV Precursor Polypeptides. The results of our previous experiments are con-

sistent with the model that Prla+b is cleaved to yield Pr3, which is
further processed to Pr4 (18). Since p30 and the other mature viral proteins can be formed during the chase experiment in the presence of cyclo-
heximide at concentrations that inhibit protein synthesis 98% (4,18), it
seems reasonable to expect that proteolytic enzymes are involved in the
processing of RLV precursor polyproteins. Therefore, several protease inhibitors of the chloromethyl ketone type were tested in RLV-infected cells
by addition of the inhibitors 5 min prior to and during the pulse-labeling
with ^{35}S-methionine. The effects of such inhibitors on precursor processing have been tested in cells infected with poliovirus (29) and Sindbis
virus (30). In these studies, TPCK (tolylsulfonyl-phenylalanyl chloromethyl ketone) was found to be effective in blocking the cleavage of viral
specific precursor polypeptides present in cells infected with either
virus. In our experiments, viral specific polypeptides were immune precipitated with anti-RLV serum absorbed with excess proteins from uninfected JLS-V16 cells (7). Treatment with TPCK (0.1 mM), an inhibitor of
chymotrypsin, resulted in the enrichment of Prla+b while simultaneously
causing a reduction of Pr3 and Pr4 (Fig. 4A and B). Prla was always increased more than Prlb. Usually, the ratio of Pr3 to Pr4 was increased by
TPCK treatment (see Fig. 4A, B, and C), indicating that the conversion of
Pr3 to Pr4 was affected also. Pr2a+b was sharply reduced in amount by
TPCK treatment, and usually several polypeptides with molecular weights in
excess of 200,000 daltons were also observed in variable amounts in the
presence of TPCK. High molecular weight polypeptides of similar molecular
weight also seem to accumulate during chase experiments in the absence of
inhibitors. The nature of these polypeptides is unknown.

To determine whether Prla+b accumulating in the presence of TPCK
was specifically precipitated by anti-RLV serum, we absorbed the anti-RLV
serum with excess RLV proteins (7), and used it to precipitate proteins
from TPCK-treated extracts. The results indicated that no significant
amount of protein was precipitated and thus most if not all the labeled
polypeptides precipitated by anti-RLV serum present in TPCK-treated cells
shared antigenic properties with viral proteins and were specifically
precipitable by the anti-RLV serum.

Comparison of the Effects of TPCK, TLCK and ZPCK on the Formation
of RLV Precursor Polyproteins. Since TPCK, a chymotrypsin inhibitor, was
effective in causing a buildup of Prla+b, it was of interest to determine
the effect of TLCK (tolylsulfonyl-lysyl chloromethyl ketone, a trypsin inhibitor) on the formation of RLV precursors. The results indicated that
TLCK (0.1 - 1.0 mM, Fig. 4C) did not enrich the pulse-labeled extract
in Prla+b. This result implies that the factor or factors involved in
the processing of Prla+b to Pr3 may be chymotrypsin-like in its specificity.
To provide further information on this point, the effects of L-ZPCK
(carbobenzyloxy-phenylalanyl chloromethyl ketone) and D-ZPCK were tested.
The former inhibits chymotrypsin whereas the latter does not. The results
indicated that both compounds at 0.1 mM caused an enrichment in Prla+b and
a reduction in Pr3 and Pr4 when they were added prior to and during the
pulse-labeling. This finding prevents any conclusion about the specificity of the enzyme involved in the cleavage of Prla+b. Since D-ZPCK inhibits thiol-type proteases (29), further work must be done on these
enzymes to check their involvement (see ref. 31 for further information).

Presence of the Reverse Transcriptase in Prla+b. Our results are
consistent with a model (18) that depicts Prla+b and Pr2a+b as primary
gene products, and together they represent the entire coding capacity (or
nearly so) of the 35S RLV genome. Prla+b differs from Pr2a+b both chemically, as determined by peptide mapping, and immunologically, as determi-

297

ed by use of monospecific sera prepared against p30 and gp69/71 (19). Since gp69/71 and p12E can account for nearly all the peptide sequences in Pr2a+b and since Pr3 only accounts for 40% of Prla+b, the most likely candidate for the precursor to the RLV reverse transcriptase (RT) is Prla+b. Purified RT from RLV grown in JLS-V9 cells was kindly provided by Dr. Takis Papas of N.C.I. This enzyme is 95-98% pure and migrated as a single band in SDS-polyacrylamide gels. Its molecular weight was estimated to about 70,000.

In an effort to determine if Prla+b contains the RT polypeptide, RLV-infected cells were treated with 0.1 mM TPCK 5 min prior to and during the pulse-labeling with ^{35}S-methionine to enrich the extract in Prla+b (Fig. 5). TPCK, as expected, caused a buildup of Prla+b (Fig. 5B) using anti-RLV serum absorbed with excess protein from uninfected cells. Anti-p30 also precipitated Prla+b in addition to Pr3 and Pr4 (Fig. 5C) whereas anti-RT serum* precipitated Prla+b but not Pr3 and Pr4 (Fig. 5D). These striking results provide evidence that Prla+b contains determinants shared by RT. The tryptic map of the candidate RT precursor (Prla+b) and RT itself will be compared to determine whether Prla+b polypeptides in fact actually do share peptide sequences with purified RT.

Recent experiments involving pulse-labeling in the absence of TPCK and using anti-RT serum absorbed with excess virion structural proteins indicated that Prla+b is cleaved in the pulse to yield RT-specific precursors Pr RT1 ($\approx$145,000 daltons) and Pr RT2 ($\approx$135,000 daltons). During the chase, the above anti-RT serum detected a third polypeptide, Pr RT3 ($\approx$85,000 daltons). In the chase the Prla+b polypeptides were not detected while Pr RT1 was strongly reduced in amount and Pr RT2 was increased. The amount of RT-specific precursors synthesized (Pr RT1, 2, and 3) was about equal in amount to Prla+b while both Prla+b and RT-specific precursors were made in amounts of 1/10 to 1/20 that of Pr3 (the structural protein precursor). Pr3 and Pr2a+b (the envelope protein precursor) were made in roughly equal amounts. These results are presented in more detail in Jamjoom et al. (31).

DISCUSSION

It is clear from the results presented here and from data previously published (4,7,18-20) that Rauscher leukemia viral structural proteins are made in infected cells by way of high molecular weight polyproteins. Fig. 6 illustrates a working model for the biosynthesis of RLV proteins. In this model, Prla+b, Pr2a+b and Pr3 are considered to be primary gene products derived by translation of 35S viral RNA. Pr3 is thought to arise by translational control mechanism in which ribosomes detach from the 35S viral messenger RNA after translating Pr3. However, the ribosome can proceed on to translate the polymerase gene in one out of 10 to 20 times to yield Prla+b. Prla+b thus is cleaved to form RT-specific proteins (Pr RT1, 2 and 3) and possibly Pr3 (31).

Viral proteins p30, p15, p12, p10 and RT are contained in Prla+b and viral proteins gp69/71 and p12E are present in Pr2a+b. Prlb is thought to be derived from Prla by proteolytic cleavage or some other post-translational alteration. Pr2a and Pr2b are assumed to have the same core polypeptide which is glycosylated to different extents during or after translation to produce either Pr2a or Pr2b. The bulk of the polypeptides p30, p15, p12 and p10 are generated by a series of cleavages of Pr3

---

*Prepared against partially purified RT by Dr. Strickland via Dr. G. Vande Woude of N.C.I.

producing Pr4, Pr5 and Pr6 in that order. Viral p10 is produced during the cleavage of Pr4 to Pr5; viral p15 is derived from the cleavage of Pr5 to Pr6. Viral p30 and p12 are produced by the cleavage of Pr6.

Recent experiments using both pactamycin treatment (23) and high salt treatment of infected cells (32) have allowed a tentative ordering of viral precursor polyproteins relative to the 5' end of the 35S viral RNA. Pulse-chase experiments carried out in the presence of 10^{-6} M pactamycin added 10-60 seconds prior to pulse-labeling with ^{35}S-methionine indicated that p30 is N-terminal to p15E. Since p30 is in the Pr1a+b and p15E is in Pr2a+b, this suggests that Pr1a+b is N-terminal to Pr2a+b. Pulse-labeling infected cells with ^{35}S-methionine after high salt treatment, which synchronizes translation of viral messenger RNA, results in Pr3 and Pr4 being labeled rapidly (within 1-2 min) and Pr2a+b being labeled later. The rapid appearance of p30 precursors suggests that the structural genes (gag) are the first polypeptides synthesized upon synchronized re-initiation and therefore are N-terminal to the reverse transcriptase in Pr1a+b. Both types of experiments can only be interpreted this way if it is assumed that the 35S viral RNA is the only messenger RNA (there being no subset messenger RNAs) and the 35S viral RNA has only one initiation site.

The model also shows the presence of one unidentified polypeptide in Pr3, termed pY. The evidence for its existence stems from tryptic mapping studies and accurate molecular weight determinations of precursor polypeptides and mature structural proteins. It is obviously not known what function pY has. It certainly is not one of the major structural proteins.

We have deduced the order of some of the polypeptides in Pr3 by comparing patterns of tryptic digests of precursors with those of p15 and p10 labeled under two sets of conditions. Tryptic digestion of proteins produces peptides containing C-terminal arginine or lysine. Labeling polypeptide with both radioactive arginine and lysine will label each tryptic peptide except the C-terminal peptide (unless it also happens to contain a C-terminal arginine or lysine). Labeling with a radioactive amino acid hydrolysate will label all tryptic peptides including the C-terminal peptide fragment. The C-terminal tryptic peptide of p15 and Pr5 were tentatively identified by this technique and found to be the same indicating that p15 is on the C-terminal end of Pr5. Since this same peptide fragment was not found in digests of Pr4, and p10 was removed from Pr4 upon cleavage to Pr5, it follows that p10 is C-terminal in Pr4 and p15 is penultimate to p10 in Pr4. Other findings suggest that p30 and p15 are adjacent thereby yielding the order shown in Fig. 6.

Gp69/71 and p15E are generated by cleavage of Pr2a+b (Fig. 6). Fucose and possibly other sugar residues are added to the subglycosylated form of gp69/71 either prior to and immediately after cleavage. Viral protein p15E is further cleaved and/or altered to form p12E.

Our results, both from cell-free (19,20) and whole cell systems (4,18) are consistent with the concept that Rauscher leukemia viral proteins result from the translation of a polycistronic messenger RNA by a mechanism in which ribosomes can initiate translation only at one site on the viral messenger RNA (19,20). It appears that two size classes of viral messenger RNAs exist (10,11), a 20S and a 35S class. The 20S class could be a subset of the 35S class in that it represents the 3' third of the 35S viral RNA. We suggest the 20S class of viral RNA is translated to yield the viral envelope proteins. We further propose that the 35S class (the viral genomic RNA) is translated to yield mainly Pr3 but in one case out of 10-20 cases Pr1a is translated. The latter (Pr1a) is cleaved to yield RT (31).

SUMMARY

Rauscher murine leukemia viral structural proteins were shown to be synthesized in infected cells by way of high molecular weight precursor polyproteins identified as Prla+b ($\approx$200,000 daltons), Pr2a+b ($\approx$90,000 daltons), Pr3 ($\approx$80,000 daltons), Pr4 ($\approx$65,000 daltons), Pr 5 ($\approx$55,000 daltons) and Pr6 ($\approx$45,000 daltons). Tryptic peptide mapping experiments have shown that p30 is contained in precursors Prla+b and Pr3 through Pr6. Viral protein p12 is also present in Pr3 through Pr6. Viral protein p15 peptide sequences are present in Pr3 through Pr5 whereas p10 is contained in Pr3 and Pr4. P10, p12, and p15, like p30, then must originate from Prla+b. Tryptic peptides of viral gp69/71 and p12E are found in Pr2a+b and not in Prla+b. Our results indicate that the viral reverse transcriptase is contained in Prla+b and in three RT-specific precursors, termed Pr RT1 ($\approx$145,000 daltons), Pr RT2 ($\approx$135,000 daltons) and Pr RT3 ($\approx$85,000). Treatment of infected cells with inhibitors of proteolytic enzymes, such as TPCK, caused a buildup of Prla+b and prevented the formation of mature structural proteins and RT. A model for the biosynthesis of Rauscher viral proteins is presented. The main feature of this model is that a translational control mechanism exists which results in synthesis of a much lower amount of RT than viral structural proteins.

ACKNOWLEDGEMENTS

We acknowledge the expert technical assistance of Mrs. Elena Leroux and Mr. James Syrewicz. This work was supported in part by a grant (CA-15495) and a contract (CP-61017) from the National Cancer Institute and by a grant from The Robert A. Welch Foundation (G-429). W. L. Karshin is a postdoctoral fellow supported by The Robert A. Welch Foundation. G. A. Jamjoom is a predoctoral fellow supported by Riyad University, Saudi Arabia.

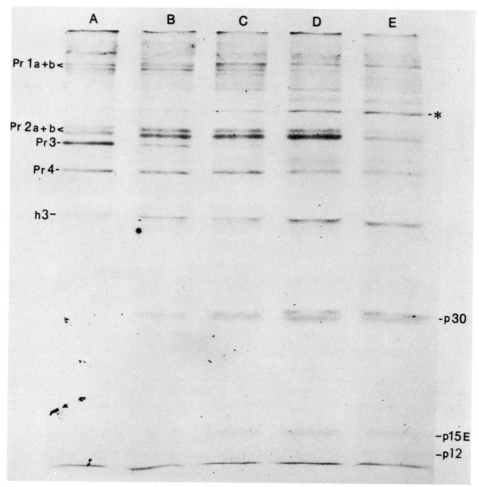

FIG. 1. Kinetics of formation and disappearance of RLV precursor polypeptides. RLV-infected JLS-V16 cells were pulse-labeled for 15 min (column A) with ^{35}S-methionine, and replicate cultures were incubated in excess non-radioactive culture fluid for 15 min (column B), 30 min (column C), 60 min (column D), and 4 hr (column E). The cytoplasmic extracts were treated with anti-RLV serum and the immune precipitates were analyzed by SDS-PAGE on a 10% slab gel. Similar amounts of radioactivity were applied to each well (9,000 cpm).

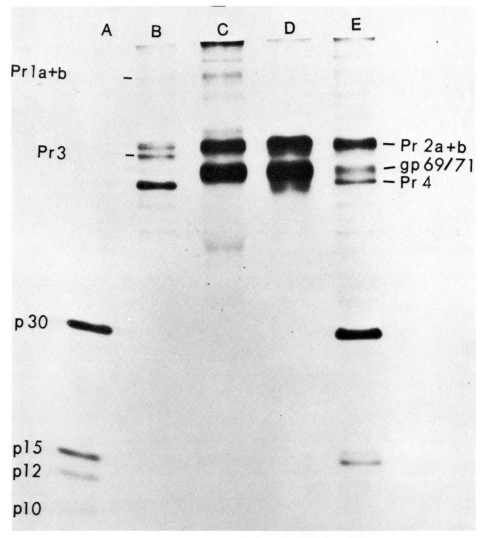

FIG. 2. Analysis of RLV-specific glycoprotein from virus-infected JLS-V16 cells. Cytoplasmic extracts from RLV-infected JLS-V16 cells were prepared in the presence of 0.5% NP-40 and DOC and immune precipitation was performed with either rabbit anti-RLV serum or goat anti-gp69/71 serum. The immune precipitates were applied to a 10% SDS polyacrylamide slab gel. After electrophoresis, the gel was fixed, treated with 2,5-diphenyloxazole (PPO), dried and finally overlaid on x-ray film for 4 days (33). Column A, purified ^{14}C-amino acid-labeled RLV produced in JLS-V5 cells; column B, anti-RLV immune precipitate of a 10 min pulse-labeling with ^{14}C-amino acid-labeled protein hydrolysate; column C, anti-RLV immune precipitate of 5½ hr labeling with ^{14}C-glucosamine; column D, anti-gp69/71 precipitate of a 5½ hr labeling with ^{14}C-amino acids followed by a 90 min chase with cold excess amino acid immune precipitated with anti-RLV serum.

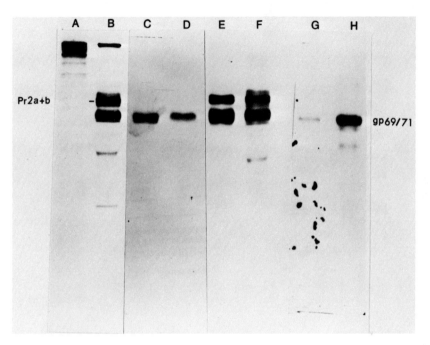

FIG. 3. SDS-PAGE of viral-specific glycoproteins from uninfected and RLV-infected JLS-V16 cells and from purified virus. Cytoplasmic extracts prepared as in Fig. 1 from uninfected cells (column A) and RLV-infected cells (column B) were labeled for 5½ hr with ^{14}C-glucosamine, and the anti-RLV immune precipitates were analyzed as in Fig. 1. Cytoplasmic extracts from RLV-infected cells were labeled with ^{3}H-fucose and the anti-gp69/71 immune precipitate (column C) or anti-RLV immune precipitate (column D) was analyzed as in Fig. 1. RLV-infected cells were labeled for 5½ hr with ^{14}C-glucosamine and the anti-gp69/71 immune precipitate (column E) or the anti-RLV immune precipitate (column F) was analyzed. Columns G and H are ^{3}H-fucose-and ^{14}C-glucosamine-labeled purified virus, respectively, obtained from RLV-infected JLS-V16 cells after a 5½ hr labeling.

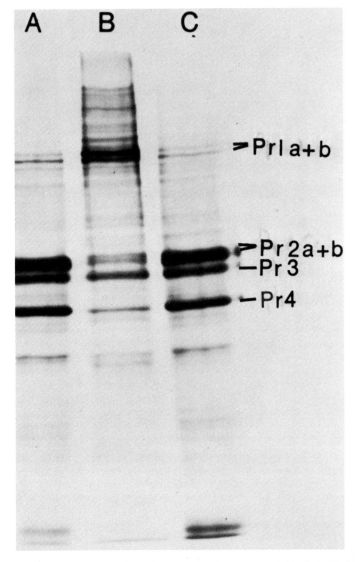

FIG. 4. Buildup of Pr1a+b by the protease inhibitor TPCK. Column A:
RLV-infected cells were incubated for 5 min at 37° in 5 ml of Hank's
balanced salt solution prior to pulse-labeling with ^{35}S-methionine for 15
min. The cytoplasmic extract was prepared as in Fig. 1 and viral specific
proteins were precipitated with anti-RLV serum absorbed with excess uninfected cell proteins (18). The proteins were analyzed by electrophoresis
on a 6-12% linear gradient slab gel of polyacrylamide in SDS. The gel
was analyzed by the flourography technique of Laskey and Mills (33).
Column B: RLV-infected cells were pretreated with 0.1 mM TPCK in Hank's
solution for 5 min at 37° prior to a 15 min pulse-labeling with ^{35}S-
methionine performed in the presence of 0.1 mM TPCK. Viral proteins were
isolated and fractionated as in A. Column C: RLV-infected cells were
treated as in B except that 0.1 mM TLCK was used.

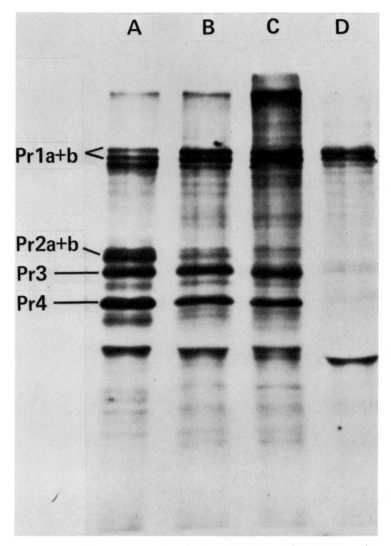

FIG. 5. Immune precipitation of extracts from TPCK-treated RLV-infected cells with antiserum that inhibits RLV reverse transcriptase. Column A: RLV-infected cells were incubated for 5 min in Hank's salt solution prior to a 15 min pulse-labeling with ^{35}S-methionine. The anti-RLV immune precipitate was analyzed on 6-12% gradient gels (Fig. 4). The anti-RLV serum was previously absorbed with excess uninfected cell proteins (18). Column B: Same as in A, except that 0.1 mM TPCK was added 5 min prior to and during the pulse-labeling. Column C: Same as B, except that anti-p30 serum was used to precipitate the proteins. Column D: Cells were treated with 0.1 mM TPCK as in B, and the proteins were precipitated by the antiserum to RT by addition of 0.03 ml of anti-RT goat serum, followed by a 30-fold excess of rabbit anti-goat IgG.

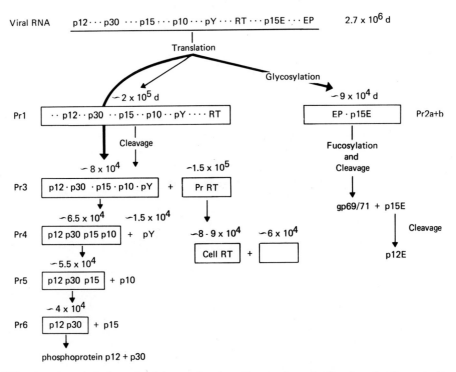

FIG. 6. A model for the biosynthesis of rauscher leukemia viral proteins.

REFERENCES

1. August, J.T., Bolognesi, D.P., Fleissner, E., Gilden, R.V., and Nowinski, R.C. A Proposed Nomenclature for the Virion Proteins of Oncogenic RNA Viruses. Virology 60: 595-601, 1974.

2. Duesberg, P.H., Martin, G.S., and Vogt, P.K. Glycoprotein Components of Avian and Murine RNA Tumor Viruses. Virology 4: 631-646, 1970.

3. Moroni, C. Structural Proteins of Rauscher Leukemia Virus and Harvey Sarcoma Virus. Virology 47: 1-7, 1972.

4. Naso, R.B., Arcement, L.J., and Arlinghaus, R.B. Biosynthesis of Rauscher Leukemia Viral Proteins. Cell 4: 31-36, 1975.

5. Ikeda, H., Hardy, Jr., W., Tress, E., and Fleissner, E. Chromatographic Separation and Antigenic Analysis of Proteins of the Oncornaviruses. V. Identification of a New Murine Viral Protein, p15(E). J. Virol. 61: 53-61, 1975.

6. Ihle, J.M., Hanna, Jr., M.G., Schaeffer, W., Hunsmann, G., Bolognesi, D.P., and Huper, G. Polypeptides of Mammalian Oncornaviruses III. Localization of p15 and Reactivity with Natural Antibody. Virology 63: 60-67, 1975.

7. Jamjoom, G., Karshin, W.L., Naso, R.B., Arcement, L.J., and Arlinghaus, R.B. Proteins of Rauscher Murine Leukemia Virus: Resolution of a 70,000 Dalton, Nonglycosylated Polypeptide Containing p30 Peptide Sequences. Virology 68: 135-145, 1975.

8. Delius, H., Duesberg, P.H., and Mangel, W.F. Electron Microscope Measurements of Rous Sarcoma Virus RNA. Cold Spring Harbor Symposia on Quantitative Biology 39: 835-843, 1974.

9. Blair, C.D., and Duesberg, P.H. Structure of Rauscher Mouse Leukemia Virus RNA. Nature 220: 396-399, 1968.

10. Fan, H., and Baltimore, D. RNA Metabolism of Murine Leukemia Virus: Detection of Virus-Specific RNA Sequences in Infected and Uninfected Cells and Identification of Virus-Specific Messenger RNA. J. Mol. Biol. 80: 93-117, 1973.

11. Schincariol, A.L., and Joklik, W.K. Early Synthesis of Virus-Specific RNA and DNA in Cells Rapidly Transformed with Rous Sarcoma Virus. Virology 56: 532-548, 1973.

12. Butterworth, B.E., Hall, L., Stoltzfus, C.M., and Rueckert, R.R. Virus-Specific Proteins Synthesized in Encephalomycarditis Virus-Infected HeLa Cells. Proc. Nat. Acad. Sci. U.S.A. 68: 3083-3087, 1971.

13. Cancedda, R., Swanson, R., and Schlesinger, M.J. Effects of Different RNAs and Components of the Cell-Free System on In Vitro Synthesis of Sindbis Viral Proteins. J. Virol. 14: 652-663, 1974.

14. Clegg, J.C.S. Sequential Translation of Capsid and Membrane Proteins Genes of Alphaviruses. Nature 254: 545-455, 1975.

15. Jacobson, M.F., and Baltimore, D. Polypeptide Cleavage in the Formation of Poliovirus Proteins. Proc. Nat. Acad. Sci. U.S.A. 51: 77-84, 1968.

16. Simmons, D.T., and Strauss, J.H. Translation of Sindbis Virus 26D RNA and 49S RNA in Lysates of Rabbit Reticulocytes. J. Mol. Biol. 86: 397-409, 1974.

17. Summers, D.F., and Maizel, Jr., J.V. Evidence for Large Precursor Proteins in Poliovirus Synthesis. Proc. Nat. Acad. Sci. U.S.A. 59: 966-971, 1968.

18. Arcement, L.J., Karshin, W.L., Naso, R.B., Jamjoom, G.A., and Arlinghaus, R.B. Biosynthesis of Rauscher Leukemia Viral Proteins: Presence of p30 and Envelope p15 Sequences in Precursor Polyproteins. Virology 69: 763-774, 1976.

19. Naso, R.B., Arcement, L.J., Karshin, W.L., Jamjoom, G.A., and Arlinghaus, R.B. A Fucose-Deficient Glycoprotein Precursor to Rauscher Leukemia Virus gp69/71. Proc. Nat. Acad. Sci. U.S.A. 73: 2326-2330, 1976.

20. Jamjoom, G.A., Naso, R.B., and Arlinghaus, R.B. Selective Decrease in the Rate of Cleavage of an Intracellular Precursor to Rauscher Leukemia Virus p30 by Treatment of Infected Cells with Actinomycin D. J. Virol. 19: 1054-1072, 1976.

21. Naso, R.B., Arcement, L.J., Wood, T.C., Saunders, T.E., and Arlinghaus, R.B. The Cell-Free Translation of Rauscher Leukemia Virus RNA Into High Molecular Weight Polypeptides. Biochim. Biophys. Acta 383: 195-206, 1975.

22. Naso, R.B., Wang, C.S., Tsai, S., and Arlinghaus, R.B. Ribosomes From Rauscher Leukemia Virus-Infected Cells and Their Response to Rauscher Viral RNA and Polyuridylic Acid. Biochim. Biophys. Acta 324: 346-364, 1973.

23. Eisenman, R., Vogt, V.M., and Diggelmann, H. The Synthesis of Avian RNA Tumor Virus Structural Proteins. Cold Spring Harbor Symposia on Quantitative Biology 39: 1067-1075, 1974.

24. Vogt, V.M., and Eisenman, R. Identification of a Large Polypeptide Precursor of Avian Oncornavirus Proteins. Proc. Nat. Acad. Sci. U.S.A. 70: 1734-1738, 1973.

25. Vogt, V.M., Eisenman, R., and Diggelman, H. Generation of Avian Myeloblastosis Virus Sctructural Proteins by Proteolytic Cleavage of a Precursor Polypeptide. J. Mol. Biol. 96: 471-493, 1975.

26. Von der Helm, K., and Duesberg, P.H. Translation of Rous Sarcoma Virus RNA in a Cell-Free System From Ascites Krebs II Cells. Proc. Nat. Acad. Sci. U.S.A. 72: 614-618, 1974.

27. Syrewicz, J.J., Naso, R.B., Wang, C.S., and Arlinghaus, R.B. Purification of Large Amounts of Murine Ribonucleic Acid Tumor Viruses Produced in Roller Bottle Cultures. Applied Microbiol. 24: 488-494, 1972.

28. Pal, B.K., McAllister, R.M., Gardner, M.B., and Roy-Burman, P. Comparative Studies on the Structural Phosphoproteins of Mammalian Type C Viruses. J. Virol. 16: 123-131, 1975.

29. Summers, D.F., Shaw, E.N., Stewart, M.L., and Maizel, Jr., J.V. Inhibition of Cleavage of Large Poliovirus-Specific Precursor Proteins in Infected HeLa Cells by Inhibitors of Proteolytic Enzymes. J. Virol. 10: 880-840, 1972.

30. Pfefferkorn, E.R., and Boyle, M.K. Selective Inhibition of the Synthesis of Sindbis Virion Proteins by an Inhibitor of Chymotrypsin. J. Virol. 9: 187-188, 1975.

31. Jamjoom, G.A., Naso, R.B., and Arlinghaus, R.B. Further Characterization of Intracellular Precursor Polyproteins of Rauscher Leukemia Virus. Virology. In press.

32. Saborio, J.L., Pong, S-S, and Koch, G. Selective and Reversible Inhibition of Initiation of Protein Synthesis in Mammalian Cells. J. Mol. Biol. 85: 211-221, 1974.

33. Laskey, R.A., and Mills, A.D. Quantitative Film Detection of [3]H- and ^{14}C in Polyacrylamide Gels by Fluorography. Eur. J. Biochem. 56: 335-341, 1975.

POLY(C)- AND POLY(G)-RICH TRACTS IN THE RNA OF ONCORNAVIRUSES

Leo A. Phillips and Roy H. L. Pang
Laboratory of Viral Carcinogenesis
National Cancer Institute
Bethesda, Maryland 20014

I. INTRODUCTION

Poly(C)-rich sequences or tracts have been detected in the viral RNA of two subgroups of picornaviruses: cardioviruses (3, 8, 19) and foot-and-mouth disease viruses (3). Recently, we have reported the detection by polynucleotide agarose affinity chromatography the presence of poly(A)-, poly(C)-, and poly(G)-rich sequences in the viral RNA of two mammalian oncornaviruses: Rauscher murine leukemia virus (MuLV) from JLS-V9 cells and murine sarcoma positive-hamster helper positive viruses (S+H+) from HTG-1 hamster tumor cells (15, 16). However, little or no poly(G)-rich tracts have been detected in the viral RNA of oncornaviruses by hybridization (7) and binding to poly(C) fiber glass filters (9).

The present studies were initiated to determine the universality or prevalence of poly(C)- and poly(G)-rich tracts in the viral RNA of leukemia and sarcoma viruses. In this communication, we present evidence for the presence of poly(C)- and poly(G)-rich tracts in the viral RNA of avian, murine, hamster, feline, and primate oncornaviruses as detected by complementary binding to polynucleotide agarose affinity columns.

II. PROCEDURES AND MATERIALS USED

A. Procedures

The procedures used in these studies have been described: extraction and isolation of viral RNA (15-18); in vitro labeling of RNA with [dimethyl-^{3}H] sulfate (6, 11, 24); enzymatic cleavage of labeled viral RNA with RNase T$_1$ (15, 16, 22) and RNase C (16, 23); and polynucleotide agarose affinity chromatography of labeled viral RNA (12, 15, 16).

B. Oncornaviruses

Virus preparations, concentrated and purified from fresh harvested supernatant fluids of infected or transformed cells by double sucrose density gradient centrifugation containing approximately 10^{11} particles/ml, were obtained from either Electro-Nucleonics Laboratories (Bethesda, Md.) or Meloy Laboratories (Springfield, Va.).

III. RESULTS

A. Poly(C)-rich Tracts in Oncornavirus RNA.

Poly(G) agarose affinity columns were used to detect the presence of poly(C)-rich tracts in [dimethyl-^{3}H] viral RNA of leukemia and sarcoma viruses. The complementary binding results of chromatogrammed untreated and RNase T_1 treated viral RNA are indicated in Table I. The binding of the majority of the viral RNA to the poly(G) agarose columns ranged from 10% to 30%, in contrast to less than 3% noncomplementary binding of [^{3}H] polynucleotides (A, G, U).

B. Poly(G)-rich Tracts in Oncornavirus RNA

Poly(C) agarose affinity columns were used to detect the presence of poly(G)-rich tracts in [dimethyl-^{3}H] viral RNA of leukemia and sarcoma viruses. The complementary binding results of chromatogrammed untreated and RNase C treated viral RNA are indicated in Table II. The binding of the majority of the viral RNA to the poly(C) agarose columns ranged from 10% to 30%, in contrast to less than 1% noncomplementary binding of [^{3}H] polynucleotides (A, C, U).

IV. DISCUSSION

A. The Universaltity of Poly(C)- and Poly(G)-rich Tracts in Oncornavirus RNA

In the present studies, we have detected by polynucleotide agarose affinity columns the presence of poly(C)- and poly(G)-rich sequences or tracts in the in vitro labeled viral RNA of avian, murine, hamster, feline, and primate oncornaviruses; thus demonstrating the universality of these tracts in the RNA of leukemia and sarcoma viruses. We have also reported previously the detection of poly(A)-, poly(C)-, and poly(G)-rich sequences in the in vivo labeled viral RNA of Rauscher-MuLV and S+H+(HTG-1) viruses by polynucleotide agarose affinity columns (15, 16) and polynucleotide fiber glass filters (17). Poly(C)-rich tracts are not unique to the viral RNA of oncornaviruses for they have also been detected in the viral RNA of some picornaviruses (3, 8, 19). To our knowledge, other investigators have not reported the presence of poly(C)-rich tracts and little or no poly(G)-rich tracts in oncornavirus RNA by hybridization (7) and 1% or less by binding studies to poly(C) fiber glass filters (9).

B. Partial Characterization of Poly(C)- and Poly(G)-rich Tracts in Oncornavirus RNA

The chain length and base composition of excised poly(C)- and poly(G)-rich tracts from the viral RNA are being determined. Although we have published partial characterization of excised poly(C)- and poly(G)-rich tracts from Rauscher-MuLV and S+H+(HTG-1) viral RNA labeled in vivo with either [^{3}H] nucleotides (A, C, G, U) or [^{32}P] phosphorous (16). The RNase T_1 excised Poly(C)-rich tracts from the RNA of Rauscher-MuLV and S+H+(HTG-1) viruses has chain lengths of circa 42 and 48 nucleotides respectively (16).

C. Possible Role(s) of the Poly(C)- and Poly(G)-rich Tracts in the RNA of Oncornaviruses

The definitive role(s) of the poly(C)- and poly(G)-rich tracts in oncornavirus RNA have not been elucidated. We have proposed a genomic stabilizing role for these tracts (15, 16). The fact that heat dissociated or subunit viral RNA binds to poly(C) and poly(G) agarose affinity columns at a greater binding efficiency than does genomic viral RNA, suggests that poly(C):poly(G) interstrand hydrogen bonding exist between the viral RNA subunits (15) as depicted in our proposed genomic model for mammalian oncornaviruses (16).

Poly(C)- and poly(G)-rich tracts may also play a role in the transcription of oncornavirus RNA because of these findings: (a) RNA-dependent-DNA polymerase (reverse transcriptase) of avian myeloblastosis virus (AMV) has been purified by poly(C) agarose affinity columns (13) because of its binding affinity for poly(C) homopolymers; (b) reverse transcriptase can be competitively inhibited in vitro by polyribo-nucleotides (1, 25); and (c) poly(rC)·(dG)$_{12-18}$ can serve as a specific template-primer for reverse transcriptase (20, 27). It has also been suggested that poly(C) may be involved in the replication of some other viruses because of these findings: (a) Encephalomyocarditis virus-infected cells contain a viral specific polymerase which can utilize poly(C) homopolymers as templates (21); and (b) poly(C) homopolymers can also serve as templates for Qβ replicase (10, 26).

D. Potential Significance of the Poly(C)- and Poly(G)-rich Tracts of Oncornavirus RNA to Cancer

If it can be determined definitively that oncornavirus RNA contains specific polynucleotide sequences or tracts which are not present in nonviral messenger RNA of human cells, then it may be possible to make sequence specific drugs against the unique viral specific polynucleotide sequences or tracts to block transcription of the viral RNA into viral DNA by reverse transcriptase and to block translation of the viral RNA into viral proteins by the cellular ribosomes, while not affecting the translation of cellular nonviral messenger RNA into cellular proteins. If this selective blocking of viral RNA transcription and translation can be accomplished, a possible molecular approach to cancer theraphy may become a reality.

V. SUMMARY

Poly(C)- and poly(G)-rich sequences or tracts have been detected by complementary binding to poly(G) and poly(C) agarose affinity columns respectively in both untreated and RNase T_1 and RNase C treated [dimethyl-^{3}H] viral RNA of <u>avian</u>, <u>mouse</u>, <u>hamster</u>, <u>feline</u>, and <u>primate</u> oncornaviruses. The possible functions(s) of these tracts have been discussed and the potential significance of the tracts as related to a possible molecular approach to cancer theraphy has been explored.

VI. ACKNOWLEDGMENTS

The authors wish to thank James J. Park for his excellent technical assistance; Dr. Raoul E. Benveniste of the Viral Leukemia and Lymphoma Section, Laboratory of Viral Carcinogenesis, National Cancer Institute for RD-114 feline and the M-7 baboon viruses; and Drs. Daniel K. Haapala, Peter J. Fischinger, and Shigeko Nomura of the Virus Control Section, Laboratory of Viral Carcinogenesis, National Cancer Institute for their stimulating discussions and suggestions.

TABLE I. Poly(G) Agarose Affinity Chromatography of Leukemia and Sarcoma Viral RNA[1]

Viral RNA[2]	Percent binding	
	Untreated	RNase T$_1$ [3]
Avian		
Schmidt Ruppin-RSV[4]	31.7	26.3
Murine		
Moloney - MuLV[5]	11.0	–
Moloney - MSV[6]	10.9	10.1
Kirsten - MuLV	31.6	27.4
Kirsten - MSV	19.9	20.2
Rauscher - MuLV	32.5	13.4
Moloney - MuLV(IC)[7]	–	23.6
Hamster		
S+H+(HTG-1)[8]	12.5	22.8
Feline		
Richard - FeLV[9]	17.0	27.6
RD-114[10]	18.5	23.3
Primate		
M-7 baboon isolate[11]	12.1	10.5

[1] Viral RNA was chromatogrammed by poly(G) agarose columns as described by Pang and Phillips (15).

[2] Viral RNA was labeled in vitro with [dimethyl-^{3}H] sulfate as described by Gaubatz and Cutler (6)

[3] [Dimethyl-^{3}H] viral RNA was treated with RNase T$_1$ (22) at a final concentration of 20 units/ml at 37°C for 30 minutes as indicated (15).

[4] RSV is Rous sarcoma virus.

[5] MuLV is murine sarcoma virus.

[6] MSV is murine sarcoma virus.

[7] MuLV(IC) is murine leukemia virus isolate obtained from the Moloney leukemia-sarcoma virus complex (4).

[8] S+H+(HTG-1) is murine sarcoma positive-hamster helper positive virus complex (5).

[9] FeLV is feline leukemia virus.

[10] RD-114 is a probable feline endogenous oncornavirus (14).

[11] M-7 is a baboon oncornavirus isolate (2).

TABLE II. Poly(C) Agarose Affinity Chromatography of Leukemia and Sarcoma Viral RNA[1]

Viral RNA[2]	Percent binding	
	Untreated	RNase C[3]
Avian		
Schmidt Ruppin - RSV[4]	37.1	16.9
Murine		
Moloney - MuLV[5]	7.3	26.6
Moloney - MSV[6]	7.3	7.5
Kirsten - MuLV	22.4	22.10
Kirsten - MSV	24.7	18.4
Rauscher - MuLV	7.6	8.0
Moloney - MuLV(IC)[7]	12.3	6.7
Hamster		
S+H+(HTG-1)[8]	8.0	11.5
Feline		
Rickard - FeLV[9]	20.8	17.5
RD-114[10]	17.2	23.2
Primate		
M-7 baboon isolate[11]	6.6	9.3

[1] Viral RNA was chromatogrammed by poly(C) agarose columns as described Pang and Phillips (15).
[2] Viral RNA was labeled _in vitro_ with [dimethyl-^{3}H] sulfate as described by Gaubatz and Cutler (6).
[3] [Dimethyl-^{3}H] viral RNA was treated with human plasma ribonuclease, RNase C (23) at a final concentration of 8 units/ml at 25°C for 30 minutes as indicated (16).
[4-11] These have been described in Table I legend.

REFERENCES

1. Beaudreau, G.S., and Riman, J. Effets de divers acides ribonucleiques (RNA) sur l'activité de la polymérase diacide désoxyribonucléique (DNA-polymérase) associée a un ribovirus oncogene. C. R. Acad. Sci. Paris, 271: 1728-1731, 1970.

2. Benveniste, R. E., Lieber, M. M., Livingston, D. M., Sherr, C. J., Todaro, G. J., and Kalter, S. S. Infectious type-C virus isolated from a baboon placenta. Nature (London), 248: 17-20, 1974.

3. Brown, F., Newman, J., Stott, J., Porter, A., Frisby, D., Newton, C., Carey, N., and Fellner, P. Poly(C) in animal viral RNAs. Nature (London), 251: 342-344, 1974.

4. Fischinger, P. J., Moore, C. O., and O'Connor, T. E. Isolation and identification of a helper virus found in the Moloney sarcoma-leukemia virus complex. J. Natl. Cancer Inst., 42: 605-622, 1969.

5. Gazdar, A. F., Phillips, L. A., Sarcoma, P. S., Peebles, P. T., and Chopra, H. C. Presence of sarcoma genome in a "noninfectious" mammalian virus. Nature New Biol., 234: 69-72, 1971.

6. Gaubatz, J., and Cutler, R. G. Hybridization of ribosomal RNA labeled to high specific radioactivity with dimethyl sulfate. Biochemistry 14: 760-765, 1975.

7. Gillespie, D., Marshall, S., and Gallo, R. C. RNA of RNA tumor viruses contain poly(A). Nature New Biol. 236: 227-231, 1972.

8. Goodchild, J., Fellner, P., and Porter, A. G. The determination of secondary structure in poly(C) tract of encephalomyocarditis virus RNA with sodium bisulphite. Nucleic Acids Research 2: 887-895, 1975.

9. Green, M., and Cartas, M.: The genome of RNA tumor viruses contains polyadenylic acid sequences. Proc. Natl. Acad. Sci. USA 69: 791-794, 1972.

10. Kamen, R. Reconstitution of Qβ replicase lacking subunit α with protein synthesis-interference factor. Eur. J. Biochem., 31: 44-51, 1972.

11. Lawley, P. D., and Shah, S. A. Methylation of ribonucleic acid by the carcinogens dimethyl sulfate, N-methyl-N-Nitrosourea and N-methyl-N'-nitro-N-Nitrosoguanidine: comparison of chemical analyses at the nucleotide and base levels. Biochem. J., 128: 117-132, 1972.

12. Lindberg, V., Persson, T., and Philipson, L. Isolation and characterization of adenovirus messenger ribonucleic acid in productive infection. J. Virol., 10: 909-919, 1972.

13. Marcus, S. H., Modak, M. J., and Cavalieri, L. F. Purification of avian myeloblastosis virus DNA polymerase by affinity chromatography on polycytidylate-agarose. J. Virol 14: 853-859, 1974.

14. McAllister, R. M., Nicolson, M., Gardner, M. B., Rongey, R. W., Rasheed, S., Sarma, P. S., Huebner, R. J., Hatanaka, M., Oroszlan, S., Gilden, R. V., Kabigting, A., and Vernon, L. C-type virus released from cultured human rhabdomyosarcoma cells. Nature New Biol., <u>235</u>: 3-6, 1972.

15. Pang, R. H. L., and Phillips, L. A. Nucleotide sequences in the RNA of mammalian leukemia and sarcoma viruses. Biochem. Biophys. Res. Commun. <u>67</u>: 508-517, 1975.

16. Phillips, L. A., and Pang, R. H. L. The detection and character-ization of polynucleotide sequences in the RNA of mammalian oncornaviruses. <u>In</u>: Proceedings of the VIIth Int'L Symp. on Comparative Research on Leukemia and Related Diseases. <u>Ed</u>: J. Clemmesen. S. Karger, AG, Basel, Switzerland (In Press).

17. Phillips, L. A., Park, J. J., and Hollis, V. W., Jr. Polyribo-adenylate sequences at the 3'-termini of ribonucleic acid obtained from mammalian leukemia and sarcoma viruses. Proc. Natl. Acad. Sci. USA <u>71</u>: 4366-4370, 1974.

18. Phillips, L. A., Hollis, V. W., Jr., Bassin, R. H., and Fischinger, P. J. Characterization of RNA from noninfectious virions produced by sarcoma positive-leukemia negative transformed 3T3 cells. Proc. Natl. Acad. Sci. USA <u>70</u>: 3002-3006, 1973.

19. Porter, A., Carey, N., and Fellner, P. Presence of a large poly(rC) tract within the RNA of encephalomyocarditis virus. Nature (London), <u>248</u>: 675-678, 1974.

20. Robert, M. S., Smith, R. G., Gallo, R. C., Sarin, P. S., and Abrell, J. W. Viral and cellular DNA polymerase: comparison of activities with synthetic and natural RNA templates. Science <u>176</u>: 780-800, 1972.

21. Rosenberg, H., Diskin, B., Oron, L., and Traub, A. Isolation and subunit structure of polycytidylate-dependent RNA polymerase of encephalomyocarditis virus. Proc. Nat. Acad. Sci. USA <u>69</u>: 3015-3019, 1972.

22. Sato-Asano, K. Studies on ribonucleases in takadiastase. II. Specificity of ribonuclease T_1. J. Biochem., <u>46</u>: 31-37, 1959.

23. Schmukler, M., Jewett, P. B., and Levy, C. C. The effects of polyamines on a residue-specific human plasma ribonuclease. J. Biol. Chem. <u>250</u>: 2206-2212, 1975.

24. Smith, K. D., Armstrong, J. L., and McCarthy, B. J. The intro-duction of radioisotopes into RNA by methylation <u>in vitro</u>. Biochem. Biophys. Acta <u>142</u>: 323-330, 1967.

25. Tuominen, F. W., and Kenney, F. T. Inhibition of the DNA polymerase of Rauscher leukemia virus by single-stranded polyribonucleotides. Proc. Natl. Acad. Sci. USA <u>68</u>: 2198-2202, 1971.

26. Weber, H., Billeter, M. A., Kahane, S., Weissmann, C., Hindley, J., and Porter, A. Molecular basis for repressor activity of Qβ replicase. Nature New Biol. 237: 166-170, 1972.

27. Weissbach, A., Bolden, A., Muller, R., Hanafusa, H., and Hanafusa, T. Deoxyribonucleic acid polymerase activities in normal and leukovirus-infected chicken embryo cells. J. Virol. 10: 321-327, 1972.

ESTABLISHMENT OF A HUMAN HEPATOMA CELL LINE WHICH PRODUCES HEPATITIS B SURFACE ANTIGEN (HB$_s$Ag)

J. Alexander, E. Bey and G. Macnab[+]

Virus Cancer Research Unit,
Poliomyelitis Research Foundation,

and

[+]Department of Serology, South African Institute for Medical Research,
P.O. Box 1038,
Johannesburg, South Africa.

INTRODUCTION

Mozambique has the highest recorded incidence of primary liver cancer (hepatocellular carcinoma)[15]. Aflatoxins have been implicated in the etiology of the disease[14, 18], however it has also been suggested that hepatitis B virus (HBV) may play a role in the initiation or promotion of liver cancer[19]. Although HBV, causative agent of serum hepatitis, is a transmissable infection, primary liver cancer does not follow the pattern of an infectious disease[22].

A laboratory investigation was undertaken in an attempt to produce cell lines derived from this tumor so that biochemical and immunological studies could be initiated using a constantly available in vitro source of material. One aim of the study was to examine cell lines derived from these tumors for the presence of virus particles and viral antigens.

We report here the establishment of a liver tumor cell line and some of the in vitro characteristics including the production of HB$_s$Ag.

PROCEDURES AND MATERIALS

Tissue Culture.

Dr. E. Geddes (Crown Mines Hospital, Johannesburg) provided us, in June 1973, with tumor specimens removed at post mortem from the liver of a 24 year old Mozambiquan male with histologically proven primary liver cancer. HB_sAg had been detected previously in his blood. The material was processed for tissue culture by conventional techniques[1] and planted into 25 cm^2 flasks (Falcon Plastics). Growth medium was Eagles minimum essential medium containing 10% fetal bovine serum and 100 ug/ml each of penicillin and streptomycin. The flasks were incubated at 37^oC and examined daily for tumor cell attachment. Once this had occurred the growth medium was renewed every 2 to 3 days. Fibroblasts contaminating the cultures were initially mechanically removed; later differential trypsinization was used. For routine passage, once fibroblast-free cultures were obtained, a trypsin-versene solution was employed (0.125% trypsin in phosphate buffered saline containing 0.05% versene and 0.05% glucose).

Chromosome Analysis.

Fresh medium containing 2 ug/ml colchicine (BDH) was added to well growing cell cultures. This was replaced 3 hours later by 0.5% sodium citrate and after 15-20 minutes the cells detached from the surface and were harvested by centrifugation. Fixation and further procedures have been described elsewhere[2]. Sixty four complete chromosome spreads were photographed and analysed.

Enzyme Studies.

Cells were assayed for glucose-6-phosphate dehydrogenase, lactic dehydrogenase, hexokinase and pyruvate kinase isozymes[5].

Electron Microscopy.

Ultrastructural examination was carried out according to the procedure described by Mollenhauer[12]. Sections were viewed in a Philips EM 300 electron microscope.

HB$_s$Ag Determinations.

Radioimmunoassay (RIA) and reverse passive hemagglutination techniques
were used (Ausria 11 and Hepnosticon, Abbot Laboratories, Hepatest,
Burroughs Welcome). Disrupted hepatoma cells and culture medium in
contact with these cells were assayed. Supernatant medium from other
human cell lines and cell cultures maintained under identical conditions
were also tested. All assays were performed under code and positive
results were confirmed by specific neutralization. For quantitative
determinations, dilutions were made from an HB$_s$Ag standard (1,000 ug/ml,
ad serotype; a gift from Dr. L.R. Overby)[11], and assayed by RIA to
generate a standard curve. Supernatant medium from hepatoma cultures
was harvested daily for 8 days (day 7 excluded) and tested for HB$_s$Ag
activity. The cell counts in each flask were determined so that the rate
of antigen production on a per cell basis could be measured. Partial
purification of HB$_s$Ag-reactive material, produced by the hepatoma cells,
was carried out using ammonium sulfate, ultracentrifugation and ultrafiltration techniques.

RESULTS

Tissue Culture.

The cell line described here developed from one of the original 14 flasks
planted. This flask initially contained 10 to 20 attached tumor cell
fragments resembling small organ cultures (20 - 100 cells per fragment).
Epithelial cells migrated from the cell clumps and within a week mitotic
cells were evident. The cells adapted slowly to in vitro conditions.
From the fourth passage the cultures were free from contaminating fibroblasts. After 20 passages (18 months in culture) the cells were considered fully adapted as they could be stored frozen, thawed and growth
reinitiated. Morphologically the cells are polygonal, vary in size and
resemble hepatocytes in culture[21] (Figure 1). At present the cells have
been in continuous culture for 30 months, the plating efficiency is 45%
and the generation time is 35 to 40 hours. The cells do not cease
growth in confluent cultures, however many cells become detached from
the surface and are dead as judged by trypan blue uptake.

Chromosome Analyses.

The chromosome pattern is male and human. A numerical chromosome analysis of 64 complete spreads showed a distribution of 52 to 61, with a mean number of 56.6. Additional chromosomes appear in C, E and F groups, and also as markers. Ninety three percent of all plates have chromosomes missing in the D group and 75% have lost more than one chromosome in the G group. In 80% of the spreads an apparent D/G fusion was identified.

Enzyme Studies.

The enzymes conform to the human pattern and the cells contain the glucose-6-phosphate dehydrogenase type A isozyme.

Electron Microscopy.

The cells contain glycogen granules. Microvilli and smooth endoplasmic reticulum are common. There is no evidence of virus particles of any type in the cells, nor is there any sign of lesions commonly associated with hepatitis-infected liver cells[10].

Hb$_s$Ag Determinations.

Trace levels were detected in washed disrupted whole cells and in cell debris precipitated from culture supernatants. Spent medium however gave high readings. Figure 2 depicts the quantitatively assayed levels of HB$_s$Ag measured in the supernatant medium over an 8 day period. The levels of antigen increase with time and the antigen is produced at approximately 500 ug/day/10^6 cells. HB$_s$Ag-activity is associated with material which sediments at 200,000 g/4 hr but not at 100,000 g/1 hr. All activity is retained by filtration through an XM 300 filter (Amicon) and the activity is precipitated in 50% saturated ammonium sulfate solutions. The material has a buoyant density in CsCl of between 1.18 and 1.2 g/cm^3. Immune electron microscopy of material prepared by the above methods shows low grade clumping of spherical particles ranging in diameter from 16 to 24 nm although the majority are 20 nm in size. No tubular forms or Dane particles have been seen.

DISCUSSION

Cultured liver tissue from patients with HB$_s$Ag in their blood has been shown to result in the presence of the antigen in the tissue culture fluid[4]. Hepatitis B core antigen (an internal component of the Dane particle) has been detected in liver slices taken from a patient with liver cell carcinoma and cirrhosis, however the antigen was present only in the cirrhotic tissue[8]. A human hepatoma cell line, established by Prozesky et. al.[16] contains no HB$_s$Ag activity and does not support the replication of HBV (Prozesky, personal communication). However the clinical association between HB$_s$Ag and primary liver cancer is well documented[9,19,20] and the patient from whose tumor this cell line was established had circulating HB$_s$Ag. The production of this antigen by a cell line derived from primary liver cancer adds some support to the suggestion that this tumor may be the end result of a process beginning with HBV infection[19], but does not rule out the possibility that other agents contribute to the initiation of the disease. Much of the previous work on the _in vitro_ production of HB$_s$Ag has begun with the infection of cells in culture[23], but the short-term nature of these experiments and the lack of a constant source of tissue culture material has not provided a standardized _in vitro_ system for the study of HBV. The cell line described here produces HB$_s$Ag-reactive material without superinfection which suggests a close association between the genetic material determining the production of HB$_s$Ag and the hepatoma cells, which may parallel the association found between the production of Epstein-Barr virus antigens and some lymphoma cell lines[7]. It is of interest that Burkitt lymphoma cases occur with high frequency in areas which are not too distant from Mozambique.

Because of the complex biochemical nature of HB$_s$Ag[6] it is unlikely that the reported molecular weight of the putative infectious particle (1.6×10^6)[17] contains sufficient genetic material to code for all the antigenic determinants associated with HBV. It has been suggested that the infectious agent may be classed among the viroids[22]. If this is so, the hepatoma cells described here may contain one or a few viroid DNA molecules but insufficient to code for the complete range of antigens. On the other hand, the suggestion that HB$_s$Ag could represent a modified cellular component[3,13], may explain the absence of any detectable virus particles in the tumor cells although HB_sAg activity in the supernatant medium is associated with small, amorphous particles. Further studies on the _in vitro_ production of HB_sAg by the hepatoma cell line may provide answers to some of these questions and may also lead to a clearer understanding of the relationship between HB_sAg and primary liver cancer.

Since it is advisable to compare this cell line with others which may subsequently become established from primary liver cancers we have designated this one PLC/PRF/5.

SUMMARY

A cell line has been established from a primary liver carcinoma and has been in continuous culture for 30 months. Morphologically the cells resemble hepatocytes and contain no viral particles. The isozyme pattern and the karyology are human. The modal chromosome number is 56.6 and markers are present. The cells produce HB_sAg which is detected predominantly in supernatant culture fluid. The levels of antigen produced are approximately 500 ng/10^6 cells/day. HB_sAg activity in culture supernatant is associated with amorphous particles ranging in size from 16 to 24 nm.

Acknowledgements

We thank Dr. E. Geddes for supplying the tumor material and the histological diagnosis, Dr. D. Balinsky for the enzyme assays and Dr. G. Lecatsas for electron microscopy. The work was supported by the South African Medical Research Council, the National Cancer Association, the South African Institute for Medical Research and the Poliomyelitis Research Foundation.

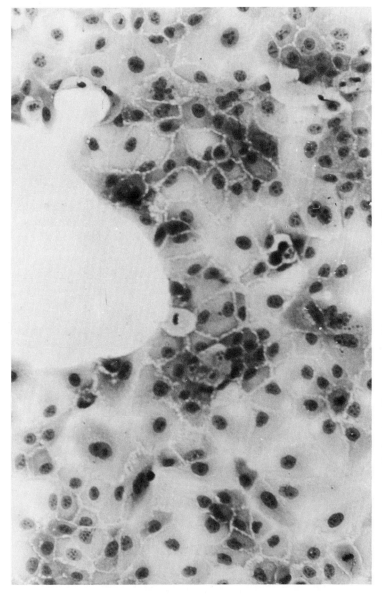

FIG. 1. Hepatoma cells, passage 20. Giemsa stained.

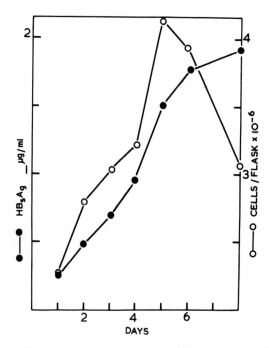

FIG. 2. Levels of HB$_s$Ag-reactive material in hepatoma cell culture supernatants over an eight day period, and the number of cells per flask. Each
point is the average recorded from 3 separate samples. Five ml supernatants were harvested from each flask.

REFERENCES

1. Alexander, J., Bey, E., Whitcutt, J., and Gear, J. Adaptation of cells derived from human malignant tumors to growth in vitro. S. Afr. J. Med. Sci. (in the press).

2. Bey, E., Alexander, J., Whitcutt, J., Hunt, J., and Gear, J. Carcinoma of the esophagus in Africans: Establishment of a continuously growing cell line from a tumor specimen. In Vitro (in the press).

3. Blumberg, B. Introduction and historical review. In Australia Antigen (J.E. Prier and H. Friedman, eds., London, Macmillan Press) pp 1-29 (1973).

4. Coyne, V., Blumberg, B., and Millman, I. Detection of Australia Antigen in human tissue culture preparations. Proc. Soc. Exptl. Biol. Med. 138, 1051-1057 (1971).

5. de Oca, F., Macy, M., and Shannon, J. Isozyme characterization of animal cell cultures. Proc. Soc. Exptl. Biol. Med. 132, 462-469 (1969).

6. Dreesman, G., Hollinger, F., and Melnick, J. Biophysical and biochemical properties of purified preparations of Hepatitis B surface antigen ($HB_s Ag$). Am. J. Med. Sci. 270, 123-129 (1975).

7. Epstein, M., Achong, B., and Barr, Y. Virus particles in cultured lymphoblasts from Burkett's lymphoma. Lancet i, 702-703 (1964).

8. Hadziyannis, S. Viral hepatitis: the agents (hepatitis B virus). Am. J. Med. Sci. 270, 208 (1975).

9. Kew, M., Geddes, E., Macnab, G., and Bersohn, I. Hepatitis B antigen and cirrhosis in Bantu patients with primary liver cancer. Cancer, 34, 539-541 (1974).

10. Krawezynski, K., Nazarewicz, T., Brzosko, W., and Nowoslawski, A. Cellular localization of hepatitis-associated antigen in livers of patients with different forms of hepatitis. J. Inf. Diseases 126, 372-377 (1972).

11. Ling, C., and Overby, L. Prevalence of hepatitis-B antigen virus antigen as revealed by direct Radioimmune Assay with 125 I-antibody. J. Immunol. 109, 834-841 (1972).

12. Mollenhauer, H., Plastic embedding mixtures for use in electron microscopy. Stain Techn. 39, 111-114 (1964).

13. Neurath, A., Prince, A., and Lippin, A. Hepatitis B antigen: antigenic sites related to human serum proteins revealed by affinity chromatography. Proc. Nat. Acad. Sci. (U.S.) 71, 2663-2667 (1974).

14. Oettlé A.G. Cancer in Africa, especially in regions South of the Sahara. J. Nat. Cancer Inst. 33, 383-439 (1964).

15. Prates, M. Malignant neoplasms in Mozambique. Br. J. Cancer 12, 177-194 (1958).

16. Prozesky, O.W., Brits, C., and Grabow, W. In "Liver", Proceedings of an International liver conference with special reference to Africa. (Saunders, S.J. and Terblanche, J., eds., Pitman Medical Books, London) pp 358-360 (1973).

17. Robinson, W., Clayton, D., and Greenman, R. DNA of a human hepatitis B virus candidate. J. Virol. 14, 384-391 (1974).

18. van Rensburg, S., van der Watt, J., Purchase, I., Pereira Coutinho, L., and Markham, R. Primary liver cancer rate and Aflatoxin intake in a high cancer area. S. Afr. Med. J. 48, 2508a-2508d (1974).

19. Vogel, C., Anthony, P., Mody, N., and Barker, L. Hepatitis-associated antigen in Ugandan patients with hepatocellular carcinoma. Lancet ii 621-624 (1970).

20. Williams, A. Hepatitis B surface antigen and liver cell carcinoma. Am. J. Med. Sci., 270, 53-56 (1975).

21. Zuckerman, A. Tissue culture of liver. In "Virus diseases of the liver". (Butterworths, London) 1970.

22. Zuckerman, A. Viral hepatitis, the B antigen and liver cancer. Cell. 1, 65-67 (1974).

23. Zuckerman, A. Tissue and organ culture studies of hepatitis B virus. Am. J. Med. Sci. 270, 197-204 (1975).

AN ELECTRONCYTOCHEMICAL STUDY OF 5'-NUCLEOTIDE PHOSPHO-
DIESTERASE IN HEPATOMA, CIRRHOSIS AND HEPATITIS

K. C. Tsou, K. W. Lo, J. E. Rhoads, and J. A. Mackie

Harrison Department of Surgical Research and Department of Surgery
School of Medicine, University of Pennsylvania
Philadelphia, Pennsylvania 19104

INTRODUCTION

Although primary hepatoma is rare in the United States, it is quite
common in Africa and Asia (1). The poor prognosis of this form of cancer
makes treatment difficult and identification of the mechanism of carcinogenesis an important task in cancer detection.

In recent years, the etiological relationship between hepatitis B and
hepatoma have been extensively studied by many laboratories. In countries
where the incidence of hepatitis is high, significantly higher incidence
of hepatitis B surface antigen (HB_SAg) have been found in the sera of
hepatoma patients (35-85%) than in the general population (2-15%) (2).
Several explanations have been offered for this observation. They include
: (a) A chain of events starting from viral hepatitis, passing through
post-necrotic scarring, nodular hyperplasia, and leading to hepatoma (3-6);
 (b) an intrinsic oncogenic potential of hepatitis B virus (6,7) or (c)
viral transformation of regenerating liver cells to develop hepatoma (3).
Continuous regeneration of liver cells are also known to occur in cirrhosis
of liver caused by diseases other than cancer (8), yet it is wellknown that
most hepatomas are associated with underlying cirrhosis (9-12). Thus,
there is a strong suggestion that the etiology of some hepatomas may be
intimately related to hepatitis B infection and cirrhosis, and that a
common marker to study these three liver diseases may be important for
such investigation.

Recently we have demonstrated that if serum proteins are separated
by polyacrylamide gel electrophoresis, there exists a common fast moving
(towards anode) isoenzyme-V of 5'-nucleotide phosphodiesterase (5'-NPDase)
in human sera of patients with hepatitis B (2), some cirrhosis (13), and
hepatoma (14,15). Hence, this enzyme could offer a useful clue to link
the etiology of hepatoma to hepatitis B related virus. Electronmicroscopic
studies have therefore been carried out on two biopsy proven human primary
hepatomas in order to search for viral-like particles related to this
etiological basis. Preliminary investigations of sera from hepatitis B
patients have also been carried out to see if the enzyme is associated
with the viral like particles that could be seen in such samples. The
results of these investigations are included in this report.

331

PROCEDURES AND MATERIALS USED

Preparation of Hepatoma Tissues for Electronmicroscopy

Hepatoma tissues from two patients were obtained at surgical removal of the tumors and were cut into 2 mm blocks immediately upon receiving, and fixed in 3% glutaraldehyde in 0.25 M sucrose at 4° C overnight. The tissues were then rinsed in 0.25 M sucrose, incubated with substrates for 5'-nucleotide phosphodiesterase as described recently (16), and /or post-fixed with 1% OsO_4 in 0.1 M phosphate buffer (pH 7.4) at room temperature for two hours, dehydrated through the various grades of alcohol, cleared in propylene oxide shortly and then embedded in Epon. Ultrathin sections were obtained with a Porter-Blum MT-2 microtome. These sections were placed on copper grids and examined with an RCA EMU-4A electronmicroscope after staining with uranyl acetate and lead citrate.

Tissue diagnosis at light microscope level were done at the Surgical Pathology Laboratory through the courtesy of Professor H. T. Enterline, and they were both classified as well-differentiated hepato-cellular carcinoma.

Testing for 5'-Nucleotide Phosphodiesterase-V (5'-NPDase-V), alpha-Fetoprotein (α-FP), and Hepatitis B Surface Antigen (HB$_S$Ag)

5'-NPDase-V was determined by polyacrylamide gel electrophoresis as described recently (14,15). α-FP was determined by counterimmunoelectro-phoresis (CIEP) and calibrated with a reference standard provided by the International Agency for Research on Cancer (Lyon, France). Rabbit anti-αFP serum was obtained from Princeton Laboratories, Princeton, N. J. HB$_S$Ag was determined by both CIEP (17) and a radioimmunoassay method (18).

Immuno-electronmicroscopy and Electrocytochemical Study on Hepatitis B Sera

Twenty µl of HB$_S$Ag positive hepatitis serum was treated with an equal volume of anti-HB$_S$Ag (Spectra Biologicals, Oxnard, California) for two hours at 37°, and then overnight at 4°. The mixture was then spun in a Coleman microcentriguge and the precipitate was washed three times with 0.9% saline. Two tubes of each serum sample were prepared. The precipitate in one tube was incubated at 37° for one hour with 100 µl of 5'-NPDase substrate solution consisting of 2 mg each of ammonium 5-iodo-indolyl 5'-thymidylate and ammonium 5-nitroindolyl 5'-thymidylate in a mixture of 2.5 ml. of 2 M NaCl and 6 ml. of 0.05 M Veronal buffer (pH 8.5), rinsed once in saline and then resuspended in 100 µl of saline (16). This suspension was then sprayed onto formvar coated copper grids, washed care-fully with a drop of deionized water, and then examined with a RCA electron microscope-4A immediately.

Some grids were also negatively stained with 3% phosphotungstic acid adjusted to pH 6.5 with 2M KOH for one minute and then rinsed three times with deionized water. The precipitate in the duplicate tubes were not incubated with substrate but were resuspended only in saline and negatively stained as above.

RESULTS

Electronmicroscopy of Hepatoma

Electronmicroscopic observation of the two hepatomas show large nuclei seen in other tumor cells. Some nuclei are also of irregular shape. At higher magnifications, clusters of virus-like particles of about 25 nm size are found in the nuclei (Fig. 1) of patient A. This patient's serum was found to be negative for HB_SAg test by RIA, but positive for 5'-NPDase-V and αFP (400 ng/ml.). Among the interesting features of the cytoplasmic organelles are an abundance of vesicular membranes, circular in shape, and often surrounding the mitochondria (Fig. 2). The mitochonria show aberrations in shape and internal structure. This feature is seen also in the cirrhotic regions of both patients.

The 5'-NPDase activity appears as a dense stain on the nuclear membrane and occasionally inside the nucleus (Fig. 1). Cytoplasmic activity can be assigned to the Golgi vesicles and plasma membrane activity appears in only a very small number of the cells. Even though the observations are limited, nuclear membrane stain and plasma membrane stain are never found in the same cell. There can also be found morphologically sometimes an extension of membrane formation in the vicinity of the nuclear envelope (Fig. 2 and inset). This cistern often contains a whirlpool like figure which seems to enclose a particle of 50 nm in size. These structures are also discernible in the cytoplasm elsewhere (Fig. 2). Even though mitotic cells are not often easy to find under the electronmicroscope, in patient A tissue, such cells can be readily seen. In these cells, mitotic spindles and the vesicles mentioned above are present. Because of the current limitation of the method, it is difficult to determine whether the 5'-NPDase activity is found in the chromosomal regions in such cells.

In the vicinity of the mitotic cells, there are observed spherical particles 88 nm in size in the intercellular space area (Fig. 3), or budding from the cell (Fig. 1). It must also be noted that it is difficult to determine whether 5'-NPDase activity is associated with these particles. While this indigogenic cytochemical method does give an increase in electrondensity in areas where there is high enzyme activity, it is not easy to use this method for areas of low enzyme activity. Such must be the case in the present art of determing enzyme activity associated with viral like particles. On the other hand, the indigo deposits surrounding the particles as a result of enzymatic hydrolysis may contribute to the slightly larger size observed under the electronmicroscope. Ma and Blackburn (19) did report recently in a hepatoma such 80 nm particles.

Because of the fact that the serum of patient B is also negative for HB_SAg and normal for αFP (10ng/ml.), but positive for 5'-NPDase-V, we had expected this sample to be negative for viral like particles. Nevertheless, the vesicular structures and the enclosed particles are seen. However, the 80 nm intercellular particles are definitely less frequently seen.

Immunoelectronmicroscopy of Hepatitis Sera

Negative staining of immune precipitate of HB_SAg positive hepatitis sera showed spherical virus-like particles, ranging in size from 38 to 49 nm, with a dense inner core (Fig. 4). The majority of these particles are about 42 nm in diameter. These particles are similar to those reported by Dane et al. (20) and others (21-23). When the negative staining is done in the presence of substrate for 5'-NPDase, larger particles (45 to 68 nm) are observed (Fig. 5). Some of these particles are oval in shape. The slightly larger size of these particles may be related to the indigo deposit as a result of the enzyme activity.

DISCUSSION

Because of the low incidence of primary hepatoma in many parts of the world, there have been few studies on both the ultrastructure (19, 24-31) and electron cytochemistry (30) of human hepatomas. It is hoped that this paper illustrates that such study is feasible.

In this study, we have demonstrated the association of the exonuclease, 5'-NPDase, in virus-like particles similar to Dane particles in hepatitis serum and other virus-like particles in human hepatoma. Phosphodiesterase activity has also recently been shown to be associated with myxo- and paramyxoviruses by biochemical assay (32).

The second aspect of this work lies in the finding of the presence of 5'-NPDase on the nuclear envelope of the tumor cells. This does not imply that the enzyme is synthesized and stored there. On the other hand, it is clear that they must exert an influence on the chromatin and perhaps affect the cell division. The appearance of this enzyme on the nuclear envelope of Morris hepatoma has also been reported from this laboratory (16,33).

The presence of spherical particles of 20-25 nm in diameter in liver cell nucleus of HB_SAg associated hepatitis has been demonstrated by a number of workers (34-41). These particles are generally believed to be the uncoated cores of the hepatitis B virus (37,38,41). The clusters of particles we observed in the nucleus of the hepatoma of patient A are probably related to these uncoated cores. It must be pointed out that this represents the first time that these particles are observed in a patient seronegative in HB_SAg.

A survey of the literature indicates that there are only two reports on the observation of virus-like particles in human primary hepatoma. Theron et al. (24) found virus-like particles about 240 nm in diameter in a South African Bantu patient. Ma and Blackburn (19) reported spherical or oval particles ranging in size from 70 to 120 nm (average 80 nm) in a hepatoma patient. These particles were found to have electron dense "nucleoid" and disperse free in the cytoplasm. The particles we observed in the intercellular space (Fig. 3) are similar in size to those reported by Ma and Blackburn (19). It is of interest to note that virus-like particles in our work are more electron-lucent in the core. Whether this was the result of different methodology as the substrate incubation step in our method would produce a more electron dense envelope remains to be further tested.

It must also be emphasized that the appearance of viral-like particles in hepatoma does not indict the role of such particles to cause cancer. However, one must bear in mind that the larger number of hepatitis cases vs. the small number of hepatoma cases would suggest that there is either no relationship between the two diseases or perhaps the host-immune response is so overwhelming that the majority of people in the hepatitis group were actually immunized against this form of viral infection. We have observed that the chronic hepatitis patients have in their sera in general higher 5'-NPDase-V isozyme. This observation supports the data we found in the association of this enzyme with the HB_SAg immune complex. We suggest therefore that 5'-NPDase may be a core protein in the virus. The hepatitis B virus has been demonstrated to be a DNA containing virus (42-44), and a virus specific DNA polymerase was found associated with the viral core (45-47). The cooperative role of this exonuclease with DNA polymerase suggests a possible function for this exonuclease in viral infection, i.e. the exonuclease helps to expose the segment of DNA to be used as template by the DNA polymerase. The close association of exonucleases with DNA polymerase in procaryotic system has been elucidated by Kornberg (48). Whether this suggestion withstands further testing with additional experimentation. should now be important. At least, one must accept that the appearance of this marker enzyme in these three groups of patients will further aid in defining interrelationships of these three groups of patients.

SUMMARY

An isozyme of 5'-nucleotide phosphodiesterase has been found in human sera of patients with hepatitis B, some cirrhosis, and hepatoma. This enzyme therefore offers a useful clue to link the etiology of hepatoma to hepatitis B related virus.

Electron microscopic studies have therefore been carried out on two biopsy proven human hepatomas in order to search for this important etiological clue. The sera of these two patients were both positive for 5'-NPDase-V, but alpha-fetoprotein levels were normal in one (10 ng/ml), and HB_SAg was negative in both sera. The presence of viral-like particles resembling those for hepatitis B described by other workers were, however, found in these two tumors. In cirrhotic livers, such particles could also be seen, but more often than not, they are found enclosed in vesicles in the cytoplasm. These findings suggest an important role for this serum marker enzyme for etiological study of liver cancer.

The association of this exonuclease with the viral particles was then tested in sera of hepatitis B patients. Using an indigogenic electron cytochemical method for the demonstration of this enzyme activity, deposits could be found on the particles obtained by the precipitation of hepatitis B serum with anti-HB_SAg. These data support the view that there may be a group of human hepatomas etiologically linked to hepatitis B associated virus, and that some cirrhosis may be a reflection of the host-immune response to the viral proliferation. A possible role for this exonuclease in hepatitis B infection is also suggested.

ACKNOWLEDGMENT

This work has been done in part with U.S. Public Health Grant CA 07339 to K. C. Tsou.

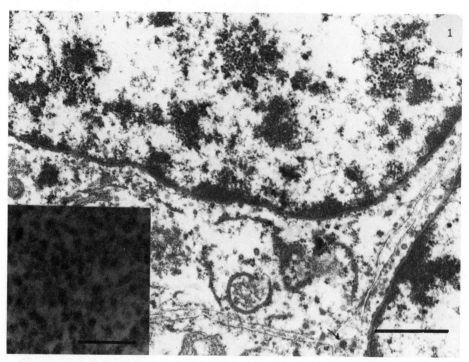

FIG. 1. Cluster of virus-like particles in nucleus of hepatoma of patient A. The nuclear membrane is highly stained for 5'-NPDase. Enzyme activities are also found in the nucleus. Note the budding of a virus-like particle (arrow) from the cell on the lower righthand corner. Scale marker = 1 μm. Inset: higher magnification of the intranuclear cluster of virus-like particles. Scale marker = 0.2 μm.

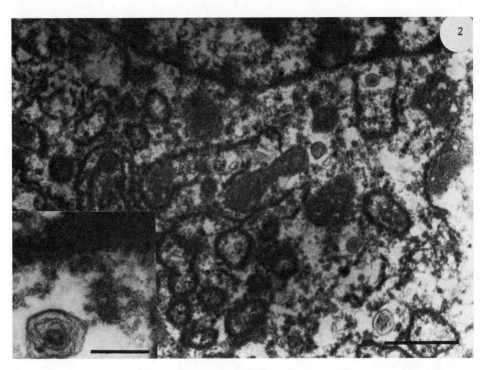

FIG. 2. Virus-like particle surrounded by "whirlpool" structure in cistern
at vicinity of nucleus. Other "whirlpool" structures are also found free
in the cytoplasm. Note the vesicular membranes enclosing the mitochondria.
Hepatoma of patient A stained for 5'-NPDase. Scale marker = 1 μm. Inset:
higher magnification of "whirlpool" structure in cistern at vicinity of
nucleus. Scale marker = 0.2 μm.

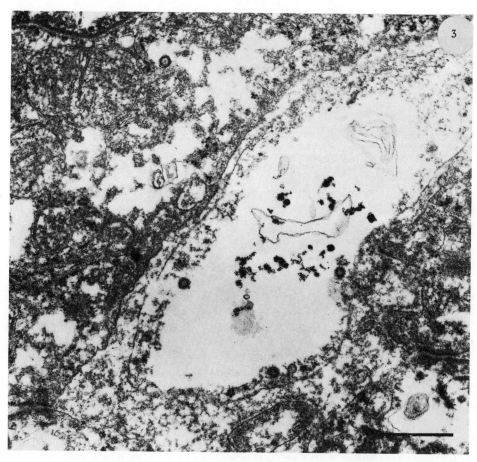

FIG 3.   88 nm particles in intercellular space of hepatoma of patient A
stained for 5'-NPDase.   Scale marker = 1 μm.

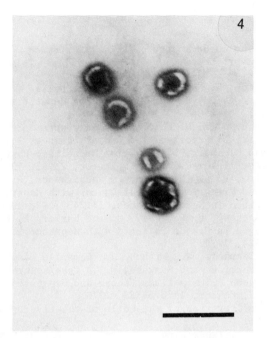

FIG. 4. Negative staining of virus-like particles of immune precipitate of HB_SAg positive hepatitis serum. Scale marker = 0.1 μm.

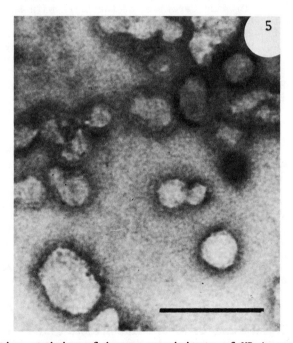

FIG. 5. Negative staining of immune precipitate of HB_SAg positive hepatitis serum after incubation with 5'-NPDase substrate. Scale marker = 0.1 μm.

REFERENCES

1. Higginson, J. The Epidemiology of Primary Carcinoma of the Liver. In: Tumors of the Liver. Eds.: G. T. Pack and A. H. Islami. Springer-Verlag, New York, pp. 38-52, 1970.
2. Tsou, K. C., McCoy, M. G., Lo, K. W. and London, W. T. 5'-Nucleotide Phosphodiesterase Isoenzyme in Patients with Hepatitis B Infection. Cancer Res., 35:2361-2364, 1975.
3. Walshe, J. M. and Wolff, H. H. Primary Carcinoma of the Liver Following Viral Hepatitis. Report of Two Cases. Lancet, 2:1007-1010, 1952.
4. Smith, J. B. and Blumberg, B. S. Viral Hepatitis, Post-Necrotic Cirrhosis and Hepatocellular Carcinoma. Lancet, 2:953, 1969.
5. Sherlock, S., Fox, R. A., Niazi, S. P. and Scheuer, P. J. Chronic Liver Disease and Primary Liver Cell Cancer with Hepatitis Associated (Australia) Antigen in Serum. Lancet, 1:1243-1247, 1970.
6. Vogel, C. L., Anthony, P. P., Mody, N. and Barker, L. F. Hepatitis Associated Antigen in Uganda Patients with Hepatocellular Carcinoma. Lancet, 2:621-624, 1970.
7. Prince, A. M., Szmuness, W., Michon, J., Demaille, J., Diebolt, G., Linhard, J., Quenum, C. and Sankale, M. A Case/Control Study of the Association Between Primary Liver Cancer and Hepatitis B Infection in Senegal. Int. J. Cancer, 16:376-383, 1975.
8. Muir, R. On Proliferation of the Cells of the Liver. J. Path. Bact., 12:287-305, 1908.
9. MacDonald, R. A. Cirrhosis and Primary Carcinoma of the Liver - Changes in their Occurrence at the Boston City Hospital 1897-1954. New Engl. J. Med., 255:1179-1183, 1956.
10. Ying, Y. Y., Ma, C. C., Hsu, Y. T., Lei, H. A., Liang, S. F., Lin, C. H. and Ku, C. Y. Primary Carcinoma of the Liver with Special Reference to Histogenesis and its Relationship to Liver Cirrhosis. Chin. Med. J. (Taipei), 82:279-294, 1963.
11. Sagebiel, R. W., McFarland, R. B. and Taft, E. B. Primary Carcinoma of the Liver in Relation to Cirrhosis. Amer. J. Clin. Pathol., 40:516-520, 1963.
12. Lin, T. Y. Primary Cancer of the Liver - Quadrennial Review. Scand. J. Gastroenterol., 5(Suppl.):223-241, 1970.
13. Tsou, K. C., McCoy, M. G., Enterline, H. T., Herberman, R. and Wahner, H. 5'-Nucleotide Phosphodiesterase Isoenzyme and Hepatic Cancer in NCI-Mayo Clinic Panel Sera. J. Natl. Cancer Inst., 51:2005-2006, 1973.
14. Tsou, K. C., McCoy, M. G. and Ledis, S. 5'-Nucleotide Phosphodiesterase Isoenzyme Pattern in the Sera of Human Hepatoma Patients. Cancer Res., 33:2215-2217, 1973.
15. Tsou, K. C., McCoy, M. G. and Lo, K. W. An Isoenzyme of 5'-Nucleotide Phosphodiesterase and alpha-fetoprotein in Human Hepatic Cancer Patient Sera. Cancer Res., 34:2459-2463, 1974.
16. Tsou, K. C. 5'-Nucleotide Phosphodiesterase. In: Electron Microscopy of Enzymes - Principles and Methods. Vol. 4. Ed.: Hayat, M. A. Van-Nostrand-Reinhold, New York. pp. 140-156, 1975.
17. Gocke, D. J. and Howe, C. Rapid Detection of Australia Antigen by Counterimmunoelectrophoresis. J. Immunol., 104:1031-1032, 1970.
18. Purcell, R. H., Wong, D. C., Alter, D. H. and Holland, P. V. A Microtiter Solid-Phase Radioimmunoassay for Hepatitis B Antigen. Appl. Microbiol., 26:278-480, 1973.
19. Ma, M. H. and Blackburn, C. R. B. Fine Structure of Primary Liver Tumors and Tumor-bearing Livers in Man. Cancer Res., 33:1766-1774, 1973

20. Dane, D. S., Cameron, C. H. and Briggs, M. Virus-like Particles in Serum of Patients with Australia-Antigen Associated Hepatitis. Lancet 1:695-598, 1970.

21. Gust, I. D., Cross, G., Kaldor, J. and Ferris, A. A. Virus-like particles in Australia Antigen Associated Hepatitis. Lancet, 1:953, 1970.

22. Solaas, M. H. Virus-like Particles in Serum of an Apparently Healthy AU/SH-Antigen Positive Blood Donor. Lancet, 2:151-152, 1970.

23. Zalan, E., Hamvas, J. J., Tobe, B. A., Kuderewko, O. and Labzoffsky, N. A. Association of Virus-like Particles with Australia Antigen in Serum of Patients with Serum Hepatitis. Canad. Med. Assocn. J., 104: 145-147, 1971.

24. Theron, J. J., Pepler, W. J. and Liebenberg, N. V. D. W. Virus-like Particles in the Cells of a Primary Carcinoma of the Liver. Nature, 194:489-490, 1962.

25. Yasutake, S. Fine Structure of Human Hepatoma. Kurume Med. J., 3: 193-204, 1962.

26. Ghadially, F. N. and Parry, E. W. Ultrastructure of a Human Hepatocellular Carcinoma and Surrounding Non-neoplastic Liver. Cancer, 19: 1989-2004, 1966.

27. Toker, C. and Trevino, N. Ultrastructure of Human Primary Hepatic Carcinoma. Cancer, 19:1594-1606, 1966.

28. Ruebner, B. H., Gonzalez-Licea, A. and Slusser, R. J. Electron Microscopy of Some Human Hepatomas. Gastroenterology, 53:18-30, 1967.

29. Creemers, J. and Jardin, J. M. Ultrastructure of a Human Hepatocellular Carcinoma. J. Microscop., 7:257-264, 1968.

30. Wills, E. J. Fine Structure and Surface Adenosine-Triphosphatase Activity of a Human Hepatoma. Cancer, 22:1046-1052, 1968.

31. O'Conor, G. T., Tralka, T. S., Henson, E. and Vogel, C. L. Ultrastructural Survey of Primary Liver Cell Carcinoma from Uganda. J. Natl. Cancer Inst., 48:587-603, 1972.

32. Pristasova, S. and Rosenbergova, M. Phosphodiesterase Activity Associated with Myxo- and Paramyxoviruses. Acta. Virol., 18:293-298, 1974.

33. Tsou, K. C., Hendricks, J., Gupta, P. D. and Lo, K. W. A New Indigogenic Method for the Light and Electron Microscopic Demonstration of 5'-Nucleotide Phosphodiesterases. Histochem. J., 6:327-337, 1974.

34. Nowostawski, A., Brzosko, W. J., Madalinski, K. and Krawczynski, C. Cellular Localization of Australia Antigen in the Liver of Patients with Lymphoproliferative Disorders. Lancet, 1:494-498, 1970.

35. Nelson, J. M., Barker, L. F. and Danovitch, S. H. Intranuclear Aggregates in the Liver of a Patient with Serum Hepatitis. Lancet, 2:773-774, 1970.

36. Scotto, J., Stralin, H. and Caroli, J. Etude de Particules D'aspect Viral et de Lesions Ultrastructuralles Variees dans des Hepatites Virales Essentiellement Graves. Rapport avec L'antigene Australia. Pathol. Biol., 19:489-496, 1971.

37. Ahmed, M. N., Huang, S. N. and Spence, L. Australia Antigen and Hepatitis: An Electron Microscopic Study. Arch. Pathol., 92:66-72, 1971.

38. Huang, S. N. Hepatitis-Associated Antigen Hepatitis. An Electron Microscopic Study of Virus-like Particles in Liver Cells. Amer. J. Pathol., 64:483-500, 1971.

39. Caramia, F., DeBac, C. and Ricci, G. Virus-like Particles within Hepatocytes of Australia Antigen Carriers. Amer. J. Dis. Child., 123: 309-311, 1972.

341

40. Almeida, J. D., Gioannini, P., Scalise, G. and Harrison, C. V. Electron Microscopic Study of a Case of Australia Antigen Positive Chronic Hepatitis. J. Clin. Pathol, 26:113-119, 1973.
41. Huang, S. M., Groh, V., Beaudoin, J. G., Dauphinee, W. D., Gutterman, R. D., Morehouse, D. D., Aronoff, A. and Gault, H. A Study of the Relationship of Virus-like Particles and Australia Antigen in Liver. Human Pathol., 5:209-222, 1974.
42. Hirschman, S. Z., Gerger, M. and Garfinkel, E. DNA Purified from Naked Intranuclear Particles of Human Liver Infected with Hepatitis B Virus. Nature, 251:540-542, 1974.
43. Overby, L. R., Hung, P. P., Mao, J. C.-H., Ling, C. M. and Kakefuda, T. Rolling Circular DNA Associated with Dane Particles in Hepatitis B Virus. Nature, 255:84-85,1975.
44. Robinson, W. S. DNA and DNA Polymerase in the Core of the Dane Particle of Hepatitis B. Amer. J. Med. Sci., 270:151-159, 1975.
45. Kaplan, P. M., Greenman, R. L., Gerin, J. L., Purcell, R. H. and Robinson, W. S. DNA Polymerase Associated with Human Hepatitis B Antigen. J. Virol., 12:995-1005, 1973.
46. Kaplan, P. M., Gerin, J. L. and Alter, H. J. Hepatitis B-Specific DNA Polymerase Activity During Post-transfusion Hepatitis. Nature, 249:762-764, 1974.
47. Krugman, S., Hoofnagle, Gerety, R. J., Kaplan, P. M. and Gerin, J. L. Viral Hepatitis, Type B. DNA Polymerase Activity and Antibody to Hepatitis B Core Antigen. New Engl. J. Med., 290:1331-1335, 1974.
48. Kornberg, A. DNA Synthesis. W. H. Freeman, San Francisco, 1974.

Chapter 4

IMMUNOLOGY

Section 1

FUNDAMENTAL IMMUNOLOGY

INCREASED INCIDENCE OF SPONTANEOUS LYMPHOMAS
IN THYMECTOMIZED MICE

Eugene A. Cornelius

Section of Nuclear Medicine
Department of Diagnostic Radiology
Yale University School of Medicine
New Haven, Connecticut

I. INTRODUCTION

The purpose of the present study was to examine the influence of
thymectomy on the incidence of spontaneous neoplasms in mice. Soon after
the explicit formulation by Thomas (1) of the idea that the immune
response is the principal defense against tumor cells, Burnet (2) elabo-
rated this concept into a theory of immunologic surveillance. Its central
theme is that the immune response destroys cancer cells while they are
still in the incipient stage of tumor formation. This theory was widely
accepted almost as fact for many years, but recently has been subjected to
critical reappraisal. Numerous reviews have been published, evaluating
the evidence pro and con. However, in view of the many different kinds of
cancer, it seems possible that the role of the immune apparatus will vary
with each. Thus the results of these experiments appear worthy of documentation.

II. PROCEDURES AND MATERIALS USED

A. Mice

(C57BL/1XA)F_1 hybrid mice [abbr. (BA)F_1] were used for most
experiments. Additional data was obtained using (SJL/JXC57BL/1)F_1 mice
[abbr. (SB)F_1].

B. Thymectomy

Mice were thymectomized (Tx) within 24 hours of birth, using a standard method (3). Control mice consisted of normal hybrids of the same age and sex.

C. Observation

Mice were observed weekly or more frequently up to 24 months of age.

D. Tumor Transplantation for Evaluation of Immunity

A lymphoma arising in a normal $(BA)F_1$ mouse was used. A 20% (weight/volume) suspension was prepared in lactated-Ringer's solution; 0.15 ml of this suspension was injected intraperitoneally into 6-day old Tx and control mice. The time of death from tumor growth was recorded.

E. Skin Grafts

Tx and control $(BA)F_1$ mice were grafted at 11 months of age with skin from 10-week old C57BL/6 mice of the same sex (non-H-2 barrier). The time of graft rejection was recorded.

F. Antiglobulin Reactions

A standard method was used (4).

G. Histological Studies

Complete necropsy studies were carried out on a group of 10 Tx and 10 control mice at 65-75 days of age. Thereafter, animals were sacrificed if moribund or if a tumor was detected clinically. Finally, 18 Tx and 20 control mice were autopsied at 24 months of age.

H. Preparation of Cell-Free Extracts of Tumors

A standard procedure was used (5). The extracts were injected into newborn B mice. These host mice were autopsied at 12-18 months of age.

I. Transplantation of Tumors Arising in Tx and Control Mice

These tumors were transplanted intraperitoneally into normal 20-day old $(BA)F_1$ mice. The dose was 0.4 ml of a 33% (weight/volume) suspension prepared in lactated-Ringer's solution.

346

III. RESULTS

A. Immunological Status of Thymectomized Mice

The transplanted lymphoma grew better in Tx mice than in normal controls. By 50 days after transplantation 35/36 (97.3%) of the Tx mice but only 7/25 (28.0%) of control mice had died as a result of tumor growth. Skin grafts were also better accepted by Tx mice. One year after grafting, 9 of 10 Tx mice demonstrated accepted grafts, whereas only 1 of 10 control mice exhibited an accepted graft.

B. Antiglobulin Reactions

Antiglobulin reactions on 25 Tx(BA)F_1 mice of various ages were uniformly negative. This group included 6 mice with anemia (hematocrit below 35%), 12 with skin lesions (see below), and 7 with tumor. Aged NZB control mice gave positive tests.

C. Clinical Findings

By 120 days, one third of Tx mice had died of the post-Tx wasting syndrome. Since deaths from this cause were infrequent thereafter, statistics of tumor incidence are based on 77 Tx mice alive at 120 days. There were 149 normal controls.

D. Tumor Incidence

The incidence of tumors is presented in Table I. Tx(BA)F_1 mice demonstrated an increased incidence of tumors, compared to normal control mice of the same age, by 8 months of age. The difference in incidence remained highly significant thereafter. At 22 months of age Tx mice had a tumor incidence rate five times that of control mice. At 24 months, the incidence of tumors in the controls had doubled over that at 22 months while in the Tx mice, the increase was less pronounced. As a result, the difference in the Tx and control groups, while significant, was not as great at 24 months as during the period from 8 to 22 months.

E. Pathological Findings

The pathological changes in Tx(BA)F_1 mice have been reported, without regard to temporal sequence (6). A rich variety of pathological changes was present - arteritis, myocarditis, synovitis, myositis, cellulitis,

347

amyloidosis, hepatic and pancreatic cellular infiltration, renal papillary necrosis, as well as mononuclear cellular infiltration of gut, ureter and skin. Lymphocytic depletion of the thymus dependent areas of lymph nodes and spleen was seen in about 10% of mice but most conspicuous was the presence of pronounced reticulum cell hyperplasia in these organs. The tumors were reticulum cell sarcomas with widespread infiltration. All of these changes have been observed during chronic graft-versus-host-reactions in $(BA)F_1$ mice (7), a model of autoimmune disease. When considered sequentially, the well-known changes of acute post thymectomy wasting were severe at 2 months but then regressed. Reticulum cell hyperplasia was maximal at 2-3 months, regressed somewhat but persisted. Arteritis, dermatitis and tumors first appeared at 4-7 months. In older Tx mice (17-23 months), tumors were highly malignant and infiltrated many organs.

Autopsy studies of Tx mice at 24 months of age confirmed the above findings of autoimmune changes (83%) and lymphomas (72%). However, the autoimmune changes were milder and the tumors, now mainly lymphosarcomas, were less widespread than in Tx mice autopsied at a younger age. Control mice of the same age demonstrated arteritis in 40%, non-thymic lymphosarcoma in 50% and thymic lymphomas in 40%. Pulmonary adenomas were slightly more frequent in the control mice; other solid tumors occurred only sporadically in both Tx and control mice.

Cell-free extracts (CFE) of tumors from Tx mice when injected into newborn B mice were associated, in 8 of 9 tumors, with a significant increase in tumor incidence in these B mice; tumor incidence for all CFE-injected mice was 19/52, compared to 2/88 for normal B mice of the same age.

Following transplantation of viable tumor into syngeneic normal $(BA)F_1$ mice, 6 of 7 tumors from normal control $(BA)F_1$ mice were accepted. By contrast, only 7 of 31 tumors arising in Tx mice were accepted.

Subsequent to these studies, 33 $Tx(SB)F_1$ and 34 normal $(SB)F_1$ mice, all females, have been followed to 18 months of age. In the interval from 10 to 14 months inclusive, tumor incidence in Tx mice was significantly higher than in controls. $Tx(SB)F_1$ mice demonstrated no autoimmune changes, and no reticulum cell hyperplasia but at 3-4 months of age had markedly enlarged spleens which demonstrated erythroblastic hyperplasia.

IV. DISCUSSION

Tx(BA)F$_1$ mice demonstrated widespread histologic changes which were practically identical to those in the same hybrid following the injection of parental strain spleen cells (7). The graft-versus-host-reaction has long been considered a model of autoimmune disease. Tx(AB)F$_1$ mice (the reciprocal hybrid) have also been found to develop antinuclear antibodies as early as 4 months of age (8). There is thus considerable support for the idea that the histologic changes in Tx(BA)F$_1$ mice have an autoimmune basis. Such mice also demonstrated a markedly increased incidence of lymphomas compared to normal control mice of the same age. This differ- ence was greatest before old age, at which time tumors became more fre- quent in normal control mice. Presumptive evidence of a subcellular oncogenic agent in the tumors of Tx mice was also obtained. Tx mice demonstrated impaired cellular immunity. Most tumors arising in Tx mice were rejected on transplantation into normal syngeneic controls, suggest- ing that the impaired cellular immunity of Tx mice permitted the growth of more strongly antigenic tumors than occur in normal mice.

It is certainly evident that neonatal thymectomy resulted in impaired cellular immunity and also in an increased incidence of lymphomas. The relationship of these changes however is not evident. The greater anti- gencity of tumors arising in Tx mice suggests that impaired immunity to tumor antigens may be responsible. Also possible is an impaired immune response to oncorna virus. A third possibility is that since the tumors were exclusively lymphoreticular, some type of derangement of this system is involved. Aged NZB mice are weak in suppressor T-cell activity with, as a result, hyperactive humoral immune responses and autoimmune disease (9). Conceivably such a mechanism may be at work in Tx(BA)F$_1$ mice. Histologically, such animals demonstrate marked plasma cellular infiltrations of many organs. Faulty immunoregulation would be a more accurate term in this instance (10). Recent studies have shown that stimulation of humoral antibody-producing cells (Bcells) is associated with replication of oncorna virus (11). The absence of an increased incidence of non-lymphoid tumors in Tx(BA)F$_1$ mice is not an argument against the concept that some type of immunological abnormality is respon- sible for more lymphomas in Tx mice. Normal (BA)F$_1$ mice had very few such tumors, even in old age, so that a genetic background of some degree of susceptibility would appear to be a necessary prerequisite.

V. SUMMARY

Neonatally thymectomized (BA)F_1 mice demonstrated impaired cellular immunity, histologic changes similar to the graft-versus-host-reaction, and a markedly increased incidence of lymphomas. Such tumors were more frequently rejected on transplantation, than tumors arising in normal (BA)F_1 control mice. Non-lymphoid tumors were not increased in incidence in Tx(BA)F_1 mice. Cell-free extracts of these tumors were oncogenic for newborn B mice. In a second hybrid, (SB)F_1, neonatal thymectomy was associated with a moderately increased incidence of lymphomas for a 4-month period. Tx(SB)F_1 mice, unlike Tx(BA)F_1 mice, demonstrated no lymphoproliferative changes and no graft-versus-host-like lesions.

TABLE I. Cumulative Incidence of Lymphomas in Tx and Control (BA)F_1 Mice

Age (mo.)	Tx mice (% tumors)	Control mice (% tumors)	P[1]
4	0.0	0.0	N.S.
8	7.8	0.7	0.01
12	9.0	2.0	0.02
16	18.0	2.0	0.001
20	32.5	5.4	0.001
22	40.3	8.1	0.001
24	47.0	16.8	0.001

[1.] Chi square test; N.S., not significant.

REFERENCES

1. Thomas, L. Reactions To Homologous Tissue Antigens In Relation To Hypersensitivity. In: Cellular and Humoral Aspects of the Hypersensitive States. Ed.: H. S. Lawrence. Hoeber-Harper, New York, pp. 529-532, 1959.

2. Burnet, F. M. The Concept Of Immunological Surveillance. Prog. Exp. Tumor Res., 13:1-27. 1970.

3. Sjodin, K., Dalmasso, A. P., Smith, J. M., and Martinez, C. Thymectomy In Newborn And Adult Mice. Transplantation, 1:521-523, 1963.

4. Cornelius, E. A., Yunis, E., and Martinez, C. Clinical, Hematologic And Serologic Features Of Parabiosis Intoxication. Transplantation, 5:112-134, 1967.

5. Cornelius, E. A. Rapid Viral Induction Of Murine Lymphomas In The Graft-Versus-Host-Reaction. J. Exp. Med., 136:1533-1544, 1972.

6. Cornelius, E. A. Induction Of Tumors and Autoimmune Changes In Thymectomized Mice. Amer. J. Roentgenol., 114:784-791, 1972.

7. Cornelius, E. A. Comparison Of Changes In The Graft-Versus-Host-Reaction And Post-Thymectomy State. Fed. Proc., 31:930, 1972.

8. Teague, P., Yunis, E. J., Rodey, G., Fish, A., Stutman, O., and Good, R. A. Autoimmune Phenomena And Renal Disease In Mice. Lab. Investig., 22:121-130, 1970.

9. Morton, R., Goodman, D., Klassen, L., Derkay, C., Gershwin, E., Squire, R., and Steinberg, A. Characteristics Of Suppressor Thymocytes In NZB Mice Related To Disease Manifestations. Fed. Proc., 35:860, 1976.

10. Schwarz, R. Another Look At Immunologic Surveillance. New Eng. J. Med., 293:181-184, 1975.

11. Ruddle, N., Armstrong, M. Y. K., and Richards, F. F. Replication Of Murine Leukemia Virus In B-Lymphocytes. Fed. Proc., 35:737, 1976.

PROTECTIVE EFFECT OF THYMECTOMY IN
A HIGH CANCER RISK POPULATION

Angelos E. Papatestas, Allan E. Kark,
Gabriel Genkins, Arthur H. Aufses, Jr.
Department of Surgery
Mount Sinai School of Medicine
New York, New York 10029 U.S.A.

INTRODUCTION

Experimental thymectomy is followed by an alteration in the incidence of tumors and a reduced occurrence of neoplasms such as mammary tumors, lymphomas and leukemias.[1]

The presence of the thymus is considered essential for the development of experimental breast cancer[2], while persistent thymic abnormalities have been linked with an increased susceptibility to neoplasia[3].

In humans, increased incidence of lymphoreticular neoplasms and breast cancer has been reported in autoimmune diseases in which presence of thymic germinal centers and/or thymomas is a frequent finding[4,5]. Decreases in lymphocytes, T-cells, IgA levels and/or abnormal cellular immune responses have also been reported in these diseases[6,7].

Patients with myasthenia gravis, a disease of auto-immune nature, have an increased incidence of extrathymic tumors prior to thymectomy with a disproportionate increase in breast cancers, lymphomas and leukemias[8,9]. Thymectomy not only results in improvement of symptoms and remission of myasthenia gravis, but preliminary data indicate that it may play a protective role against the high cancer risk associated with this disease[8]. A restoration of cellular immune competence following transcervical thymectomy has been reported in uremic patients[10].

The current report investigates further the cancer risk in myasthenia gravis in relation to thymic pathology, the

353

differences in cancer incidence between patients with and without thymectomy, and the role of thymectomy in altering the risk of oncogenesis.

MATERIAL AND METHODS

The records of 2000 patients with myasthenia gravis (MG) registered at The Mount Sinai Hospital, (M.S.H.), New York City and at The New End Hospital, (N.E.H.), London, England, were reviewed. Patients were separated into groups according to sex, presence or absence of a thymoma and according to whether or not they had undergone thymectomy (Table 1).

There were 139 patients with extrathymic neoplasms in the entire population. However, 9 patients, all women, had presented with more than one extrathymic primary, and the total number of extrathymic neoplasms was 149. The most common primary sites are shown in Table 2. Breast cancer was the most frequent neoplasm in women with non-thymomatous myasthenia gravis in all periods of observation (Table 3).

The risk of cancer development was evaluated separately in the periods of observations after the onset of myasthenia and prior to thymectomy and the period of observation following thymectomy. Since both hospitals were referral centers, where patients from widely scattered geographic areas were referred for evaluation and treatment, direct comparison of cancer risk with a regional cancer registry would be arbitrary. Yet in order to compare the relative risk between the different groups of patients and in the various periods of observation, a point of reference had to be selected. The Connecticut Cancer Registry age and sex specific rates[11] utilized in the previous study of cancer risk in myasthenia gravis[8], were selected as such a reference point.

The risk of oncogenesis in each study group was evaluated by counting the patient-years of observation in each decade of life, computing the expected numbers of neoplasms from the sex and age specific rates and comparing the expected with the observed numbers for the entire group.

The significance of the observed differences between observed and expected numbers was tested under the Poisson assumption[12].

We have attempted to identify low and high cancer risk subgroups according to severity of disease, thymic pathology and timing of thymectomy.

In patients with non-thymomatous myasthenia gravis, comparison of risk of oncogenesis was made between patients who were operated shortly after the onset of symptoms of disease and those who had thymectomy after a long delay. The former group has a lower percentage of germinal centers and reaches clinical remission after a shorter interval following thymectomy, when compared to the latter group[6]. The risk of oncogenesis following thymectomy was also evaluated separately in the symptomatic period and the period after the onset of remission.

Severity of disease was taken into consideration in a direct comparison between pre- and post-thymectomy risk, since the severity of disease determines the indication for operation, and patients with ocular myasthenia gravis are not referred for thymectomy[6]. In this particular comparison, 'the patient-years of observation accumulated in patients with ocular myasthenia were excluded.

A comparison of cancer risk between the two hospital series was also made. Study of the risk of oncogenesis prior to thymectomy, was not possible for the British Series, since essentially only patients referred for thymectomy were followed at the N.E.H. In fact, 84% of the patients referred to N.E.H. had had thymectomies as compared to 34% of patients at M.S.H.

RESULTS

There was a total of 18,993 patient-years of observation from both hospitals of which 13,706 were after the onset of myasthenia gravis, but prior to thymectomy and 5,289

following thymectomy, women had 12,503 years of observation
of which 3,885 were following thymectomy.

In myasthenic women a significant increase in relative
cancer risk was present prior to thymectomy both in those
with non-thymomatous myasthenia gravis and those with
associated thymomas. Following thymectomy, the relative
risk decreased, and there was no difference from the
expected numbers (Table 4).

In myasthenic men the relative risk prior to thymectomy
was also higher than that observed following to thymectomy,
but there were no significant differences in the relative
risk. In both sexes patients with thymomas had a higher
relative risk than those without thymomas (Table 4).

The relative cancer risk was then compared in women with
non-thymomatous generalized myasthenia gravis only, since
patients with purely ocular disease were not referred for
thymectomy. The relative cancer risk prior to thymectomy was
significantly increased in all categories, regardless of
severity of disease, but patients in the more severe clinical
categories (III, and IV) of the Osserman Clinical Classification[13] had a higher relative risk (Table 5).

Following thymectomy, a marked decrease in the relative
risk (ratio of observed to expected) neoplasms was noted in
the period of observation after the onset of remission.
Indeed this was the only study group where the numbers of
observed neoplasms was smaller than the expected number.
A small, but not significant difference in relative cancer
risk between the two hospitals were noted in the post-
thymectomy period. The relative risk for the entire post-
thymectomy period was lower at N.E.H. O/E = 1.14, while the
risk for the symptomatic period was slightly higher,
O/E = 1.710. The decrease in the relative risk for the
period of remission at the N.E.H. was significant at P = 0.05,
(one-tailed test for significance of decrease).

Since remission occurs earlier and more frequently in
patients operated upon early in the course of the disease,

cancer risk following thymectomy was evaluated prior to thymectomy.

The evaluation was made with M.S.H. patients only. Six of the 9 (66%) neoplasms occurring following thymectomy in patients without thymomas, occurred in those patients in whom thymectomy was delayed for five or more years after the onset of symptoms. They represented only 26% of all patients who had thymectomy.

DISCUSSION

While the role of the thymus and the effects of thymectomy in experimental oncogenesis have been extensively investigated[1,2,3], there is a remarkable paucity of information on this subject in relation to human oncogenesis.[8]

From the available reports however, it would appear that the presence of thymic pathology is associated with an increased frequency of extrathymic neoplasms[5,8,14,15] while thymectomy is not followed by an increased risk of oncogenesis[8,15]. On the contrary, it appears that thymectomy may play a protective role, similar to that observed in experimental tumors[1,2,17,18].

The availability of a large number of patients who underwent thymectomy for the treatment of myasthenia gravis, provided the opportunity for an investigation of the thymic role and the effects of thymectomy in oncogenesis in humans.

The present report provides evidence that there is an increased risk of oncogenesis in myasthenic patients prior to thymectomy. Women are at a higher risk than men (Table 4). It appears that the risk is also proportionate to the severity of thymic pathology. Patients with thymomas have a higher relative risk than patients with non-thymomatous myasthenia gravis (Table 4). Within the latter group, a higher relative cancer risk was present in the subgroups where many germinal centers is a frequent finding, (i.e. , women, patients with long duration of disease, patients with severe symptoms). Although only this indirect evaluation of the role of thymic germinal centers in the risk of oncogenesis was possible, the consistency of the pattern is remarkable.

Thymectomy was followed by a reduction of the oncogenetic risk. It would appear that its protective role was more pronounced in populations where the operation was performed early in the course of the disease, since these are the groups that reach early remission.[7,19] The timing of thymectomy is known to affect cancer risk in experimental oncogenesis.[18]

There are several observations that could explain that increased risk associated with the presence of the thymus in myasthenia gravis and the protective effect of thymectomy. An immunosuppressive substance similar to that found in patients with advanced neoplasms has been isolated from the stoma of human thymus.[20] Decreased IgA[6], decreased lymphocytes[7], decreased androgens[7], decreased progesterone[21], and increased carcinoembryonic antigen levels have been reported in myasthenic patients prior to thymectomy. All these parameters have been associated with an increased risk of oncogenesis in general or specifically for breast cancer[7,22,23,24]. Most of these parameters are also associated with the presence of thymic germinal centers[7,22]. A correlation in the existing abnormalities of these parameters in patients with myasthenia gravis has been observed following thymectomy[7,22]. It would appear that those abnormalities are not specific for myasthenia gravis, but are common in patients with autoimmune disease in which thymic pathology and a higher risk of cancer is a frequent finding[4,5,6,25].

If further studies confirm the protective effect of thymectomy against the high cancer risk associated with thymic pathology, the availability of the transcervical approach with its negligible morbidity[19] should facilitate the application of the procedure to populations in whom the presence of the thymus may play an oncogenetic role.

SUMMARY

The risk of extrathymic cancer and the effects of thymectomy in oncogenesis were studied in 2000 patients with
myasthenia gravis, of whom 189 had undergone thymectomy.
A total of 149 neoplasms were recorded in the entire
population. Identification of high cancer risk subgroups
was made. The relative cancer risk was high in patients
who did not have thymectomy, while a decrease was noted
following thymectomy. An association between cancer risk
and thymic pathology was noted. Patients with thymomas
and those with many germinal centers had the highest
relative risk. The increase in the relative cancer risk was
significant in women prior to thymectomy. The post-
thymectomy decrease in cancer risk was more marked in
patients who were operated early after the onset of disease
and those who had reached remission. The observed numbers
of neoplasms in the period of observation after the onset
of remission were lower than expected, while in all other
periods observed numbers were higher than expected. These
findings indicate that thymectomy may have a protective
effect against the high cancer risk associated with thymic
abnormalities.

TABLE I. Sex Distribution and Thymectomy Status of 2000
Patients with Myasthenia Gravis

| | MOUNT SINAI HOSPITAL | | | NEW END HOSPITAL | | |
| | ALL | SEX | | ALL | SEX | |
		MEN	WOMEN		MEN	WOMEN
MG NO THYMOMA						
NO THYMECTOMY	1109	513	596	38	8	30
T-T THYMECTOMY	111	17	94	211	60	151
T-C THYMECTOMY	297	98	99	—	—	—
ALL	1517	628	889	249	68	181
MG WITH THYMOMA						
NO THYMECTOMY	53	20	33	11	4	7
T-T THYMECTOMY	97	46	51	47	20	27
T-C THYMECTOMY	26	13	13	—	—	—
ALL	176	79	97	58	24	34
TOTALS	1693	707	986	307	92	215

TABLE II. Location of Primary Neoplasma in Patients with
Myasthenia Gravis

PRIMARY LOCATION	WOMEN	MEN	ALL
BREAST	37	1	38
COLORECTAL	11	9	20
SKIN	9	7	16
LEUKEMIA	8	3	11
LUNG	8	3	11
PROSTATE	–	9	9
SARCOMA	3	4	7
UTERUS	5	–	5
CERVIX	5	–	5
LYMPHOMAS	4	–	4
OTHER LOCATIONS	11	12	23
ALL	101	48	149

TABLE III. 149 Extrathymic Neoplasms in 2000 Patients with
Myasthenia Gravis

	MYASTHENIA GRAVIS WITHOUT THYMOMA		THYMOMATOUS MYASTHENIA GRAVIS		ALL PATIENTS WITH MYASTHENIA GRAVIS	
	MSH	NEH	MSH	NEH	MSH	NEH
PERIOD PRIOR TO THE ONSET OF MYASTHENIA GRAVIS						
MALE	4		2		6	
FEMALE	25(15)		2		27(15)	
TOTAL	29		4		33	
PERIOD AFTER THE ONSET OF MYASTHENIA GRAVIS AND PRIOR TO THYMECTOMY						
MALE	34	1	1		35	1
FEMALE	47(15)	2(1)	9(1)		56(16)	2(1)
TOTAL	81	3	10		91	3
PERIOD FOLLOWING THYMECTOMY						
MALE	3		1	2(1)	4	2
FEMALE	3(3)	9(2)	2	2	5(3)	11(2)
TOTAL	6	9	3	4	9	13
ALL YEARS						
MALE	41	1	4	2(1)	45	3(1)
FEMALE	75(33)	11(3)	13(1)	2	88(34)	13(3)
TOTAL	116	12	17	4	133	16

* NUMBERS IN PARENTHESIS INDICATE BREAST CARCINOMAS.

TABLE IV. Extrathymic Neoplasms Following Onset of Myasthenia Gravis

	PRE-THYMECTOMY		POST-THYMECTOMY	
WOMEN	EXP	OBS	EXP	OBS
NON-THYMOMAS O/E (RELATIVE RISK)	23.16 2.11^+	49	9.85 1.21	12
THYMOMAS O/E (RELATIVE RISK)	1.75 5.14^+	9	1.74 2.29	4
MEN				
NON-THYMOMAS O/E (RELATIVE RISK)	26.17 $1.33^§$	35	3.76 $0.79^§$	3
THYMOMAS O/E (RELATIVE RISK)	0.31 $3.22^§$	1	0.96 $3.12^§$	3

+   P < 0.01

§   N.S.

TABLE V. Extrathymic Neoplasms in Non-Thymomatous Myasthenia Gravis

RELATION TO SEVERITY OF DISEASE				
PRE-THYMECTOMY			POST-THYMECTOMY	
M.S.H.			M.S.H. & N.E.H.	
	WOMEN	RATIO O/E	WOMEN	RATIO O/E
ALL GENERALIZED MG E O	20.00 42	2.10^{+}	9.85 12	$1.21^{\S}$
IIA & IIB E O	15.04 30	1.99^{+}		
III & IV E O	4.96 12	$2.41^{\#}$		
SYMPTOMATIC E O			7.58 12	$1.58^{\S}$
REMISSION E O			2.27 0	$-^{\S}$

BIBLIOGRAPHY

1. Allison, A.C., Taylor, R.A. Observations on Thymectomy and Carcinogenesis. Cancer Res., 27:703-707, 1967.

2. Yunis, E.J., Martinez, E., Smith, J., Stutman, I., Good, R.A. Spontaneous Mammary Adenocarcinoma in Mice: Influence of Thymectomy and Reconstitution with Thymus Grafts or Spleen Cells. Cancer Res., 29:174-177, 1969.

3. Miller, J.F.A.P. The Thymus In Relation to Neoplasia. In: Modern Trends in Pathology. Ed.: T. Crawford, Appleton Century Crofts, New York, 2: 160-175, 1967.

4. Miller, D.G. The Association of Immune Diseases and Malignant Lymphomas. Ann. Intern. Med., 66:507-521, 1967.

5. Itoh, K., Maruchi, N. Breast Cancer in Patients with Hashimoto's Thyroiditis. Lancet, II:1119-1121, 1975.

6. Behan, P.I., Simpson, J.A., Behan, W.M.H. Decreased Serum IgA in Myasthenia Gravis. Lancet, I:593-594, 1976.

7. Papatestas, A.E., Genkins, G., Horowitz, S., Kornfeld, P. Thymectomy in Myasthenia Gravis, Pathologic, Clinical and Electrophysiologic Correlations. Ann. N.Y. Acad. Sci., (In Press).

8. Papatestas, A.E., Osserman, K.E., Kark, A.E. The Relationship Between Thymus and Oncogenesis. A Study of the Incidence of Non-Thymic Malignancy in Myasthenia Gravis. Brit. J. Cancer, 25:635-645, 1971.

9. Papatestas, A.E., Genkins, G., Kark, A.E. Thymus Transplantation in Leukemia and Malignant Lympho-granulomatosis. Lancet, II:795, 1973.

10. Birkeland, S.A., Moesner, J., Julie, F., Kemp, E., Sorenson, H.R. Thymectomy as Immunosuppression in Uremic Patients. Transplantation, 19:373-381, 1975.

11. Cancer Registry of Connecticut, Connecticut State Department of Health, Hartford, Connecticut, 1963.

12. Bailar, J.C., III, Ederer, F. Significance Factors for the Ratio of a Poisson Variable to its Expectation. Biometrics, 20:639-643, 1964.

13. Osserman, K.E. Myasthenia Gravis. Grumme Stratton, 1958.

14. Ferguson, F.R. A Critical Review of the Clinical Features of Myasthenia Gravis. Proc. Roy. Soc. Med., 55:49-52, 1962.

15. Souadjian, J.B., Silverstein, M.N., Titus, J.L. Thymoma and Cancer. Cancer,22:1221-1225, 1968.

16. Vessey, M.P., Doll, R. Thymectomy and Cancer. Br. J. Cancer, 26:53-58, 1972.

17. Martinez, C. Effect of Early Thymectomy on Development of Mammary Tumors in Mice. Nature, 203:1118, 1964.

18. Nagaya, H. Thymus Function in Spontaneous Lymphoid Leukemia I. Premature Leukemogenesis in "young" thymectomiezed mice bearing "old" thymus grafts. J. Immunol., 111:1048-1051, 1973.

19. Papatestas, A.E., Genkins, G., Kornfeld, P., Horowitz, S., Kark, A.E. Transcervical Thymectomy in Myasthenia Gravis. Surgery, Gynecology & Obstetrics, 140:535-540, 1975.

20. Davis, R.C., Cooperband, S.R., Mannick, J.A. A Natural Inhibitor of Lymphocyte Stimulation Produced by Human Thymus. Surg. Forum, 20:244-245, 1969.

21. Greene, R., Schrire, I. Myasthenia Gravis: Studies in Progesterone Metabolism. In: Myasthenia Gravis. The Second International Symposium Proceedings. Ed.: H.R. Viets. Charles C. Thomas., Springfield, Illinois, 282-290, 1961.

22. Papatestas, A.E., Kim, U., Genkins, G., Kornfeld, P., Horowitz, S.H., Aufses, Jr., A.H. The Association of CEA and Peripheral Lymphocytes; Diagnostic and Prognostic Significance. Surgery, 78:343-348, 1975.

23. Bulbrook, R.D., Hayward, J.L. Abnormal Urinary Steroid Excretion and Subsequent Breast Cancer. A Prospective Study in the Island of Guernsey. Lancet, 1:519-522, 1967.

24. Sherman, B.M., Korenman, S.G. Inadequate Corpus Luteum Function: A Pathophysiological Interpretation of Human Breast Cancer Epidemiology. Cancer, 33:1306-1311, 1974.

25. Gordon-Nesbitt, D.S., Malka-Abbo, S., Sloper, J.C., Sinclair, L. Myasthenia Gravis, Hypothyroidism and Abnormality of Lymphocyte Functions. Lancet, 1:150, 1976.

T-LYMPHOCYTE CELL DIVISION: A REQUIREMENT
FOR THE TUMOR SPECIFIC IMMUNE RESPONSE IN VITRO

Robert L. Lundak, Gale A. Granger and
Marvin S. Kaplan

Department of Molecular Biology and Biochemistry
University of California, Irvine
Irvine, California

and

Veterans Administration Hospital
Long Beach, California

INTRODUCTION

There is substantial evidence that T-lymphocytes proliferate in the
presence of allogeneic cells in a mixed lymphocyte response (MLC)
(Wilson and Nowell, 1971; Zoschke and Bach, 1971; and Anderson, et al.,
1973), and are a result of the recognition by the responder cell of
membrane specificities on the stimulator cells. The level of this mixed
lymphocyte response has been shown to be influenced by both nonspecific
serum factors and non-lymphoid cells (Peck, et al., 1973). It has also
been shown that lymphocytes may be allogeneically stimulated to produce
T-lymphocyte cytotoxic cells which are specific for the sensitizing cells
(Lundak and Raidt, 1973; Wagner and Feldmann, 1972). The direct relationship between proliferation in MLC responses and cytotoxic cell development has been established. The induction of tumor specific T-lymphocyte
cytotoxic cells in vitro has been reported by several investigators.
This study was conducted to examine the role of cell division in the
production of syngeneic (tumor specific) cytotoxic T-cells in vitro.

PROCEDURES AND MATERIALS USED

Mice

Two to three month old male C57Bl/6J mice were used in all experiments.
Stocks were obtained from Jackson Laboratories, Bar Harbor, Maine.

Stimulator Cells

P-815-X2 mastocytoma cells (DBA/2J) were used as the stimulating tumor
antigen. These cells were maintained by serial passage in RPMI 1640
medium (Gibco), supplemented with 10% calf serum. The tumor was passed
through DBA/2J mice every 90 days by interperitoneal injection of 5×10^6
cells suspended in 0.1 Hank's balanced salt solution (BSS). Passed DBA

mastocytoma tumor was harvested 14 days later by withdrawing peritoneal fluid and starting new cultures. Irradiated DBA mastocytoma tumor cells (DBA_{m-x}) used as antigen were prepared by washing twice in Hanks balanced salt (HBS), resuspended to 1×10^7 cells/ml in a 2.0 volume, then irradiated with 1250 rad x-ray (5 mA, 100 kV, 0.1 mm Cu filter at six inches) followed by washing three times and resuspending in HBS at 3.3×10^6 cells/ml.

Cell Suspensions

Spleens were removed from DBA mice killed by cervical dislocation and teased apart in BSS using sterile technique. Cell aggregates were allowed to settle out in conical centrifuge tubes held upright in ice for 10 min. The supernatant containing mostly single cells was centrifuged at 800 x g for 10 min at $4^{\circ}C$. The packed cells were resuspended in culture media at a culture density of $1.3-1.7 \times 10^7$ cells/culture.

^{3}H-Thymidine Pulse Technique

^{3}H-Thymidine of high specific activity was used to kill dividing cells as described elsewhere (Dutton and Mishell, 1967). Briefly, 20 μC of tritiated thymidine (27 C/mM) in 30 μl of media was added to cultures for various 24 hr time periods. The pulse was terminated by the addition of 100 μg of cold thymidine in 90 μl of media to each culture. (See Table 1)

5-Bromodeoxyuridine (BUdR) Pulse Technique

Elimination of dividing cell populations using BUdR and visible light was also employed as described by Puck (Puck and Kao, 1967). Briefly, 10^{-5} M BUdR (final culture concentration) was added to each culture at various 24 hr time periods. Twelve hours later, these cultures were exposed to 40-watt fluorescent lamps at a distance of two inches for one hour. These cultures were incubated for 12 hr as described, and then removed, washed three times in media, and resuspended in new media for the remainder of the five day incubation period. (See Table 2)

Culture System

The Mishell-Dutton system was used. Briefly, 1.3×10^7 to 1.7×10^7 viable nucleated spleen cells in 2.0 ml of media were stimulated with syngeneic tumor cells (DBA_{m-x}) at various densities. Cultures were gassed, 5% CO_2 and 95% air, and fed with a nutritional cocktail as described elsewhere (Mishell and Dutton, 1967). Following the culture period (usually five days), cells were recovered by scraping the dishes with a plastic policeman, washed once with HBS and resuspended at 1×10^7 viable cells/ml in HBS for assay.

Chromium Release Assay

Cultured DBA mastocytoma cells were used as target cells in the assay. The target cells were labeled with ^{51}Cr as described by Brunner (Brunner, et al., 1968). The labeled tumor target cells were resuspended in minimal essential medium (MEM) to a concentration of 1×10^5/ml, and 1.0 ml of target cells was placed in 10 x 25 mm flat-bottomed tubes, 1.0 ml of cultured spleen cells at a concentration of 1×10^7 was added to three replicate tubes and incubated without rocking at $37^{\circ}C$ in 5% CO_2, 95% air for 15 hr. Following incubation, tubes were centrifuged at 1500 x g for 15 min, and 0.8 ml of supernatant was carefully removed. The radioactivity of the cell pellet and the supernatant were counted in a well type gamma counter (Tracerlab). The results were expressed as percent specific kill.

Method of Statistical Analysis

Specific kill figures were analyzed employing Student's t test. The values on the figures represent the geometric means of replicate sets; bars indicate one standard deviation.

RESULTS

Several parameters significantly influence the *in vitro* primary syngeneic immune response and the subsequent ^{51}Cr assay. These include time of primary cell culture stimulator cell done and ^{51}Cr assay incubation time.

Kinetics of the Syngeneic Response In Vitro

Cultures of DBA spleen cells were stimulated with 1×10^5 irradiated tumor cells (DBA_{m-x}) at time 0 hours. Replicate cultures of immunized and non-immunized spleen cells were assayed one hour following preparation of cultures and every 24 hr for six days. T-killer cells were first detected at 72 hr and increased to a maximum at 5 days (Fig. 1). The day 6 decrease appeared to be due to pH changes in culture and exhaustion of culture ingredients. All subsequent experiments were assayed on day 5.

Affect of Antigen Doses on the Syngeneic Response in Vitro

DBA/2 spleen cell cultures were sensitized with various doses of DBA_{m-x} cells from 10 through 10^6 cells per culture dish. All cultures were assayed against 51 Cr-labeled DBA mastocytoma cells on Day 5. Maximum cytotoxicity developed when 10^5 DBA cells were used (Fig. 2), however, as few as 100 tumor cells could stimulate a detectable lymphocyte cytotoxic response. All subsequent cultures were sensitized with 10^5 $DBA_{(m-x)}$ cells.

Kinetics of the ^{51}Cr-Release Assay

Specific kill as assayed by ^{51}Cr release is a time dependent event. Significant ^{51}Cr release can be detected as early as 5 hr after incubation of immunized DBA spleen cells on ^{51}Cr labeled DBA cells (Fig. 3). Maximum release is observed by 15 hr of incubation. All culture results reported were assayed for 15 hr.

369

The Effect of Hot Thymidine and BUdR Pulse on the Generation of Cytotoxic T-Cells In Vitro

DBA spleen cells ($1.3-1.7 \times 10^7$) were stimulated at time 0 hr with 1×10^5 DBA_{m-x} cells and cultures were "pulsed" with 20 μC ^{3}H-thymidine per culture for successive 24 hr periods, starting at time 0 and continuing through day 5. Following the 24 hr pulse, 100-fold excess of cold thymidine was added to block pulse. All cultures were assayed on day 5 for cytotoxicity. Elimination of dividing cells during the first 24 hr of culture did not affect the production of cytotoxic lymphocytes on day 5 (Fig. 4), indicating that cell division during the initial 24 hr was not necessary for the development of the cytotoxic response on day 5. Elimination of the dividing cell population during 24-48, 48-72 and 72-96 hr resulted in partial loss of cytotoxicity in day 5 cultures. Cultures which were "pulsed" from 96-120 hr developed control levels of cytotoxic cells on day 5. The addition of cold thymidine at the same time as the ^{3}H-thymidine pulse resulted in cytotoxic cells at the same level as the control cultures, indicating that the hot thymidine was not nonspecifically toxic.

Cultures were pulsed with BUdR as described for 24 hr and assayed on day 5. The results of BUdR pulses are shown (Fig. 4) and are the same as those obtained using ^{3}H-thymidine.

Removal of macrophages from spleen cell cultures at time 0 resulted in cultures which could be completely pulsed out to background levels.

DISCUSSION

The development of syngeneic cytotoxic T-cells in vitro has been shown to be a time dependent event. The first 24 hr appears to be an amitotic recognition and induction period followed by 72 hr of mitotic activity. The development of normal cytotoxicity in cultures pulsed from 96-120 hr indicates an efficient mitotic control in vitro which results in rapid cessation of cell division after 96 hr, and that once division has ceased, the T-lymphocyte cytotoxic cell is committed and specific for the stimulating tumor antigen.

Removal of adherent (macrophage) cells from the cultures at time 0 removed the non-pulsable background cytotoxicity. It appears that macrophages from spleen cultures become sensitized to the tumor antigen and develop significant levels of cytotoxicity but do not require a proliferative cycle as do the lymphocytes.

TABLE I. Protocol for ^{3}H-Thymidine Pulse Experiments

Culture	Hours in Culture					Assay ↓
	0	24	48	72	96	120
1	^{3}H-TD	cold TD ——————————————————→				
2		^{3}H-TD	cold TD ——————————————→			
3			^{3}H-TD	cold TD ——————————→		
4				^{3}H-TD	cold TD —→	
5					^{3}H-TD ——→	
6	^{3}H-TD + cold TD	——————————————————————————→				
7		^{3}H-TD + cold TD	——————————————————————→			
8			^{3}H-TD + cold TD	——————————————————→		
9				^{3}H-TD + cold TD	——————→	
10					^{3}H-TD + cold TD	—→
11	Media only	———————————————————————————				

371

TABLE II. Protocol for BUdR Pulse Experiments

Culture	0	12	24	36	48	60	72	84	96	108	Assay ↓ 120
1	BUdR	Light	Wash								→
2			BUdR	Light	Wash						→
3					BUdR	Light	Wash				→
4							BUdR	Light	Wash		→
5									BUdR	Light	→
6	Media alone										→

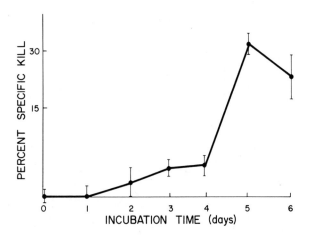

FIG. 1.   Kinetics of the syngeneic in vitro response of 1 x 10^7 DBA/2 spleen cells to 1 x 10^5 DBA/2 irradiated mastocytoma tumor cells (DBA_{m-x}). Values represent the geometric mean of two replicates in five different experiments $\pm$ one standard deviation (S.D.).

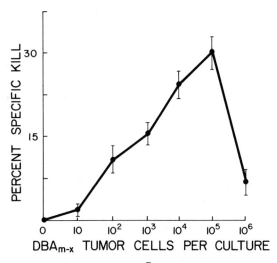

FIG. 2.   In vitro response of 1.5 x 10^7 DBA/2 spleen cells to various numbers of $DBA_{(m-x)}$ tumor cells.   Values represent the geometric mean of two replicates in three different experiments $\pm$ 1 S.D.

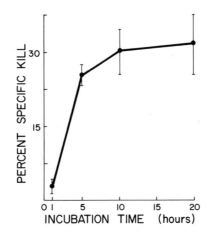

FIG. 3. Kinetics of the in vitro ^{51}Cr cytotoxic release assay. DBA/2 spleen cell cultures were immunized with 1 x 10^5 DBA $_{(m-x)}$ tumor cells and harvested for assay on day 5 of culture. The spleen to tumor cell ratio was 100:1.

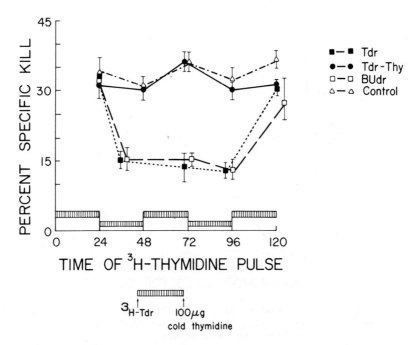

FIG. 4. Effect of ^{3}H-thymidine and BUdR pulse on successive 24 hr culture periods. All cultures were assayed on day 5. Values represent the mean of two replicates in three experiments.

REFERENCES

Anderson, L. C., S. Nordling, and P. Hayry. 1973. Allograft immunity *in vitro*. VI. Autonomy of T lymphocytes in target cell destruction. Scand. J. Immunol. 2:107.

Brunner, K. T., J. Mauel, J. C. Cerottini, and B. Chapuis. 1968. Quantitative assay of the lytic action of immune lymphoid cells on ^{51}Cr labeled allogeneic target cells *in vitro*; inhibition by isoantibody and by drugs. Immunology 14:181.

Dutton, R. W., and R. I. Mishell. 1967. Cell populations and cell proliferation in the *in vitro* response of normal mouse spleen to heterologous erythrocytes: analysis of the hot pulse technique. J. Exp. Med. 126:443.

Lundak, R. L., and D. J. Raidt. 1973. Cellular immune response against tumor cells. I. *In vitro* immunization of allogeneic and syngeneic mouse spleen cell suspensions against DBA mastocytoma cells. Cell. Immunol. 9:60.

Mishell, R. I., and R. W. Dutton. 1967. Immunization of dissociated spleen cell cultures from normal mice. J. Exp. Med. 126:423.

Peck, A. B., E. Katz-Heber, and R. E. Click. 1973. Immune responses *in vitro*. IV. A comparison of the protein-free and mouse serum-supplemented mouse mixed lymphocyte interaction assays. Eur. J. Immunol. 3:516.

Puck, T. T., and F. Kao. 1967. Genetics of somatic mammalian cells, V. Treatment with 5-bromodeoxyuridine and visible light for isolation of nutritionally deficient mutants. Proc. Natl. Acad. Sc. 58:1227.

Wagner, H., and M. Feldman. 1972. Cell-mediated immune response *in vitro*. I. A new *in vitro* system for the generation of cell-mediated cytotoxic activity. Cell. Immunol. 3:405.

Wilson, D. B., and P. C. Nowell. 1971. Quantitative studies on the mixed lymphocyte interaction in rats: Tempo and specificity of the proliferative response and the number of reactive cells from immune donors. J. Exp. Med. 133:422.

Zoschke, D. C., and F. H. Bach. 1971. Specificity of allogeneic cell recognition by human lymphocytes *in vitro*. Science (Wash. D.C.) 172:1350.

CORYNEBACTERIUM PARVUM - INDUCED PROTECTION AGAINST
DEVELOPMENT OF METASTASES OF A MURINE MAMMARY CARCINOMA

Luka Milas and H. Rodney Withers

Central Institute for Tumors and Allied Diseases, Zagreb
Yugoslavia, and M.D. Anderson Hospital and Tumor Institute,
Houston, Texas, U.S.A.

INTRODUCTION

The presence of tumor cells in the circulation is not
necessarily followed by the appearance of metastases. The
process of development of metastases, starting with the detachment of cells from a primary tumor and ending with the growth
of secondary deposits, is under the influence of many factors
such as blood turbulance, blood coagulability or trauma (8).
In addition to these nonimmunological factors, immunological
antitumor reaction may also influence metastatic spread of
tumors. In experimental animals, more immunogenic tumors give
rise to metastases less frequently than do the weak antigenic
tumors (10). Furthermore, tumors which do not normally metastasize do so if they are grown in immunosuppressed animals
(6,7). In contrast to immunosuppression, procedures which
augment immunologically specific and nonspecific antitumor
resistance reduce development of metastases (3,14,20). Particularly effective in this respect were treatments of animals
with BCG (3) or anaerobic acrynebacteria (20) which nonspecifically stimulate the reticuloendothelial system.

Our earlier studies showed that treatment of mice with
Corynebacterium granulosum (CG) or C. parvum (CP) induces a
significant protection against tumor cells injected intravenously (11). In the present study we have investigated the
effect of these bacteria on the spontaneous development of
pulmonary metastases of a syngeneic mammary carcinoma in mice.

PROCEDURES AND MATERIALS USED

Three month old specific-pathogen-free mice of the inbred
C3Hf/Bu strain were used. All mice in separate experiments
were of the same sex.

The tumor was a spontaneously developed mammary carcinoma;
it is fairly immunogenic for its syngeneic C3Hf/Bu hosts and
it regularly metastasizes to the lung (12). Single cell sus-

pensions were prepared from this tumor by a mechanical method
(12). Primary tumors were generated by injecting 4.4×10^5 or
5×10^5 viable carcinoma cells intramuscularly into the right
legs or subcutaneously into the right flanks of animals. When
tumors in the legs grew to 9 mm in diameter they were surgically removed or inactivated by 6000 rads of gamma-rays. Surgical
and radiation procedures are described in detail elsewhere(16).
The number of metastases in the lung was determined 28 days
after surgery or radiation. In the case of subcutaneously
growing tumors, the number of metastases was determined at the
time of death of animals.

Formalin-killed CG (Batch 5197) was generously supplied
by the late Professor M. Raynaud, Institute Pasteur, Garches,
France and CP (Batch PX 378) by Doctor J.K. Whisnant, Burroughs Wellcome Research Laboratories, Research Triangle Park,
N.C., USA. The bacteria were injected into mice intravenously
or intraperitoneally.

RESULTS

Mice were injected subcutaneously with 5×10^5 tumor cells
and then 3, 7 or 14 days later they were treated intraperitoneally with 0.5 mg CG. This bacterium slowed the growth of tumors and prolonged the survival of recipients. At the time
of death all mice had metastases in the lung (Table I). While
untreated mice had median number of metastases 295, the number
of metastases in mice treated with CG was 3 to 4 times lower.

In the following experiment we studied the effect of CP
on development of metastases in mice whose primary tumors were
removed by surgery or inactivated by local irradiation. CP
is similar to CG in its lymphoreticular stimulating (1,11) and
antitumor adjuvant properties (11). Tumors in the right legs
were generated by injection of 4.4×10^6 mammary carcinoma
cells. They were amputated or irradiated with 6000 rads, single dose, when they grew to 9 mm in diameter. This radiation
dose caused the complete regression of all irradiated tumors
in 19 days. Two days before or after the amputation or irradiation of tumors the mice were given intravenous injections
of 0.25 mg of CP. Twenty-eight days after amputation or irradiation the mice were sacrificed and the number of lung
colonies determined. Most of untreated mice as well as most
of those treated with CP had metastases in the lung (Table II).
The median number of metastases in mice whose tumors were surgically removed was 7. This number was significantly reduced
if CP was administered before amputation. However, this bacterium given after surgery did not influence development of
metastases. Local irradiation of primary tumors facilitated
the metastatic growth; median number of metastases in this
group was 21 ($P < 0.05$). While administration of CP before
irradiation prevented the harmful effect of irradiation, administration of this bacterium after irradiation exhibited no
effect.

DISCUSSION

The results presented in this paper show that CG and CP
induced a resistance against development of spontaneous pulmonary metastases in mice bearing subcutaneously or intramuscularly growing primary tumors. The mechanisms of this resistance to neoplasia is not clearly understood. Anaerobic
corynebacteria stimulate the reticuloendothelial system on
proliferation, in particular they stimulate macrophages. Macrophages from mice treated with CP (18) or CG (2) are capable of destroying or inhibiting proliferation of tumor cells
in vitro in immunologically nonspecific manner. That this
type of response to tumors may also be opperative in vivo,
shows our earlier observation that the whole body irradiation
with 200 to 800 rads does not effect antitumor resistance
induced in mice with CG (15). Radioresistance of CP-induced
antitumor response was reported by Bomford and Olivotto (4).
These investigators also observed that the arrest in the lung
of tumor cells injected intravenously is decreased in mice
treated with CP shortly before tumor cell injection which resulted in a fewer number of lung metastases. The effectiveness of preoperative and preirradiation treatment with CP
in our studies could be partly explained by a reduced arrest
in the lung of tumor cells released into the circulation by
primary tumors. Tumor cells which already settled in the
lung could have been destroyed by nonspecifically activated
macrophages. Olivotto and Bomford found that lung macrophages from CP-treated mice inhibit growth of tumor cells in
vitro (18).

Nonspecific antitumor response is not the only one to
which the antimetastatic effect of CP could be ascribed.
Since mammary carcinoma used in the present study is immunogenic (12), it is to be expected that the specific antitumor
response will also be mounted as it has already been demonstrated in other tumor models both in vivo (22) and in vitro
(9).

CP given two days after tumor amputation did not affect
development of metastases. Proctor et al. (19) reported that
CP reduced the number of spontaneous pulmonary metastases of
a rat ethionine-induced hepatoma if given 7 and 14 days
after surgical removal of the primary tumor, but it was without effect when given before surgery. Nonefficiency of post-
operative treatment with CP in the present studies could be
explained in the way that this bacterium was applied too
early after surgery, at the time when the immune system depressed by the operative procedure had not yet recovered, and
could not immunologically respond to the bacterium. We have
previously reported that CP is not effective in mice whose
immune system was suppressed by the whole body irradiation
(13).

Facilitation of metastases by local irradiation of primary tumors was an unexpected observation of this study.
Usually, irradiation of tumors causes an augmentation of antitumor immunity (5, 21). The reasons for the phenomenon observed in this study are not known. It may be that radiation

caused the release of high amounts of tumor antigens into circulation which can block cytotoxic antitumor activity of immune lymphocytes. Other factors that might have contributed to this harmful effect of local irradiation were discussed elsewhere (17). However, an important finding was that treatment of mice with CP before local irradiation prevented the radiation-induced facilitation of development of lung metastases.

SUMMARY

Corynebacterium parvum (CP) and C. granulosum (CG), potent nonspecific stimulators of the reticuloendothelial system, were studied for their ability to induce resistance to the metastatic spread of tumors. Primary tumors were generated by transplanting mammary carcinoma cells subcutaneously into the flank or intramuscularly into the leg of syngeneic C3Hf/Bu mice. Intraperitoneal injection of CG, 3, 7 or 14 days after subcutaneous transplantation of tumor cells induced 3- to 4-fold reduction in the number of lung metastases determined at the time of death of animals. Nine mm primary tumors in the legs of mice were surgically removed or inactivated by 6000 rads of gamma-irradiation. Four weeks later majority of these animals had lung metastases. Development of metastases was inhibited if mice were given intravenous inoculations of CP 2 days before, but not 2 days after, surgery or irradiation.

TABLE I. Effect of CG on Development of Spontaneous Pulmonary
Metastase of a Mammary Carcinoma in C3Hf/Bu Mice

Days CG was given (0.5 mg intraperitoneally) after subcutaneous injection of 5×10^5 mammary carcinoma cells	Metastases in the lung			
	Mice with metastases/ total mice	Median No of metastases	Range	P (Mann-Whitney U-test)
No treatment	10/10	295	147 - >300	
3	9/9	112	40 - 218	< 0.002
7	9/9	106	27 - >300	< 0.02
14	9/9	74	22 - 297	< 0.002

TABLE II. Effect of CP on Development of Spontaneous Pulmonary Metastases of a Mammary Carcinoma in C3Hf/Bu Mice

Treatment	Mice with metastases/ total mice	Median No of metastases	Range
I Amputation (Day 0)	12/15	7	0-125
II Amputation plus CP on day -2	9/16	1	0-11
III Amputation plus CP on day 2	14/16	11	0->300
IV Tumor irradiation with 6000 rads (Day 0)	15/17	21	0->300
V Tumor irradiation plus CP on day -2	13/17	3	0-50
VI Tumor irradiation plus CP on day 2	17/17	18	1->300

Tumors in the legs were generated by injection of 4.4×10^5 carcinoma cells and were amputated or irradiated with 6000 rads when grew to 9 mm in diameter. The dose of CP was 0.25 mg and it was given intravenously. Statistical evaluation of the number of lung metastases (Mann-Whitney U - test): II versus I, $P < 0.01$; IV versus I, $P < 0.05$; V versus IV, $P < 0.01$

References

1. Adlam, C., and Scott, M.T. Lympho-reticular stimulatory properties of Corynebacterium parvum and related bacteria. J. Med. Microbiol., 6:261-274, 1973.

2. Bašić, I., Milas, L., Grdina, D.J., and Withers, H.R. In vitro destruction of tumor cells by macrophages from mice treated with C. granulosum. J. Natl. Cancer Inst., 55:589-596, 1975.

3. Bast, R.C., Zbar, B., Borsos, T., and Rapp, H.J. BCG and cancer. New England J. Med., 290:1413-1420, 1458-1469, 1974.

4. Bomford, R., and Olivotto, M. The mechanisms of inhibition by Corynebacterium parvum of the growth of lung nodules from intravenously injected tumor cells. Int. J. Cancer, 14:226-235, 1974.

5. Crile, G., Deodhar, S.D. Role of preoperative irradiation in prolonging concomitant immunity and preventing metastases in mice. Cancer, 27:629-634, 1971.

6. Eccles, S.A., and Alexander, P. Macrophage content of tumors in relation to metastatic spread and host immune reaction. Nature, 250:667-689, 1974.

7. Fidler, I.J. Immunologic factors in experimental metastases formation. Int. J. Radiat. Oncol. Biol. Phys., 1:93-96, 1975.

8. Fisher, B., and Fisher, E.R. Biological aspects of cancer-cell spread. In: Proceedings of the Fifth National Cancer Conference, Eds.: American Cancer Society, Inc., and National Cancer Institute. J.B. Lippincott Co., Philadelphia, pp. 105-122, 1964.

9. Fisher, B., Wolmark, N., and Coyle, J. Effect of Corynebacterium parvum on cytotoxicity of regional and nonregional lymph node cells from animals with tumors present or removed. J. Natl. Cancer Inst., 53:1793-1801, 1974.

10. Kim, U. Metastasizing mammary carcinomas in rats: Induction and study of their immunogenicity. Science, 167: 72-74, 1970.

11. Milas, L., Gutterman, J.U., Hunter, N., Bašić, I., Mavligit, G., Hersh, E.M., and Withers, H.R. Immunoprophylaxis and immunotherapy for a murine fibrosarcoma with C. granulosum and C. parvum. Int. J. Cancer, 14:493-503, 1974.

12. Milas, L., Hunter, N., Bašić, I., Mason, K., Grdina, D.J., and Withers, H.R. Nonspecific immunotherapy of murine tumors with C. granulosum. J. Natl. Cancer Inst., 54:895-902, 1975.

13. Milas, L., Hunter, N., Bašić, I., and Withers, H.R. Protection by Corynebacterium granulosum against radiation - induced enhancement of artificial pulmonary metastases of a murine fibrosarcoma. J. Natl. Cancer Inst., 52:1875, 1974.

14. Milas, L., Hunter, N., Mason, K., and Withers, R.H. Immu-
    nological resistance to pulmonary metastases in C3Hf/Bu
    mice bearing syngeneic fibrosarcoma of different sizes.
    Cancer Res., 31:61-71, 1974.

15. Milas, L., Hunter, N., and Withers, H.R. Corynebacterium
    granulosum - induced protection against pulmonary metastas-
    es of a syngeneic fibrosarcoma in mice. Cancer Res., 34:
    613-620, 1974.

16. Milas, L., Hunter, N., and Withers, H.R. Concomitant im-
    munity to pulmonary metastases of a murine fibrosarcoma:
    Influence of removal of primary tumor by radiation or sur-
    gery, of active specific immunization and treatment with
    Corynebacterium granulosum. Int. J. Radiat. Oncol., Biol.
    and Phys. In Press.

17. Milas, L., Mason, K., and Withers, H.R. Therapy of spon-
    taneous pulmonary metastases of a murine mammary carcinoma
    with anaerobic corynebacteria. Cancer Immunol. Immunother.
    Submitted.

18. Olivotto, M., and Bomford, R. In vitro inhibition of tu-
    mour cell growth and DNA synthesis by peritoneal and lung
    macrophages from mice injected with Corynebacterium par-
    vum. Int. J. Cancer, 13: 478-488, 1974.

19. Proctor, J., Rudenstam, C.M., and Alexander, P. Increas-
    ed incidence of lung metastases following treatment of
    rats bearing hepatomas with irradiated tumour cells and
    the beneficial effect of Corynebacterium parvum in this
    system. Biomedicine, 19:248-252, 1973.

20. Scott, M.T. Corynebacterium parvum as an immunotherapeu-
    tic anticancer agent. Seminars Oncol., 1:367-378, 1974.

21. Suit, H.D., Kaštelan, A. Immunologic status of host and
    response of a methylcholanthrene-induced sarcoma to local
    X-irradiation. Cancer, 26:232-238, 1970.

22. Yuhas, J.M., Toya, R.E., and Wagner, E. Specific and non-
    specific stimulation of resistance to the growth and me-
    tastasis of line 1 lung carcinoma. Cancer Res., 35:242-
    244, 1975.

INDUCTION OF RESISTANCE TO L1210 LEUKEMIA IN CD2F$_1$ MOUSE
USING L1210 CELLS TREATED WITH GLUTARALDEHYDE
AND CONCANAVALIN A

Tateshi Kataoka, Shigeru Tsukagoshi and Yoshio Sakurai

Cancer Chemotherapy Center
Japanese Foundation for Cancer Research
Kami-Ikebukuro, 1-37-1, Toshima-ku, Tokyo 170, Japan

Introduction

Many experimental procedures have been used to immunize laboratory
animals to syngeneic transplantable tumors. Tumor cells modified in vitro
are often used as an immunogen (3). It is, however, desirable to know
prior to inoculation whether modified cells are transplantable. In the
previous communication, it was reported that transplantability of L1210
mouse leukemic cells treated with glutaraldehyde was inversely related to
cell agglutinability measured in vitro by concanavalin A. It was however, noted that leukemic cells treated with as low as 0.013% glutaraldehyde which were not agglutinable by concanavalin A and therefore no more
malignant were not immunogenic either although their cell surfaces were
close to those of intact cells from immunological and physicochemical
points of view (4).

In the present communication, it is reported that further modification was made on glutaraldehyde-treated leukemic cells to make them
immunogenic and that multiple inoculations of concanavalin A-bound leukemic cells induced immune resistance in CD2F$_1$ mice.

Materials and Methods

L1210 and P388 mouse leukemic cells were collected from ascites of
DBA/2Cr male mice 4 to 5 days after i.p. inoculation of 1 to 3x10^6
cells. BALB/c x DBA/2CrF$_1$ (hereafter referred to as CD2F$_1$) male mice
kindly supplied by DR and D, National Cancer Institute were used for
experiments. Immunogenic cells were prepared by incubating for 30 min at
ice-cold temperature in the presence of glutaraldehyde (4) and for another 1 h in the presence of concanavalin A (Miles Laboratory, Kankakee,
Ill.). Thus-treated cells are referred to as G-ConA-L1210 cells. CD2F$_1$
mice were given i.p. inoculations of immunogenic cells. Challenges were
made by i.p. inoculating 1x10^3 intact leukemic cells or 0.0008%G-ConA
(330 mcg/ml)-L1210 cells (1x10^6). None of non-treated mice survived
any of these inoculations.

Results

Immunogenicity of 0.013%G- and 0.2%G-ConA (330 mcg/ml)-Ll210 cells was examined in terms of effect of concentration of glutaraldehyde. $CD2F_1$ mice were given i.p. inoculation of these immunogenic cells (1×10^6) and one month later challenged with 1×10^3 intact Ll210 cells. None of the mice preimmunized with either of above immunogenic cells survived. However, if the challenge was made by 0.0008%G-ConA (330 mcg/ml)-Ll210 cells (1×10^6) with which all of non-treated mice were killed within 15 days, 10 to 20% of the mice preimmunized with 0.013%G-ConA-Ll210 cells but not with 0.2%G-ConA-Ll210 cells survived. And these survivors were resistant to the subsequent inoculation of intact Ll210 cells (1×10^3). These results indicate that 0.013% glutaraldehyde was superior to 0.2% glutaraldehyde in terms of preservation of the tumor associated antigen without difference in suppression of malignancy of the tumor. This is consistent with the previous result showing that 0.013%G-Ll210 cells were susceptible to immune lysis using rabbit anti Ll210 cell sera and guinea pig sera as a source of complement and also susceptible to sonication to the same extent as intact cells whereas 0.2%G-Ll210 cells were resistant to these treatments. In the following experiments, therefore, 0.013% glutaraldehyde was used.

To induce the immune mice resistant to direct inoculation of intact Leukemic cells, G-ConA (330 mcg/ml)-Ll210 cells (1×10^6) were inoculated to mice three times at two week intervals. One month later they were challenged with intact Ll210 cells (1×10^3). Ten to 20% of the immunized mice survived the challenge. None of the mice immunized with G-Ll210 cells survived indicating the requirement of ConA for induction of immune resistance. No further increase of survival incidence was obtained with G-ConA (2.6 mg/ml)-Ll210 cells under the same experimental condition. It is likely that ConA binding sites on cell surface were saturated in the presence of 330 mcg/ml Con A (5).

To increase survival incidence, mice were immunized three times with G-ConA (330 mcg/ml)-Ll210 cells (8×10^6) at half a week intervals. Three weeks later, they were challenged with intact Ll210 cells (1×10^3). The result is shown in Table. Over 50% of the mice survived. The specificity of induced resistance was evidenced by the fact that none of immunized mice under the same experimental condition survived inoculation of P388 mouse leukemic cells (1×10^3) although Ll210 leukemia was more malignant than P388 leukemia in terms of resultant mean survival days of non-treated mice after inoculation (11.5 days and 17.2 days respectively).

Discussion

At the present moment it is not clear how inoculation of ConA-bound tumor cells leads to induction of immune resistance. However, it should be noted that intact EL-4 mouse lymphoid leukemia cells were lysed by spleen cells collected from the mice preimmunized with irradiated and ConA treated EL-4 cells (5). Further experiments will clarify the role played by ConA.

With regard to significance of glutaraldehyde treatment, it will be discussed from three points of view. First, glutarldehyde suppressed transplantability of leukemic cells so that immunization was made safely without killing animals. Secondly, cell-bound ConA molecules that were required for immunogenic cells would be liberated through endocytosis (7) unless cells were pretreated with glutaraldehyde. Thirdly, tumor transplantation antigen was preserved in G-L1210 cells if concentration of glutaraldehyde was sufficiently low.

Other investigators have shown that tumor cells treated with glutaraldehyde or formaldehyde were sufficiently immunogenic to induce the resistant mice (1) (2). This was not the case with L1210 leukemia. This discrepancy is open to further experiments although it is probable that L1210 leukemia used in this study was less immunogenic and more malignant (6).

Summary

Preimmunization with L1210 mouse leukemia treated with glutaraldehyde and concanavalin A induced L1210 leukemia-specific immune resistance in BALB/c x DBA/2CrF$_1$ mice measured by survival incidence after challenge with the intact or modified leukemic cells of less malignancy. For the preparation of immunogenic cells incubation with both of glutaraldehyde and ConA was required. Multiple immunizations by large inoculum dose at short intervals induced higher immune resistance.

Acknowledgement

We are grateful to DR&D, National Cancer Institute for supply of DBA/2Cr and CD2F$_1$ male mice. This research was supported in part by a Grant-in-Aid for Cancer Research from the Ministry of Education, Science and Culture, Japan.

TABLE

Specificity of immune resistance induced by glutaraldehyde- and ConA-treated L1210 cells. Mice were immunized three times with 0.013%G-ConA (330 µg/ml)- L1210 cells (0.8×10^7) at half a week intervals. Three weeks later they were challenged with L1210 cells or P388 cells. Survivors were counted one month later.

Challenging Inoculum	No. of Survivors/Total
L1210 cells 1×10^2	7/10
1×10^3	6/10
1×10^4	4/10
P388 cells 1×10^3	0/9

References

1. Bekesi, J.G., St.-Arneault, G. and Holland, J.F. Increase of Leukemia L1210 Immunogenicity by _Vibrio cholerae_ Neuraminidase Treatment. Cancer Research, 31: 2130-2132, 1971.

2. Frost, P. and Sanderson, C.J. Tumor Immunoprophylaxis in Mice Using Glutaraldehyde-treated Syngeneic Tumor Cells. Cancer Res., 35: 2646-2650, 1975.

3. Hersh, E.M., Gutterman, J.U., and Mavligit, G. Immunotherapy of Cancer in Man, pp. 74-78. Charles C. Thomas, U.S.A. 1973.

4. Kataoka, T., Tsukagoshi, S., and Sakurai, Y. Transplantability of L1210 Cell in BALB/c x DBA/2F$_1$ Mice Associated with Cell Agglutinability by Concanavalin A. Cancer Res., 35: 531-534, 1975.

5. Martin, W.J., Wunderlich, J.R., Fletcher, F., and Inman, J.K. Enhanced Immunogenicity of Chemically-Coated Syngeneic Tumor Cells. Proc. Natl. Acad. Sci., 68: 469-472, 1971.

6. Mihich, E. Combined Effects of Chemotherapy and Immunity Against Leukemia L1210 in DBA/2 Mice. Cancer Res., 29: 848-854, 1969.

7. Unanue, E.R., Perkins, W.D. and Karnovsky, M.J. Ligand-induced Movement of Lymphocyte Membrane Macromolecules. I. Analysis by Immunofluorescence and Ultrastructural Radioautography. J. Exptl. Med. 136: 885-906, 1972.

Section 2

CELL MEDIATED IMMUNITY

ANTI-TUMOUR CELL MEDIATED IMMUNITY AND 'BLOCKING'
FACTOR (ANTIBODY) IN PROSTATIC CANCER

Richard J. Ablin*, Rashid A. Bhatti, Gailon R. Bruns, and
Patrick D. Guinan

Divisions of Immunology* and Urology, Cook County Hospital,
Chicago, Illinois

INTRODUCTION

Studies derived from a rather broad base of experimental
and clinical investigation have brought forth a substantial
body of evidence of the participation of immunobiologic phenomena in the resistance of the host to malignancy. Initially
receiving little attention, the diverse behavior of the natural history of prostatic cancer suggests that host resistance
may play a significant role in the pathogenesis of this disease (14). This together with the identification of the participation of parameters of cellular and humorally-mediated
immunologic responsiveness in prostatic cancer, recently reviewed (4), has provided evidence and impetus for continued
investigation of the role of immunobiologic factors in diseases of the prostate and of the possible implementation of
immunotherapy in patients with prostatic cancer (3).
Recent interest in immunologic studies of the patient
with prostatic malignancy has focused in the main on evaluation of the cellular aspects of immunologic responsiveness.
Such studies have, with exception of recent reports from this
laboratory employing inhibition of leukocyte migration by extracts of prostatic tissue (9,10,13), relied upon evaluation
of non-specific parameters. While the results derived from
evaluating non-specific parameters of cellular responsiveness
have, other than demonstrating that prostatic cancer patients
possess aberrations of immunocompetence (8,11,16,17,19,26,28,
29), which become depressed further following therapy (7,12,
18,30), not only shown no correlation with the clinical extent of disease but do not provide a means for evaluating host
responsiveness to tumour.
As one means of evaluating cellular immunity, inhibition
of leukocyte migration by prostatic tissue extracts has provided some indication of host responsiveness to tumour (9,10,
13). However, technical difficulties with this assay (13)
have directed attention to other in vitro tests for evaluation
of host responsiveness to tumour at the cellular level. For
this purpose modification of the recently described leukocyte

391

adherence inhibition (LAI) test (23) has been employed as an alternate method to evaluate the presence of anti-tumour immunity in patients with prostatic cancer.

Suppression of cellular responsiveness by serum from prostatic cancer patients (6,11,17,19,26), although observed through evaluation of non-specific parameters, and the concomitant abrogation or reduction of this suppression in association with a favorable clinical response following cryotherapy of the prostate (3) also prompted study of the interference ('blocking') of anti-tumour immunity by serum of the patients evaluated.

PROCEDURES AND MATERIALS USED

Patients.

Eight patients with a histologic diagnosis of adenocarcinoma of the prostate stage D, ranging in age from 62 to 75 years were evaluated. Staging was in accord with conventional protocol (31). All patients were receiving conventional treatment at the time of evaluation.

Specimens.

Tissues were obtained at surgery. In the case of prostatic tissue this was at the time of transurethral resection. Twenty ml. of heparinized blood and 10 ml clotted blood were obtained from each patient. Normal human serum as a source of homologous serum was obtained from healthy adult volunteers.

Tissue Extracts.

Extracts were prepared by solubilization of tissues in hypertonic (3M) KCl employing a modification of the method of Meltzer (27) and Brannen et al. (15). Finely minced tissue trimmed of extraneous material was washed in phosphate buffered saline (PBS) pH 7.2, and lyophilized. The resulting lyophilizate was pulverized with mortar and pestle, resuspended in 10 ml of 3M KCl in 0.005M potassium phosphate buffer pH 7.4, per gram wet weight of original tissue, and left overnight at 4°C with intermittent agitation. The KCl tissue suspension was then centrifuged at 40,000 g for 60 min. after which the supernate was dialyzed overnight at 4°C against deionized water. The supernate was then recentrifuged at 40,000 g for 15 min. to remove the gelatinous precipitate formed during dialysis and passed through a 0.45 mμ Nalgene filter into a sterile Nalgene filter flask. The filtrate was lyophilized and reconstituted to one tenth of its original volume in sterile PBS.

The protein concentration of extracts so prepared as determined by the Lowry method (25) ranged from 1.0 to 3.8 mg/ml

Cells and Sera.

Peripheral blood lymphocytes (PBL) were obtained by centrifugation of the leukocyte-rich plasma of heparinzed blood on a Ficoll-Isopaque gradient. Following washing in minimal essential medium, PBL were resuspended in RPM1 1640 medium containing 100 units/ml penicillin G and 100 µg/ml streptomicin at a concentration of 2×10^7 cells/ml.

Sera were heat inactivated at 56°C for 30 min. prior to use.

Leukocyte Adherence Inhibition Test.

Employing a modification of the LAI test (23) three cultures of equal volumes (0.1 ml) of the patient's PBL plus:

   (i)   Homologous serum of a blood type identical to that of the patient under evaluation. This was the control and contained no tumour ex tract, permitting establishment of a baseline of normal adherence. Tumour extract (as a source of antigen), employed in (ii) and (iii) described below, was replaced by the same volume of medium.

   (ii) Homologous serum + autologous tumour extract.

   (iii) Autologous serum + autologous tumour extract.

were initially prepared and incubated at 37°C for 30 minutes with intermittent shaking. Each culture mixture was then introduced independently into each of the two chambers of Standard Neubauer haemocytometers, i.e., one culture/haemocytometer, thereby permitting duplicate cell counts/culture and incubated at 37°C for 60 minutes in a humid atmosphere. The total number of cells in each chamber were then counted microscopically at a magnification of 400x in predetermined areas. In the present study, 8 squares (0.2mm x 0.2mm) were counted in each chamber of the haemocytometer. Cover slips were floated off, each haemocytometer gently immersed in Hanks' solution at 37°C, slowly withdrawn, and again immersed and withdrawn. Each chamber of the haemocytometer then received one drop of Hanks' solution and was covered with a clean coverslip The number of remaining "adherent" cells were counted in the same squares of the haemocytometer examined previously and the mean % of adherent cells for each culture determined.

A standard deviation of ± 10.25% adherence between the cell counts for each chamber of the haemocytometer/culture was obtained with this method.

Investigation of the cross-reactivity and tissue specificity of sensitized PBL and 'blocking' factor was carried out by incubation of cultures of the patient's PBL and autologous serum with extracts of allogeneic tumour and non-tumourous tissues of prostatic and non-prostatic origin.

Patients with prostatic cancer were evaluated for the presence of anti-tumour cell mediated immunity and for the ability of their serum to interfere ('block') this immunity employing the LAI test. An example illustrating the manner of
approach in employing the LAI test in this study is shown in
Table I.

Initially a baseline of normal % adherence as a control
was determined by culturing the patient's PBL in medium and
homologous serum in the absence of tumour extract. The patient's PBL were then cultured with homologous serum and autologous tumour extract. As shown in the example (Table I), 8%
adherence obtained in such cultures was reduced compared to
the normal baseline of 65% adherence obtained in the absence
of tumour extract. This difference in % adherence suggested
that an interaction of extract (antigen) with presumably sensitized PBL had occurred.* In contrast to the interaction of
antigen and PBL in the presence of homologous serum, culturing
of the patient's PBL with autologous serum and tumour extract
resulted in an increase in the % adherence from 8 to 60, the
latter approximating the % adherence obtained in the absence
of extract. This difference in % adherence suggested the absence of the interaction of antigen and sensitized cells. Absence of a detectable reaction between tumour extract and autologous PBL, presumed to be sensitized on the basis of their
interaction with extract in the absence of autologous serum
was suggested to be due to the presence of a factor(s) in the
patient's serum interfering ('blocking') with this interaction.

Further application of the method of LAI for evaluation
of cross-reactive tumour immunity of sensitized PBL and the
specificity of serum 'blocking' factor(s) employed in this
study are also illustrated in Table I.

When sensitized PBL and autologous serum were reacted
with an allogeneic prostatic tumour extract of the same tumour
type, reactivity, i.e., interaction of cells and extract, was
observed as indicated by the low % adherence obtained in comparison with that in the control, i.e., in the example given,
17% vs. 65%. This cross-reactivity indicated that the patient's lymphocytes were also sensitized to antigens apparently shared in common within tumours of the same type. Observation of a lower % adherence when the tumour extract was allogeneic with respect to the patient's PBL rather than autologous, i.e., 17% vs. 8%, suggested that cross-reactive immunity
to allogeneic tumour was less. In contrast to the high % adherence observed when PBL and autologous serum were reacted
with an autologous tumour extract, i.e., 60%, indicating the
absence of an interaction of antigen and cells and the presence of 'blocking', a low % adherence, i.e., 17%, was

---

*The possibility that the observed reduction in the % of ad-
hering cells was attributable to toxic effects of the tumour
extract on PBL rather than their interaction was not apparent
as determined by trypan-blue dye exclusion.

observed when the tumour extract was allogeneic with respect
to cells and serum. This interaction of antigen and cells in
the presence of serum previously demonstrated to interfere
with the reactivity of autologous PBL and tumour extract suggested the absence of 'blocking' and the apparent specificity
of the serum 'blocking' factor(s) for autologous PBL and tumour extract.

Following the example illustrating the application of the
LAI test and interpretation of the results shown in Table I,
the presence of anti-tumour immunity; serum 'blocking' factor;
antigenic cross-reactivity of this immunity and specificity of
'blocking' factor(s) in patients with prostatic cancer were
evaluated.

As shown in Table II, cell-mediated responsiveness of PBL
to autologous tumour and the presence of serum 'blocking' factor were observed in six patients.

Antigenic cross-reactivity of immunity with allogeneic extracts prepared from tumours of the same type and the specificity of 'blocking' factor of the reactions for autologous
tumour were further evaluated in five of the six patients.
Two patients (G.E. and J.T.) were evaluated with two allogeneic extracts. In each case, cross-reactivity between the
patient's PBL previously observed to react with autologous tumour was observed with allogeneic tumour. Cross-reactivity
with allogeneic tumour, as shown in Table II, appeared to be
less than that observed with autologous tumour in three patients (G.E., W.G. and J.T.) and greater in two (J.F. and
W.H.). Comparison of the degree of cross-reactive immunity
present in two patients (R.C. and S.T.) to that observed with
autologous tumour was not possible as the latter was not
evaluated.

In contrast to cross-reactive immunity, the apparent absence of 'blocking' when the patient's serum was allogeneic
with respect to the extract, i.e., to interfere with the interaction of sensitized PBL and allogeneic prostatic tumour
extract, as indicated from the low % adherence in each of the
patients evaluated (Table II), implied that the serum fac-
tor(s) was specific for interference of the interaction of
autologous PBL and tumour extract.

Studies to ascertain the tissue-specificity of anti-tumour immunity disclosed the presence of reactivity of PBL with
extracts of benign prostatic tissue in two patients (R.C., 32%
adherence and S.T., 33% adherence) and normal bladder in one
(G.E., 6% adherence). Evaluation of one patient (J.T.) with
extract of carcinomatous kidney (renal cell carcinoma) showed
no reactivity (51% adherence).

DISCUSSION

Modification of the LAI test has provided further evidence suggestive of the presence of anti-tumour cell mediated
immunity in patients with prostatic cancer previosuly observed
by inhibition of leukocyte migration (9,10,13). Serum from

the patients evaluated was observed to interfere ('block') with anti-tumour immunity as observed through its inhibitory effect on the interaction of sensitized PBL and autologous tumour antigen. This effect of autologous serum may be analogous to 'blocking' observed in colony inhibition and lymphocyte cytotoxicity tests (24) and may be indicative of one means by which the potential effects of sensitized PBL are inhibited in vivo.

Lymphocytes reactive with extract preparations of autologous tumour were also observed to react with allogeneic extracts prepared from tissue of the same tumour type. Cross-reactive immunity between individual tumours, within a given tumour type is in keeping with observations employing LAI in evaluation of patients with other tumours, e.g., breast, colon and melanoma (23).

Specificity studies of anti-tumour immunity disclosed reactivity of sensitized PBL with benign prostatic tissue (two patients) and with normal bladder (one patient). No reactivity was observed in one patient evaluated with kidney extract prepared from a patient with renal cell carcinoma.

In the two patients showing cross-reactivity of their PBL with benign prostatic tissue, it is perhaps of interest to mention that the % adherence was greater than that observed when the same PBL were reacted with malignant prostatic tissue extracts. This suggested that while reactivity was observed with benign tissue, that the degree of sensitization and immunity was greater to malignant tissue.

Similar cross-reactivity, however, occurring at the humoral level, where: (i) antisera from animals immunized with extracts of carcinomatous prostatic tissue reacted with benign prostatic tissue extracts (1) and (ii) serum from patients with benign prostatic hypertrophy and carcinoma of the bladder yielded immunofluorescent staining patterns similar to those observed with prostatic cancer patients (5) has been observed. Thus, evidence of some degree of reactivity with tissues other than malignant prostate, however so slight, suggests that this immunity might best be referred to as "anti-tumour associated immunity".

In contrast to cross-reactive immunity, the observed 'blocking' effect of serum on immunity appeared to be specific for interference of the interaction of sensitized PBL and autologous tumour, as 'blocking' was not observed when the serum was allogeneic to the tumour extract. The suggestion of the specificity of 'blocking' factor for autologous tumour in prostatic cancer patients is somewhat unique in comparison to observations in other tumours and will require confirmation.

It has been suggested (22) that the reactions observed in the LAI test, may be related to the interaction of antigen with sensitized PBL as, e.g., in inhibition of macrophage or leukocyte migration as related to the liberation of 'lymphokines' which in turn alter the adhering properties ("stickiness") of indicator macrophages or leukocytes (20). We may envisage that PBL, including indicator macrophages, cultured in the presence of homologous serum and absence of antigen, maintain their adhesive properties and stick to the glass surface of the haemocytometer. Re-encounter of sensitized PBL with specific antigen, i.e., in cultures of cells, tumour extract and homologous serum, leads to the liberation of 'lymphokines', altering their adhesive properties such that cells reacting with antigen no longer stick to the glass surface. When sensitized cells and specific antigen are cultured in the presence of serum possessing 'blocking' factor (antibody), interaction of antigen with sensitized cells and the liberation of 'lymphokines' is prevented. The cells, thus maintain their adhesive properties sticking to the glass surface as indicated by the high % adherence observed.

Contrary to the above mechanism, recent studies (21) suggest that no evidence was obtained that a factor analogous to migration inhibitory factor or to other 'lymphokines' was released. Rather, it has been suggested (21) that interaction of sensitized PBL with tumour antigen, produces cell surface alterations inhibiting attachment of the cells to glass.

Studies are in progress to elucidate the immunoglobulin nature of the observed serum 'blocking' factor (antibody), alterations of its reactivity as related to tumour stage and clinical responsiveness, as well as further evaluation of the tissue-specificity of sensitized PBL from prostatic cancer patients and from patients with other malignancies. It will be particularly interesting to evaluate and compare the antigenic diversity of extracts of carcinomatous prostatic tissue [previous studies of which have suggested malignant tissue to be antigenically deficient with respect to normal and benign (1)] and the sensitivity of autologous and allogeneic lymphocytes with their reactivity to extracts of normal and benign prostatic tissue. Pending the outcome of such studies, the identification of a prostatic tumour-specific or tumour-associated antigen is a possibility in view of the present preliminary observations.

SUMMARY

Antigen-induced leukocyte adherence inhibition has been employed to investigate the presence of anti-tumour cell mediated immunity in patients with adenocarcinoma of the prostate. Interference ('blocking') of this immunity by homologous and autologous serum was also evaluated. Peripheral blood lymphocytes (PBL) from patients with prostatic cancer reacted to varying degrees with 3M KCl extracts of autologous and allogeneic prostatic tumours when cultured in the presence of homologous serum. When sensitized PBL and tumour extract were cultured in autologous serum inhibition ('blocking') of the interaction of PBL and antigen was observed. 'Blocking' was not observed when the tumour extract was allogeneic with respect to the origin of PBL and serum. Cross-reactivity between individual tumours within a given tumour type is in keeping with observations of anti-tumour immunity in patients with other tumours. Observations suggestive of a specificity of 'blocking' for autologous tumour only is somewhat unique and will require further confirmation. In view of the small patient population evaluated, the preliminary nature of these observations is stressed.

TABLE I

Example Illustrating Application of the Leukocyte Adherence
Inhibition Test for the Detection of Anti-Tumour Cell-Mediated
Immunity; Serum 'Blocking' Factor (Antibody); Antigenic Cross-
Reactivity and Specificity of Serum 'Blocking' Factor
(Antibody) in Patient with Prostatic Cancer

Patient's Leukocytes plus:	Mean % Adherence	Explanation
Homologous Serum	65	Normal adherence (Control)
Homologous Serum + Autologous Tumour Extract	8	Cells reactive with autologous extract indicating immunity.
Autologous Serum + Autologous Tumour Extract	60	Serum 'Blocking'
Autologous Serum + Allogeneic Tumour Extract	17	Cells reactive with allogeneic extract indicating cross-reactive immunity but absence of 'blocking' by autologous serum demonstrating specificity of serum 'blocking' factor for autologous tumour.

TABLE II

Anti-Tumour Immunity; Serum 'Blocking' Factor (Antibody);
Antigenic Cross-Reactivity and Specificity of 'Blocking'
Factor (Antibody) in Patients with Prostatic Cancer

Patient's Leukocytes plus:	Mean % Adherence Obtained with Patient:							
	R.C.	G.E.	J.F.	W.G.	W.H.	T.R.	J.T.	S.T.
Homologous Serum	50	65	47	35	66	53	27	72
Homologous Serum + Autologous Tumour Extract	NE[1)	8	31	10	17	34	7	NE
Autologous Serum + Autologous Tumour Extract	NE	60	70	23	72	57	15	NE
Autologous Serum + Allogeneic Tumour Extract	27	23,17[2)	17	12	5	NE	13,28[2)	21

[1) NE = Not evaluated.

[2) Evaluated with two different extracts.

REFERENCES

1. Ablin, R.J. Immunologic studies of normal, benign and malignant human prostatic tissue. Cancer, $\underline{29}$:1570-1574, 1972.

2. Ablin, R.J. Immunotherapy for prostatic cancer. Previous and prospective considerations. Oncology, $\underline{31}$:177-202, 1975.

3. Ablin, R.J. Alpha$_2$-globulin and prostatic cancer: Alteration in level and immunosuppressive properties prior to and following cryoprostatectomy. IRCS Med. Sci., $\underline{4}$:60, 1976.

4. Ablin, R.J. Immunobiology of the Prostate. Experimental, Clinical and Therapeutic Considerations. In Tannenbaum, M. (Ed.): Urological Pathology, Vol. 1, Lea and Febiger, Philadelphia, In press, 1976.

5. Ablin, R.J. Serum antibody in patients with prostatic cancer. Brit. J. Urol., Submitted, 1975.

6. Ablin, R.J., Bruns, G.R., Guinan, P.D., and Bush, I.M. Migration-inhibitory effect of serum from patients with prostatic cancer. Oncology, $\underline{30}$:423-428, 1974.

7. Ablin, R.J., Bruns, G.R., Al Sheik, H., Guinan, P.D., and Bush, I.M. Hormonal therapy and alteration of lymphocyte proliferation. J. Lab. Clin. Med., $\underline{87}$:227-231, 1976.

8. Ablin, R.J., Bruns, G.R., Guinan, P.D., and Bush, I.M. Evaluation of cellular immunologic responsiveness in the clinical management of patients with prostatic cancer. I. Thymic dependent lymphocytic blastogenesis. Urol. int., Submitted, 1976.

9. Ablin, R.J., Bush, I.M., Bruns, G.R., and Guinan, P.D. Continuing evaluation of the use of inhibition of leukocyte migration for in vitro studies of cellular responsiveness in patients with prostatic cancer(Abstract). Clin. Res., $\underline{23}$:485A, 1975.

10. Ablin, R.J., Guinan, P.D., John, T., Sadoughi, N., and Bush, I.M. Evaluation of cellular immunologic responsiveness in the clinical management of patients with prostatic cancer(Abstract). American Urological Association, Inc., 69th Annual Meeting, St. Louis, Mo., 1974.

11. Ablin, R.J., Guinan, P.D., Bruns, G.R., Sadoughi, N., and Bush, I.M. Serum proteins in prostatic cancer. II. Effect on in vitro cell-mediated immunologic responsiveness. Urology, $\underline{6}$:22-29, 1975.

12. Ablin, R.J., Guinan, P.D., Sadoughi, N., Bruns, G.R., and Bush, I.M. Perturbations of host resistance in patients with prostatic cancer following cryosurgery and trans-urethral resection(Abstract). IX European Surgical Congress, Amsterdam, The Netherlands, p. 131, 1975.

13. Ablin, R.J., Guinan, P.D., Bruns, G.R., John, T., Sadoughi, N., and Bush, I.M. Evaluation of cellular immunologic responsiveness in the clinical management of patients with prostatic cancer. III. Inhibition of leukocyte migration. J. Urol., Submitted, 1976.

14. Ashley, D.J.B. On the incidence of carcinoma of the prostate. J. Path. Bact., 90:217-224, 1965.

15. Brannen, G.E., Gomolka, Diana M., and Coffey, D.S. Specificity of cell membrane antigens in prostatic cancer. Cancer Chemotherapy Rep., 59:127-138, 1975.

16. Brosman, S., Hausman, M., and Shacks, S. Immunologic alterations in patients with prostatic carcinoma. J. Urol., 113:841-845, 1975.

17. Bruns, G.R., Ablin, R.J., Guinan, P.D., Nourkayhan, S., and Bush, I.M. Reduced lymphocytic blastogenesis in prostatic cancer(Abstract). Clin. Res., 22:610A, 1974.

18. Catalona, W.J., Potvin, C., and Chretien, P.B. Effect of radiation therapy for urologic cancer on circulating thymus-derived lymphocytes. J. Urol., 112:261-267, 1974.

19. Catalona, W.J., Tarpley, J.L., Chretien, P.B., and Castle, J.R. Lymphocyte stimulation in urologic cancer patients. J. Urol., 112:373-377, 1974.

20. Dumonde, D.C. 'Lymphokines': Molecular mediators of cellular immune responses in animals and man. Proc. Roy. Soc. Med., 63:899-902, 1970.

21. Grosser, N., and Thomson, D.M.P. Cell-mediated antitumor immunity in breast cancer patients evaluated by antigen-induced leukocyte adherence inhibition in test tubes. Cancer Res., 35:2571-2579, 1975.

22. Halliday, W.J., and Miller, Susan. Leukocyte adherence inhibition: A simple test for cell-mediated tumour immunity and serum blocking factors. Int. J. Cancer, 9:477-483, 1972.

23. Halliday, W.J., Maluish, A., and Isbister, W.H. Detection of antitumour cell mediated immunity and serum blocking factors in cancer patients by the leucocyte adherence inhibition test. Brit. J. Cancer, 29:31-35, 1974.

24. Hellström, I., Sjögren, H.O., Warner, G., and Hellström, K.E. Blocking of cell-mediated tumor immunity by sera from patients with growing neoplasms. Int. J. Cancer, 7: 226-237, 1971.

25. Lowry, O.H., Rosebrough, N., Farr, A., and Randall, R. Protein measurement with the Folin phenol reagent. J. Biol. Chem., 193:265-275, 1951.

26. McLaughlin, III, A.P., and Brooks, J.D. A plasma factor inhibiting lymphocyte reactivity in urologic cancer patients. J. Urol., 112:366-372, 1974.

27. Meltzer, M.S., Leonard, E.J., Rapp, H.J., and Borsos, T. Tumor-specific antigen solubilized by hypertonic potassium chloride. J. Nat'l. Cancer Inst., 47:703-709, 1971.

28. Robinson, M.R.G., Nakhla, L.S., and Whitaker, R.H. Lymphocyte transformation in carcinoma of the prostate. Brit. J. Urol., 43:480-486, 1971.

29. Robinson, M.R.G., Nakhla, L.S., and Whitaker, R.H. A new concept in the management of carcinoma of the prostate. Brit. J. Urol., 43:728-732, 1971.

30. Robinson, M.R.G., Nakhla, L.S., Shearer, R., Trott, P., and Rigby, C.C. Lymphocyte transformation and the prognosis of prostatic cancer. XVI Congress of the International Society of Urology, Vol. 2, pp. 177-188, 1973.

31. Scott, W.W., and Schirmer, H.K.A. Carcinoma of the Prostate, p. 1143. In Campbell, W.W. and Harrison, H.W. (Eds.): Urology, W.B. Saunders Co., Philadelphia, 1970.

RELATIONSHIP BETWEEN T-LYMPHOCYTE BLASTOGENESIS, SERUM BLOCKING FACTORS AND PROGNOSIS IN CANCER

Charles H. Antinori, Joseph A. Buda, Frederic P. Herter, Anthony P. Molinaro, Keith Reemtsma, Nicole Suciu-Foca

Columbia University,
College of Physicians and Surgeons
New York, N.Y., U.S.A.

I. INTRODUCTION

The major role of thymus dependent lymphocytes (T-cells) in the immunological defense against cancer is indicated by the observation that impairment of T-cell functions as occurring with increasing age, immuno-suppressive treatments or congenital thymus deficiencies is accompanied by a significant increase in the incidence of malignacies. While a breakdown of immunological surveillance might well account for the escape from immune destruction of cells undergoing neoplastic differen-tiation, progressive tumor growth per se appears to further suppress T-cell reactivity. Evidence to this effect derives both from in vitro and in vivo studies which indicate that depression of T-cell responses parallels progression of neoplastic disease. The hypotheses were advanced that cellular immune deficiencies in cancer are caused by an intrinisic defect of T-lymphocytes or that the immunological function of these cells is inhibited by humoral blocking factors (1).

We have challenged this second hypothesis by testing the effect of sera from cancer patients on the responsiveness of autologous lymphocytes and of lymphocytes from normal individuals to PHA and to allogenic cells. Since MLC and PHA responsiveness (2) are the most reliable functional markers for cells mediating the cellular immune response (T-lymphocytes), it was assumed that, if blocking factors are present in cancer sera, they should lead to inhibition of in vitro blastogenesis as displayed by normal lymphocytes.

II. PROCEDURES AND MATERIALS USED

A. Subjects. Sera and heparinized blood were obtained from patients with cancer of the gastrointestinal tract, breast, lung and extremities. Criteria of patient selection included no prior chemotherapy, irradiation or blood transfusions. Lymphocytes and sera from healthy controls were simultaneously tested.

B. Preparation of Lymphocyte Suspensions. Lymphocyte suspensions were ob-tained from venous blood by the Ficoll-Isopaque gradient purification method. Cells were suspended and washed 3 times in RPMI 1640 medium supplemented with penicillin, streptomycin and glutamine. Cultures were

set up in microtest plates as described previously (1). All cells were tested in parallel in the presence of autologous serum and of a pool of homologous serum which was obtained from a panel of healthy male volunteers. Sera were added directly to the culture wells at a final concentration of 25% (v/v). Cells were incubated for 5 days in a humidified 5% CO_2 atmosphere, then labelled with tritiated thymidine (1μCi per culture), and harvested automatically. Triplicate cultures were used for each reaction. Thymidine incorporation was measured by liquid scintillation counting and expressed as the mean of CPM in triplicate cultures.
C. MLC Test. Responding lymphocytes from each subject were cultured with a mixture of mitomycin-treated stimulating cells obtained from a standard panel of 10 HLA different individuals. Each culture contained $1x10^5$ responding lymphocytes and $2x10^5$ stimulating lymphocytes in a total volume of 0.25 ml. of medium.
D. PHA Test. Cultures containing $2x10^5$ lymphocytes were challenged with purified PHA (Burroughs-Wellcome Phytomitogen MR 68) at a final concentration of 5 mcg per ml.
E. Determination of Serum Blocking Activity. The ability of each serum to support in vitro lymphocyte blastogenesis was screened on a panel of responding lymphocytes obtained from 10 healthy staff members. Responding lymphocytes from the panel members were challenged in parallel cultures with the standard stimulating cell mixture and with PHA. The percent inhibition of blastogenesis produced by the tested serum was calculated from the baseline values obtained in pooled male AB serum (1,3,4).

III. RESULTS

A. Relationship between Lymphocyte Reactivity in MLC and PHA Tests and Survival of Patients with Cancer. Results obtained by testing the PHA and MLC responsiveness of lymphocytes from cancer patients and of normal controls in autologous and normal homologous serum were grouped according to the extent of tumor growth at the time of testing and to the patient's survival for more than one year or less than one year (Table 1). Sera depressing the blastogenic response below 50% of the values obtained in pooled normal homologous serum were considered positive for inhibitory factors.

Lymphocyte reactivity in both PHA and MLC tests was significantly lower in patients who survived for less than one year than in those with longer survival. Impairment of lymphocyte reactivity in these patients was particularly evident when autologous rather than pooled normal homologous serum was used for testing.

Patients with localized cancer, as well as 1-year survivors from the group with regional or distant spread at the time of testing showed a lower incidence of inhibitory sera and higher rates of lymphocyte blastogenesis.
B. Effect of Serum from Cancer Patients on MLC and PHA Reactivity of Lymphocytes from Normal Subjects. Table 2 summarizes the results obtained by testing the effect of sera from cancer patients and normal controls on the MLC and PHA reactivity of lymphocytes from a constant panel of 10 healthy volunteers.

There was a significant increase in the frequency of sera with lymphocyte suppressive activity in patients surviving for less than one year as compared to patients with longer survival. The lymphocyte suppressive effect, as reflected in the incidence of sera reducing blastogenesis by more than 50%, was better visualized in MLC than in PHA tests.

The negative correlation between survival of the patient and serum inhibitory activity was seen in all groups of cancer patients, regardless of the primary site of the tumor.

IV. DISCUSSION AND SUMMARY

Our present investigations demonstrate that lymphocytes from cancer patients have a decreased ability to respond to in vitro stimulation with allogenic cells and with PHA. Data obtained by testing the effect of sera from cancer patients on autologous lymphocytes and on normal homologous lymphocytes clearly indicate that cancer sera contain lymphocyte suppressive factors (1,3).

The incidence of strongly inhibitory sera was significantly increased in patients surviving for less than one year as compared to those in earlier stages and/or with longer survival, particularly when tested in MLC.

The positive correlation between strong inhibitory activity and rapid evolution of the tumor suggests the possible prognostic value of the MLC inhibition test and its potential use in basing therapy on immunologic evidence. If further confirmed, the availability of a simple method for studying in vitro the interference between serum blocking factors and T-lymphocytes opens a new approach to the immunological evaluation of cancer patients. In view of the possible therapeutic manipulation of the level of serum inhibitory factors in a variety of clinical conditions such as cancer, autoimmune diseases, and transplantation (1,3,4,5), the isolation and characterization of this factor becomes a major challenge which now lies ahead of us.

TABLE I. Relationship between Lymphocyte Reactivity in MLC and PHA Tests and Survival of Cancer Patients

Subjects	Survival	No. of subjects	MLC reactivity (CPM x 10^3 + SE) autologous serum	normal serum	Per cent inhibitory sera	MLC reactivity (CPM x 10^3 +SE) autologous serum	normal serum	Incidence of inhibitory sera %
Normal controls		60	25 ±4	25 ±5	0	23 ±2	24 ±3	0
Patients with cancer:								
Localized	1 Year	40	18 ±3	22 ±3	26	17 ±2	20 ±3	10
Regional spread	>1 Year	29	14 ±2	20 ±3	14	14 ±2	18 ±3	10
	< 1 Year	15	3 ±1	11 ±2	68	5 ±1	8 ±2	45
Distant spread	>1 Year	32	14 ±3	21 ±4	20	12 ±2	14 ±2	18
	< 1 Year	14	7 ±2	12 ±3	54	7 ±2	11 ±2	50

TABLE II. Effect of Serum from Cancer Patients on MLC and PHA Reactivity of Lymphocytes from Normal Subjects

Serum Donors	Survival	MLC Test No. inhibitory sera/total	(%)	PHA Test No. inhibitory sera/total	(%)
Normal controls		0/60	(0%)	0/60	(0%)
Patients with Cancer:					
Localized	1 Year	10/40	(25%)	4/40	(10%)
Regional spread	> 1 Year	5/29	(17%)	3/29	(10%)
	< 1 Year	10/15	(66%)	6/15	(40%)
Distant spread	> 1 Year	7/32	(21%)	7/32	(21%)
	< 1 Year	9/14	(64%)	5/14	(36%)

TABLE III. Relationship Between Primary Site of the Tumor, Serum Inhibitory Activity and Survival

Primary site of the tumor	Patients survival for: More than one year No. patients with MLC inhibitory sera/total patients (%)		Less than one year	
Breast	9/46	(20%)	6/10	(60%)
Gastro-intestinal	9/38	(24%)	9/14	(64%)
Lung	1/4	(25%)	2/2	(100%)
Extremities	3/13	(23%)	2/3	(67%)
Total	22/101	(22%)	19/29	(65%)

REFERENCES

1. Suciu-Foca, N., Buda, J.A., McManus, J., Thiem, T., and Reemtsma, K. Impaired Responsiveness Of Lymphocytes And Serum Inhibitory Factors In Patients With Cancer. Cancer Res., 33: 2373-2377, 1973.
2. Good, R.A. Structure-Function Relations In The Lymphoid System. Clin. Immunol., 1: 1-28, 1972.
3. Suciu-Foca, N., Buda, J.A., LoGerfo, P., Moulton, A., Weber, C., Wheeler, B., and Reemtsma, K. Serum Inhibitory Factors In Cancer Oncology. 29: 219-226, 1974.
4. Suciu-Foca, N., Buda, J.A., Thiem, T., Almojera, P., Reemtsma, K., Inhibition Of Mixed Leukocyte Culture Reactivity By Sera From Haemodialysis Patients And Transplant Recipients As An Indicator Of Isoimmunization. Lab. Invest. 31: 1-5, 1974.
5. Suciu-Foca, N., Buda, J.A., Thiem, T., and Reemtsma, K. Impaired Responsiveness Of Lymphocytes In Patients With Systemic Lupus Erythematosus. Clinical Exp. Immunol., 18: 295-301, 1974.

A SERUM INHIBITOR OF CELL MEDIATED IMMUNOLOGICAL FUNCTIONS
IN HEALTHY MICE AND POSSIBLE CORRELATIONS WITH C-TYPE VIRAL
EXPRESSION AND SPONTANEOUS NEOPLASIA

James G. Krueger and Rex C. Moyer

Thorman Cancer Research Laboratory
Trinity University
San Antonio, Texas 78284 U.S.A.

I. INTRODUCTION

The responsiveness of peripheral lymphocytes in various mouse strains
has previously been measured using an unpurified preparation of the mitogen phytohemagglutinin (Heiniger et al., 1975). It has been suggested that
the lack of response of lymphocytes from certain inbred mouse strains may
be attributable to inhibition by serum factors (Heiniger et al., 1973;
Heiniger et al., 1975). However, inhibitors have heretofore not been described in healthy, virgin mice. Factors in serum which inhibit cell-
mediated immunological functions such as phytohemagglutinin responsiveness have been described for leukemias (Abell et al., 1970; Humphrey and
Lankford, 1973; Humphrey et al., 1975) and for other types of neoplasia
(Hellström et al., 1971; Sample et al., 1971).

If serum factors interfere with immunological surveillance against
neoplastic cells (Burnet, 1970), it is possible that inhibitors could be
present before the neoplastic transformation. This paper presents data
suggesting an inhibitor of cell-mediated immunological functions in the
serum of healthy DBA/2J mice possessing latent C-type leukemia virus.
The inhibitor reduces phytohemagglutinin responsiveness of peripheral and
splenic lymphocytes and the inhibitor prevents the stimulation of DBA/2J
splenic lymphocytes by soluble tumor associated antigen from a syngeneic
mammary carcinoma.

II. PROCEDURES AND MATERIALS USED

A. Mice

Virgin female mice 10 to 14 weeks of age from the following inbred
strains were used: A/J, AKR/J, C57BL/6J, C57BL/10J, C57L/J, C57BR/cdJ,
DBA/2J, PL/J, and SWR/J. In addition, the congenic resistant strain
B10.D2/oSn--H-2^d and the F_1-hybrid C57BL/6J x DBA/2J (hereafter called
B6D2F$_1$) were used. Mice were obtained from production colonies of the
Jackson Laboratory, Bar Harbor, Maine, USA, at 5 to 7 weeks of age.

Animals were maintained in our laboratory and were age-matched in parallel experiments. C57BL/6 x DBA/2 F_2 (hereafter called B6D2F$_2$) mice used for genetic analysis were bred in our laboratory from B6D2F$_1$ parents.

B. Medium

RPMI 1640 containing 100 IU penicillin per ml, 100 µg streptomycin per ml, and 2 mM glutamine obtained from Grand Island Biological Company (GIBCO), Grand Island, N. Y., USA, was used for all experiments. In specified experiments the medium was supplemented with 15% fetal calf serum (GIBCO), or with 10% autologous mouse serum and 5% fetal calf serum.

C. Mouse Sera

Mice were bled either from the retro-orbital sinus or from the tail vein. Blood was allowed to clot at room temperature for 20 minutes and the serum was separated by centrifugation at 2000 x g for 30 minutes. Sera were used fresh or stored at -20°C.

D. Tumors

Two tumor lines were used as a source of soluble tumor associated antigen: BW10232, a mammary adenocarcinoma, which arose spontaneously in C57BL/6J mice at the Jackson Laboratory and has been maintained in subcutaneous transplant since 1958; and CaD2, a mammary adenocarcinoma which arose spontaneously in DBA/2J mice and has been maintained in subcutaneous transplant since 1960. The tumor lines were obtained in tumor-bearing mice from the Jackson Laboratory and were passed in subcutaneous transplant at least 3 times in our laboratory before use in experiments.

E. Purified Phytohemagglutinin and ^{3}H-Phytohemagglutinin

Purified phytohemagglutinin was obtained as a lyophilized powder from Burroughs Wellcome, Triangle Park, N. C., USA. Tritium labeled ([3]H-) phytohemagglutinin was prepared by exposing 10 mg of the powder to 3 Ci tritium gas for a period of 21 days (Wilzbach, 1957). The tritium labeling was performed by New England Nuclear Corporation, Boston, Mass., USA. Final specific activity was 2.2 mCi per mg. Phytohemagglutinin and ^{3}H-phytohemagglutinin were diluted to a concentration of 1 mg per ml with sterile H_2O and stored at -20°C for a maximum of 6 months. Phytohemagglutinin and ^{3}H-phytohemagglutinin were diluted to final working concentrations with medium.

F. Lymphocyte Microculture From Whole Blood

Microculture of whole blood modified from Heiniger et al. (1973) was used to assess lymphocyte blastogenic response to phytohemagglutinin. Fifty µl heparinized whole blood was introduced into 12 mm x 75 mm plastic tubes containing 500 µl serum-free medium and phytohemagglutinin. The cultures were incubated for 52 hours in a humidified atmosphere of 5% CO_2 and 95% air. The cultures were pulsed with 0.5 µCi ^{3}H-thymidine, (2.0 Ci/mM, New England Nuclear Corporation, Boston, Mass., USA) 22 hours

410

prior to harvesting. The cultures were harvested by extraction onto glass fiber filters (Reeve Angel, No. 934AH) with a vacuum sampling manifold (Millipore, No. 3025) followed by washes with 15 ml of 0.14 M NaCl, 6% perchloric acid, and 70% ethanol. The filters were solubilized in 1 ml NCS tissue solubilizer (Amersham/Searle) and the amount of ^{3}H-thymidine incorporated was determined by scintillation counting. The counts per minute of the incorporated ^{3}H-thymidine were corrected for quench and the results were expressed in disintegrations per minute (DPM). Results were also expressed as a stimulation index (SI) which is the ratio of mean DPM in phytohemagglutinin-treated cultures to the mean DPM in control cultures.

G. Culture of Purified Peripheral Lymphocytes

Lymphocytes were separated from heparinized whole blood by the Ficoll-Hypaque technique (Bφrum, 1968; Ting and Morris, 1971; Thorsby and Bratile, 1970). A standard preparation of the Ficoll-Hypaque solution was obtained from Nyegaard and Co., Oslo, Norway. Purified lymphocytes were cultured in medium supplemented with either 15% fetal calf serum or 10% autologous mouse serum and 5% fetal calf serum. Culture and harvesting were performed as with whole blood cultures.

H. Splenic Lymphocyte Culture

Spleens were removed from animals which had been sacrificed by cervical dislocation. The spleens were minced with scissors into Hank's balanced salt solution and gently homogenized once in a glass homogenizer. The cells were centrifuged at 400 x $\underline{g}$ and resuspended in medium to the desired concentration. The cell viability as measured by trypan blue dye exclusion was >97%. Splenic lymphocytes were cultured in medium supplemented with 15% fetal calf serum or 10% autologous mouse serum plus 5% fetal calf serum. After 30 hours incubation, cells treated with phytohemagglutinin or tumor associated antigen were pulsed with 0.5 μCi ^{3}H-thymidine for 22 hours prior to harvesting and were extracted onto glass fiber filters. Splenic lymphocytes treated with ^{3}H-phytohemagglutinin were harvested by centrifugation at 1000 x $\underline{g}$ for 10 minutes followed by 2 washes with 0.14M NaCl. The cell pellet was dissolved in NCS tissue solubilizer, and the ^{3}H-phytohemagglutinin uptake was determined.

I. Preparation of Tumor Associated Antigen From Tumor Cells

Low ionic strength membrane extracts containing soluble tumor associated antigens were prepared from tumor cell lines BW10232 and CaD2 by a method modified from Oren and Herberman (1970). Solid tumors were removed from several mice and homogenized. The tumor cells were packed by centrifugation at 2000 x $\underline{g}$ and immediately plunged into liquid nitrogen. The cells were thawed at 37°C and suspended in 0.14 M NaCl. The extraction procedure consisted of incubating the disrupted cells in saline solutions of decreasing ionic strength. The disrupted cells were mixed in the saline solution on a magnetic stirrer for 30 minutes at 4°C, and centrifuged for 10 minutes at 2000 x $\underline{g}$. The cell debris was extracted 3 times with 0.14 M NaCl, twice with 0.07 M NaCl, and twice with 0.035 M NaCl. All supernatants were pooled and centrifuged at 10,000 x $\underline{g}$ for 30 minutes to remove insoluble material. The resultant supernatant was centrifuged at

411

105,000 x g for 60 minutes to remove insoluble material. The resultant pellets were then dialyzed against 2000 volumes of 0.14 M NaCl, pH 5.5, at 4°C for 48 hours. The protein content of the dialyzed material was determined by the method of Lowry et al. (1952).

III. RESULTS

A. Phytohemagglutinin Responsiveness and C-Type Viral Expression

The response of peripheral lymphocytes to phytohemagglutinin was measured by a culture of whole blood using 7.5 μg phytohemagglutinin per culture. This amount of phytohemagglutinin produced near-maximal stimulation of lymphocytes in C57BL/6J mice (Figure 1). Table II shows the strain variation in response of peripheral lymphocytes for 9 inbred mouse strains at 14 weeks of age. Testing for response of peripheral lymphocytes to phytohemagglutinin at 10 weeks of age showed that some high responding strains, e.g., C57BL/10J showed a lower response (Table I). Little change has been observed in animals older than 14 weeks and the low responders do not develop the ability to respond at a later age (unpublished data). The A/J, AKR/J, DBA/2J, PL/J, and SWR/J inbred strains responded insignificantly to phytohemagglutinin with a stimulation index less than 3. Three of the above low responders, DBA/2J, AKR/J, and PL/J, show C-type virus expression throughout their lives (Table II). The PL/J and AKR/J strains have extremely high incidence of spontaneous leukemia (>80%), while the DBA/2J strain carries latent C-type leukemia virus (Heiniger, personal communication). The high-responders--C57BL/6J, C57BL/10J, C57L/J, and C57BR/cdJ--show no C-type expression in young animals. Only the C57BR/cdJ shows some C-type expression in older animals. Thus all animals with simultaneous C-type expression exhibited low phytohemagglutinin responsiveness in peripheral lymphocytes. To further investigate the low phytohemagglutinin responsiveness of peripheral lymphocytes, the DBA/2J strain was chosen as the low responder, and for control experiments the C57BL/6J strain was chosen as the high responder. Selection of these strains was based partly on the dominance of the low response in DBA/2J x C57BL/6J F_1 mice.

B. Phytohemagglutinin Responsiveness of Purified Peripheral Lymphocytes

Peripheral lymphocytes purified from whole blood of DBA/2J and C57BL/6J were cultured to determine if the low phytohemagglutinin responsiveness of DBA/2J peripheral lymphocytes was attributable to the whole blood culture technique. Purified lymphocytes from both strains cultured in the presence of 10% autologous mouse serum and 5% fetal calf serum (Figure 2) exhibited a pattern of response similar to the whole blood dose-responses. While the net incorporation of ^{3}H-thymidine was higher in the purified peripheral lymphocytes, the net response of DBA/2J lymphocytes was only 40% of the C57BL/6J net response. The DBA/2J stimulation index was only 20% of the C57BL/6J stimulation index. DBA/2J lymphocytes showed the same level of response in 15% fetal calf serum, while the C57BL/6J lymphocytes exhibited a much lower response without autologous serum (Table III).

C. Response of Splenic Lymphocytes to Phytohemagglutinin

Five x 10^5 splenic lymphocytes were cultured in medium supplemented with 15% fetal calf serum. Lymphocytes from DBA/2J and C57BL/6J showed good phytohemagglutinin responsiveness. Splenic lymphocytes from both strains incorporated equally high amounts of ^{3}H-thymidine in response to phytohemagglutinin stimulation and the peak response was produced with the same amount of phytohemagglutinin per culture (Figure 3). These data suggest that the low PHA responsiveness of DBA/2J peripheral lymphocytes was not due to an intrinsic defect in the ability of the cells to respond to the mitogen.

D. Inhibition of Allogeneic C57BL/6J Lymphocytes by DBA/2J Serum

Lymphocytes from C57BL/6J and DBA/2J whole blood were cultured as previously described with 7.5 µg phytohemagglutinin per culture. To the C57BL/6J cultures, 50 µl (approximately 10%) serum from DBA/2J were added. DBA/2J lymphocytes were cultured with the same amount of C57BL/6J serum. DBA/2J serum reduced the response of high responding C57BL/6J lymphocytes by 80% (Table IV). The addition of 50 µl serum from the allogeneic high responder C57L/J did not produce any inhibition in response of lymphocytes to phytohemagglutinin. Xenogeneic fetal calf serum produced only about 10% inhibition of response on C57BL/6J lymphocytes. Fetal calf serum did not produce any inhibition of DBA/2J lymphocytes, while C57BL/6J serum did produce some inhibition of the DBA/2J lymphocytes. Analysis of the reduction in phytohemagglutinin responsiveness produced by the various sera by 2α - T-test showed that the only significant inhibition was produced by DBA/2J serum.

E. Inhibition of Splenic Lymphocytes by Serum

Five x 10^5 splenic lymphocytes were incubated for 30 minutes in medium containing 10% autologous mouse serum and 5% fetal calf serum. After the incubation, the lymphocytes were stimulated with 1 µg phytohemagglutinin, a dose which produced near-maximal stimulation of splenic lymphocytes. DBA/2J serum reduced the phytohemagglutinin responsiveness of syngeneic lymphocytes by over 50% (Table V), while C57BL/6J serum caused an insignificant reduction in the phytohemagglutinin responsiveness of syngeneic lymphocytes.

F. Effects of Syngeneic Serum on Uptake of ^{3}H-Phytohemagglutinin by Splenic Lymphocytes

Five x 10^5 splenic lymphocytes were incubated for 30 minutes in media supplemented with either 15% fetal calf serum or 10% autologous mouse serum and 5% fetal calf serum. One µg ^{3}H-phytohemagglutinin was added to each culture and the amount incorporated after 1 hour and 12 hours was measured. After 1 hour, DBA/2J lymphocytes incubated in 15% fetal calf serum bound more ^{3}H-phytohemagglutinin than C57BL/6J lymphocytes, but the change in incorporation after 12 hours was approximately the same (Table VI), which agrees with the similar lymphocyte response in 15% fetal calf serum to phytohemagglutinin

413

stimulation (Figure 3). After 1 hour, C57BL/6J serum produced a 420% increase in uptake of ^{3}H-phytohemagglutinin and after 12 hours a 56% increase in ^{3}H-phytohemagglutinin incorporation. After 1 hour the DBA/2J serum caused a 25% reduction in the uptake of ^{3}H-phytohemagglutinin and after 12 hours an 83% reduction in uptake. These data suggest that the inhibitory serum factor in DBA/2J does not prevent initial binding of ^{3}H-phytohemagglutinin to the cell surface, but in some manner the serum inhibitor prevents the phytohemagglutinin from stimulating cell division.

G. Effects of Serum on Response of Splenic Lymphocytes to Syngeneic Tumor Associated Antigen

Five x 10^5 splenic lymphocytes were cultured either in media supplemented with 15% fetal calf serum or 10% autologous mouse serum and 5% fetal calf serum. Lymphocytes were treated with membrane extracts rich in tumor associated antigen with amounts ranging from 10 to 10^{-3} μg protein per culture. Lymphocytes were taken from animals not previously sensitized to the antigen to eliminate the possibility of introducing active virus from the membrane extracts into healthy animals. C57BL/6J serum caused over a 100% increase in response of syngeneic lymphocytes to BW10232 tumor associated antigen (Figure 4). DBA/2J serum reduced the response of syngeneic lymphocytes to CaD2 tumor associated antigen by 75%, yielding essentially no response in the autologous serum.

H. Genetic Analysis of Low Phytohemagglutinin Responsiveness

The F_1-hybrid B6D2F_1 shows an inhibited response similar to the DBA/2J parent. The stimulation index of the B6D2F_1 was found to be 4.2 using purified phytohemagglutinin, which agrees with the low response obtained in B6D2F_1 animals by Heiniger et al. (1975). This suggests that the low phytohemagglutinin responsiveness is due to a dominant gene or genes from the low responding parent, DBA/2J. Since the parental strains showed a wide difference in response at 10 weeks of age, the response of B6D2F_2 mice was measured in 10 week old animals. Figure 5 shows the net phytohemagglutinin responsiveness of 46 virgin female F_2 mice measured by net ^{3}H-thymidine incorporation. About 40% (18/46) show low responsiveness, with the highest incorporation value of >9000 disintegrations per minute, while the other animals show varying degrees of responsiveness to phytohemagglutinin. If the F_2 data is analyzed by the stimulation index, 50% (23/46) show low phytohemagglutinin responsiveness (stimulation index $\leq$ 4.1), while the other animals also show varying degrees of responsiveness, range: 5.5 - 17.7, mean: 10.4.

The phytohemagglutinin responsiveness of B10.D2/oSn--H-2^{dd} is low. The net response is 1549 disintegrations per minute (stimulation index = 3.0) compared to age matched C57BL/10J mice which have high responsiveness (net response 60,400 disintegrations per minute; stimulation index, 20.7). The B10.D2/oSn mice are congenic with C57BL/10J mice except for the H-2 locus, which is congenic with DBA/2J.

IV. DISCUSSION

Peripheral lymphocyte phytohemagglutinin responsiveness measured in 9 inbred strains of mice showed both high and low responsiveness of peripheral lymphocytes. The strains showing high responsiveness were

414

C57BL/6J, C57BL/10J, C57L/J, and C57BR/cdJ. The strains showing low responsiveness were A/J, AKR/J, DBA/2J, PL/J, and SWR/J. Three of the low responders--AKR/J, DBA/2J, and PL/J--show C-type virus expression throughout their lives. No mice with simultaneous C-type expression were found to be high responders. Heiniger et al. (1975), using male mice and phytohemagglutinin from another source, found that mice simultaneously expressing the C-type genome exhibited either high or low phytohemagglutinin responsiveness in peripheral lymphocytes. The lack of response of peripheral lymphocytes in our system does not seem to be based on differences in the age of the animals, for the low responders do not develop the ability to respond at an older age (Krueger and Moyer, in press). Further investigation into the low responsiveness in DBA/2J peripheral lymphocytes showed that the low responsiveness was not related to the culture technique, to a time shift in stimulation, or to the dose of phytohemagglutinin employed.

While the DBA/2J peripheral lymphocytes in DBA/2J showed low phytohemagglutinin responsiveness, the splenic lymphocytes in DBA/2J showed a high phytohemagglutinin responsiveness. Splenic lymphocytes from DBA/2J and C57BL/6J, a high responder, showed equally high levels of ^{3}H-thymidine incorporation after stimulation by phytohemagglutinin and the lymphocytes showed a peak response with the same dose of phytohemagglutinin. The high response of splenic lymphocytes in DBA/2J suggested that some extrinsic factor was involved in the low response of peripheral lymphocytes.

Several experiments showed that cell-mediated functions of lymphocytes could be inhibited by serum from the low responder DBA/2J. Serum from DBA/2J, the low responder, reduced the phytohemagglutinin responsiveness of peripheral lymphocytes from C57BL/6J by 80%. Allogeneic and xenogeneic sera from other sources did not produce significant inhibition of responsiveness. Within a syngeneic system, serum from DBA/2J reduced the phytohemagglutinin responsiveness of syngeneic splenic lymphocytes by 53%, while serum from C57BL/6J insignificantly reduced the response of syngeneic splenic lymphocytes. This again suggests an inhibitor in the DBA/2J serum. In experiments testing the amount of ^{3}H-phytohemagglutinin incorporated by DBA/2J and C57BL/6J splenic lymphocytes in the presence of syngeneic serum, the C57BL/6J serum caused large increases in the amount of ^{3}H-phytohemagglutinin bound by splenic lymphocytes. The DBA/2J serum completely prevented the incorporation of ^{3}H-phytohemagglutinin into syngeneic lymphocytes even though more ^{3}H-phytohemagglutinin had bound to the cell surface by 1 hour. This suggests that the DBA/2J serum in some way prevents splenic lymphocytes from being stimulated by phytohemagglutinin.

Experiments were also designed to test effects of serum on lymphoblastogenesis to a specific antigen. Soluble tumor associated antigens from mammary adenocarcinomas CaD2, a DBA/2J tumor, and BW10232, a C57BL/6J tumor, produced lymphoblastogenesis in splenic lymphocytes from syngeneic hosts. Serum from C57BL/6J caused over 100% increase in the response of syngeneic lymphocytes to the BW10232 tumor associated antigen. Serum from the low responder DBA/2J prevented any response of syngeneic splenic lymphocytes to the CaD2 tumor associated antigen. These data suggest that the DBA/2J serum contains an inhibitor which causes a decrease in cell-mediated immunological functions. This inhibitor may be responsible for the low response of peripheral lymphocytes to phytohemagglutinin. Since the inhibitor prevented lymphocyte response to a tumor associated antigen from a syngeneic mammary tumor, it would seem possible that this serum factor could deter immunological surveillance if a neoplastic clone should arise. Since DBA/2J possess latent C-type virus for leukemia, it would seem possible that an inhibitor produced in this way could be another route of escape from immunological surveillance. Since the virus is latent in the DBA/2J strain, this type of mouse may be a good model for further work on the inhibitor. Before any conclusions can be drawn concerning possible immunological inhibitors produced in animals before neoplastic transformation, it will be necessary to perform extensive characterizations of the inhibitor found in the DBA/2J serum, of inhibitors found in leukemic sera (Nelson, 1972), and of inhibitors found associated with other types of neoplasia (Sjörgen et al., 1971; Nimberg et al., 1975; and Hellström and Hellström, 1975).

If an inhibitor in serum is responsible for the low phytohemagglutinin responsiveness of DBA/2J peripheral lymphocytes, how can the high phytohemagglutinin responsiveness of splenic lymphocytes be explained since serum also reaches the spleen? One possibility is that different subpopulations of lymphocytes exist in the peripheral blood and spleen, or that the peripheral lymphocytes are in contact with a greater amount of serum. In C57BL/6J mice carrying the BW10232 tumor, the phytohemagglutinin responsiveness declines from a stimulation index of 10 to less than 2 during the growth of the tumor. When the peripheral lymphocyte response is at its lowest, the splenic lymphocytes still possess full phytohemagglutinin responsiveness. Fifty µl (9%) serum from a tumor-bearing animal added to a whole blood culture of peripheral lymphocytes from non-tumor bearing C57BL/6J reduces the phytohemagglutinin responsiveness by over 80% to a stimulation index of 2 (unpublished data). This also suggests that a serum factor might affect peripheral lymphocytes to a greater extent than splenic lymphocytes, since the tumor bearing animals possessed full phytohemagglutinin responsiveness of splenic lymphocytes. The inhibition of normal lymphocyte phytohemagglutinin responsiveness by serum from the tumor bearing animal suggests that the low responsiveness of peripheral lymphocytes may prove to be useful in isolating and characterizing this inhibiting serum factor.

The genetics of the low phytohemagglutinin responsiveness appear to be somewhat complicated. In $B6D2F_1$ mice the phytohemagglutinin responsiveness is low, suggesting a dominant gene or genes in the DBA/2J parent. In $B6D2F_2$ mice, no simple gene assortment is seen (Figure 5), especially since some responses are higher than the C57BL/6J "high response." The assortment of genes in the F_2 would indicate multiple genes influencing phytohemagglutinin responsiveness. But in B10.D2/oSn--$H-2^{dd}$ mice, which carry the genetic background of the high responding C57BL/10J except for the H-2 complex of DBA/2J, the phytohemagglutinin responsiveness is low. The low response of the congenic mice suggests that genes associated with the $H-2^{dd}$ locus can produce the low responsiveness, but the F_2 gene distribution suggests multiple genes. Perhaps genes controlling degrees of responsiveness rather than inhibition are responsible for the number of genes influencing responses in F_2 animals.

V. SUMMARY

Phytohemagglutinin responsiveness of peripheral lymphocytes in a whole blood culture was measured by ^{3}H-thymidine uptake in 9 inbred strains of mice. High and low phytohemagglutinin responsiveness were seen in different strains, though lymphocytes were taken from young, age-matched, sex-matched healthy mice. Of the 9 strains, 4 showed high phytohemagglutinin responsiveness and 5 showed low phytohemagglutinin responsiveness. All mouse strains which at less than 6 months of age spontaneously elicited properties characteristic of latent C-type viral genome expression were low responders to phytohemagglutinin. The possibility that low phytohemagglutinin responsiveness was caused by some type of immunological inhibitor was investigated using DBA/2J mice, low responders, and C57BL/6J mice, high responders. The low phytohemagglutinin responsiveness in DBA/2J mice was not related to a dose-response factor, to a time shift in response to phytohemagglutinin, nor to age-related responsiveness. Splenic lymphocytes showed good phytohemagglutinin responsiveness, thus ruling out the possibility of an intrinsic cellular defect in DBA/2J mice. Serum from the low responder reduced the phytohemagglutinin responsiveness of syngeneic splenic lymphocytes, and in the presence of DBA/2J serum, splenic lymphocytes failed to actively incorporate ^{3}H-phytohemagglutinin. Serum from C57BL/6J showed no significant inhibiting effect on allogeneic or syngeneic lymphocytes. Splenic lymphocyte response to soluble tumor associated antigens from the DBA/2J transplantable mammary carcinoma CaD2 and the C57BL/6J transplantable mammary carcinoma BW10232 was also measured. High responder serum increased the response of C57BL/6J splenic lymphocytes to syngeneic tumor associated antigens by over 100%. Low responder serum totally prevented the response of DBA/2J splenic lymphocytes to syngeneic tumor associated antigens. Data suggest that the ability of lymphocytes to perform cell-mediated functions may be inhibited by factors contained in the serum of healthy mice. Genetic analysis of the low phytohemagglutinin responsiveness is also discussed.

VI. ACKNOWLEDGMENTS

We thank R. E. Paque, D. E. Thor, and M. P. Moyer for their helpful advice and comments. We also thank H. J. Heiniger for valuable preliminary results before publication of his 1975 paper on murine lymphocyte phytohemagglutinin responsiveness. Technical assistance provided by R. Brian Stumhoffer is greatfully acknowledged. This work was supported in part by a grant from Morrison Trust.

TABLE I. Phytohemagglutinin Responsiveness of Peripheral Lymphocytes from 10 Week Old Mice

Strain	Phytohemagglutinin Response[a]	Control Response[a]	Net Response[a]	SI[b]
A/J	5.3	2.8	2.5	1.9
AKR/J	3.3	1.2	2.1	2.7
C57BL/6J	16.8	1.7	15.1	10.0
C57BL/10J	8.2	1.6	6.7	5.3
C57BR/cdJ	67.5	2.3	65.2	28.8
DBA/2J	5.0	2.9	2.1	1.7

[a]Disintegrations Per Minute (DPM) x 10^3
[b]SI, stimulation index

TABLE II. Phytohemagglutinin Responsiveness of Peripheral Lymphocytes from 14 Week Old Mice

Strain	Phytohemagglutinin Response[a]	Control Response[a]	Net Response[a]	SI[b]	C-Type Expression[c]	Tumorigenesis[d]
A/J	5.0	2.8	2.1	1.8	---	---
AKR/J	11.9	4.1	7.8	2.9	+++	+++
C57BL/6J	10.9	1.1	9.7	9.5	---	---
C57BL/10J	63.5	3.1	60.4	20.7	---	---
C57L/J	48.8	1.7	47.0	28.5	---	---
C57Br/cdJ	67.5	2.3	65.2	28.8	+-[e]	---
DBA/2J	5.6	2.5	3.1	2.1	+++	---
PL/J	5.1	1.7	3.4	2.9	+++	+++
SWR/J	6.7	3.8	2.8	1.7	---	---

[a]Disintegrations Per Minute (DPM) x 10^3, rounded to nearest 0.1
[b]SI, stimulation index
[c]C-type virus expression in young animals (< 6 months) from H. J. Heiniger, personal communication, 1975.
[d]Levels of spontaneous tumorigenesis, +++ indicates very high incidence of leukemia, H. J. Heiniger, personal communication, 1975.
[e]Some C-type expression in animals older than 6 months.

419

TABLE III. Phytohemagglutinin Responsiveness of Peripheral Lymphocytes from C57BL/6J and DBA/2J[a]

Strain	Phytohemagglutinin Response	Control Response	Net Response	Stimulation Index
DBA/2J	14,700	3,400	11,300	4.3
C57BL/6J	16,100	2,200	14,100	8.0

[a]Lymphocytes were purified from whole blood by the Ficoll-Hypaque technique and grown in medium supplemented with 15% fetal calf serum

TABLE IV. Effect of Allogeneic and Xenogeneic Sera on Phytohemagglutinin Responsiveness of Peripheral (Whole Blood) Lymphocytes

Lymphocyte type	Serum[a]	PHA[b]	% Change Over Normal Response	Significance[d]
C57BL/6J	----	10,850	----	----
C57BL/6J	DBA/2J	2,066	−81.0	++
C57BL/6J	C57L/J	13,148	+21.2	N.S.
C57BL/6J	FCS[c]	9,411	−13.3	N.S.
DBA/2J	----	5,631	----	----
DBA/2J	C57BL/6	2,993	−46.9	N.S.
DBA/2J	FCS	4,850	−13.9	N.S.

[a]9-10% serum added to normal whole blood culture
[b]Phytohemagglutinin responsiveness, disintegrations per minute of incorporated ^{3}H-thymidine.
[c]FCS, fetal calf serum
[d]Significance of change over normal response as analyzed by 2α-T-test; ++ is significant (p<0.05); N.S. is not significant.

TABLE V. Effect of Autologous Mouse Serum on Phytohemagglutinin Responsiveness of Splenic Lymphocytes

	Strain	Response in Fetal Calf Serum[a]	Response in Autologous Serum	% Change	Significance[b]
PHA	C57BL/6	22,753	18,351	-19.4	N.S.
control	C57BL/6	2,031	1,672	-17.7	N.S.
PHA	DBA/2	33,224	15,687	-52.8	++
control	DBA/2	2,905	1,559	-46.3	++

[a] ^{3}H-thymidine incorporation, disintegrations per minute
[b] Significance of change in response as analyzed by 2α-T-test;
++ is significant (p<0.05); N.S. is not significant

TABLE VI. Effects of Autologous Mouse Serum from DBA/2 and C57BL/6 on Uptake of ^{3}H-phytohemagglutinin by Splenic Lymphocytes

Strain (Lymphocyte Type)	Uptake After 1 Hour[a]	After 12 Hours	% Change in Uptake[b]
C57BL/6			
+fetal calf serum	9,579	26,792	+179
+autologous serum	49,839	42,036	-15
% Change in Uptake[c]	+420	+56	
DBA/2			
+fetal calf serum	67,445	200,093	+196
+autologous serum	50,539	33,084	-34
% Change in Uptake[c]	-25	-83	

[a] Uptake expressed in disintegrations per minute (DPM) of incorporated ^{3}H-phytohemagglutinin
[b] Change in ^{3}H-phytohemagglutinin uptake from 1 to 12 hours of culture
[c] Change in ^{3}H-phytohemagglutinin uptake by autologous mouse serum

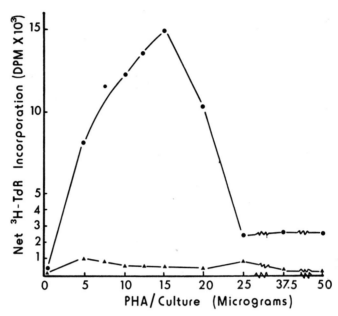

FIG. 1. Phytohemagglutinin dose-response for peripheral lymphocyte whole blood cultures from DBA/2J (▲) and from C57BL/6J (●).

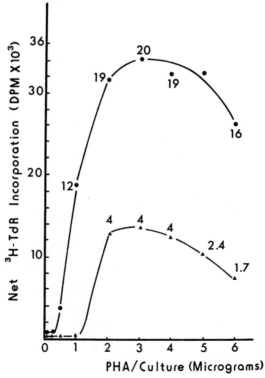

FIG. 2. Phytohemagglutinin dose-response for lymphocytes purified from whole blood by the Ficoll-Hypaque technique. The lymphocytes are from DBA/2J (▲) and C57BL/6J (●).

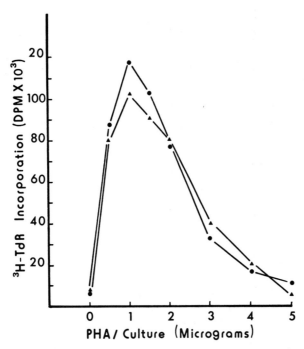

FIG. 3. Phytohemagglutinin dose-response for splenic lymphocytes from
DBA/2J (▲) and from C57BL/6J (●).

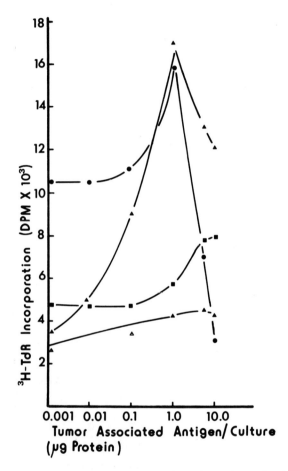

FIG. 4. Response of splenic lymphocytes from healthy animals to soluble tumor associated antigen from syngeneic mice carrying mammary adenocarcinomas. (■) is the response of C57BL/6J lymphocytes to BW10232 tumor associated antigen in medium with fetal calf serum only, while (●) is the response of C57BL/6J lymphocytes to BW10232 tumor associated antigen in medium with 10% C57BL/6J serum. (▲) is the response of DBA/2J lymphocytes to CaD2 tumor associated antigen in medium with fetal calf serum only, while (△) is the response of DBA/2J lymphocytes to CaD2 tumor associated antigen in medium with 10% DBA/2J serum.

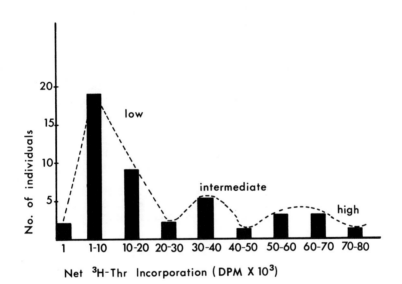

FIG. 5. Lymphocyte phytohemagglutinin responsiveness in 46 virgin female B6D2F$_2$ mice. Responsiveness measured with a whole blood culture with 7.5 µg phytohemagglutinin per culture.

VII. REFERENCES

1. Abell, C.W., Kamp, C. W., and Johnson, L.D. Effects Of Phytohemagglutinin And Isoproterenol On DNA Synthesis In Lymphocytes From Normal Donors And Patients With Chronic Lymphocytic Leukemia. Cancer Res., 30: 717-723, 1971.

2. Børum A. Separation Of Leucocytes From Blood And Bone Marrow. Scand. J. Clin. Lab. Invest., 21 Suppl. 97, 1968.

3. Burnet, F.M. Immunological Surveillance. Pergamon, Oxford, 1970.

4. Cantor, H., and Asofsky, R. Synergy Among Lymphoid Cells Mediating The Graft-Versus-Host Response III. Evidence For Interaction Between Two Types Of Thymus-Derived Cell. J. Exptl. Med., 135: 764-779.

5. Heiniger, H.J., Wolf, J.M., Chen, H. W., and Meier, H. A Micro-Method For Lymphoblastic Transformation Of Mouse Lymphocytes From Peripheral Blood. Proc. Soc. Exptl. Biol. Med., 143: 6-11, 1973.

6. Heiniger, H.J., Taylor, B.A., Hards, E.J., and Meier, H. Heritability Of The Phytohemagglutinin Responsivenss Of Lymphocytes And Its Relationship To Leukemogenesis. Cancer Res., 35: 825-831, 1975.

7. Hellström, I., Sjögren, O., Warner, G., and Hellström, K.E. Blocking Of Cell-Mediated Tumor Immunity By Sera From Patients With Growing Neoplasms. Int. J. Cancer, 7: 226-237, 1971.

8. Hellström, I., and Hellström, K. E. Cytotoxic Effect of Lymphocytes From Pregnant Mice On Cultivated Tumor Cells. I. Specificity, Nature Of Effector Cells, Blocking By Serum. Int. J. Cancer, 15: 1-16, 1975.

9. Humphrey, G.B., and Lankford, J. Inhibition Of Normal Lymphocyte Transformation By Leukemic Serum. Exp. Hematol., 1: 276, 1973.

10. Krueger, J.G. and Moyer, R.C. Strain Distribution And Serum Inhibition of Mouse Lymphoblastic Response To Phytohemagglutinin In Vitro. Proc. Gulf Coast Mol. Biol. Conference: Texas J. Sci., 26: 5, 1975. In Press.

11. Lowry, O.H., Rosebrough, N.J., and Farr, A.L. Protein Measurement With The Folin Phenol Reagent. J. Biol. Chem., 193: 265, 1952.

12. Nelson, D. S. Mouse Serum Factor Depressing Lymphocyte Transformation. Experientia, 28: 1227-1228, 1972.

13. Nimberg, R. B., Glasgow, A. H., Menzoian, J. O., Constantian, M. B., Cooperband, S. R., Mannick, J. A., and Schmid, K. Isolation Of An Immunosuppressive Peptide Fraction From The Serum Of Cancer Patients. Cancer Res., 35: 1489-1494, 1975.

14. Oren, M. E., and Herberman, R. B. Delayed Cutaneous Hypersensitivity Reactions To Membrane Extracts Of Human Tumor Cells. Clin. Exp. Immunol., 9: 45-56, 1971.

15. Sample, W. F., Gertner, H. R., and Chretien, P. B. Inhibition Of Phytohemagglutinin-Induced In Vitro Lymphocyte Transformation By Serum From Patients With Carcinoma. J. Nat. Cancer Instit., 46: 1291-1297, 1971.

16. Segal, S., Cohen, I. R., and Feldman, M. Thymus-Derived Lymphocytes: Humoral And Cellular Reactions Distinguished By Hydrocortisone. Science, 1975: 1126-1128, 1972.

17. Sjögren, H.O., Hellström, I., Bansal, S. G., and Hellström, K. E. Suggestive Evidence That The "Blocking Antibodies" Of Tumor-Bearing Individuals May Be Antigen-Antibody Complexes. Proc. Nat. Acad. Sci. USA, 68: 1372-1375, 1971.

18. Stobo, J. D., and Paul, W. E. Functional Heterogeneity Of Murine Lymphoid Cells. III. Differential Responsiveness Of Cells To Phytohemagglutinin And Conconavalin A As A Probe For T Cell Subsets. J. Immunol., 110: 362-375, 1973.

19. Ting, A., and Morris, P. J. A Technique For Lymphocyte Preparation From Stored Heparinized Blood. Vox Sang., 20: 561, 1971.

20. Thorsby, E., and Bratlie, A. A Rapid Method For Preparation Of Pure Lymphocyte Suspensions. In: P. I. Terasaki (ed.), Histocompatibility Testing 1970. Munksgaard, Copenhagen, p. 655, 1970.

21. Waksal, S. D., St. Pierre, R. L., Hosteller, J. R., and Fold, R. M. Brain-Associated-Theta Antiserum: Differential Effects On Lymphocyte Subpopulation. Cellular Immunol., 12: 66-73, 1974.

22. Wilzback, K. E. Tritium-Labeling By Exposure Of Organic Compounds To Tritium Gas. J. Am. Chem. Soc., 79: 1013, 1957.

NATURAL CELL-MEDIATED CYTOTOXICITY IN MAN

Mitsuo Takasugi, Donna Akira, Yoko Mullen, Julie Takasugi,
and Robert Ivler

Department of Surgery, University of California,
Los Angeles, California   90024

I. INTRODUCTION

Although natural cell-mediated cytotoxicity has been observed previously in human and animal systems by most investigators, it was usually ignored as background. Recently, the reaction has received considerable attention because of its possible role in interfering with
the detection of tumor-associated cell-mediated specificities (1-3) and
by the proposal from several investigators relating its specificity to
viruses (4-6). If natural cytotoxicity in mice is directed toward leukemia viruses (4) or to endogenous viruses (5,6), the existence of strong
natural cytotoxicity in man has important implications to parallel studies of such viruses in man.

Natural cytotoxicity is observed with effector cells from healthy,
untreated individuals as well as patients (1,2). The reactions are mediated by a class of lymphocytes different from conventional T or B cells
(7-9) which have been called N cells in humans (7) and in mice (9). In
human systems, the Fc receptors play an important role in the reaction
with cytotoxicity being inhibited by aggregated IgG (7) or by Ag-Ab
complexes.

When natural cytotoxicity is tested across different species,
reactivity is partially limited to that species. When testing is confined to human effectors on human target cells, most of the reactivity
observed appears to be nonselective, that is, the resultant cytotoxicity
is determined to a large extent by the relative strength of the effectors and the sensitivity of the target cells. However, some specificity

429

is detected. In the following study, we report our initial results regarding the specificity of natural cytotoxicity by human effector cells.

II. PROCEDURES AND MATERIALS USED

A. Assays for Cell-Mediated Cytotoxicity

1. THE MICROASSAY FOR CELL-MEDIATED IMMUNITY. The assay and the methods for isolating effector cells and for calculating the mean reduction titer (MRT) score have been described (2). Human peripheral blood lymphocytes and spleen lymphocytes from mice and rats were used as effector cells.

2. ^{51}CHROMIUM RELEASE AND THE COMPETITION ASSAY. Cultured target cells were labeled by incubating 0.5×10^6 cells with 0.05 ml ^{51}Cr (2 ul/ml) for 1 hr. The cells were washed 3 times and 5000 target cells in 5 ul were mixed with 200,000 effector cells in a total volume of 0.2 ml in the wells of a sterile microtiter V plate. Cells were incubated overnight and then centrifuged at 2000 RPM for 10 min. 100 ul media was collected and counted in a gamma scintillation counter.

The competition assay was modified from the method described by Ortiz de Landazuri and Herberman (10). Inhibition of specific cell-mediated cytotoxicity was performed by the addition of 150,000 unlabeled target cells as competitors to the regular test. Inhibition was assessed by the difference in cytotoxicity in tests performed with and without competitors.

Percent cytotoxicity was calculated as follows:

$$\text{Percent cytotoxicity} = \frac{\text{Test count - minimum count}}{\text{Maximum count - minimum count}} \times 100$$

The minimum count was obtained for the labeled cells in medium; the maximum count from labeled cells in distilled water.

B. Target Cells

The following target cells were used:

	Identification	Source	Reference
Human:	372 or Mel80	cervix	1,2,7
	497 or SKLMS 1	leiomyosarcoma	1,2,7

Human	Identification	Source	Reference
(cont.)	548	breast	1,2,7
	696 or 2T	osteosarcoma	1,2,7
	917	melanoma	7
	1042	osteosarcoma	7
	G11	breast	1,2
	T24	bladder	11
	MeWo	melanoma	11
	RD	osteosarcoma	12
Mouse:	AM1	methylcholanthrene-induced in A/J	
	Sa 1	benzanthracene-induced in A strain	13
	L cells	fibroblast line C3H	
	SC-1		14
	Balb/c 3T3		
	NIH Swiss 3T3		
Rat:	LS	spontaneous tumor in Lewis strain	
	FMF1	methylcholanthrene-induced tumor in Fisher strain	
	FMM2	"	
	FMM3	"	

(Targets SC-1, RD, Balb/c 3T3 are NIH Swiss 3T3 were received from Dr. V. Klement and M. Gardner, University of Sourthern California.)

C. The Interaction Analysis

The interaction analysis (15) was used to determine specific reactivity. In testing human lymphocytes on cultured human target cells, there is an especially strong reactivity against most target cells which gives it the appearance of nonselectivity. Specific activity must be differentiated from this nonselective cytotoxicity. The nonselective cytotoxicity was estimated from the average reactivity for each effector and target by the application of the 2-way analysis of variance (16). The interaction analysis emphasizes the difference between the estimated nonselective effect and the observed result and uses this difference as a measure of specificity. Application of this analysis is more appropri-

431

ate for differentation of 2 separate effects as specific T cell cytotoxicity and a less selective N cell cytotoxicity as observed in cell-
mediated lympholysis (17). In the application of the analysis to the
specificity of natural cytotoxicity through direct cytotoxicity, the
analysis provides a level of cytotoxicity which can be accounted for
nonselectively and which must be surpassed before specificity can be
detected.

The interaction analysis was applied as follows:

Test results (T) = % cytotoxicity for each effector target combi-
    nation.

Average results for effector cells (E_A) = average test results for
    each effector against different targets (average for a row).

Average results for target cells (T_A) = average test results for
    a target cell with different effectors (average for a column).

Overall average (O_A) = average for all tests.

Then:

Specific cytotoxicity = $T - E_A - T_A + O_A$;
Nonspecific cytotoxicity = $E_A + T_A - O_A$.

Correlations were calculated with biomedical programs from the UCLA
computer services.

IV RESULTS

When natural cytotoxicity was tested across species using effector
cells from man, mouse, and rat on target cells from these species, a
specificity relating to each species became apparent. Table I shows
these results with scores for each effector tested against each target
cell. The first figure is the observed MRT score from the microassay,
the second is the expected nonselective cytotoxicity calculated from the
average reactivity of the effector and the average sensitivity of the
target. This score provides an estimate of the cytotoxicity assuming
that no specific activity occurred. The third score is the difference
between the observed and the expected nonselective activity, in this
case, an assessment of detectable specific activity.

Effector cells from individual 115719 were specifically positive
for the 5 human target cultures and negative for the mouse and rat lines.
Effector cells from a Lewis rat were negative on human target cells,
positive for 5 of 6 mouse cultures, and 2 of 4 rat targets. Distinction

432

between mouse and rat lines for species specificity was more difficult than with human cultures reflecting the closeness of the 2 species. Although the relationship is not perfect, the results are reproducible and we concluded that species differences could be detected through natural cytotoxicity.

The detection of specificity within a species, as in testing for human tumor specificities, is much more difficult. Since testing patients and controls on cultured tumor cells gives very little information on the actual specificities involved, we decided to first investigate and identify the target antigens on cultured tumor lines. A preliminary study of the antigens on target cell lines was initiated on 4 target lines; 372, 497, 548, and 1042. We soon realized that 4 targets were insufficient and targets 696, 917, G11, T24, and MeWo were added while 1042 was dropped from the panel.

Altogether 240 persons including 108 cancer patients, 112 healthy individuals, and 20 persons with other or unknown diseases were tested in the study in groups of 4 against the 8 target lines. The interaction analysis was applied to the results for each set to distinguish specific effects. The results from this study were specific cytotoxic scores against the 8 target lines by each effector cell tested.

To identify target antigens on the cell lines, each target was compared for similarities in reactivity with every other target line. Two methods of chi-square and coefficient of correlation analyses were used to make comparisons. For the analysis by chi-square, specific cytotoxicity greater than 5 was considered positive. The results of comparison between target 548 and 696 are shown in Table II. A chi-square of 8.38 was achieved which was significant with a probability of less than 0.01.

A complete comparison by chi-square analysis for all the cell lines is given in Table III. Significantly positive correlations were observed between target 548 and 696, between 696 and 917, and between 372 and G11. We concluded from these results that targets 548, 696, and 917 shared common specificities, the relationship between 548 and 917 having barely missed significance. This group designated TA 1 (target antigen 1) and the 372-G11 combination called TA 2 are distinct since they are negatively correlated with respect to each other. Line 497 behaved more like TA 1 (target antigen 1) and the 372-G11 combination called TA 2 are

433

distinct since they are negatively correlated with respect to each other. Line 497 behaved more like TA 1 than TA 2 cells.

Table IV shows the same data analyzed by coefficient of correlation. Of the TA 1 group only 548 and 917 were significantly correlated. Targets 548 and 696 were also positively correlated but not significantly so. The other significant correlation was between G11 and 372 confirming the chi-square analysis. In view of the preliminary nature of this study, we considered a sharing of common specificities among 548, 696, 917, and possibly 497 and also between 372 and G11. Our inability to clearly define the specificities may be due to more than one specificity being carried by each target cell or by technical difficulties.

To support the existence of common antigenicity, inhibition studies were performed against TA 1 cells using TA 1 cells and another cell as competitors. Table V shows these results using 4 cell lines; 548, 696, G11, and MeWo. Natural cytotoxicity against targets 548 and 696 was specifically inhibited by 548 and 696 but not MeWo, supporting the validity of common target antigens for the TA 1 cells detected by direct cytotoxicity.

IV. DISUCUSSION

Although background cytotoxicity, which was at times very strong, has been previously observed in tests of cellular immunity, this effect received little attention until the interference it caused in the detection of specificity became so obvious it could not be ignored. Much of what is reported as histologic type specificity is no more than differences in background or in natural cytotoxicity. With the development of better understanding for lymphocyte subclasses and the observation that a population of cells other than T cells mediated this effect and the possibility that specificity was related to viruses, interest has been refocused on this phenomenon. Studies from mice (4,5,8,9) and man (7) and now rats indicate that very similar reactions occur within the three species and that the differences observed may be only superficial.

When testing effectors and targets across species, natural cytotoxicity was primarily directed to targets from that species, that is, it was species specific. However, this was a loose relationship with considerable reactivity across species. The rather loose species specificity of natural cytotoxicity reminds one of the relationship between different viruses and their host species. However, the direct relationship between target specificities and viruses has not been established in humans and specificities other than those related to viruses have not been excluded. The exact nature of target antigens for natural cytotoxicity needs to be investigated further.

The general impression that one achieves when testing different persons on many targets, is that the cytotoxicity is mostly nonselective (7). However, indications of some specificity have been detected by most investigators. When a patient appeared to be reacting specifically against a target tumor cell, it was used to support the concept of specificity for "histologic" types of cancer. Similar patterns of reactivity are observed with normal healthy persons and patients with other diseases. If sufficient numbers of patients and controls are tested, support for histologic type specificity fades. We felt it would be more appropriate to find and identify the specificities involved for natural cytotoxicity and then to determine its relationship to disease, genetics, and/or other causes of cytotoxicity.

The interaction analysis allowed us to exclude nonselective effects and examine selective reactivity. We were able to determine by chi-square and coefficient of correlation analyses that certain target cultures reacted alike and we concluded that the cell lines shared common target specificities. Lines 548, 696, and 917 appear to share a common specificity which has been designated as TA 1. Cells from this group do compete with each other and they inhibit natural cytotoxicity of labeled TA 1 cells. Although natural cytotoxicity appears nonselective since most target cells are killed, on closer examination, differences between target cells can be detected by direct cytotoxicity.

If one tests by inhibition with competitor cells, the specificity becomes even clearer. The paradox between an overall nonselectiveness by N cells and clear specificity by competitive inhibition of natural cytotoxicity needs examination. Nonselective reactions can be caused by killing of all target cells nonspecifically or by a family of cells which includes specific effector cells for each of the target cells. The specificity by competitive studies supports the latter explanation.

The major problem in cell-mediated cytotoxicity is the need for better definition of what is natural cytotoxicity and also of acquired immune cytotoxicity and ways of differentiating between the two effects.

Acquired immune cytotoxicity implies the introduction of antigen to the responder or, at least, some knowledge that the responder has experienced contact with it. Knowledge about the antigen is _perhaps_ a major difference between the two reactions. The specificity of immune cytotoxicity is quite limited and the reactions appear to be mediated by T cells. Natural cytotoxicity is mediated by N cells and little is known about how and why the cytotoxic cells are generated and always present. N cells, as a total entity, have wider specificity for a variety of target cells. Further studies in natural cytotoxicity are sorely needed, not only for better understanding of this interesting and important phenomenon, but also to improve understanding of immune cytotoxicity.

V. SUMMARY

When effector cells from man, mouse, and rat were tested for natural cytotoxicity on target cultures from man, mouse and rat, a loose species specificity was observed. When tests were confined to man, the overall appearance of the reactivity was rather nonselective. However, on closer examination some specificity is detected. Over 200 persons were tested on 8 cultured target lines and the results were analyzed for selective and nonselective cytotoxicity by the interaction analysis. Target lines were compared for similarity in reactivity which suggested sharing of antigens. Two groups with common antigens were identified.

TABLE I. Species Specificity of Natural Cytotoxicity

| | MRT Scores with Effector Cells | | | | | | | | | Average for Observed Results |
| Target Cells | Human 115719 | | | Mouse A/J | | | Rat Lewis | | | |
	Obs[a]	Exp[b]	Spec[c]	Obs	Exp	Spec	Obs	Exp	Spec	
Human										
497	63	31	32	10	29	-19	4	19	-15	26
548	85	37	48	6	35	-29	6	35	-19	32
696	56	27	29	8	25	-17	1	15	-14	22
917	67	33	84	17	31	-14	0	21	-21	28
RD	88	47	41	29	45	-16	8	35	-27	42
Mouse										
AM1	42	63	-21	56	61	-5	76	51	25	58
SA1	38	61	-23	53	59	-6	78	49	29	56
L	34	68	-34	79	66	13	75	56	19	63
SC-1	59	68	-9	76	66	10	55	56	-1	63
Balb/c 3T3	61	67	-6	61	65	-4	63	35	8	62
NIH 3T3	4	35	-31	45	33	12	42	23	19	30
Rat										
LS	1	29	-28	44	27	17	28	17	11	24
FMT1	1	19	-18	32	17	15	10	7	3	14
FMM2	12	23	-11	43	21	22	0	11	-11	18
FMM3	17	25	-8	43	23	20	0	13	-13	20
Average	42			40			30			37

[a] = Observed

[b] = Expected

[c] = Specific

TABLE II. Chi-Square Analysis of Results on Targets 548 and 696

	Target 548	
	+	-
Target 696 +	18[a]	20
-	19	74

Chi-square = 8.38

P < 0.01

[a] Specific cytotoxic scores from the interaction analysis greater than 5 were considered positive.

TABLE III. Chi-Square of Specific Cytotoxicity Between Target Cell Lines

Target Lines	Target Lines							
	548	696	917	G11	372	T24	MeWo	1042
497	0.7	0.4	-0.0	-3.3	-11.8[a]	1.7	-1.1	-5.1[a]
548		8.4[a]	3.4	-0.8	-15.2[a]	-3.0	-3.0	-1.3
696			5.2[a]	-2.1	-3.2	-5.1[a]	-3.8	-0.7
917				-14.1[a]	-10.1[a]	0.0	-5.2[a]	-0.1
G11					8.1[a]	-2.5	0.5	
372						-0.4	+0.6	+0.4
T24							+0.3	

[a] P < .05

438

TABLE IV. Coefficient of Correlation Analysis of Specific Cytotoxicity Between Target Cell Lines

Target Lines	Target Lines							
	548	696	917	G11	372	T24	MeWo	1042
497	-0.01	-0.04	-0.08	-0.33[a]	-0.47[a]	+0.01	-0.23[a]	-0.40[a]
548		+0.22	+0.24[a]	-0.19	-0.45[a]	-0.41[a]	-0.39[a]	-0.34[a]
696			+0.03	-0.31[a]	-0.41[a]	-0.38[a]	-0.39[a]	-0.18
917				-0.30[a]	-0.42[a]	0.13	-0.29[a]	-0.11
G11					+0.23[a]	-0.32[a]	-0.05[a]	
372						+0.14	+0.08	+0.01
T24							0.05	

[a] $p < .05$

TABLE V. Specific Inhibition by Competition of Natural Cytotoxicity Percent Specific Inhibition

Competitor Cells	Target Cells			
	548	696	G11	MeWo
696	16	15	-19	-5
917	20	12	-5	-12
G11	-1	8	3	-6
MeWo	-12	-4	4	4

REFERENCES

1. Takasugi, M., Mickey, M.R., and Terasaki, P.I. Reactivity of Lymphocytes from Normal Persons on Cultured Tumor Cells. Cancer Res. 33:2898-2902, 1973.

2. Takasugi, M., Mickey, M.R., and Terasaki, P.I. Studies on Cell-Mediated Immunity to Human Tumors. J. Natl. Cancer Inst., 53: 1527-1538, 1974.

3. Oldham, R.K., Djeu, J.Y., Cannon, G.B., Servorski, D., and Herberman, R.B. Cellular Microcytotoxicity in Human Tumor Systems: Analysis of Results. J. Natl. Cancer Inst., 55:1305-1318, 1975.

4. Kiessling, R., Klein, E., and Wigzell, H. "Natural" Killer Cells in the Mouse. I. Cytotoxic Cells with Specificity for Mouse Maloney Leukemia Cells. Specificity and Distribution According to Genotype. Eur. J. Immunology 5:112-117, 1975.

5. Herberman, R.B., Nunn, M.E., and Lavrin, D.H. Natural Cytotoxic Reactivity of Mouse Lymphoid Cells Against Syngeneic and Allogeneic Tumors I. Distribution of Reactivity and Specificity. Int. J. Cancer, 16:216-229, 1975.

6. Hirsch, M.E., Kelley, A.P., Profitt, M.R., and Black, P.H. Cell-Mediated Immunity to Antigens Associated with Endogenous Murine C-Type Leukemia Viruses. Science, 187:959-961. 1975.

7. Kiuchi, M. and Takasugi, M. The Nonselective Cytotoxic (N Cell). J. Natl. Cancer Inst., (In press).

8. Kiessling, R., Klein, E., and Wigzell, H. "Natural" Killer Cells in the Mouse. II. Cytotoxic Cells with Specificity for Mouse Moloney Leukemia Cells. Characteristics of the Killer Cell. Eur. J. Immunol., 5:117-121, 1975.

9. Herberman, R.B., Nunn, M.E., Holden, H.T., and Lavrin, D.H. Natural Cytotoxic Reactivity of Mouse Lymphoid Cells Against Syngeneic and Allogeneic Tumors. II. Characterization of Effector Cells. Int. J. Cancer, 10:230-239, 1975.

10. Ortiz de Landazuri, M., and Herberman, R.B. Specificity of Cellular Immune Reactivity to Virus-Induced Tumors. Nature (New Biol.), 238:18-19, 1975.

11. Bean, M.A., Bloom, B.R., Herberman, R.B., Old, L.J., Oettgen, H.F., Klein, G., and Terry, W. Cell-Mediated Cytotoxicity for Bladder Carcinoma: Evaluation of a Workshop. Cancer Res., 35:2902-2913, 1975.

440

12. McAllister, R.M., Melnyk, J., Finklestein, J.Z., Adams, E.C., Jr., and Gardner, M.B. Cultivation in vitro of Cells Derived from a Human Rhabdomyosarcoma. Cancer, 24:520-526, 1969.

13. Kaliss, N. Immunological Enhancement of Tumor Homografts in Mice: A Review. Cancer Res., 18:992-1003, 1958.

14. Hartley, J.W., and Rowe, W.P. Clonal Cell Lines from a Feral Mouse Embryo Which Lacks Host-Range Restrictions for Murine Leukemia. Virology, 15:128-134, 1975.

15. Takasugi, M., and Mickey, M.R. Interaction Analysis of Selective and Nonselective Cytotoxicity. J. Natl. Cancer Inst. (In press).

16. Snedecor, G.W. Statistical Methods. The Iowa State College Press, Ames, Iowa, p. 214-317, 1937.

17. Takasugi, M., Akira, D., and Mickey, M.R. Specific and Non-specific Effects in Cell-Mediated Lympholysis. In: Histocom-patibility Testing, 1975. Ed.: F. Kissmeyer-Nielsen, Munksgaard, Copenhagen, pp. 827-834, 1975.

IMPAIRMENT OF ALLOGENIC CYTOTOXICITY IN PATIENTS WITH CANCER

Nicole Suciu-Foca, Anthony P. Molinaro, Frederic P. Herter, Joseph Buda, Charles H. Antinori and Keith Reemtsma

Columbia University,
College of Physicians and Surgeons
New York, New York, U.S.A.

I. INTRODUCTION

The ability of lymphocytes to recognize allogenic transplantation antigens in the mixed lymphocyte culture test (MLC) and to acquire in vitro cytotoxic activity against allogenic targets can be used as functional markers for T-lymphocytes (3,4). We have evaluated the cellular (T-cell mediated) immune response of 40 patients with cancer and of 40 normal controls by determining the blastogenic and cytotoxic responses displayed by their lymphocytes following in vitro stimulation with mitomycin-inhibited lymphoblastoid B-cell lines (LBC). LBCs of B-cell origin have been used in our investigations in view of their properties of inducing strong MLC activation and allogenic cytotoxicity.

II. PROCEDURES AND MATERIAL USED

Heparinized blood samples were obtained from 40 patients with non-lymphoid malignancies who had a negative history of transfusions, chemotherapy and radiotherapy and from 40 healthy volunteers.

A. Preparation of Effectors

Lymphocyte suspensions were prepared by flotation on Ficoll-Isopaque as previously described (3). The medium used was RPMI 1640 (GIBCO-Grand Islands Biologicals, N.Y.) supplemented with pooled heat inactivated normal human serum (25% v/v) penicillin, streptomycin and glutamine. MLC-activated lymphocytes as well as non-activated cells from each individual were simultaneously tested in cytotoxicity assays. For this fresh lymphocyte suspensions, (1×10^5/well) were dispersed (horizontally) in two complete rows of Microtest II plates.

One of the rows contained lymphocytes to be used as non MLC activated effectors. The second row contained lymphocytes which were MLC activated by adding to each well 1×10^5 mytomicin inhibited LBC. Stimulating cells (in RPMI 1640 supplemented with 25% human serum) were used as a mixture composed of equal numbers of cells from three different LBC.

The killing ability of both sensitized and non-sensitized effectors was tested following 5 days of incubation at 37°C in a 5% CO_2 humidified atmosphere.

B. Preparation of Targets

Three established cell lines (HEF,HE2,HEL) derived from human embryo and the HeLa human tumor cell line were used as targets. Tissue culturing was carried out in MEM with 20% fetal calf serum, antibiotics and mycostatin. Labelling of target cells with tritiated proline was performed as described by Bean (1).

C. Microcytotoxicity Test

3H-Proline labelled target cells from each of the four different lines were individually added (vertically, i.e. column-wise) to triplicate cultures of sensitized and non-sensitized responding cells from the same donor. Equal numbers of reactions with lymphocytes from cancer subjects and normal controls were included on each tray. Cultures were incubated for 18 hours at 37°C. At the end of the incubation time, the medium was aspirated from the wells, and the adhering cells were washed 3 times with calcium and magnesium free phosphate buffered saline. Cells were detached from the bottom of the wells by treatment with 0.5% pronase solution and harvested automatically as previously described (4). Residual radio-label activity was measured by liquid scintillation counting. Mean cpm of triplicate cultures were calculated for each reaction. Cytotoxicity acquired following MLC activation by each effector was calculated for the four different targets from the following formula:

$$1- \frac{\text{(Mean CPM in triplicate cultures with MLC activated effectors)}}{\text{(Mean CPM in triplicate cultures with non-sensitized effectors)}} \times 100$$

D. Determination of MLC reactivity (MLCR)

The blastogenic response displayed by lymphocytes from each subject in MLC with LBC was evaluated following 5 days of incubation by determining the rate of tritiated thymidine incorporation per 1×10^5 responding lymphocytes, as previously described (3).

III. RESULTS

Results obtained by testing the MLCR and the cytotoxic activity acquired by lymphocytes from normal subjects and from cancer patients are summarized in Table 1.

Patients with cancer showed lower capacity to respond in MLC against LBC as compared to normal controls. The ability of MLC activated lymphocytes to destroy allogenic targets was also decreased as reflected by the lower mean values as well as by the lower percent cytotoxicity against any of the individual targets. The statistical significance of these differences results from a two by two comparison between cancer patients and

444

healthy controls with respect to the number of responders showing arbitrarily selected "normal" values for MLCR (more than 35,000 cpm/10^5 lymphocytes) and for cytotoxicity (more than 45% killing/10^5 MLC activated
lymphocytes):

	MLCR (cpmx10^3)		Cytotoxicity	
	≤ 34	≥ 35	$\leq 44\%$	$\geq 45\%$
Normal	4	36	5	35
Cancer	28	12	21	19
	$\chi^2 = 30$	$p < 0.005$	$\chi^2 = 14.7$	$p < 0.005$

Impairment of the recognition as well as of the cytotoxic capacity of
lymphocytes from cancer patients appears to parallel the progression of the
disease. The stage dependency of these defects is shown in Table 2, which
demonstrates that while lymphocytes from patients with tumors confined to
the primary site display a rather normal pattern of MLC and cytotoxic responses, the strength of both types of reactions decreases significantly in
patients with regional and distant spread.

Analysis of paired results obtained in MLC and cytotoxicity testings
showed that the degree of lymphocyte cytotoxicity was directly related to
the magnitude of the MLC response induced by LBC (correlation co-efficient
0.569; $p < 0.001$).

IV. DISCUSSION AND SUMMARY

Our present investigations demonstrate that lymphocytes from cancer
patients have a decreased capacity to recognize and become immunized in
vitro against allogenic antigens. This conclusion derives from the observation that the strength of cytotoxic responses is directly related to that
of the blastogenic response in MLC and that the cytotoxic activity acquired
by lymphocytes from cancer patients following stimulation with LBC is significantly lower than that of normals.

Cytotoxicity acquired following stimulation with pooled cells from
three HLA-D different lymphoblastoid B-cell lines showed no specificity for
any particular target, but rather appeared to reflect the immune potential
of the responders. Weak and strong responders could easily be distinguished by the degree of cytotoxicity acquired to each target and this was
accurately reflected in the mean cytotoxicity of each individual tested.
The cytotoxic potential of lymphocytes from patients with regional spread
and with metastatic disease was lower than that found in patients with
tumors confined to the primary site.

This observation suggests that serial determination of MLC induced
cytotoxicity in patients with cancer might be of prognostic value.

Our data are consistent with previous observations indicating that the
ability of lymphocytes to display cytotoxic activity in vitro on allogenic
target cells and to become immunized to cultured human tumor cells is
lower in cancer patients than in normal controls (2,5).

Our observation that the decreased cytotoxic potentialities of lymphocytes from cancer patients parallels the progression of the disease,
suggests that this abnormality is an effect of the disease rather than an
expression of the breakdown of the immunological surveillance mechanism
allowing malignancies to occur. It is conceivable that impairment of self-
nonself discriminatory capacity, as possibly reflected in decreased allogenic recognition ability, preceeds and eventually leads to the inability
of lymphocytes from cancer patients to acquire and efficiently display cell
mediated immunigy against tumor specific neo-antigens.

TABLE I. Reactivity of Lymphocytes from Normal Subjects and Cancer Patients in MLC and Cytotoxicity Tests

Subjects	No. of subjects	MLCR cpm ± SE	% Cytotoxicity for: Target 1	Target 2	Target 3	Target 4	Average % cytotoxicity
Normal	40	67203 ±5619	57 ±4.90	73 ±3.59	70 ±3.5	57 ±4.61	64 ±3.5
Cancer	40	33055 ±4972	35 ±4.61	46 ±4.61	51 ±4.76	33 ±4.46	42 ±4.15

TABLE II. Relationship between Extent of Tumor Growth and Lymphocyte Reactivity

Extent of tumor growth	No. of patients	MLCR cpm ±SE	% Cytotoxicity for: Target 1	Target 2	Target 3	Target 4	Average % cytotoxicity
Primary site	10	51705±8847	56 ±10	65 ±64	68 ±7	49 ±9	60 ±6.12
Regional spread	16	31974±6515	37 ±6.7	47 ±7.75	52 ±8	29 ±9	36 ±7.25
Distant spread	14	18246±7849	17 ±10	27 ±11	34 ±15	16 ±8.5	24 ±10

REFERENCES

1. Bean, M.A., Pees, H., Rosen, G., and Oettgen, H.F. Prelabelling Target Cells With 3H-Proline As A Method For Studying Lymphocyte Cytotoxicity. Natl. Cancer Inst. Monogr. 37: 41-48, 1973.
2. Sharma, B., and Terasaki, P.I. Immunization Of Lymphocytes From Cancer Patients. J. Natl. Cancer Inst. 52: 1925-1926, 1974.
3. Suciu-Foca, N., Buda, J.A., McManus, J., Thiem, T., and Reemtsma, K. Impaired Responsiveness Of Lymphocytes And Serum Inhibitory Factors In Patients With Cancer. Cancer Res., 33: 2373-2377, 1973.
4. Suciu-Foca, N., Buda, J.A., Herter, F., Molinaro, A., Broell, J., and Reemtsma, K. Impaired Cytotoxicity Of Lymphocytes From Patients With Cancer. J. Surgical Oncol. 8: 75-81, 1976.
5. Takasugi, M., Mickey, M.R., and Terasaki, P.I. Reactivity Of Lymphocytes From Normal Persons On Cultured Tumor Cells. Cancer Res., 33: 2898-2908, 1973.

Section 3

HUMORAL IMMUNITY

HUMORAL IMMUNE RESPONSE IN BREAST CARCINOMA PATIENTS

Engikolai C. Krishnan, William R. Jewell, Loren J. Humphrey

Department of Surgery
University of Kansas Medical Center
College of Health Science Center
Kansas City, Kansas 66103 U.S.A.

I. INTRODUCTION

It has been shown by flourescein conjugated anti-immunoglobulin reagents that various human and animal tumors are coated in vivo with
immunoglobulin and by indirect radioimmunoassay (17,18,21,26). Immunoglobulins have been detected in acid eluates of animal tumors (25,35)
and in human tumors (19,30). It is also shown that the eluates occasionally contain antibodies against sarcomas (5) and melanoma (9,23).
Estimated amounts of IgG on tumor cells are of the order 10^5 molecules/
cell. The lack of cytotoxicity of the immunoglobulin raises the possibility that Ig on tumor cells could be bound by a non-immunologic phenomenon. There have been reports (29,31) that human malignant tumors
absorb erythrocytes sensitized with IgG antibodies. The attachment of
these molecules was selectively more when in a complexed form compared
to native IgG.

In this report we present results of three different studies with
breast carcinoma: a) Quantitative estimates of Immunoglobulin G associated with breast carcinoma tumor cells by radioimmunoassay technique,
b) Fc receptor activity in various breast carcinoma tissues by closed
chamber technique using sensitized sheep erythrocytes, and c) Results
of reactivity of breast carcinoma patients with breast carcinoma antigen.
Although the intent of these studies was not to specifically correlate
the separate parameters, the results indicate the possibility of an existing interrelationship.

The existence of humoral response may play an important role in
host survival. This study was directed towards establishing the presence
of IgG on human breast carcinoma cells which is presumably antibody directed against tumor antigen or components associated with tumor, to
study the possible attachment of these immunoglobulin to tumor cells in
a nonimmunological fashion and to evaluate the humoral immune response
in human breast cancer patients with respect to prognosis.

II. PROCEDURES AND MATERIALS USED

A. Tumor and Cell Suspension

Breast tissue samples from malignant tumors were obtained during
surgery. Tissue was thoroughly minced with tris scissors and suspended

449

in Hank's balanced salt. To remove coarse particles the suspension was allowed to settle at 4°C for 5 minutes. The suspension was then filtered through a gauze. The cells in the filtrate were washed and .5 to 2×10^6 cells were used to determine the amount of IgG on tumor cells. Tissue not used immediately was embedded in phosphate buffered saline pH 7.2 (PBS) and stored at -70°C in plastic bags.

B. Serum and Serum Fractination

Normal human serum was pooled from healthy donors. Immunoglobulin G (IgG) was isolated from serum by filtering through gel as described (8) and then treating twice with the chloride form of DEAE sephadex (4). The purified preparation produced a single IgG line in agar diffusion and immunoelectrophoresis when tested against antisera to whole human serum. The IgG line of the purified preparation made a line of identity with that produced by the commercial antiserum (Hyland) to IgG. Antiserum to human IgG was produced by subcutaneous injection of 200mg IgG in complete Freund's adjuvant at multiple sites every other week for 10 weeks. The rabbits were bled after the last injection. Antiserum specific to human IgG were also purchased from Hyland Laboratories, Costa Mesa, California, U.S.A.

C. Radioimmunoassay for Quantitation of IgG

The assay is essentially the same as described earlier (16,19). Briefly, the optimum ratio of specific antiserum to a constant amount of labeled and unlabeled IgG was determined by testing an increasing series of dilutions of antiserum required to precipitate the maximum amount of labeled IgG. Diluent was normal rabbit serum 1:50 in 0.05 Molar Borate buffer, pH 8.4. To obtain a standard curve, 0 to 800ng of unlabeled human IgG was preincubated with rabbit anti-human IgG of appropriate dilution as determined above. After 24 hours of incubation at 4°C ^{125}I-labeled IgG was added, and the incubation was continued for another 24 hours. The binding of ^{125}I-labeled IgG in presence of different amounts of unlabeled IgG was calculated and a standard curve constructed.

To determine the quantity of IgG on the tumor cell surface, a known number of cells were incubated in triplicate with the antiserum of the same dilutions as used to obtain the standard inhibition curve. The amount of ^{125}I-labeled IgG that this absorbed antiserum can precipitate was found. By referring to the standard inhibition curve, the amount of IgG on the tumor cell surface was determined.

D. Detection of Fc Receptors

The procedure to detect Fc receptors using tissue sections was the same as described earlier, using a closed chamber technique (32). Detailed technique has been described for tumor tissue sections (34). Indicator cells (E) were sheep erythrocytes sensitized with various amounts of corresponding rabbit IgG antibodies (A) expressed as agglutinating units. One agglutinating unit is defined as the amount of the highest dilution of antiserum which agglutinates an equal amount of a 1% suspension of sheep erythrocytes. For sensitization, equal amounts of E and dilutions of A were mixed and left at room temperature for 30 minutes. After washing three times the EA were resuspended to 1% and layered on cryostat sections of frozen tissue on large cover glasses. The slide covers were incubated in wet chambers with the EA applied using microculture slides with a single concavity allowing the EA to settle on the cover glass. After 30 minutes at room temperature the slides were turned cover glass up, and left for detachment from the glass and non-reactive tissue. The degree of hemadsorption (3+, 2+, 1+, etc.) was recorded microscopically when the glass around the tissue was free of erythrocytes.

E. Antigen

Breast carcinoma tissues were obtained at surgery and autopsy and preserved at -70°C. The detailed antigen preparation has been described earlier (13). Briefly, tissue was minced in 0.25 Molar sucrose in medium A to make a 20% V/V homogenate. First, the coarse particles were removed by centrifugation at 5,000xg for 15 minutes; the supernatant was again centrifuged at 102,000xg for 75 minutes. This supernatant was concentrated to one-half the original tumor volume using Amicon VM-10 filter. This was used as antigen.

F. Immunodiffusion

Immunodiffusion was performed as described by Ouchterlony (22). All experiments were carried out in 1% agarose in phosphate buffered saline pH 7.2. Plates were read after 24 to 72 hours.

III. RESULTS

A. IgG on Tumor Cells

Cells in suspension from each of the tumors were tested for the presence of IgG bound to the cell surface. The mean values of parallel determinations in two tests are shown in Table I. In all the cells tested, IgG was found to a variable degree. In three instances the cells were incubated with low pH Glycine-HCl buffer and the eluates were tested for IgG content. IgG could not be completely recovered in the eluates. In three (II,IV,VI) tumors the same tissues were used for Fc receptor activity and IgG. Tumor VI which showed maximum Fc receptor activity had minimum IgG on the cell surface. In some of the experiments the breast carcinoma tissue was washed with PBS extensively and eluated with 15% NaCl. The eluation contained IgG and consumed complement in an indirect complement assay. On the other hand, similarly treated normal breast tissue eluates did not consume complement. Also, in addition to IgG, Fab and Fc fragments of IgG were found in most cases. In some instances IgM and IgA were also found.

B. Fc Receptors in Tissue

Individual tumor tissues showed different degrees of reactivity in tests using EA. Though the degree of reactivity was graded on a relative scale by evaluating the reactivity at different levels of sensitization of sheep erythrocytes. Reactivity is considered both by observing the density of the adherence of EA and by various levels of sensitization. The reactivity at weaker sensitization is considered higher than tissue that reacts only at stronger sensitization. By this evaluation it can be seen that tumor #9 had the highest overall reactivity whereas normal breast tissues could be considered to be weakest in Fc reactivity (Table II). This reactivity is enhanced by treating with neuraminidase. Also, the reactivity could be completely blocked by using anti-lymphocyte serum.

451

C. Reactivity of Breast Carcinoma Patients' Sera

Serum from 438 patients were examined by double gel diffusion for reactivity against breast carcinoma Ag. Out of these, 154 were diagnosed as breast carcinoma, 218 were fibrocystic disease, and 66 were fibro-adenoma. Antibody to breast carcinoma antigen was found in 20 breast cancer patients, 16 with fibrocystic disease, 8 with fibroadenoma. More than 80% of patients with metastases to auxillary lymph nodes and no detectable antibody to breast carcinoma antigen had expired or had recurrence within two years. On the other hand 80% of patients with positive sera in the positive lymph node group were alive without evidence of recurrence at two years.

IV. DISCUSSION

Reports of Pilch and Riggins (24) and Morton (21) show that the titer of circulating antibodies increases after primary tumor has been removed. Jewell and Hunter (15) in an animal model have shown that the turnover of circulating IgG was higher in tumor hosts compared to normal animals. These findings suggest that either antibodies are absorbed in vivo by tumor cells or that the antigen released by tumor neutralizes antibody by forming antigen-antibody complex. After removal of the tumor, these antibodies would be in excess since the source of antigen has been removed. From our work and from the reports of other inves-tigators, it appears that the tumor cells are coated with immunoglobulins in vivo. Whether these globular molecules are in fact antibodies specifically directed against tumor cells or antibodies attached to tumor cells by non-immunological mechanisms is unclear. The alternatives are not mutually exclusive. The fact that tumor cells have a higher affinity for IgG(Fc) of complexed antibodies (20) strengthens the view that Ig molecules could be attached to tumor cells non-immunologically. We have observed fragments of IgG(Fab) and IgG(Fc) along with aggregated IgG in tumor eluates. Independently, in support of this interpretation, Fish and coworkers (7) reported that eluated fragments of degraded IgG had a higher affinity for tumor cells than native IgG molecules.

The quantitative estimation of IgG on each tumor cell is 10^5 molecules. Consequently, the tumor cells should have been lysed if the classical Ag-Ab reaction were to occur against tumor cells.

These IgG molecules, if attached non-specifically to tumor cells, may block antigenic determinants on the surface of the tumor cells. This type of antigenic blocking could signify a mechanism of non-recognition of antigenic tumor. It has been shown (31) that receptors for the Fc end of antibody molecules are similar in tumor and lymphoid cells. The presence of complexed and/or degraded immunoglobulin in the tumor host complicates the issue since these molecules could inhibit the host re-activity at the target level as well as at the affector level.

In this regard it has been suggested (1,28) that the effectors abrogating lymphocyte-mediated destruction of tumor cells in vitro are complexes of tumor antigen and specific antibody. It is possible that metabolic turnover of the tumor membrane could release antigen from the tumor cell surface. These antigen molecules could form antigen-antibody complexes in the tumor mass vicinity which reattach to the tumor surface non-specifically. These immunoglobulins may undergo degradation by tumor-associated lysosomal enzymes. It has been reported (35) that xenogenic anti-tumor antibodies lost the ability to mediate complement-dependent cytotoxicity following a treatment with lysosomal enzymes extracted from corresponding tumor tissue. Romsdahl and Cox (27) demonstrated that in human sarcoma eluates free IgG(Fab) was found in excess of Fc fragment and suggested that IgG(Fab) lacking the Fc end could make lymphoid cells incapable of mediating lymphotoxicity.

The crucial observation of this communication is that patients with positive antibody activity had improved prognosis. It is tempting to postulate that the antibodies which we are detecting in breast carcinoma patients' sera is directed against blocking antibody molecules. These autoantibodies could be helping patients by eliminating the blocking effect and facilitating lymphocytotoxicity. The antibody that we are observing may be the same unblocking antibody that has been reported in several other cytotoxicity systems (2,3,10,11). Further investigations are underway attempting to elaborate the humoral response mechanism of breast carcinoma patients.

V. SUMMARY

Fresh malignant breast carcinoma cells were tested for Immunoglobulin G, using an indirect radioimmunoassay technique. Twenty-two different breast carcinoma tissues were tested for Fc receptor activity using sheep erythrocytes sensitized by rabbit IgG antibodies. Reactivity of breast carcinoma patients' sera against breast carcinoma antigen was evaluated from the point of prognosis.

The amount of IgG on breast carcinoma tumor cells varied from <100ng to 800ng per million cells. Fc receptor activity was found in all tumor tissues tested to a variable degree. The results also show that the patients with positive antibody had better prognostic sign compared to patients with negative antibody.

TABLE I. Immunoglobulin G Detected on Various Fresh Breast Carcinoma Cells

Patient Identification	IgG/10^6 cells	IgG in Tumor Eluates/10^6 cells	Fc Receptor Activity
J.W.	280	70	ND
V.E.	590	200	+
E.C.	460	ND	ND
C-1	>800;400	ND	F+
C-2	496	ND	ND
L-1	<100	ND	+++
C-3	<100	8	ND
T-1	860	ND	ND
Cultured Breast Carcinoma Cells	0	0	ND

TABLE II. FC Receptor Activity on Various Tissues at Different Sensitization

Patient Ident.	SRBC Sensitized to Limits of Agglutination								Unsensitized	Comments
	4	2	1	1/2	1/4	1/8	1/16	1/32		
M.R.	2+	3+	3+	3+	3+	3+	1+	-	-	Diffuse
V.E.	3+	3+	3+	1+	1+	-	-	-	-	F++
A.L.	3+	3+	3+	3+	2+(F)	1+(F)				-
L.B.	1+	1+(F)	1+	-	-	-	-	-	-	Focal
M.C.	3+	2+	1+(F)	1+(F)	-	-	-	-	-	-
A.W.	2+	2+	2+(F)	2+(F)	1+(F)	-	-	-	-	-
M.R.	3+	3+	3+	2+	2+	1+(F)	1+(F)	1+(F)		Focal
F.D.	3+	3+	3+	2+	2+	2+	2+	2+		Focal
P-1	3+	3+	3+	2+	1+	1+(F)		-	-	Diffuse
V-1	3+	3+	3+	3+	3+	3+	1+	1+	-	
A.G.	3+	3+	3+	2+	2+	1+	1+	1+	-	
A.G.-2	1+	1+	1+	1+	1+	1+(F)	1+(F)	1+(F)	-	Focal
J.A.	3+	3+	2+	1+	1+	1+	1+	-	-	Focal
C.B.	3+(F)	3+(F)	2+(F)	1+(F)	1+(F)	1+(F)	1+(F)	1+(F)	-	Focal
H.K.	3+	3+	3+	2+	1+	1+	1+	1+	-	
L.S.	3+	3+	2+	1+	1+	1+	1+	-	-	
L.H.	3+	3+	2+	2+	1+	-	-	-	-	-
Normal Breast	-	-	-	-	-	-	-	-	-	
Muscle	2+	2+	-		-	-	-	-	-	
Liver	3+	3+	2+	1+	1+	-	-	-	-	
Kidney	1+(F)	1+(F)	-	-	-	-	-	-	-	Focal
Placenta	3+	3+	3+(F)	3+(F)	3+(F)	2+(F)	1+(F)	-	-	Focal

TABLE III. Antibody in Sera of Patients with Breast Disease

Type of Breast Disease	No. of Sera Tested	No. of Sera with Positive Ab
Carcinoma	154	20
Fibrocystic	218	16
Fibroadenoma	66	8
Total No. Tested	438	44

REFERENCES

1. Baldwin, R.W., Price, M.R. & Robin, R.A.: Blocking Of Lymphocyte Mediated Cytotoxicity For Rat Hepatoma Cells By Tumor-Specific Antigen-Antibody Complexes. Nature; New Biology 238(84):185-187,1972.

2. Bansal, S.C. and Sjögren, H.O.: "Unblocking" Serum Antibody In Vitro In The Polyoma System May Correlate With Antitumor Effect Of Antiserum In Vivo. Nature (London) New Biology 233:76-78, 1971.

3. Bansal, S.C. and Sjögren, H.O.: Counteraction Of The Blocking Of Cell-Mediated Tumor Immunity By Inoculation Of Unblocking Sera And Splenectomy; Immunotherapeutic Effect On Primary Polyoma Tumors In Rats. Int. J. Cancer 9:490-509, 1972

4. Baumstark, J.S., Laffin, R.J. and Bardawil, W.A.: A Preparative Method For The Separation Of 7 s Gamma Globulin From Human Serum. Archives of Bio Chem and Bio Phys. 108:514-522, 1964.

5. Elber, F.R. and Morton, D.L.: Immunologic Response To Human Sarcomas, Relation Of Antitumor Antibodies To The Clinical Course. In: Progress in Immunology. Ed.: B. Amos. Academic Press Inc., New York, 951-957, 1970.

6. Estes, N.C., Morse, P.A., Humphrey, L.J.: Antibody Studies Of Sera From Patients With Breast Cancer. Surgical Forum XXV:121-123, 1974.

7. Fish, F., Witz, I.P., and Klein, G.: Tumor-Bound Immunoglobulins: The Fate Of Immunoglobulin Disappearing From The Surface Of Coated Tumor Cells. Clin. Exp. Immunol. 16:355-365, 1974.

8. Flodin, P. and Killander, J.: Fractionation Of Human Serum Protein By Gel Filtration. Bio. Chem. Bio Phys. ACTA 63:403-410, 1962.

9. Gupta, R.K. and Morton, D.L.: Suggestive Evidence For In Vivo Binding Of Specific Antitumor Antibodies Of Human Melanomas. Cancer Res. 35:58-62, 1975.

10. Hellstrom, I. and Hellstrom, K.E.: Colony Inhibition Studies On Blocking And Non-Blocking Serum Effects On Cellular Immunity To Moloney Sarcoma. Int. J. Cancer 5:195-201, 1970.

11. Hellstrom, I. and Hellstrom, K.E.: Serum Mediated Inhibition Of Cellular Immunity To Methylcholanthrene-Induced Murine Sarcomas. Cellular Immunology 1:18-30, 1970.

12. Humphrey, L.J.: Studies On Hemadsorption By Murine Tumors. Doctoral Thesis, 1967.

13. Humphrey, L.J., Estes, N., Morse, P., et al: Serum Antibody In Patients With Breast Disease: Correlation With Histopathology. Ann. Surg. 180(1):124-129, 1974.

14. Humphrey, L.J., Estes, N.C., Morse, P.A., Jewell, W.R., Boudet, R.A., Hudson, M.J.K.: Serum Antibody In Patients With Mammary Disease. Cancer 34:(4)1516-1520, 1974

15. Jewell, W.R., and Hunter, L.: Kinetic Studies Of Hyperimmune 7s Globulins In Allogeneic Rats Bearing Walker 256 Tumors. J. Surgical Onc. 3(1)9-15, 1971.

16. Jewell, W.R. and Krishnan, E.C.: Quantitative Radioimmunoassay Of Immunoglobulins On The Surface Of Human Tumor Cells. J. of Surgical Research 16:424-427, 1974.

17. Klein, E., Klein, G., Nadkarni, J.S., Nadkarni, J.J., Wigzell, H., Clifford, D.P.: Surface IgM-Kappa Specificity On A Burkitt Lymphoma Cells In Vivo And In Derived Culture Lines. Cancer Res. 28:1300-1310 1968.

18. Klein, G., Clifford, P., Henle, G., Henle, W., Geering, G., Old, L.J.: EBV Associated Serological Patterns In Burkitt Lymphoma Patients During Regression And Recurrence. Int. J. Cancer 4:416-421, 1969.

19. Krishnan, E.C. and Jewell, W.R.: Quantitation Of Elutable Immuno-globulin G (7s) From Fresh Malignant Human Tumor Cells Surface. Transplantation Proc. VII(1)541-544, 1975.

20. Krishnan, E.C., Jewell, W.R. and Tønder, O.: Receptor On Human Malignant Tumor Cells Which Selectively Bind Complexed Antibodies. Proceedings of XI International Cancer Congress, Panel 10, 1974.

21. Morton, D.L., Eilber, F.R., Milmgren, R.A.: Immune Factors In Human Cancer; Malignant Melanomas, Skeletal And Soft Tissue Sarcomas. Progr. Exp. Tumor Res. 14:25-42, 1971.

22. Ouchterlony, O.: Antigen Antibody Reaction In Gel. Arkive Kem., 26:14-21, 1948.

23. Phillips, T.M., Lewis, M.G.: A Method For Elution Of Immunoglobulin From The Surface Of Living Cells. Rev. Europeene Etudes Clin. 16:1052-1053, 1971.

24. Pilch, Y.H., Riggens, R.S.: Antibodies To Spontaneous And Methyl-cholanthrene Induced Tumors In Inbred Mice. Cancer Res. 26:871-875, 1966.

25. Ran, M., and Witz, I.P.: Tumor Associated Immunoglobulins; The Elution Of IgG2 From Mouse Tumors. Intern. J. Cancer 6:361-372, 1970.

26. Romsdahl, M.M. and Cox, I.S.: Characterization Of Human Sarcoma Tumor Associated Immunoglobulins And Proteins. Proceedings of American Association of Cancer Res. 16:661, March, 1975.

27. Romsdahl, M.M., Cox, I.S.: Evidence For Enhancing Antibodies In Human Sarcomas. Proc. American Assn. Cancer Res. 12:66, 1971.

28. Sjögren, H.O., Hellström, I, Bansal, S.C., Hellström, K.E.: Suggestive Evidence That The "Blocking Antibodies" Of Tumor-Bearing Individuals May Be Antigen-Antibody Complexes. Proc. National Acad. Of Scie (Wash.) 68:1372-1375, 1971.

29. Thunold, S., Abeyounir, C.J., Milgram, F., and Wilebsky: Anti-globulin Factors In Serum And Tissue Of Cancer Patients. Int. Allergy 38:260-268, 1970.

30. Thunold, S., Tønder, O., and Larson, O.: Immunoglobulins In Eluates Of Malignant Human Tumors. ACTA Pathol. Microbiol. Scand. Suppl. 236:97-100, 1973.

31. Tønder, O., Humphrey, L.J., Morse, P.A.: Further Observations On Fc Receptors In Human Malignant Tissue And Normal Lymphoid Tissue. Cancer 35(3):580-587, 1975.

32. Tønder, O, Milgram, F., and Witebsky, E.: Mixed Agglutination With Tissue Section. J. Ex. Med. 119:265-274, 1964.

33. Tønder, O., Morse, P.A. and Humphrey, L.J.: Similarities Of Fc Receptors In Human Malignant Tissue And Normal Lymphoid Tissue. J. of Immunology 113(4)1162-1169, 1974.

34. Tønder, O., and Thunold, S.: Receptors For Immunoglobulins In Human Malignant Tissue. Scand. J. Immunol. 2:207-215, 1973.

35. Witz, I., Yagi, Pressman, D.: IgG Associated With Microsomes From Autochonous Hepatomas And Normal Lives Of Rats. Cancer Res. 27:2295-2299, 1967.

36. Witz, I.P., Levy, H.J., Keisari, Y. and Izsak, F.C.: Tumor Bound Immunoglobulins: Their Possible Role In Circumventing Anti-Tumor Immunity. Johns Hopkins Med. J. Suppl. 3:289.

IMMUNOGLOBULIN LEVELS IN BREAST FLUIDS OF
WOMEN WITH BREAST CANCER

Nicholas L. Petrakis, Marie Doherty, Rose Lee, Lynn Mason,
Stella Pawson, and Robert Schweitzer*

G. W. Hooper Foundation
and the Department of International Health
University of California School of Medicine
San Francisco, California 94143
and the
*Breast Screening Center of Northern California
Merritt Hospital
Oakland, California 94609

Recently, we reported that nipple aspiration of human breast-duct
fluid can be employed in cytological, biochemical and epidemiological
studies of breast cancer (6,7,13). These studies have indicated that the
biochemical composition of the fluid closely resembles that of colostrum
and milk (12) and that breast fluids of adult nonpregnant women contain
high concentrations of immunoglobulin.

Because in several recent reports authors have suggested that immune
disturbances may be present in women with breast cancer (2,4,9,15,17,18,20,
21,24), we studied the immunoglobulin levels in breast fluid and serum
from women with normal breasts, benign breast disease and breast cancer.
Strikingly high elevations of IgM and marked variations in IgA levels were
found in the breast fluids of some women with breast cancer, which may be
of diagnostic, prognostic, and etiologic importance.

MATERIALS AND METHODS

Breast fluids were aspirated from the nipple with a modified breast
pump technique consisting of a suction-cup device placed over the nipple
and attached to a 10 cm^3 syringe (13). Retraction of the syringe created
a negative pressure in the cup, which in most of the Caucasian women yielded fluid at the nipple surface. The fluid was collected in capillary tubes

that were sealed at both ends and frozen until studied in the laboratory. A blood sample was obtained from each woman for comparison with the breast fluid.

The amounts of IgA, IgG, and IgM in breast fluid and plasma were determined by using Laurell rocket electrophoresis on Millipore Biomedia®* electro agar slides with one μl of sample. The slides are agarose gels containing monospecific IgA, IgG and IgM antiserum from rabbit or goat. Results were expressed as mg of immunoglobulin per 100 ml of breast fluid or plasma. Rocket electroimmunoassay enhances the reaction rate between antigen and antibody and makes measurement of the end point more precise in comparison with the Mancini technique.

Sick and healthy women were seen at Moffitt Hospital and the Ambulatory Care Center of the University of California, San Francisco, the Northern California Breast Screening Center at Merritt Hospital, Oakland, California, and at a screening program conducted with the members of the Marin Mastectomy Services, Marin County, California.

Three groups of women were studied: (1) 55 with normal breasts, (2) 95 with benign breast disease, and (3) 29 with breast cancer (9 had newly diagnosed primary breast cancer and 20 had a prior mastectomy, but no clinical evidence of recurrence). Diagnoses of normal breasts and breasts with benign disease were made by palpation and mammography. In some women, the diagnosis of benign breast disease was established by biopsy. All new diagnoses of breast cancer were based on histologic examination at operation. An attempt was made to correlate the degree of mononuclear infiltration in the histological specimens with the immunoglobulin findings.

Results are given in terms of "breasts" rather than patients. Fluid was obtained in 70% of the women, but not always from both breasts (13).

RESULTS

Mean levels and standard errors for immunoglobulins found in breast fluid and plasma samples from the three groups are shown in Table I.

Normal Breasts and Breasts with Benign Disease

Mean immunoglobulin levels in fluids from normal breasts and those with benign disease resemble those reported for colostrum (10). Mean IgA

---

*Obtained from Millipore Biomedica, 15 Craig Road, Acton, Massachusetts 01720.

levels of breast fluids were markedly elevated above those for plasma, whereas the reverse was found for IgG and IgM, where mean plasma levels were higher than for breast fluids.

Primary Breast Cancer and Prior Mastectomy

PLASMA LEVELS OF IMMUNOGLOBULINS

Mean plasma levels of IgA were significantly lower in patients with breast cancer in comparison to those with normal and benign-disease breasts (see Table I) ($p = .02-.001$). There was no statistically significant difference in mean IgG plasma levels between the three groups, except in women with a prior mastectomy; they had a significantly lower mean level of IgG ($p = .02$). Mean IgM levels did not differ significantly between the three groups.

A possible relationship between age and plasma immunoglobulin levels was investigated. A statistically significant positive correlation was found only for IgA in normal women with normal breasts; their IgA levels increased with age (Table II).

IgA AND IgG BREAST FLUID LEVELS

No statistically significant differences were noted between mean IgA and IgG levels in the breast fluids from all groups. However, the mean IgA level in breast fluids was elevated above plasma levels in all groups (see Table I). The reverse was found for IgG, whose highest mean level occurred in plasma, and not in breast fluids. Distribution of individual values is shown in Figures 1 and 2. No relationship was found between age and breast fluid immunoglobulin levels.

IgM LEVELS OF BREAST FLUIDS

Mean levels of IgM were similar in breast fluids from normal and benign-disease breasts; mean breast fluid levels were lower than plasma levels in all groups. A striking elevation of the mean level of IgM was found in breast fluids from cancerous and prior-mastectomy breasts in comparison with corresponding plasma levels. Figure 3 shows the distribution of IgM values for breast fluid from the three groups. Ninety-five percent of the individual values for IgM from normal and benign-disease breasts were under 400 mg/100 ml, with most under 100 mg/100 ml. The others were as high as 900 mg/100 ml. Six of nine patients with newly diagnosed breast cancer and 5 of 15 with a prior mastectomy had significantly high levels of IgM ranging from 800 to 16,000 mg/ml.

461

ABSENCE OF IMMUNOGLOBULINS IN BREAST FLUIDS

In many samples of breast fluid, IgA, IgG and IgM could not be detected. Ten of 30 cancerous breasts (33%) lacked IgA, compared to 5 of 81
(6.1%) normal breasts (p < .001), and 9 of 160 (5.6%) benign-disease
breasts (p = .001). Nine of 31 (29%) cancerous breast fluids and 33 of
84 (39%) normal fluids lacked IgG, which is not significant. However,
breasts with benign disease lacked IgG in only 32 of 156 (21%) samples, a
significant difference from normal breasts (p < .001). IgM was absent
in 56 of 85 (66%) of normal breasts, 93 of 154 (60%) of benign-disease
breasts and in 15 of 30 (50%) cancerous breasts. These differences, however, are not statistically significant (Table III).

HISTOLOGIC AND CYTOLOGIC CORRELATIONS

There was no consistent relationship between the histology of the
biopsy sample, cytology of the breast fluid, and the levels of immunoglobulins. However, because of the few specimens available, further
studies are necessary to evaluate possible correlations.

DISCUSSION

These studies indicate that the concentration of IgM increases
significantly in breast fluids in many women with breast cancer or prior
mastectomy, In addition, a large number of these women lack IgA in their
breast fluids. At present we can only speculate about the meaning of
these findings.

Roberts and associates (18) studied the immunoglobulin content of
extracts of breast tumors and adjacent normal breast tissue. They found
that one-third of cancerous breast tissue extracts contained higher
concentrations of IgM than adjacent normal breast tissue, and that the
concentrations of IgA and IgG were reduced in extracts of cancer tissue.
Rowinska-Zakrewska and associates (20) and Roberts and associates (17)
reported that serum IgA levels were elevated in patients with breast cancer
in comparison with those of normal women. They also found that serum IgG
levels were significantly reduced. In contrast, our results on plasma
revealed a decrease in IgA levels in women with breast cancer, and a reduction in IgG levels only among women with prior mastectomy. We also
found no major relationship between age and plasma immunoglobulin levels.

Recently, Lentino (9) reported that serum IgM levels were elevated
in breast cancer patients with sinus histiocytosis in regional lymph nodes.
Also, serum IgG values were increased in breast cancer patients with axil-

lary metastases. Evidently, further studies are needed to clarify the contradictory findings of studies on serum immunoglobulins in breast cancer.

In a related study, Richters and Kaspersky (16) found the proportion of IgM-positive lymphocytes increased in tumor-positive lymph nodes in primary breast cancer, but not in tumor-negative nodes. Low levels of both IgG- and IgM-positive lymphocytes were present in the cancer tissue itself. Important alterations in the IgM-related components of the immune system likely occur in many women with breast cancer.

The function of immunoglobulins in breast fluid secretions of non-pregnant women is unknown. In addition to their presence in serum, immuno-globulins exist in other sites (23): IgA is found in saliva, tears, milk, and in the secretions of the gastrointestinal and respiratory tracts and of other mucous membranes. Serum IgA probably is derived from lymphocytes in the Peyer's patches of the intestinal tract. Lesser concentrations of IgG and IgM are also present in these secretions. IgA is transferred from the blood into glandular secretions probably by the production of secre-tory piece by the epithelial cells, which may protect IgA from enzymatic degradation. Strober and associates (22) have suggested that the presence of secretory piece may initiate the selective proliferation of IgA cells. Absence of IgA in breast fluid but not in plasma may represent a local deficiency or qualitative alteration of secretory piece produced by breast alveolar cells.

Recurrent infections have been reported in IgA deficiency, which might mean that IgA may play a role in immunity to bacterial and viral infections (1). However, Koistenin recently challenged this view because no patients had infections in the presence of IgA deficiency (8). IgA deficiency has been associated with a variety of other diseases including malignancies (3). As we found in our study, 33% of fluids from cancerous breasts lacked IgA compared to 5% for normal and benign-disease breasts. The significance of the absence of IgA in breast fluids and its role, if any, in the pathogenesis of breast cancer is unknown.

We also do not know why IgM concentrations are elevated in breast fluids of cancer patients. Moderate to high elevations in serum IgM levels may occur in association with bacterial infections; however, no evi-dence of breast infection was present in our patients. Marked elevations of serum IgM, comparable to our breast fluid findings, have been found in children with immune-deficiency diseases, and in the jejunal secretions of adults with coeliac disease (5,19). It has been conjectured that these high levels of IgM might be a compensatory response to a quantitative decrease in IgA or to a qualitative impairment of IgA and IgG production or function.

The elevations of breast fluid IgM and absences of IgA seen here may represent a locally aberrant immune response of mononuclear cells to tumor-specific antigens secreted into the breast fluids of many women with breast cancer. Possibly qualitative and quantitative deficiencies exist in local IgA immunoglobulin secretion or production similar to that for immune-deficiency diseases. For example, two of the fluids from cancerous breasts with extreme elevations of IgM (6,000 and 16,000 mg/100 ml) had no detectable IgA. Roberts (18) suggested that breast cancer may arise from an alteration in response to prolonged autoimmune stimulation of the epithe- lium by secretory products. This hypothesis is supported by studies, which indicate that exogenously derived substances are readily secreted into breast fluids and may possibly affect glandular function and morphol- ogy of the breast (11,14). The ability of the secreted substances to provoke local immunological responses in the breast is under investigation.

We will continue to study the diagnostic and prognostic implications of our findings. It may be significant that 33% of women with prior mastectomy and 5% of those with benign-disease and normal breasts had elevated levels of IgM. Lentino (6) also reported that patients with elevated serum IgM levels had markedly better 5-year survival rates than those who did not. However, as no clinical details are given, it is likely that the author relates improved prognosis to the reported longer surviv- al of breast cancer patients with nodal sinus histiocytosis. Prospective studies of women at breast screening centers may provide information on the clinical significance of the observed variations in immunoglobulin con- tent of human breast secretions.

SUMMARY

Investigations were made of the immunoglobulin levels of nipple aspirates of breast fluid and plasma of women with normal breasts, benign breast disease and breast cancer by using rocket immunoelectrophoresis. We found that concentrations of IgM are markedly increased in breast fluids of many women with breast cancer and prior mastectomy (33%), but in few women with normal and benign-disease breasts (5%). In addition, many women with breast cancer (33%) lacked IgA in their breast fluids. In view of numerous reports of immune disturbances associated with breast cancer, the present findings may have diagnostic and etiologic significance.

ACKNOWLEDGMENTS

This work was supported by Public Health Service Grant CA 13556 and Contract CB 33882 from the National Cancer Institute and by a gift from Mrs. Viola K. Schroeder. We would also like to thank the Marin Mastectomy Services in Marin County, California, for their help.

TABLE I. Immunoglobulin Levels in Breast Fluid and Plasma

Condition of Breasts	IgA			IgG			IgM		
	X	SE	(N)	X	SE	(N)	X	SE	(N)
Normal									
Breast fluid	1709 ±	168	(86)	249 ±	61	(84)	66 ±	16	(85)
Plasma	247 ±	23	(55)	1063 ±	60	(55)	194 ±	15	(52)
Benign disease									
Breast fluid	1784 ±	132	(160)	214 ±	31	(157)	84 ±	14	(155)
Plasma	279 ±	81	(95)	1116 ±	52	(93)	189 ±	12	(89)
Cancer									
Breast fluid	1620 ±	593	(12)	258 ±	104	(11)	1629 ±	580	(11)
Plasma	114 ±	14	(9)	1059 ±	181	(9)	189 ±	40	(9)
Prior Mastectomy									
Breast fluid	1968 ±	567	(20)	254 ±	85	(20)	2150 ± 1115		(20)
Plasma	168 ±	26	(20)	861 ±	78	(20)	152 ±	20	(20)

TABLE II. Correlation Coefficients for Plasma Immunoglobulin Levels and Age

Condition of Breasts	IgA	(N)	IgG	(N)	IgM	(N)
Normal	0.28*	(55)	0.02	(55)	0.17	(52)
Cancer	-0.22	(29)	-0.19	(29)	-0.18	(29)

*p = .05

TABLE III. Absence of Immunoglobulin in Breast Fluids

Condition of Breasts	IgA			IgG			IgM		
	Absent	Total	%	Absent	Total	%	Absent	Total	%
Normal	5	81	6.1	33	84	39	56	85	66
Benign disease	9	160	5.6	32	156	21*	93	154	60
Cancer	10	30	33.3*	9	31	29	15	30	50

*p < .001

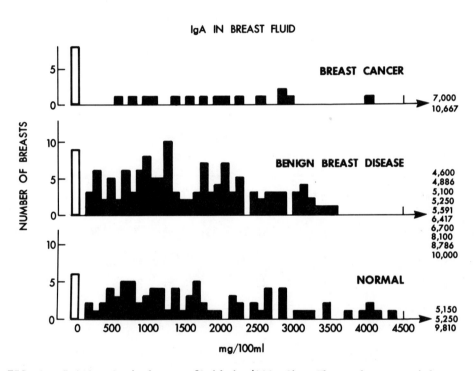

FIG. 1.   IgA levels in breast fluid (mg/100 ml).   The numbers at right are values above the scale drawn on graph and the empty bar indicates an absence of IgA.

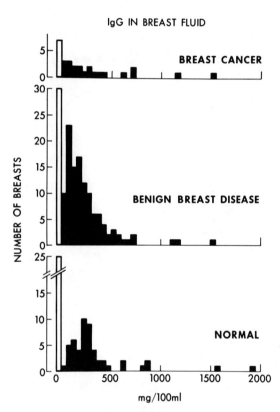

FIG. 2. IgG levels in breast fluid (mg/100 ml). The empty bar indicates an absence of IgG.

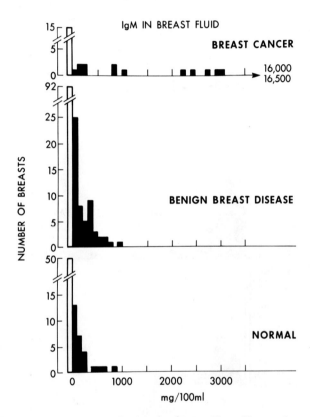

FIG. 3. IgM levels in breast fluid (mg/100 ml). The numbers at right are values above the scale drawn on graph and the empty bar indicates an absence of IgG.

REFERENCES

1. Ammann, A.J., and Hong, R. Selective IgA Deficiency. Presentation Of 30 Cases And A Review Of The Literature. Medicine, 50:223-236, 1971.

2. Edynak, E.M., Lardis, M.P., and Vrana, M. Antigenic Changes In Human Breast Neoplasia. Cancer, 28:1457-1461, 1971.

3. Gatti, R.A., and Good, R.A. Occurrence Of Malignancy In Immunodeficiency Diseases. A Literature Review. Cancer, 28:89-98, 1971.

4. Harris, J.P., Caleb, M.H., and South, M.A.: Secretory Component In Human Mammary Carcinoma. Cancer Res., 35:1861-1864, 1975.

5. Hobbs, J.R., Hepner, G.W., Douglas, A.P., Crabbé, P.A., and Johansson, S.G.O. Immunological Mystery of Coeliac Disease. Lancet, 2:649-650, 1969.

6. King, E.B., Barrett, D., King, M.-C., and Petrakis, N.L. Cellular Composition Of The Nipple Aspirate Specimen Of Breast Fluid. I. The Benign Cells. Am. J. Clin. Pathol., 64:728-738, 1975.

7. King, E.B., Barrett, D., and Petrakis, N.L.: Cellular Composition Of The Nipple Aspirate Specimen Of Breast Fluid. II. Abnormal Findings. Am. J. Clin. Pathol., 64:739-748, 1975.

8. Koistenen, J. Selective IgA Deficiency In Blood Donors. Vox Sang., 29:192-202, 1975.

9. Lentino, J.A. Immunological Studies In Breast Cancer. Allergologia et Immunopathologia, 3:279-288, 1975.

10. Michael, J.G., Ringenback, R., and Hottenstein, S. The Antimicrobial Activity Of Human Colostral Antibody In The Newborn. J. Infect. Dis., 124:445-448, 1971.

11. Petrakis, N.L. Genetic Cerumen Type, Breast Secretory Activity And Breast Cancer Epidemiology. Presented at National Cancer Institute Conference on The Genetics of Human Cancer, Orlando, Florida, December 1-4, 1975. In Press.

12. Petrakis, N.L. Analysis Of Breast Secretions Obtained By A Breast Pump. Presented at First Breast Cancer Task Force Working Conference of The National Cancer Institute, Williamsburg, Va., February 5-7, 1973.

13. Petrakis, N.L., Mason, L., Lee, R., Sugimoto, B., Pawson, S., and Catchpool, F. Association Of Race, Age, Menopausal Status, And Cerumen Type With Breast Fluid Secretion In Nonlactating Women, As Determined By Nipple Aspiration. J. Natl. Cancer Inst., 54:829-834, 1975.

14. Petrakis, N.L., Beelen, T., Castagnoli, N., Craig, J., and Grunenke, L. Detection Of Nicotine And Its Metabolites In Breast Fluid Of Nonlactating Women. Presented at Annual Meeting of American Society for Mass Spectroscopy, Houston, Texas, May 25-30, 1975.

15. Priori, E.S., Seman, G., Dmochowski, L., Gallager, H.S., and Anderson, D.E. Immunofluorescence Studies On Sera Of Patients With Breast Carcinoma. Cancer 28:1462-1471, 1971.

16. Richters, A., and Kaspersky, C.L. Surface Immunoglobulin Positive Lymphocytes In Human Breast Cancer Tissue And Homolateral Axillary Lymph Nodes. Cancer, 35:129-133, 1975.

17. Roberts, M.M., Bathgate, E.M., and Stevenson, A. Serum Immunoglobulin Levels In Patients With Breast Cancer. Cancer, 36:221-224, 1975.

18. Roberts, M.M., Bass, E.M., Wallace, I.W.J., and Stevenson, A. Local Immunoglobulin Production In Breast Cancer. Br. J. Cancer, 27:269-275, 1973.

19. Rosen, F.S., Kevy, S.V., Merler, E., Janeway, C.A., and Gitlin, D. Recurrent Bacterial Infections And Dysgammaglobulinemia. Deficiency Of 7S Gamma-Globulins In The Presence Of Elevated 19S Gamma-Globulins. Pediatrics, 28:182-195, 1961.

20. Rowinska-Zakrewska, E., Lazar, P., and Burtin, P. Dosage des immunoglobulines dans le sérum des cancéreux. Ann. Inst. Pasteur, 119:621-625, 1970.

21. Springer, G.F., Desai, P.R., and Scanlon, E.F. Blood Group MN Precursors As Human Breast Carcinoma-Associated Antigens and "Naturally" Occurring Human Cytotoxins Against Them. Cancer, 37:169-176, 1976.

22. Strober, W., Krakauer, R., Klaeveman, H.L., Reynolds, H.Y., and Nelson, D.L. Secretory Component Deficiency. A Disorder Of The IgA Immune System. N. Engl. J. Med., 294:351-356, 1976.

23. Tomasi, T.B., Jr., and Bienenstock, J. Secretory Immunoglobulins. Adv. Immunol., 9:1-96, 1968.

24. Whittaker, M.G., Rees, K., and Clark, C.G. Reduced Lymphocyte Transformation In Breast Cancer. Lancet, 1:892-893, 1971.

NATURAL AUTOANTIBODIES CYTOTOXIC FOR THYMOCYTES IN THE SERA OF NORMAL AND LEUKEMIC AKR MICE

Michael Schlesinger, James F. Holland, and J. G. Bekesi

Department of Neoplastic Diseases
Mount Sinai School of Medicine
100th Street and Fifth Avenue
New York, New York 10029

INTRODUCTION

Autoantibodies to thymus cells are known to occur in the serum of normal, non-immunized mice of a number of inbred strains (1,2), although there are striking differences in the titer of such autoantibodies among various strains (3,4). In the present study, the serum of mice of the AKR strain was found to contain a high titer of autoantibodies which, in the presence of complement, are cytotoxic for autologous thymus cells. This strain is characterized by a high incidence of "spontaneous" leukemias, developing from thymus-derived lymphocytes. A number of observations indicate that autoimmune phenomena may participate in the process leading to the formation of leukemias (5). It was of interest, therefore, to characterize the nature of the thymic autoantibodies detectable in the serum of AKR mice, and to determine their relationship to the leukemias appearing in these mice.

The present study describes preliminary observations on naturally occurring autoantibodies present in the serum of AKR mice, which react either with thymus cells or with neuraminidase-treated leukemia cells. The effect of the development of spontaneous leukemias and of chemotherapy on the appearance of autoantibodies to thymus cells was analyzed.

MATERIALS AND METHODS

Sera were obtained by bleeding of mice from the para-orbital venous complex. The bloods were kept at room temperature for three to five hours prior to separation of the sera. The sera used for cytotoxic tests either were freshly isolated sera or were thawed following storage at -20°C. The guinea-pig serum employed for the cytotoxicity tests was purchased from GIBCO (Grand Island Biological Company). It was absorbed with washed and packed homogenates of AKR brain, to remove the cytotoxicity of normal guinea-pig serum for mouse thymus cells.

The sera tested were obtained from non-immunized mice of various strains. AKR mice used as serum donors were either free of leukemia ("pre-leukemic") or had been diagnosed as having lymphatic leukemia. Some of the sera from leukemic mice were obtained a day after the mice received a course of chemotherapeutic treatment. This consisted of two i.p. injections of cytoxan (cyclophosphamide) 9 days apart, at a dose of 100 mg/kg and 200 mg/kg, respectively.

The target cells in most of the cytotoxicity tests were untreated thymus cells of AKR mice. In some tests neuraminidase-treated leukemia cells were used. The leukemia cells were harvested from the enlarged mesenteric lymph nodes of AKR mice with spontaneous leukemia. Suspensions of leukemia cells were incubated for 45 minutes at 37°C with Vibrio cholerae neuraminidase (Behringwerke) at a concentration of 25 to 35 units of neuraminidase per 2.5×10^7, suspended in 1.0 ml of sodium acetate buffer, according to the procedure of Bekesi, et al.(6).

Cytotoxicity tests were performed in flat-bottomed microcytotoxicity plates (Falcon Plastic Co., Oxnard, California). Each well contained 0.050 ml of serially diluted mouse serum, 0.050 ml cell suspension (10^6 cells/ml), and 0.050 ml of a 1:3 dilution of absorbed complement. The plates were incubated for an hour at 37°C and the proportion of dead cells was determined after the addition of trypan blue.

RESULTS

The sera of normal AKR mice were found to exert a cytotoxic effect only on thymus cells but not on lymphocytes of either the lymph nodes or the spleen (Figure 1). The toxicity of the sera of AKR mice was as strong as that of the sera of mice of the 129 strain (Figure 1). The cytotoxic effect of AKR serum depended on the presence of active guinea-pig complement. Fractionation of AKR serum on a Sephadex G-200 column indicated that the autoantibody activity was restricted to the IgM fraction. The autoantibodies were heat-labile, since heating to 56°C for 20 minutes abolished their activity.

474

The activity of AKR sera on thymus cells could be completely removed by absorption with homogenates of various tissues of normal AKR mice (brain, kidney, liver, spleen and thymus) and by AKR leukemia cells. The cytotoxic activity of thymus autoantibodies could be inhibited by various simple sugars. Of the sugars tested, those that inhibited the autoantibodies to the greatest degree were D-mannose, methyl D-mannopyranoside, and L-fucose. Autoantibody activity was completely inhibited by these sugars at concentrations of 2.5 mM or less. D-galactose and lactose were only weak inhibitors of the toxicity of thymic autoantibodies.

In some experiments, the sera of normal AKR and C_3H mice were tested in parallel for their cytotoxic effect on AKR thymus cells and on neuraminidase-treated AKR leukemia cells. AKR sera showed a strong cytotoxic effect on both target cells (Figure 2). The sera of C_3H mice regularly displayed a strong cytotoxic activity on neuraminidase-treated leukemia cells (Figure 3). In contrast, most batches of C_3H sera tested either showed a weak cytotoxic effect on AKR thymus cells or none at all (Figure 3). An additional indication that autoantibodies to thymus cells are different from those which react with neuraminidase-treated leukemia cells was obtained in studies on the inhibition of these antibodies with sugars. D-galactose and lactose, which hardly affected the activity of thymic autoantibodies were found to be potent inhibitors of the toxicity of AKR and C_3H normal sera for neuraminidase-treated leukemia cells. On the other hand, potent inhibitors of the toxic activity of thymic autoantibodies such as L-fucose and D-mannose had no effect on the toxicity of normal mouse sera for neuraminidase-treated leukemia cells.

The sera of all normal AKR mice examined contained autoantibodies cytotoxic for thymus cells, although the cytotoxic titer of the sera of individual mice varied somewhat (Figure 4). In contrast, the majority of the sera of mice with spontaneous lymphatic leukemia had no demonstrable thymic autoantibodies (Figure 4). The sera of leukemic mice lacking thymic autoantibodies were found to be capable of inhibiting the cytotoxic activity of the autoantibodies present in the sera of normal AKR sera. Preliminary fractionation procedures indicate that the inhibitory factor present in the serum of leukemia mice is not a simple sugar but rather a glycoprotein.

Leukemic AKR mice, whose sera did not show any autoantibody activity, received chemotherapeutic treatment. A day after the completion of the treatment schedule, the sera of about half of the treated mice contained thymic autoantibodies (Figure 4). Preliminary observations indicate the the presence of thymic autoantibodies can serve as an indicator for the prognosis of treated mice. The survival of the treated leukemic mice which possessed thymic autoantibodies was somewhat longer than that of the leukemic mice which lacked thymic autoantibodies following chemo-therapy.

DISCUSSION

The serum of preleukemic mice of the AKR strain was found to contain autoantibodies to thymus cells and to neuraminidase-treated AKR leukemia cells. Naturally occurring autoantibodies to thymocytes [1-4] and to neuraminidase-treated cells [7-9], have been studied extensively by a number of investigators. The present study indicates that the two types of autoantibodies are distinct entities, since they may appear indepen-dently in the serum of various inbred strains of mice. The sera of AKR mice contained both types of autoantibodies, whereas the sera of C_3H mice regularly contained autoantibodies to neuraminidase-treated cells but usually had only a low or negligible titer of autoantibodies to thymus cells. Another indication that the two types of autoantibodies are distinct, is the finding that although both are inhibitable by simple sugars, the pattern of inhibition by various sugars was different. Auto-antibodies to thymus cells were highly inhibitable by L-fucose, D-mannose, and ⍺-methyl-D-mannopyranoside, while D-galactose and lactose were only weak inhibitors. In contrast, the cytotoxic activity of AKR serum to neuraminidase-treated leukemia cells was only inhibitable by D-galactose and lactose, whereas the other sugars tested had no effect.

The possible functions of naturally occurring autoantibodies is not known at present. Only in the NZB strain, which suffers from a variety of autoimmune derangements, have pathogenetic properties been attributed to the thymic autoantibodies present in the sera of these mice [3]. Evidence was presented [10] that autoantibodies in the sera of NZB mice, which react with thymus cells and T-lymphocytes, cause a gradual deple-tion of T-lymphocytes from the peripheral organs of these mice [11]. It is conceivable that in mice of the AKR strain autoantibodies to thymus cells may play a role in the formation of leukemia from thymus-derived lymphocytes. Immune stimulation of lymphocytes has been shown to cause

activation of the MuLV (12,13). Possibly, the attachment of autoantibodies to the peripheral T-lymphocytes of AKR mice may trigger a similar
process. Another possibility to be considered is that a common derangement of the immune surveillance mechanism may lead both to the appearance
of autoantibodies to thymus cells and the leukemia formation. Finally,
AKR mice like other mice exposed to the MuLV are known to form antibodies
to antigens associated with this virus (14,15). It has been suggested
that the production of autoantibodies in NZB mice is triggered by infection with C-type viruses (16,17) and it can be suggested therefore that
the MuLV triggers a similar chain of events in AKR mice.

In most mice tested, the development of clinically detectable leukemia was associated with the disappearance of autoantibodies to thymus
cells. Following chemotherapy these autoantibodies reappeared in about
half of the leukemic mice. The mechanism by which the development of
leukemia eliminates autoantibodies to thymus cells is not clear. Leukemic
cells could remove thymic autoantibodies by specific absorption. In vitro
absorption experiments indicate, however, the leukemic cells have the
same capacity for absorption of thymic autoantibodies as normal peripheral
lymphocytes. The fact that the serum of leukemic mice is capable of
inhibiting the activity of autoantibodies to thymus cells opens the
possibility that the disappearance of autoantibodies may be related to an
increased concentration of a distinct glycoprotein in the serum of leukemic mice. A third possibility is that as part of the generalized immunosuppressive effects of murine leukemia (18,19), the progressive growth of
leukemia inhibits the production of autoantibodies. Whatever the mechanisms leading to the disappearance of autoantibodies in leukemic mice and
their reappearance following chemotherapy, it is obvious that the level
of autoantibodies to thymus cells may serve as an indicator of the leukemic tumor load to which the AKR mouse is exposed. It may thus serve as
guideline for the clinical stage of the leukemic animal and its responsiveness to treatment.

SUMMARY

The sera of mice of the high leukemic AKR strain were found to contain natural autoantibodies which, in the presence of guinea-pig complement, are cytotoxic for thymus cells but not for lymph-node or spleen
cells. These naturally occurring autoantibodies could be removed by

absorption with lymphocytes from AKR thymus, spleen or lymph-nodes, and by homogenates of AKR liver, kidney or brain. The autoantibodies are of the IgM class, and heat-labile. Their cytotoxic activity could be inhibited by a number of simple sugars, D-mannose, methyl-D-mannopyranoside and L-fucose being the most potent inhibitors. AKR sera also contain natural autoantibodies cytotoxic for neuraminidase-treated AKR leukemia cells. The activity of these antibodies was inhibitable only by D-galactose and lactose.

In the majority of AKR mice bearing spontaneous leukemias no auto-antibodies to thymus cells could be detected. Some leukemic mice, whose sera did not contain thymic autoantibodies, were treated with two i.p. injections of cytoxan. One day after the last injection the serum of about half of the mice was again found to contain thymic autoantibodies.

Autoantibodies to thymus cells could play a role in the pathogenesis of T-cell leukemias, or their appearance may reflect a derangement of normal homeostatic mechanisms in these mice. The presence or absence of thymic autoantibodies in the serum of leukemic AKR mice undergoing chemo-therapy may be an indication of the leukemia load to which these animals are exposed.

ACKNOWLEDGMENT

This study was supported by Special Cancer Virus Program NCI-NO1-CP 43225.

478

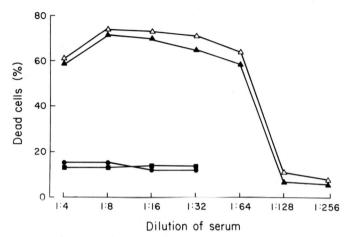

FIG. 1. The cytotoxic effect of sera from normal mice of the AKR and 129
strains. Filled Symbols: results obtained with AKR serum. Open symbols:
results obtained with 129 serum. The target cells in the cytotoxicity
tests were thymus cells (triangle), lymph-node cells (circle), or spleen
cells (square).

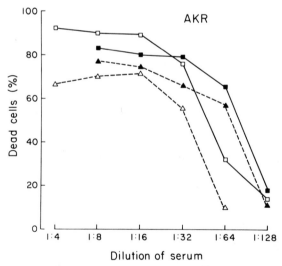

FIG. 2. Cytotoxicity tests with two different batches of AKR serum. The
results obtained with one batch are shown as filled symbols, while the results
obtained with the second batch are shown as open symbols. The target cells
(triangle) or neuraminidase-treated leukemia cells (square).

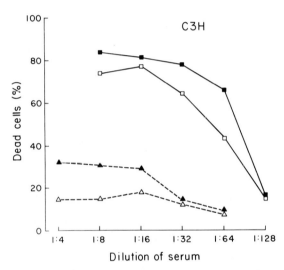

FIG. 3. Cytotoxicity tests with two different batches of C3H serum. The
results obtained with one batch are shown as filled symbols, while the
results obtained with the second batch are shown as open symbols. The
target cells in the cytotoxicity tests were either thymus cells (triangle)
or neuraminidase-treated leukemia cells (square).

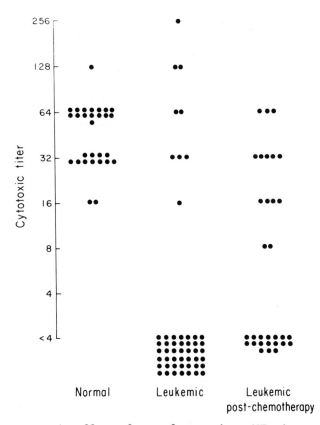

FIG. 4. The cytotoxic effect of sera from various AKR mice on syngeneic thymus cells. Sera were obtained from normal mice, untreated leukemic mice, or leukemic mice receiving chemotherapy. Each circle represents the cytotoxic titer obtained in tests with the serum of a single mouse.

REFERENCES

1. Schlesinger, M. Nature 207:429, 1965.

2. Raff, M.C. Israel J. Med. Sci. 7:724, 1971.

3. Shirai, T. and Mellors, R.C. Clin. Exp. Immunol. 12:133, 1972.

4. Martin, W.Y. and Martin, S.E. Nature 254:716, 1975.

5. Melief, C.J.M. and Schwartz, R.S. In: Cancer, a comprehensive treatise ed. F.F. Beker, Plenum Press, New York 1:121, 1975.

6. Bekesi, J.G., Roboz, J.P., Zimmerman, E. and Holland, J.F. Cancer Res. 36:631, 1976.

7. Sanford, B.H., and Codington, J.F. Tissue Antigens 1:153, 1971.

8. Ray, P.K., Gewurz, H., Simmons, R.L. Clin. Exp. Immunol. 11:441, 1972.

9. Rosenberg, S.A. and Schwarz, S. J. Nat. Cancer Inst. 52:1151, 1974.

10. Shirai, T., Yoshiki, T. and Mellors, R.C. J. Immunol. 110:517, 1973.

11. Stutman, O. J. Immunol. 109:602, 1972.

12. Armstrong, M.Y.K., Ruddle, N.H., Lipman, M.B. and Richards, F.F. J. Exp. Med. 137:1163, 1973.

13. Hirsch, M.S., Ellis, D.A., Black, P.H., Monaco, A.P. and Wood, M. Science 180:500, 1973.

14. Oldstone, M.B., Aoki, T. and Dixon, F.J. Proc. Nat. Acad. Sci. 69:134, 1972.

15. Nowinski, R.C., and Kaehler, S.L. Science 185:869, 1974.

16. Mellors, R.C., Shirai, T., Aoki, T., Huebner, R.J., Krawczynski, K. J. Exp. Med. 133:113, 1971.

17. Levy, J.A. Amer. J. Clin. Path. 62:258, 1974.

18. Metcalf, D. and Mouldi, R. Int. J. Cancer 2:53, 1967.

19. Ceglowski, W.S. and Friedman, H. J. Nat. Cancer Inst. 40:983, 1968.

SUPPRESSION OF ENDOGENOUS TYPE C MURINE VIROGENE EXPRESSIONS
WITH VIRUS SPECIFIC HYPERIMMUNE IMMUNOGLOBULIN (IgG)

Robert J. Huebner*, Raymond V. Gilden**, Robert Toni**
Paul R. Hill*, and Roy W. Trimmer*

*Laboratory of RNA Tumor Viruses
National Cancer Institute
Bethesda, Maryland 20014

**Frederick Cancer Research Center
Frederick, Maryland 21701

INTRODUCTION

Leukemia and other cancers produced in experimental animals by
horizontal transmission of exogenous type C oncornaviruses can be prevented
by prior administration of potent type-specific viral vaccines (1-5)
and by immune gamma globulin (5). On the other hand, attempts to
suppress type C virus infections after the virus was fully expressed
and/or when viral-induced tumors are already established have not been
successful (6-7). This was not unexpected since attempts to reverse
established infections with prophylactic vaccines from all past experience
would be expected to fail. Indeed, in some cases enhancement of both
infection and disease can be anticipated.

Because naturally occurring type C viruses in mice are genetically
transmitted, the prospects for suppressing virus replication and neoplasia
at first consideration seemed rather poor. However, long-term studies
of endogenous ecotropic type C virus expresssions during embryogenesis
and during early and late postnatal life in a number of inbred and
crossbred mice, some of which had been given chemical carcinogens,
suggested that immunological suppression of endogenous virus might
be possible (8-13).

Certain mouse strains and crossbred mice noted for their high levels
of virus and leukemia expressions, such as AKR's, were found to have
relatively low virus expressions during the first few days of postnatal

life (14), thus providing opportunities to produce specific immunity prior to virus expression. However, in order to suppress virus in AKR mice, efforts had to be undertaken by 7 days of age since high levels of virus were found in visceral and bone marrow tissues after one week of age. On the other hand, relatively low virus expressors such as C57BL/6, BALB/c, C57L/J, NIH Swiss, SWR/J, and particularly certain crossbred strains producing low amounts of detectable virus during early life remained relatively poor virus expressors in maturity. However, when leukemia and other cancers reached their peak occurrence, generally at 16 to 24 months of age (15,16), virus expressions, particularly p30 and infectious virus, also reached quite significant levels. Parenthetically, it should be pointed out that strains which ordinarily express only xenotropic viruses (MuX) at low levels, such as C57L, NZB, 129/J, SWR and NIH Swiss, also develop lymphoma and other tumors late in life when the MuX expressions appear to be more extensively expressed (6,10). Although a direct etiological link between virus expression and cancer must still be conclusively proven, a number of studies have shown that high levels of endogenous ecotropic virus expression are frequently correlated with the occurrence of spontaneous cancer in a number of strains and crossbred lines of mice (10,17). It seemed to us that the most direct way to prove an etiological role for the endogenous viruses would be to use the classical approach of prevention of viral replication in the host by means of active vaccines or passive immunoglobulin (IgG). In recent reports (18,19) we described significant and prolonged suppression of type C oncornavirus expressions in a number of crossbred and backcross mice known to normally have high levels of virus and tumor expressions by type-specific vaccines (Table I and Legend).

Our chief purpose in this report is to present information showing that passive IgG antibodies directed against the endogenous ecotropic oncornaviruses also suppressed the normally high levels of endogenous type C viral expression in AKR mice and (BALB/c x AKR) x AKR backcross progeny. The suppression of virus persisted for significant periods during postnatal and early mature life. Unfortunately, our current experiments require continuing observation before definitive effects on the incidence of cancer can be made available. In any event, successful suppression of the natural Akv-1 virogene expression represents not only a highly significant observation, but also provides excellent opportunities for determining in definitive fashion the roles of type C oncornaviruses in the etiology of spontaneous cancer and possibly also in environmentally induced cancer.

PROCEDURES AND MATERIALS USED

Mice. Pregnant AKR and BALB/c mice were acquired from The Jackson Laboratory, Bar Harbor, Maine, and the Frederick Cancer Research Center, Frederick, Maryland, respectively.

Assays for Type C Virus in Tail Tissues. The tail virus assay was that described by Lilly et al. (16) and by Huebner et al. (18). At specified ages (Tables I and II) the 2 cm terminal segments of tails were cut off each test and control mouse with a sharp scissors. The extracts, 2% by volume, were lightly centrifuged, sonicated and tested for infectious virus by the XC method using the continuous passage SC-1 cell. Viral titers were expressed as the number of plaque forming units per 0.4 ml of 2% extracts.

Virus Preparations Used for IgG Production. Spleen extract virus containing the radiation leukemia virus (RadLV), originally from Lieberman and Kaplan (20), were grown in SC-1 cells (21). These cells, replicating high titers of RadLV, were used for large scale virus production. The fluids derived from these cultures were clarified by filtration through a 1.2 μ pore size membrane filter (Millipore Corp.). Virus was then concentrated by continuous flow centrifugation with isopycnic banding in 20-50% wt/wt tris-buffered sucrose gradients. Peak fractions based on absorption at 280 nm and on p30 antigen content were rebanded by rate zonal centrifugation. The choice of rotor depended on fluid volumes as described by Olpin et al. (22).

Preparation of Neutralizing Antibody and IgG. Castrated male goats 1 and 1-1/2 years of age (Denver Serum Co., Denver, Pa.) were immunized intramuscularly at 1-2 week intervals with 1.0 - 3.0 mg of purified virus mixed with equal parts of Freund's Complete Adjuvant. Animals were bled at 10-day intervals beginning 2 weeks after the third inoculation. When 0.5 liters of serum were accumulated (usually 4 sequential bleedings), pools were made for fractionation. The globulin fraction of the pooled sera was prepared by addition of an equal volume of saturated ammonium sulfate and stirring for 1 hour at room temperature. The precipitate was collected by centrifugation at 5,000 rpm for 20 minutes and resuspended in 1/2 the original volume in phosphate buffered saline (PBS). After dialysis against PBS at 4°C for 48 hours with several buffer changes, the resulting globulin solution was filtered through a 0.45 μ filter and dispensed in 2.0 to 5.0 ml aliquots under sterile conditions.

The IgG preparations were tested for neutralizing capacity in the XC test using the SC-1 cell as the susceptible cell system, and the AKR, Rauscher leukemia virus (RLV), MSV(AKR) and MSV(AT124) were utilized as the test viruses. The sera were titrated at 1:100 dilution through 1:3200 versus generally 60 to 80 AKR plaques and/or 50-60 MSV foci.

Those IgG preparations having neutralizing antibody titers of 1:800 to 1:1600 based on 70% to 100% inhibition in each dilution were used for virus suppression tests in the AKR and backcross mice (see below). Comparable antiviral IgG prepared against RLV and xenotropic viruses provided little or no suppression of the ecotropic AKR or GLV viruses and were available as control antisera.

Experimental Design. Newborn AKR and BALB/c x AKR backcross mice were given their first inoculation of RadLV IgG on the day of birth. Subsequent inoculations were given at 3 or 4 day intervals. The number of inoculations varied from 5 in AKR to 8 in the backcross mice (Table II). Controls remained uninoculated or were inoculated with IgG to RLV, a heterotypic strain of type C virus that does not cross react to any significant degree in neutralization tests with AKR virus. The mice, even as newborns, tolerated the goat IgG in a dosage schedule given subcutaneously as follows:

For IgG experiments in AKR mice

Day 0	0.05 ml
Day 3	0.05 ml
Day 7	0.05 ml
Day 10	0.10 ml
Day 14 or 15	0.10 ml

For the IgG experiment in (BALB/c x AKR) x AKR

Day 0	0.05 ml
Day 3	0.05 ml
Day 7	0.10 ml
Day 10	0.20 ml

Day 15	0.30 ml
Day 20	0.30 ml
Day 25	0.30 ml
Day 30	0.50 ml

RESULTS AND DISCUSSION

AKR Experiments. Table II illustrates the effects of the antiviral IgG in 3 separate experiments. While more than 4 logs of infectious virus were demonstrated in all AKR controls when tested at 18 to 34 days of age, the immunized mice revealed titers of $< 10^{1.0}$ to $10^{2.6}$ at these same periods. The tails of all immunized and control mice (at least several litters) for each test were assayed in the XC test.

(BALB/c x AKR) x AKR Experiment. Profound suppression of type C virus expressions by IgG were also observed in the progeny of immunized (BALB/c x AKR) x AKR backcross mice. The reduction of virus to $< 10^{1.0}$ in the tails of all immunized mice tested (several litters) at 50 days of age suggests that future immunizations continued beyond 14 to 20 days may provide profound suppression of virus for longer periods than have so far been explored in the AKR experiments.

Lilly et al. (17) recently reported that the Akv-1 and Akv-2 viral genes and the regulating genes Fv-1 and H-2 each determine rates of leukemogenesis in the (BALB/c x AKR) x AKR backcross. Thus those progeny mice segregating with the $Fv-1^b$ gene developed, as expected, low virus expressions $(< 10^{2.0})$ in their tissues at 40+ days and low leukemia rates later in life, while those containing the viral permissive $Fv-1^n$ gene developed much higher viral titers $(10^3$ or $>)$ which correlated with higher rates of leukemia. Unfortunately our experiment requires a year or more of observation before significant leukemogenesis can be expected in the test or control groups; however, several hundred backcross mice are being monitored for observation. This experiment may prove to be particularly valuable in that it may make it possible to determine the effects of two critical factors in restricting oncogenesis in the same host: (a) gene regulation, and (b) antiviral immunity. It is important, however, to note that while IgG produced almost total virus suppression at 50 days of age in the BALB/c x AKR backcross mice (Table II), the vaccinated backcross mice showed little or no significant reduction in virus titers compared with that of controls; this was true at 30 to 40 days of age as well as at the 113 day period

shown in Table I. Thus, in this backcross the passive IgG may provide
more protection than the active vaccine.

Although more time will be required to determine the effects of
longer term immunizations on subsequent virus titers and on the incidence
of leukemia, the profound reduction of natural virus expression for
20 to 30 days after final immunization suggests that the clonal cells
producing the Akv-1 gene-determined virus were either inactivated or
otherwise seriously restricted in their ability to produce viruses.
Rowe and his associates (23) have noted that infectious virus is ordinarily produced in only a proportion of AKR cell clones established in
tissue culture. Also studies by Meier et al. (10), Lilly et al. (17),
and Heiniger et al. (24) of crossbred and congenic mice revealed that
well-defined genetic factors mentioned above which control the segregation
of high and low levels of ecotropic infectious virus expression detected
at 30 to 50 days of age represent specific determinants that correlated
with high or low incidences of spontaneous leukemias later in life.
As of this writing only a few leukemias have been observed in our initial
AKR experiments: at 240 days, 1 of 36 (2.7%) of the vaccinated mice,
and 5 of 27 (18.5%) of the controls developed leukemia. Although significant, these data cannot be regarded as definitive at this early stage.

COMMENTS

Possible toxic reactions on the part of goat IgG antibodies and
reactions with the alloantigens of mouse cells have been assessed
repeatedly in the XC SC-1 mouse cell test system; thus far we have
not observed significant effects on the SC-1 cells. Price et al. (25)
observed some reduction in the efficiency of plating of rat cells after
treatment with IgG preparations; the effects, however, were equivalent
in both infected and control cells, and were produced by heterotypic
as well as homologous IgG. In vivo, the mice tolerated the IgG inoculations surprisingly well even as newborns and no toxic deaths or anaphylactic
reactions have been observed after 10 or more immunizations. While
this might be attributable to the induction of tolerance in the mice
inoculated as newborns, we have not observed serious reactions even
when the inoculations were started in mature mice. Thus it seems likely
that virus suppression by IgG might very well be continued for periods
longer than that shown in Table II. Immunization experiments now in
the planning stage include attempts to employ vaccines and IgG separately

and together to suppress virus and tumor expressions in mice that ordinarily have low virus expressions in early life, yet significant incidences of cancer later in life, particularily when given carcinogens. This approach would be applicable to certain well-known inbred strains of mice and might also be useful in attempts to suppress the late cancers that occur in rats and hamsters and cancers which might be induced in primates. Of course this would require appropriate IgG and/or vaccine reagents specific for known endogenous viruses.

Prevention of disease is preferable and generally more successful than therapy. Furthermore, virtually all successful immunizations were developed in experimental animals prior to trials in humans. Should it prove possible to achieve successful prevention of animal cancers with the use of artificially induced immunity, similar approaches aimed at prevention of cancer in man could then be considered.

TABLE I. Titers (Long Range) of Type C Virus in 2% Tail Extracts of Vaccinated and Control F_1 Progeny and Backcross Mice

Experiment	Age (Days)	Vaccinees	Controls
F_1 Progeny			
1. SWR/AKR	41-58	$<10^{1.0}-10^{3.1}$	$>10^{4.6}$
	309-321	$10^{3.9}-10^{4.4}$	$>10^{5.4}$
2. C57L/AKR*	30	$<10^{1.0}$	$10^{4.1}-10^{4.6}$
	125	$10^{2.5}-10^{2.6}$	$10^{4.4}$
3. NIH/AKR	40	$<10^{1.0}$	$10^{4.9}$
	80	$10^{1.5}-10^{1.7}$	$10^{3.7}-10^{4.0}$
4. BALB/c/AKR	76	$<10^{1.0}$	$10^{1.5}-10^{4.1}$
	113	$10^{1.8}-10^{2.1}$	$10^{3.9}$
Backcrosses			
(C57L x AKR) x AKR 117		$10^{1.9}-10^{3.6}$#	$10^{5.1}$##
(BALB/c x AKR) x AKR 113		$<10^{1.0}-10^{3.6}$†	$<10^{1.0}-10^{3.6}$††

*2% tail extracts from vaccinees when tested undiluted gave titers of $10^{0}-10^{0.3}$.

#Mean = $10^{3.2}$

##Mean = $10^{5.1}$

†Mean = $10^{3.0}$

††Mean = $10^{3.4}$

LEGEND - TABLE I

Preparation of Killed and Live Vaccines. Banded and concentrated
(1000-fold) Gross leukemia virus (GLV) was inactivated in the frozen
state by irradiation from a 55 MEV,S band traveling wave electron linear
accelerator (18). The samples revealed no infectious virus or radio-
activation. The live vaccine was shown to produce high level neutralizing
antibodies to GLV in sera of vaccinated females which completely prevented
sarcomas when challenged with MSV(GLV) live vaccine. This "live vaccine"
was 100% lethal within 10-12 days when given to unvaccinated F_1 mice at
10 days of age. However, progeny of mice vaccinated with the killed
banded vaccine were in virutally all cases resistant.

MSV(GLV) as Live Vaccine. MSV(GLV) was produced by serial passage
in NIH Swiss mice. The vaccine preparation consisted of 10X concentrated
modified Moloney procedure extracts (26) with focus- and sarcoma-inducing
titers of 10^3 logs.

Experimental Design and Strategy. The low virus expressors C57L,
SWR/J, NIH Swiss and BALB/c were bred to the high expressor AKR/J males
after immunization with 3 to 6 injections of killed vaccine. The main
objective basically was to use the banded killed vaccine to produce
extensive antiviral immunity to GLV that would persist in young females
during pregnancy and protect F_1 mice against a single large challenge
dose of MSV(GLV) at 10 days of age, the latter representing a live
challenge vaccine. The tail virus titers were assayed in the XC test
according to the same protocol for the IgG AKR experiments described in
this paper.

TABLE II. Passive Type-specific (IgG) Suppression of Endogenous Virus in Tails of AKR and (BALB/c x AKR) x AKR Backcross Mice

Experiment	No. of Immunizations	Day of Age Tested	Immunized (Log Range)	Controls (Log Range)
1. AKR	5	18	$<10^{1.0}$	$10^{4.1}$
		25	$<10^{1.0}$	$10^{4.1}$
		32	$<10^{1.0}-10^{2.3}$	$10^{4.2}$
2. AKR	5	24	$<10^{1.0}$	$10^{4.1}$
		33-34	$<10^{1.0}-10^{2.3}$	$10^{4.1}$
3. AKR	5	34	$10^{2.6}$	$10^{4.6}$
4. (BALB/c x AKR) x AKR	8	50	$<10^{1.0}$	$10^{1.0}-10^{4.0}$

In AKR experiments, the number of mice tested ranged from 15 to 32 in test and controls; in (BALB/c x AKR) x AKR backcross at 50 days 8 immunized and 8 control mice were tested.

In Experiment 3, total amount of IgG given was 0.3 ml as compared to 0.7 ml in Experiments 1 and 2.

REFERENCES

1. Friend, C., and Rossi, G. B. Transplantation Immunity and the Suppression of Spleen Colony Formation by Immunization with Murine Leukemia Virus Preparations (Friend). Int. J. Cancer, $\underline{3}$: 523-529, 1968.

2. Fink, M. A., and Rauscher, F. J. Immune Reactions to a Murine Leukemia Virus. I. Induction of Immunity to Infection with Virus in the Natural Host. J. Nat. Cancer Inst., $\underline{32}$: 1075-1082, 1964.

3. Ioachim, H. L., Gimovsky, M. L., and Keller, S. E. Maternal Vaccination with Formalin-Inactivated Gross Lymphoma Virus in Rats and Transfer of Immunity to Offspring. Proc. Soc. Exp. Biol. Med., $\underline{144}$: 376-379, 1973.

4. Kirsten, W. H., Stefanski, E., and Panem, S. Brief Communication: An Attenuated Mouse Leukemia Virus. I. Origin and Immunization. J. Nat. Cancer Inst., $\underline{52}$: 983-985, 1974.

5. Hunsmann, G., Moennig, V., and Shaefer, W. Properties of Mouse Leukemia Viruses. IX. Active and Passive Immunization of Mice against Friend Leukemia with Isolated Viral GP_{71} Glycoprotein and Its Corresponding Antiserum. Virology, $\underline{66}$: 327-329, 1975.

6. Huebner, R. J. Unpublished Data.

7. Whitmire, C. E. Unpublished Data.

8. Huebner, R. J., Kelloff, G. J., Sarma, P. S., Lane, W. T., Turner, H. C., Gilden, R. V., Oroszlan, S., Meier, H., Myers, D. D., and Peters, R. L. Group-Specific Antigen Expression During Embryogenesis of the Genome of the C-Type RNA Tumor Virus: Implications for Ontogenesis and Oncogenesis. Proc. Nat. Acad. Sci. USA, $\underline{67}$: 366-376, 1970.

9. Peters, R. L., Hartley, J. W., Rabstein, L. S., Whitmire, C. E., Spahn, G. J., Turner, H. C., and Huebner, R. J. Prevalence of the Group-Specific (gs) Antigen and Infectious Virus Expressions of the Murine C-Type RNA Viruses During the Life Span of BALB/cCr Mice. Int. J. Cancer, $\underline{10}$: 283-289, 1972.

10. Meier, H., Taylor, B. A., Cherry, M., and Huebner, R. J. Host-Gene Control of Type C RNA Tumor Virus Expression and Tumorigenesis in Inbred Mice. Proc. Nat. Acad. Sci. USA, $\underline{70}$: 1450-1455, 1973.

11. Meier, H., Myers, D. D., and Huebner, R. J. Genetic Control by the hr-Locus of Susceptibility and Resistance to Leukemia. Proc. Nat. Acad. Sci. USA, $\underline{63}$: 759-766, 1969.

12. Whitmire, C. E. Virus-Chemical Carcinogenesis: A Possible Viral Immunological Influence on 3-Methylcholanthrene Sarcoma Induction. J. Nat. Cancer Inst., $\underline{51}$:473-478, 1973.

13. Tung, J-S., Vitetta, E. S., Fleissner, E., and Boyse, E. A. Biochemical Evidence Linking the G_{IX} Thymocyte Surface Antigen to the gp69/71 Envelope Glycoprotein of MuLV. J. Exp. Med., 141: 198-226, 1975.

14. Rowe, W. P., and Pincus, T. Quantitative Studies of Naturally Occurring Murine Leukemia Virus Infection of AKR Mice. J. Exp. Med., 135: 429-436, 1972.

15. Peters, R. L., Rabstein, L. S., Spahn, G. J., Madison, R. M., and Huebner, R. J. Incidence of Spontaneous Neoplasms in Breeding and Retired Breeder BALB/cCr Mice Throughout the Natural Lifespan. Int. J. Cancer, 10: 273-282, 1972.

16. Huebner, R. J., Todaro, G. J., Sarma, P., Hartley, J. W., Freeman, A. E., Peters, R. L., Whitmire, C. E., Meier, H., and Gilden, R. V. "Switched-Off" Vertically Transmitted C-Type RNA Tumor Viruses as Determinants of Spontaneous and Induced Cancer: A New Hypothesis of Viral Carcinogenesis. In: Defectiveness, Rescue and Stimulation of Oncogenic Viruses. Second International Symposium on Tumor Viruses. Editions du Centre National de la Recherche Scientifique, Paris, pp. 33-57, 1970.

17. Lilly, F., Duran-Reynals, M., and Rowe, W. Correlation of Early Murine Leukemia Virus Titer and H-2 Type with Spontaneous Leukemia in Mice of the BALB/c x AKR Cross: A Genetic Analysis. J. Exp. Med., 141: 882-889, 1975.

18. Huebner, R. J., Gilden, R. V., Lane, W. T., Toni, R., Trimmer, R. W., and Hill, P. R. Suppression of Murine Type C Virogenes by Type-Specific Oncornavirus Vaccines. Prospects for Prevention of Cancer. Proc. Nat. Acad. Sci. USA, 73: 620-624, 1976.

19. Huebner, R. J., Gilden, R. V., Lane, W. T., Trimmer, R. W., and Hill, P. R. Suppression of Endogenous Type C RNA Virogene Expression in Mice by Serotype-Specific Viral Vaccines: Progress Report. In: Proceedings of Second Conference on Modulation of Host Resistance in the Prevention or Treatment of Induced Neoplasias. Ed.: M. A. Chirigos. Raven Press. In Press.

20. Lieberman, M., and Kaplan, H. S. Leukemogenic Activity of Filtrates from Radiation-Induced Lymphoid Tumors of Mice. Science, 130: 387-388, 1959.

21. Hartley, J. W., and Rowe, W. P. Clonal Cell Lines from a Feral Mouse Embryo which Lack Host-Range Restrictions for Murine Leukemia Viruses. Virology, 65: 128-134, 1975.

22. Olpin, J., Oroszlan, S., and Gilden, R. V. Biophysical-Immunological Assay for Ribonucleic Acid Type C Viruses. App. Microl, 28: 100-105, 1974.

23. Rowe, W. P., Hartley, J. W., Lander, M. R., Pugh, W. E., and Teich, N. Noninfectious AKR Mouse Embryo Cell Lines in which Each Cell has the Capacity to be Activated to Produce Infectious Murine Leukemia Virus. Virology, 46: 866-876, 1971.

24. Heiniger, H. J., Huebner, R. J., and Meier, H. Effect of Allelic Substitutions at the Hairless Locus on Endogenous Ecotropic Murine Leukemia Virus Titers and Leukemogenesis. J. Nat. Cancer Inst., 56: 110-111, 1976.

25. Price, P. J., Bellew, T. M., King, M. P., Freeman, A. E., Gilden, R. V., and Huebner, R. J. Prevention of Viral-Chemical Co-carcinogenesis In Vitro by Type-Specific Anti-Viral Antibody. Proc. Nat. Acad. Sci. USA, 73: 152-155, 1976.

26. Moloney, J. B. Biological Studies on a Lymphoid-Leukemia Virus Extracted from Sarcoma 37. I. Origin and Introductory Investigations. J. Nat. Cancer Inst., 24: 933-951, 1960.

TOLERANCE AND PREVENTION OF TUMOR GROWTH IN IMMUNE DEFICIENT MICE

N. Allegretti, M. Taradi and B. Malenica

Department of Physiology, University of
Zagreb Faculty of Medicine and Central
Institute for Tumors and Allied Diseases,
Zagreb, Yugoslavia

INTRODUCTION

Results have been reported /14,15/ that chemical carcinogens,
injected in mice of the same strain, induce tumors with different tumor specific transplantation antigens /TSTA/. A tumor induced by a single injection of a chemical carcinogen
displays, more or less, only one TSTA in their cells. It is
hard to believe that a chemical carcinogen given in a single
injection would in affected cells exert identical changes
responsible for the development of the tumor with the identical TSTA expressed in its cells. On the contrary, it can
be assumed that a single cell /or a clone of identically
changed cells/ gave rise to the tumor development. It should
be questioned about the ways and means by which the neigh-
bouring tumorous cells with dissimilar TSTA were eliminated.
It is improbable that the immune reaction would give preference to the subsistence of the one clone of carcinogen-af-
fected cells. Otherwise, chemical carcinogens would not give
rise to the development of tumors with different TSTA in one
strain of mice /or in one single organism/. It appears, accordingly, that some nonimmunological surveillance mechanisms
might also act in preventing /or allowing/ the tumor development.

The purpose of the present study was to provide evidence of
some nonimmunological mechanisms capable of preventing the
development of transplantable tumors in mice. The mixtures
of cells of two tumors, both of them tolerated by recipient
mice, were injected. The outgrowth of a tumor formed predominantly of one kind of cells would give evidence of the
assumed mechanisms.

Thymectomized, lethally irradiated mice reconstituted with
the syngeneic normal bone marrow cells /TIR mice/ were shown
to be nonspecifically tolerant to the xenogeneic rat tumor
/2,11/. In these T-cell deficient mice it was impossible to

induce any immunological response at all. Therefore, they were expected to exert no immunological response to any component of the injected mixture of rat and transplantable mouse tumor cells. In another model two tumors with different TSTA, induced by a chemical carcinogen in mice of the same strain, were used. These two tumors happened to show the same virulence as proved by the growth rate and death appearance of mice. It was felt that the immune system of normal mice would show no significant preference to any of the two syngeneic tumors if injected as a mixture of cells.

Any change in the virulence or in the incidence of any component of the injected tumor cell mixture would, accordingly, speak in favor of the assumed nonimmunological cellular interaction.

PROCEDURES AND MATERIALS USED

/a/ Animals. CBA mice of both sexes were used. They were of different age as required by the experiment.

Nonspecifically tolerant mice were obtained by thymectomy, lethal irradiation and reconstitution with syngeneic bone marrow cells. Another group of thymectomized, lethally irradiated mice were reconstituted with the syngeneic bone marrow cells deriving from the normal mice having rejected the xenogeneic tumor.

Rats were of the WVM strain, littermate bred from an ancestor Wistar pair.

/b/ Tumors. Yoshida ascites sarcoma /YAS/ has been passaged at this Department for more than 10 years. It is transplantable in all strains of rats but not in normal mice. Ehrlich ascites tumor /EAT/ has also been passaged in this Department over the same period. It is transplantable in all strains of mice. In an extremely large number of cells EAT can sometimes grow in the rat's abdominal cavity. In this study TIR mice were inoculated subcutaneously with a mixture of YAS and EAT cells.

One milligram of 20-methylcholanthrene /MCA//Fluka AG., Buchs SG/ in seed oil was given subcutaneously per CBA mouse. After about 12 to 14 weeks of latency a fibrosarcoma appeared at the injection site. The minced tumor tissue corresponding to 5 million tumor cells was subcutaneously transplanted into normal CBA mice. The remains of tumors were kept in a vessel with liquid nitrogen. Transplant generation F_1 of MCA tumors, were further transplanted in the same way and checked for the growth rate, death appearance and antigenicity. Two fibrosarcomas MCAA and MCAB of the F_1 transplant generation of about an equal growth rate and death appearance and dissimilar antigenicity were used in experimental procedures. They were kept in a vessel with the liquid nitrogen before use. Mice were subcutaneously inoculated also with a mixture of F_1 transplant generation of MCAA and MCAB cells.

Care was taken to perform all tumor manipulations and procedures in aseptic conditions.

/c/ Immunization. CBA mice were injected intraperitoneally twice with 1×10^6 YAS cells two weeks apart. After one week their bone marrow cells were harvested and used for the reconstitution of thymectomized, lethally irradiated syngeneic mice /TIR-anti-YAS mice/.

Immunization of CBA mice with fibrosarcomas was induced by the subcutaneous inoculation of a minced tumor corresponding to 5 million tumor cells. After about two weeks the tumor knot was excised and after 1 week more the animal used for testing the antigenicity of the unknown developed tumor.

/d/ Thymectomy. Mice were thymectomized at the age of 3 to 4 weeks. The operation was performed by sucking out the mice thymus. All operation sites were inspected at necropsy.

/e/ Irradiation. A Philips X-ray therapeutic device was used for the total body irradiation of mice. Irradiation constants were: 200 kV, 15 mA; 0.5 mm Cu and 1.0 mm Al filters; focal distance to target 40 cm; irradiation dose 100 R/56 sec; total irradiation dose 900 R measured in air. Mice were irradiated in a plastic box 3 to 4 weeks after thymectomy.

/f/ Cell transfer. Bone marrow cells of normal or anti-YAS immunized CBA mice were obtained from femurs and tibias after squeezing the tissue suspended in physiological buffered saline /PBS/ through a nylon gauze filter and blowing it through a No. 16 needle. The cells were washed once by centrifugation and resuspension. Reconstitution of irradiated mice was performed within 4 hours after irradiation. Spleens were dissected suspended in PBS, squeezed through a nylon gauze filter and blown through a No. 16 needle several times. Cells were washed three times by centrifugation and resuspension. Care was taken to do all cell manipulations under aseptic conditions.

/g/ Scoring of tumor virulence. The cell suspension of tumor outgrowth of YAS and EAT cell inoculated singly or of the mixture inoculated in TIR mice was transferred intraperitoneally in normal mice and rats. Death appearance were compared with those in animals inoculated with the known number of tumor cells.

The outgrowths of MCAA and MCAB tumors were scored according to their growth rate indicated by the slope b and the latency period /horizontal distance/. The size of the tumor was determined by multiplying the longest diameter /a/ by their diameter vertical half the length of a /b/ and by the

average of both /a + b//2. Their dissimilar antigenicity was
detected by transferring the tumor outgrowth in mice preimmunized with MCAA or MCAB. The antigenicity of the tumor
knots outgrown from a mixture of MCAA and MCAB cells was determined in two ways: by inoculating the mixture in the mice
preimmunized with MCAA or MCAB cells, or by inoculating MCAA
or MCAB tumor cells in mice preimmunized with the outgrown
tumor mixture cells. Preimmunization with the outgrown tumor
mixture was performed in the same way as that with the MCAA
and MCAB tumors.

/h/ Skin-grafting. Full thickness rat skin grafts
1 x 2 cm deprived of the adjacent adipose particles were put
in the corresponding defect on the flank of recipient mice.
Dressings were removed 6 days after transplantation and the
grafts were inspected daily. The first day of complete
breakdown when only scar tissue remained was scored as the
day of rejection.

RESULTS

I. YAS and EAT cells inoculated in TIR mice

T-cell deficient TIR mice inoculated intraperitoneally or
subcutaneously with 50 million YAS cells cannot inhibit YAS
cell multiplication or induce rejection of the xenogeneic
tumor tissue. As shown in Table I, TIR mice inoculated either intraperitoneally or subcutaneously succumb to death
caused by 50 million YAS cells.

Mixtures of EAT and YAS cells in a ratio of 1:99, 25:75 and
50:50 million, were given subcutaneously to TIR mice. It was
hoped that the mouse tumor would be privileged to grow in
its own specific environment and the ratio of cells was,
therefore, chosen to be in favor of the xenogeneic YAS cells.
After two weeks the mice were killed, tumors dissected,
their cells teased apart, and 10 million tumor cells were
injected into rats or mice intraperitoneally.

As shown in Table II, the growth of YAS in xenogeneic T-cell
deficient mice induced no significant biological change of
the tumor. Transfer of the tumor intraperitoneally back to
normal rats induced their dying after 7 to 10 days, just as
it did to rats receiving YAS cells from normal rats. Normal
mice rejected the transferred tumor. Intraperitoneal transfer to normal mice and rats of tumor cells from T-cell deficient, TIR mice, inoculated subcutaneously with a mixture
of EAT and YAS cells showed a significant impairment of
both tumor cells. The mice receiving cells from the outgrowth of tumor mixtures died markedly later than those injected with as few as 100000 EAT cells from normal donors.
Rats receiving cells of the same origin died later than
those receiving 100 YAS cells from normal rats.

TIR mice can resist the YAS inoculum differing, however, strongly from the above described effect. Table III shows two models in which TIR mice can resist the YAS inoculum. In the first model thymectomized, lethally irradiated mice do not allow the xenogeneic tumor to take when reconstituted with bone marrow cells of anti-YAS immune syngeneic donors /TIR-anti-YAS mice/. Tumor outgrowths persisted for a long time before having disappeared completely. No scar tissue was formed. TIR-anti-YAS mice displayed somewhat higher rat skin rejection ability in comparison with TIR mice. Two third of mice TIR-anti-rat skin showed a prompt rejection of subcutaneously inoculated YAS. The rejection was similar to the skin graft rejection by forming scar tissue. As expected there was a prompt rejection of rat skin in mice TIR-anti--rat skin. In the second model, addition of normal spleen cells almost simultaneously with YAS cells induced rejection of tumor. Spleen cells of TIR and TIR-anti-YAS mice displayed no such activity. All the described qualities of immune manifestations were not noticed in the outgrowths of tumor mixtures.

It can be summarized that impairment of YAS and EAT cells having grown as a mixture in T-cell deficient mice cannot be ascribed to the immune or any other host activity since the resistance of TIR mice to YAS has a different manifestation and can be induced in another way.

II. Two syngeneic methylcholanthrene induced fibrosarcomas /MCAA and MCAB/ inoculated in normal mice

As shown in Fig. 1 minced fibrosarcomas MCAA and MCAB of the F_1 transplant generation corresponding to 5×10^6 cells inoculated subcutaneously separately in normal syngeneic CBA mice display growth patterns which exhibit no difference at all. The growth was recorded only until the first appearance of death to avoid misleadings which might have resulted from the omission of the largest tumor data. Both tumors developed the same growth patterns also if simultaneously inoculated separately into two flanks of a single mouse.

Fibrosarcomas MCAA and MCAB showed distinct TSTAs as presented in Table IV. Immunity to a particular tumor specifically lowered the tumor take and growth in mice by 70 to 80%. This was sufficient to distinguish two TSTAs.

Mice were inoculated with a mixture of two minced tumors corresponding each to 2.5×10^6 tumor cells. The growth rate of the mixed tumor did not differ from that of singly inoculated tumors. The knots produced by the tumor mixture were excised to be treated for the presence of either of the two TSTAs in mice immunized to MCAA and MCAB, respectively. Tumor mixture knots were also used for the immunization for another set of mice. The growth and take of MCAA and MCAB tumors in these mice was used for the identification of TSTAs in tumor cells in the outgrowth of the inoculated tumor mixture. Table IV presents also the results of both ways of tumor identification. Immunization of CBA mice to MCAA fibrosarcoma inhibits in the recipient mice the growth of the corresponding tumor only, leaving MCAB and mixture outgrowth unimpaired. However, immunization to MCAB induces the impairment of corresponding MCAB tumor as well as of the mixture outgrowth. Moreover, the tumor appearance in mixture outgrowth injected mice was greatly delayed as if a very low number of MCAA tumor cells /less than 25000 cells/ were injected alone /Fig. 2/. In addition CBA recipient mice immunized to the tumor mixture outgrowth showed a stronger impairment of the MCAB tumor take and growth than of the MCAA tumor. Accordingly the tumor mixture consisted mainly of MCAB tumor cells. It may, therefore, be concluded that MCAA fibrosarcoma was inhibited in growth in the syngeneic host if grown in a mixture with MCAB fibrosarcoma cells.

DISCUSSION

The intention to provide evidence of nonimmunological mechanisms preventing the take and growth of transplantable tumors means, among others, to draw attention to cell incompatibilities which prevent their adhesion - a property essential for morphogenesis. In the experiments presented two tumors differing in antigenic properties were inoculated into mice as a mixture of cells. Care was taken to make the immune activity of the host irrelevant to any tumor growth.

Thymectomized, lethally irradiated bone marrow reconstituted /TIR/ mice were shown to be nonspecifically tolerant to the allogeneic skin and xenogeneic tumor /2,4,5,6,11,12/. They were shown to be unimmunizable /1/ unless reconstituted with the bone marrow of immunized syngeneic donors or unless given simultaneously with the immunogen some small amount of the syngeneic spleen cells. The impairment of mouse EAT and rat YAS if grown mixed in TIR mice can in no instance be related to the immune response of the host. It is justifiable to think of a mutual incompatibility and impairment of EAT and YAS cell. Local environmental incompatibility between tumors and host environment in TIR mice seems to have a minor influence upon tumor growth. It may therefore be concluded that it is incompatibility between EAT and YAS tumors that lies at the bottom of their impairment which was clearly visible when the outgrowth cells were transferred in normal environment i.e. the mouse and rat abdominal cavity.

Immunologically fully competent CBA mice were hosts of two syngeneic methylcholanthrene induced fibrosarcomas, MCAA and MCAB. Strong impairment of the MCAA tumor growth could hardly be explained as influenced by the host. Either tumor, grown separately in the same host displayed an almost identical growth rate. It may be concluded once again that intercellular incompatibility between two fibrosarcomas is to be ascribed the impairment of the MCAA tumor growth.

Adhesive selectivity in cellular interactions appears important in the control of embryonic growth, in differentiation and, particularly in, morphogenesis /9,10/. This cell and tissue affinity, well known in embriology and differentiation studies, has given no adequate weight in surveillance hypotheses. Yet unicellular organism were shown to have a distinct affinity to identical /self/ or similar determinants. Sponges were the first to be shown to display disaggregation and specific aggregation phenomena in decalcinated and recalcinated sea water /7/. Ingenious experiments with Botryllus /3/ have shown that cells can not aggregate unless having some membrane surface determinant in common. Similar results are obtained with Hydra viridis /16/. It should be noted that parts of several Hydras put together successively give information to the first one about the transplanted mass. Separation between the first and the second transplant then occurs. Corrals show the nontake /or rejection/ of the dissimilar transplants /18/. Echinodermata also display the rejection /or nontake/ of dissimilar transplants /8/. All these lower animals have nodifferentiated immunological system, so that the rejection /or nontake/ of dissimilar transplants can be explained as the effect of nonadhesivity due to the strong dissimilarity. The principle of communication between identical determinants /9/ and its later elaboration are today the basis of morphogenesis and of the formation of organs in higher more differentiated animals /13/.

There is no reason to believe that this fundamental cellular principle of identical or similar cell communication or recognition has been extinguished in higher animals. Even more erroneously appears the belief that the immune system has developed from the above principle. The immune cell does not communicate but with the dissimilar "complementary" determinant. Therefore it appears untenable to believe that the immune system has developed from the above principle of the recognition of identical or similar determinants of cell surfaces responsible for selective adhesion. For this reason the results obtained could be explained as being due to the degree of incompatibility between the cells of two tumors, and of the degree of incompatibilities between surrounding and tumor cells. The imagined outcome could be the impairment of one or both tumors as deduced from the principles of the thermodynamics of cell arrangement /17/. This would, however, require a revision of our views of allograft rejection mechanisms.

SUMMARY

Besides intraperitoneally, Yoshida ascites sarcoma /YAS/ can grow also as a subcutaneous solide tumor if given thymectomized, lethally irradiated, syngeneic bone marrow reconstituted /TIR/ CBA mice. These mice injected subcutaneously with a mixture of YAS and Ehrlich ascites tumor /EAT/ develop a solid tumor. The outgrowths of the YAS and EAT

mixture display a well expressed growth retardation if transferred intraperitoneally to normal rats and mice, respectively. A mixture of two methylcholanthrene mice fibrosarcomas
/MCAA and MCAB/ injected subcutaneously in normal mice gives
preference of growth to one of them /MCAB/. The virulence of
both fibrosarcomas was almost identical differing only in the
tumor specific transplantation antigen /TSTA/. The mutual
tumor cell interactions are considered to be responsible for
the impairment of both or only one of the tumor given in immunologically irrelevant hosts.

ACKNOWLEDGMENT

This work has been supported by the Research Fund of Croatia

TABLE I. Deaths in Thymectomized, Irradiated Syngeneic Bone Marrow Reconstituted Mice /TIR/ Inoculated Intraperitoneally or Subcutaneously with Yoshida Ascites Sarcoma /YAS/ Cells

Recipient mice	Inoculated YAS cells / x 10^{-6}/	Dead/inoculated recipient mice	Death appearance after YAS inoculation /days/
Normal	1 i.p.	0/20	
	50 i.p.	0/20	
	50 s.c.	0/25	
TIR	1 i.p.	11/16	11,13,16x2,17x2, 19,20x2,21,22
	50 i.p.	16/16	10,13x4,14x5, 15x2,16x2,17x2
	50 s.c.	16/16	14,17,18x4,19, 20x3,26,31,32, 34,35,37

TABLE II. Death of Mice and Rats Inoculated Intraperitoneally with 10 x 10^6 Cells of Tumor Outgrowths Resulting from Subcutaneous Inoculation of TIR[a] Mice with Different Mixtures of EAT and YAS Cells[b]

Tumor recipients	Tumor donors	Intraperitoneally inoculated cells of subcutaneous tumor outgrowths	Dead/ inoculated recipient mice	Death appearance after tumor inoculation /days/
Mice	Normal rats[c]	YAS	0/10	
	Normal mice	EAT	8/8	11x3,13x2, 15x2,16
	TIR[a] mice	YAS	0/12	
	TIR mice	Mixture[b] 1:99	9/9	32,33,35x5, 38x2
	TIR mice	Mixture 25:75	5/5	25,28,31,35x2
	TIR mice	Mixture 50:50	4/4	24,25,26,38
Rats	Normal rats	YAS	12/12	5x3,6x5,7x2, 8x2
	Normal mice	EAT	0/20	
	TIR mice	YAS	5/5	6,7,9,10x2
	TIR mice	Mixture 1:99	12/12	10x2,11,12x2, 13x2,15,17x2, 22x2
	TIR mice	Mixture 25:75	6/6	10,11x2,12,13, 17
	TIR mice	Mixture 50:50	11/12	10x5,11x3, 12x3

[a]Thymectomized, irradiated, syngeneic bone marrow reconstituted mice

[b]TIR mice tumor donors were subcutaneously injected 100 x x 10^6 tumor cells of EAT and YAS cells mixture 1:99, 25:75 or 50:50

[c]Normal mice and rats inoculated subcutaneously 15 days before with 10 x 10^6 EAT and YAS cells, respectively.

TABLE III. Rejection of the Xenogeneic Tissue by TIR[a] Mice

Recipient	Xenogeneic tissue grafted	Rejected/ grafted	Rejection time /days/
TIR	YAS[b] s.c.	0/16[c]	
TIR	Rat skin graft	8/10	20x3,21,22,36x3
TIR-anti-YAS[d]	YAS s.c.	9/9	29x2,35x3,40x2,49, 53 /probably non take/
TIR-anti-YAS	Rat skin graft	7/7	17x3,18x3,19
TIR-anti-rat skin	YAS s.c.	6/9	18x3,22x3
TIR-anti-rat skin	YAS i.p.	0/9[c]	
TIR-anti-rat skin	Rat skin graft	5/5	12,14x4
TIR+normal spleen cells[e]	YAS s.c.	16/16	
TIR+TIR spleen cells[e]	YAS s.c.	0/10[c]	
TIR+ TIR-anti-YAS spleen cells[e]	YAS s.c.	0/10[c]	

[a]Thymectomized, lethally irradiated, syngeneic bone marrow reconstituted

[b]50 x 10^6 Yoshida ascites sarcoma cells

[d]Reconstitution was done with the bone marrow from syngeneic mice which rejected the intraperitoneal inoculum of YAS

[e]30 x 10^6 spleen cells were injected intravenously about simultaneously with xenogeneic tissue grafted

TABLE IV. Identification[a] of Tumor Cells in Outgrowths of MCAA[b] and MCAB[b] Minced Tumor Mixture

Tumor recipient	Inoculated tumor	Tumor take[c] and growth/ inoculated	Tumor take and growth %
Normal	MCAA	21/21	100
	MCAB	20/20	100
	Mixture outgrowth	20/20	100
Immunized to MCAA	MCAA	2/10	20
	MCAB	9/9	100
	Mixture outgrowth	16/16	100
Immunized to MCAB	MCAA	10/10	100
	MCAB	3/11	27
	Mixture outgrowth	8/12	67
Immunized to mixture outgrowth	MCAA	4/9	44
	MCAB	2/10	20

[a]Mixture outgrowth was inoculated subcutaneously into CBA mice preimmunized to MCAA or MCAB fibrosarcoma or both fibrosarcomas were singly inoculated into CBA mice preimmunized with the mixture outgrowth. Immunization performed by excising a tumor knot 14 days after minced tumor inoculation. The inoculum of minced tumor contained about 5×10^6 tumor cells.

[b]MCAA and MCAB fibrosarcomas of the F_1 transplant generation of 20-methylcholanthrene induced tumors.

[c]All mice with tumor take and growth died with a tumor of excessive size.

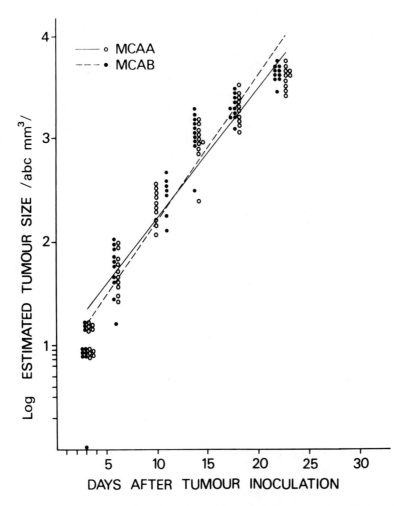

FIG. 1. Growth pattern of methylcholanthrene fibrosarcomas MCAA and MCAB in CBA mice. Minced tumor corresponding to 5 x 10^6 tumor cells was inoculated.

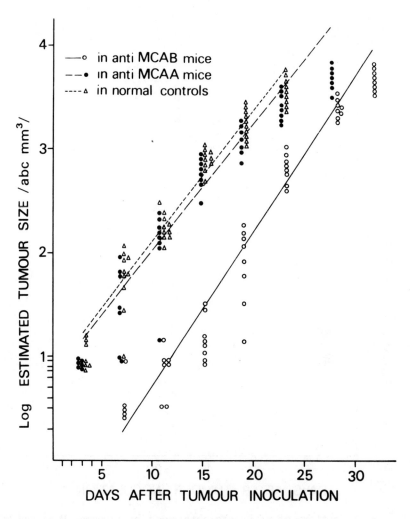

FIG. 2. Growth pattern of outgrowths from the two fibrosarcomas MCAA and
MCAB in mice immunized to either tumor. Minced tumor corresponding to
5 x 10⁶ outgrowth cells was inoculated.

REFERENCES

1. Allegretti, N. and Marušić, M. Immune reactivity in thymectomized, lethally irradiated and syngeneic bone marrow reconstituted mice and rats. Exp.Hematology /in press/

2. Allegretti, N., Marušić, M., Čulo, F. and Andreis, I.
   The growth of xenogeneic tumour in mice depleted of T-
   -lymphocytes. Proc.Iug.Immunol.Soc., 3: 98-100, 1974.

3. Burnet, F.M. "Self-recognition" in colonial marine forms
   and flowering plants in relation to the evolution immunity. Nature, 232: 230-236, 1971.

4. Castro, J.E. Human tumours grown in mice. Nature New
   Biology, 239: 83-84, 1972.

5. Cobb, L.M. and Mitchley, B.C.V. The growth of human tumours in immune deprived mice. Europ.J.Cancer, 10: 473-
   -476, 1974.

6. Franks, C.R., Perkins, F.T. and Holmes, T.J. Subcutaneous
   growth of human tumours in mice. Nature, 243: 91, 1973.

7. Galtsoff, P. Regeneration after dissociation. /An experimental study on sponges/. I. Behaviour of dissociated
   cells of Microciona prolifera under normal and altered
   conditions. J.Exp.Zool., 42: 183-222, 1925.

8. Hildemann, W.H. and Dix, T.G. Transplantation reactions
   of tropical australian Echinoders. Transplantation, 15:
   624-633, 1972.

9. Holtfreter, J. Gewebsaffinität, ein Mittel der embryonal
   Formbildung. Arch.Exp.Zellforsch.Gewebezücht., 23: 169-
   -209, 1939.

10. Holtfreter, J. Studien zur Ermittlung der Gestaltungs-
    faktoren in der Organentwicklung der Amphibien II. Dyna-
    mische Vorgänge in einigen mesodermalen Organanlagen.
    Arch.Entwicklungsmech.Organism., 139: 110-190, 1939.

11. Marušić, M., Allegretti, N. and Čulo, F. Yoshida ascites
    sarcoma grown in mice. Int.Arch.Allergy Appl.Immunol.,
    49: 568-572, 1975.

12. Miller, J.F.A.P., Smith, S.M.A. and Cross, A.M. Role of
    the thymus in the recovery of the immune mechanism in
    the irradiated adult mouse. Proc.Soc.Exp.Biol.Med., 112:
    785-792, 1963.

13. Moscona, A.A. Surface specification of embryonic cells:
    Lectin receptors, cell recognitions and specific cell
    ligands, In: The Cell Surface in Development. Ed.: A.A.
    Moscona. John Wiley & Sons, New York, pp. 67-99, 1974.

14. Prehn, R.T. and Main, J.M. Immunity to methylcholanthre-
    ne induced sarcomas. J.Nat.Cancer Inst., 18: 769-788,
    1957.

15. Prehn, R.T. Analysis of antigenic heterogenicity within
    individual 3-methylcholanthrene-induced mouse sarcomas.
    J.Nat.Cancer Inst., 45: 1039-1045, 1970.

16. Shostak, S. Graft rejection and the regulation of length in <u>Hydra viridis</u>. In: Contemporary Topics in Immuno-biology, Vol. 4. Invertebrate Immunology. Ed.: E.L. Cooper. Plenum Press, New York, pp. 127-139, 1974.

17. Steinberg, M.S. The problem of adhesive selectivity in cellular interactions. In: Cellular Membranes in Development. Ed.: M. Locke. Academic Press, New York, pp. 321--366, 1964.

18. Theodor, J.L. Distinction between "self" and "not-self" in lower invertebrates. Nature, <u>227</u>: 690-692, 1970.

Section 4

IMMUNOCOMPETENCE AND HUMAN CANCER

SO-CALLED IMMUNOSUPPRESSION STIMULATES THE PROLIFERATION OF CELLS (ESPECIALLY NEOPLASTIC) BY NON-SPECIFIC MEANS

Frederick D. Dallenbach
Institute of Experimental Pathology
German Cancer Research Center
Heidelberg, Germany

INTRODUCTION

One of the strong supports for the theory that human tumors may be immunogenic is the observation that a high percentage of patients given chronic immunosuppressive therapy develop cancers (1,2,3,4,5). That relationship suggests that when the normal defense mechanisms of immunity are impaired, malignant cells arising by spontaneous mutation and bearing foreign antigens go unrecognized, multiply, and invade. Presumably immune surveillance is lost.

Other factors, however, unrelated to lost immunosurveillance could induce an increased proliferation of cells. For instance, in earlier studies we found (6) that immunosuppression of one-sided nephrectomized rats stimulated regeneration of the remaining kidney. Ausinsch and Richard (7) also reported enhancement of compensatory renal growth after immunosuppression with antilymphocyte globulin and cyclophosphamide. Other investigators (8, 9) have observed that after thymectomy the regeneration of a partially resected liver was depressed.

To learn more about how immunosuppression acts on proliferating cells, we had to turn to a different model of cellular regeneration. To avoid an effect of the cellular immune system, thereby excluding a possible immune surveillance, we isolated proliferating tumor cells in millipore chambers (10, 11), implanted these in animals and counted the increase in cells at intervals during and after treating the animals with immunosuppressive agents. The present paper represents a report of our results.

PROCEDURES AND MATERIALS

The cells we used for our several sets of experiments were local strains of Walker carcinoma, HeLa carcinoma, and hamster melanoma. We placed either 500 or 1000 of each strain in millipore chambers (10, 11) made with millipore filters with openings either 0.2 or 0.45 micron. We planted the cell-bearing chambers intraperitoneally in groups of 20 animals (either Sprague-Dawley rats or golden hamsters three months old) of both sexes. Half of the animals received immuno-suppressive therapy (12) induced by cyclophosphamide (dose 30 mg daily per kg body weight), dexamethasone (daily dose 0.1 mg) and/ or rabbit anti-rat lymphocyte gamma globulin (1 mg./ day). The control half of the animals received normal saline solution injected like the immunosuppressive agents. After three, six, and fourteen days we removed the chambers from the animals, fixed them with Zenker's solution, opened them and stained and counted the numbers of tumor cells covering their inner surfaces. To prove that immuno-suppression had been effective, we examined the thymus, spleen and lymph nodes (Table I) of all 240 animals studied.

RESULTS

As Graphs I and II show, the tumor cells in the chambers of both male and female animals receiving immunosuppres-sive therapy were consistently more numerous than in those of the control animals. An analysis with Student's t-test proved the differences in numbers to be significant.

DISCUSSION

To obtain significant results we had to use young ani-mals. No differences between sexes were found however. The tumor cells chosen for such studies must grow well on sur-faces and depending on the experimental plan, must flourish in xenogeneic hosts. From the profound involution of the thymus and lymph nodes it was apparent the immunosuppressive agents had been effective. As our counts of the tumor cells in the millipore chambers indicate, even when tumor cells are separated from contact with immune cells, immunosuppression still stimulates their proliferation. Since the cells are isolated, the stimulating effect cannot be due to impaired immunity (loss of immunosurveillance) against presumably immunogenic tumor cells. The metabolic changes and disturbances induced by the immunosuppressive agents we used are extremely complex (12). The control of cellular proliferation appears to be even more complicated (13). Just how immunosuppressive therapy stimulates the proliferation of tumor cells remains unclear. Several possible factors are listed in Table 2. Stimulation might come from increased function of the pituitary or adrenals (14). It may also, we suggest, represent a non-specific increase of nutriments that tumor cells need for DNA synthesis and proliferation. Our suggestion is supported by the results of others (15, 16, 17), especially those of Rieke (15), who proved in radioautographs that tumor cells transplanted into the peritoneal cavity can reutilize DNA released from lymphocytes labelled with tritiated thymidine. Perhaps the lysis of immune cells and the involution of the lymphatic tissues occurring in immunosuppression liberates abundant amounts of DNA byproducts and other substances needed by cells able to proliferate. Tannenbaum's discovery (18) many years ago that well fed rats develop more tumors than underfed may perhaps be explained by similar metabolic phenomena.

SUMMARY

Our aim was to learn how immunosuppression stimulates proliferating tissues. When we implanted millipore chambers containing tumor cells into young rats and hamsters and treated these with immunosuppressive agents, the tumor cells proliferated faster than in the control animals. Our results indicate that immunosuppression can stimulate growth of tumor cells but by means other than loss of immune surveillance.

**Table I. Morphological Studies to Prove
Immunosuppressive Effect**

Weights: total body
 kidney
 thymus
 spleen

Histology: thymus
 kidney
 spleen
 lymph nodes

Table II

Factors Influencing Cell Regeneration

A. Hormones: hypophyseal
 thyroid
 adrenal
 thymic
 "growth factor"

B. Thymic involution-"trephocyte
 effect"

C. Age of animal

D. Nutritional state

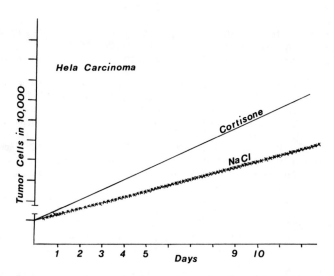

GRAPH I. Immunosuppression stimulates growth of tumor cells in intra-peritoneal millipore chambers. (Significance: p < 0.05, Student's t-test.)

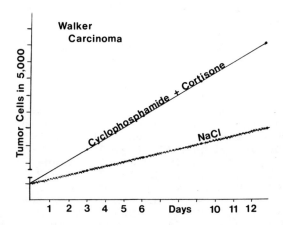

GRAPH II. Immunosuppression stimulates growth of tumor cells in intra-peritoneal millipore chambers (p < 0.05, Student's t-test.)

REFERENCES

1. Burnet, F. M. The Concept Of Immunological Surveillance. Prog. Exp. Tumor Res., 13: 1-27, 1970.
2. McKhann, C.F. Primary Malignancy In Patients Undergoing Immunosuppression For Renal Transplantation. Transplant.8: 209-212, 1969.
3. Good, R.A. Relations Between Immunity and Malignancy. Proc. Nat. Acad. Sci. 69: 1026-1032, 1972.
4. Penn, I., and Starzl, T.E. Immunosuppression And Cancer. Transplant. Proc. 5: 943-947, 1973.
5. Melief, C.J.M., and Schwartz, R.S. Immunocompetence And Malignancy. In: Cancer I - A Comprehensive Treatis. Etiology: Chemical and Physical Carcinogenesis. Ed.: Frederick F. Becker. Plenum Press, New York and London, pp. 121-159, 1975.
6. Dallenbach, F.D., and Bauz, R. The Effect Of Immunosuppression On Compensatory Renal Hyperplasia In Rats. Abstr. 73., 10th Intern. Congress, Intern. Acad. Path. Hamburg, Sept. 17, 1974.
7. Ausinsch, B., and Richard, G.A. The Enhancement Of Compensatory Renal Growth By Antilymphocyte Globulin. Ped. Res. 6: 415, 1972.
8. Dukor, P., and Miller, J.F.A.P. Leberregeneration nach partieller Hepatektomie bei thymektomierten Mäusen. Naturwiss. 52: 189, 1965.
9. Fachet, J., Stark, E., Palkovits, M., and Vallent, K. Der Einfluss der Thymektomie auf die Leberregeneration nach partieller Hepatektomie. Ztsch. f. Zellforsch. 60: 609-614, 1963.
10. Algire, G.H., Borders, M.L., and Evans, V.J Studies Of Heterografts In Diffusion Chambers In Mice. J. Natl. Cancer Inst. 20: 1187-1201, 1958.
11. Bartlett, G.L., and Prehn, R.T. An Improved Design For General Purpose Diffusion Chambers. Transplant. 7: 225-227, 1969.
12. Bach, J.F. The Mode Of Action Of Immunosuppressive Agents. Vol. 41 - Frontiers of Biology, North-Holland Publishing Co., Amsterdam, 1975.
13. Sheppard, J.R., and Bannai, S. Cyclic AMP and Cell Proliferation. In: Control of Proliferation in Animal Cells. Eds.: Bayard Clarkson and Renate Baserga. Cold Spring Harbor Laboratory, pp. 571-579, 1974.
14. Green, H.N., and Whitely, H.J. Cortisone And Tumour Growth. Brit. Med. Jour. 2: 538-540, 1952.
15. Rieke, W.O. The In Vivo Reutilization Of Lymphocytic And Sarcoma DNA By Cells Growing In The Peritoneal Cavity. J. Cell Biol. 13: 205-216, 1962.
16. Bryant, B.J. Reutilization Of Leukocyte DNA By Cells Of Regenerating Liver. Exp. Cell Res. 27: 70-79, 1962.
17. Fichtelius, K.E., and Bryant, B.J. On The Fate Of Thymocytes. In: The Thymus in Immunobiology. Eds.: Robert A. Good and Ann E. Gabrielsen. Harper and Row, New York-Evanston-London, pp. 274-286, 1964.
18. Tannenbaum, A. The Genesis And Growth Of Tumors. III. Effects Of A High Fat Diet. Cancer Res. 2: 468-475, 1942.

PHYTOHEMAGGLUTININ SKIN TEST IN CANCER PATIENTS: A PARAMETER FOR DETECTING CELLULAR IMMUNODEFICIENCY DURING ANTICANCER THERAPY

Saburo Sone, Kentaro Yata and Eiro Tsubura

Third Department of Internal Medicine
Tokushima University School of Medicine
Kuramoto-cho, Tokushima 770, Japan

1. INTRODUCTION

Phytohemagglutinin (PHA),obtained from Phaseolus vulgaris,is a non-specific mitogen of thymus-derived lymphocytes (T-cells) in vitro[17],and responses to it are not dependent on prior exposure to an antigen in the environment. This in vitro response to PHA appears to be correlated with the capacity of the host to give a skin reaction of delayed type hyper-sensitivity. The first clinical trial on the skin reaction to PHA was reported by Schrek and Stefani[32]. Thereafter,the PHA skin test has been used for detecting congenital cellular immunodeficiency in infants and children[5,6,25,30]. However,there have been no reports on changes in skin reactivity to PHA in patients with neoplasmas during anticancer therapy. This stimulated us to evaluate the clinical value of the PHA skin test in patients with neoplasmas.
Cellular immunity is known to play an important role in the host defense mechanism against neoplasmas,and impaired immunity has been noted in certain patients with neoplasmas[2,15,24,26,33,36]. On the other hand, it has been reported that anticancer therapies,such as chemotherapy and immunotherapy, are valuable in treatment of some cancer patients, and remission or prolonged survival can now be achieved by suitable therapy[19,22,27-29,31,37]. Recently,change in the immunological status of patients with neoplasmas during therapy was recognized to be more important for the ultimate prognosis than the status before therapy[12,21]. In fact,patients with neoplasmas who change from immunoincompetence to immunocompetence are likely to have a relative good prognosis.

With the current trend toward increasing use of anticancer therapy, it seems important to establish a simple,generally applicable method for use as a repeatble test of cellular immunocompetence. The methods most widely used at present for repeated tests of cellular immunity are measurement of the total T-cells in peripheral blood, in vitro lymphocyte transformation and delayed type hypersensitivity to dinitrochlorobenzene (DNCB)[2,8,12,14,16,21,26]. However,these tests have several disadvantages,such as that they require complicated techniques and that they are difficult to standardize. If the PHA skin test proved reliable as a test of cellular immunocompetence, it would have the advantages of speed,simplicity and economy. Accordingly,we investigated the clinical application of the PHA skin test for use instead of other immunological tests for assessing immunodeficiency in patients with neoplasmas, and we also compared the PHA skin test with other in vitro and in vivo tests of cellular immunity.

2. PROCEDURES AND MATERIALS USED

Subjects

Skin reactivity to PHA was examined in 69 normal subjects (average age 32,age range 18-62) and 149 patients with various kinds of cancer, excluding lymphoreticular malignancies (average age 51,age range 21-81). For comparing the PHA skin test with age, 301 adults of various ages without malignancies or general debility were tested. To examine the correlation between the results of the PHA skin test and those of other in vitro and in vivo tests, the PHA skin test was performed simultaneously with the following tests:

a) An in vitro test on lymphocyte transformation in 87 subjects,that is 26 normal subjects and 61 cancer patients (i.e. 25 cases of lung cancer, 14 of gastric cancer, 6 of hepatoma, 3 of cancer of the breast and 13 others).

b) Measurement of the number of T-cells (lymphocyte count x fraction of lymphocytes forming rosettes) in 82 subjects,that is 24 normal subjects and 58 cancer patients (i.e. 35 cases of lung cancer, 10 of gastric cancer , 3 of hepatoma, 3 of cancer of the larynx and 7 others).

c) Measurement of delayed cutaneous hypersensitivity to purified protein derivative (PPD) in 177 cancer patients (i.e. 76 cases of gastric cancer, 48 of lung cancer, 24 of cancer of the breast, 9 of cancer of the colon and rectum, 6 of esophageal cancer, 6 of uterine cancer and 8 others).

d) Measurement of delayed hypersensitivity to DNCB in 35 cancer patients
(i.e. 14 cases of lung cancer, 11 of gastric cancer, 5 of hepatoma and
cancer of the gall bladder and 5 others).

Sequential evaluation of host immunocompetence was studied in 17 patients
with nonlymphomatous malignancies (i.e. 11 cases of lung cancer, 3 of
hepatoma and 3 others), and in 8 patients with lymphoreticular malignancies
,namely 3 cases of acute leukemia, one of chronic leukemia and 4 of
reticulum cell sarcoma of stages II and III[11].

Skin tests

Purified phytohemagglutinin (PHA,Wellcome Reagents Ltd.,Beckenham
England.,Lots K-7644,K-8463 and K-9347) was diluted in sterile saline to
a concentration of 0.05mg per ml, and kept frozen untill just before use.
Subjects were injected intradermally in different parts of the forearm with
5 µg of PHA, and with 0.05 µg of purified protein derivative (PPD) (Japan
BCG Laboratory,Tokyo,Japan) both in a volume of 0.1 ml. The average of the
two main diameters of the erythema and the induration were recorded 24 hr
and 48 hr after the injection. The skin reaction to 5 µg of PHA was
regarded as positive when the diameter of the area of erythema was 25 mm
or more 24 hr after the injection. Delayed cutaneous hypersensitivity to
2,4-dinitrochlorobenzene (DNCB)(Nakarai Chemical,Ltd,Kyoto.,Japan) was
examined in 35 cancer patients. For this DNCB was dissolved in acetone at
a concentration of 2 %. Occlusive adhesive plaster with gauze of 1.5 cm
diameter for the patch test (Torii Pharmaceutical Co,Ltd.,Tokyo.,Japan)
was used for sensitization and challenge with DNCB. The adhesive plaster
with gauze soaked in the 2 % solution of DNCB (0.025ml) was applied to the
volar surface of the forearm after cleasing the area with acetone solution.
The adhesive plaster was removed after 48 hr and 10 to 14 days later the
DNCB skin response was regarded as positive if spontaneous flare-up
(erythema and induration) was seen at the site of sensitization. If the
response was not positive, the subject was challenged in a different site
with 0.1 % DNCB in acetone (0.025ml) on occlusive adhesive plaster 2 weeks
after immunization and the DNCB skin response was regarded as positive if
erythema and induration had developed at the site of challenge after 48
hr. The PHA skin test was made at the times of sensitization and challenge
with DNCB, and was regarded as positive when the PHA skin response was
positive at both times.

T-cell counts

Lymphocytes were obtained from peripheral blood by the method of Bøyum[7]. Heparinized venous blood was subjected to "Conray/Ficoll 400" gradient centrifugation, and the lymphocytes obtained were used both to count rosette formation and for lymphocyte culture. To examine rosette formation with sheep red blood cells (SRBC), the lymphocytes were collected by centrifugation at 1,000 rpm for 10 min and suspended at a concentration of 3×10^6 cells/ml in fetal calf serum (PCS) (Grand Island Biological Company, N.Y., U.S.A.). A mixture of 0.1 ml of the cell suspension and 0.1 ml of a 1 % suspension of SRBC in Eagle's MEM was incubated in a small test tube at 37° for 15 min. Then the mixture was centrifuged at 1,000 rpm for 5 min. The precipitate of lymphocytes and SRBC was left in the test tube undisturbed at 4° for 1 hr and then examined in a hemocytometer and the number of rosettes among 300 cells was measured. The total number of T-cells was expressed as the count of lymphocytes collected x the fraction of lymphocytes forming rosettes[38].

Lymphocyte culture

Lymphocyte culture were prepared as described previously[34]. Each culture contained 10^6 lymphocytes/2 ml MEM supplemented with 20 % FCS. Duplicate cultures were stimulated by addition of 1 µl of phytohemagglutinin-P (Difco Laboratory, Detroit, Mich., U.S.A.). Two days later 1 µCi tritiated (^{3}H) thymidine (Daiichi Pure Chemicals Co.,Tokyo,Japan) was added. The cells were incubated for a further 24 hr, and harvested. Their blastogenic response was examined by measuring ^{3}H-thymidine incorporation and recorded as counts per min (cpm) per 10^6 lymphocytes.

2. RESULTS

PHA skin test in various groups

Results of the PHA skin test in normal controls and patients with cancer are shown in Table I. In normal subjects, erythema and induration developed after intradermal injection of 5 µg of PHA, reaching a maximum after 24 hr. A positive response to PHA was arbitrarily defined as development of an area of erythema with a mean diameter of 25 mm or more 24 hr after the injection of PHA, because erythema is generally easier to measure than induration. No individuals developed a scar or necrosis at the site of injection, and the only local reaction other than induration and erythema was itching. The skin reactivity of cancer patients was less than that of the control group and among 68 cancer patients under anticancer therapy, only 24 (35.3%) showed a positive reaction.

Skin reactivity to PHA of subjects of different ages without malignancies

The skin reactivity to PHA was measured in 301 subjects of various ages of more than 15 years. The subjects were arbitrarily divided into various age groups and the mean ($\pm$ S.E) for each group was calculated. As shown in Fig.1, the skin reactivity to PHA was similar in elderly individuals to that in younger adults.

Skin reactivity to PHA in repeated tests

The PHA skin test was repeated 4 times at intervals of a few weeks on 21 patients without malignancies who initially showed a positive response. Their responses were similar in successive tests (Table II).

Sequential skin tests with PHA on clinical cases during therapy

Sequential PHA skin tests were made on 17 patients with nonlymphomatous malignancies and 8 patients with lymphoreticular malignancies during anti-cancer therapy. The relationship between the serial skin reactivities to PHA and the subsequent prognosis in cases of nonlymphomatous cancer is shown in Fig.2. All cases showed a gradual decrease in skin reactivity to PHA and almost all cancer patients showed markedly depressed reactivity to PHA for at least 35 days before death.

Fig.3,4,5 and 6 show the effects of various types of chemotherapy to induce remission on the skin reactivity to PHA in patients with leukemia. Two patients,as shown in Figs.3 and 4,with negative skin reactivity to PHA and impaired blastogenesis of lymphocytes on admission developed normal responses to PHA both in vitro and in vivo during therapy to induce remission. Immediately after an intermittent intensive chemotherapy,such as DCP (daunomycin,cytosine arabinoside and prednisolone) and DCMP (daunomycin,cytosine arabinoside,6-mercaptoprine and prednisolone),the PHA skin reactivity was markedly suppressed,but it began to return to normal within a few days after each intensive therapy. As a result of a sequential combination chemotherapy,such as VAMP (vincristine,methotrexate, 6-mercaptoprine and prednisolone), the PHA skin reactivity gradually became positive (Fig.3). In these cases,the results of the in vitro lymphocyte stimulation test were paralleled with those of PHA skin test in cases during remission. However,the results of these tests in vivo and in vitro were not parallel in a case of acute lymphocytic leukemia who failed to show remission (Fig.5): in this case the skin reactivity to PHA remained negative during treatment to induce remission, but lymphocyte blastogenesis in vitro increased to the normal level during chemotherapy.

On the other hand,in a patient with chronic myelogenous leukemia treated with a single dose of busulfan, inhibition of skin reactivity to PHA was delayed,though slight,after the end of the therapy (Fig.6). This result showed the accumulative effect of busulfan on the depression of host immunocompetence. This case who recovered the skin reactivity after the therapy,showed a good clinical course. The effects of sequential combination chemotherapy on the skin reactivity to PHA in four patients with reticulum cell sarcoma are shown in Fig.7. The maintenance or recovery of host immunocompetence,as judged by the PHA skin test,suggests that a sequential chemotherapy,such as VEMP (vincristine,cyclophosphamide,6-mercaptoprine and prednisolone),is effective in these cases. These results indicated that changes in immunological reactivity of the host were related to the disease itself,and to the type and dose of anticancer agents used.

Correlation of in vivo and in vitro PHA responses

As shown in Fig.8, cancer patients showed impaired reactivities to PHA in vivo and in vitro. The cancer patients receiving anticancer therapy showed particularly low reactivities in both tests. There was a good correlation between the responses to PHA in vivo and in vitro ($P < 0.001$)

Correlation between the PHA skin test and the number of peripheral T-cells

The number of cells forming rosettes with SRBC (T-cells)[38] was measured in peripheral blood samples from 24 normal subjects and 58 cancer patients. As shown in Fig.9, there were fewer T-cells in the specimens from cancer patients than in those from normal subjects. There was a less significant correlation between the PHA skin test and the total number of T-cells ($P < 0.05$).

Correlation of PHA and PPD skin responses

The PHA and PPD skin tests were performed simultaneously in 177 cancer patients,of whom 118 were untreated and 59 under therapy. As shown in Table III,the responses to both PHA and PPD were less in cases under therapy than in untreated cases. In 125 (70.6%) of the 177 cases there was a significant correlation (P < 0.01) between the qualitative responses (positive or negative) in the two tests. But in the other cases the responses were qualitatively different and the reactivity to PPD was observed to depend upon the degree of prior exposure to this compound.

Correlation between PHA and DNCB skin responses

The correlation of the PHA and DNCB skin responses was examined in 35 cancer patients (Table IV). As described in the methods, a positive PHA skin response was arbitrarily defined as a skin response with erythema of 25 mm diameter or more both at the times of sensitizing and on challenge with DNCB. Positive responses to both PHA and DNCB were observed in 12 cases (34.3%) and negative responses to both in 17 cases (48.6%). A spontaneous flare-up phenomenon was observed in 5 of 12 cases who showed a positive response to DNCB. Thus a qualitative correlation between the responses in the two tests was observed in 29 (82.9%) of the 35 cancer patients (P < 0.01). Slight discrepancies between the results in these tests were seen in 6 cases (17.1%), but all the cases who showed a negative response to DNCB showed a positive response to PHA.

3. DISCUSSION

The skin test with PHA has been used mainly in infants and children by several investigators[5,6,25,30]. Studies in normal subjects have shown that erythema and induration develop 24 hr after intradermal injection of PHA. We also observed this reaction in healthy adults, and preliminary studies indicated that 5 μg of purified PHA injected intradermally produced maximum erythema after 24 hr with optimal discrimination. To assess the immunocompetence of the subjects, we measured the diameter of erythema after 24 hr because this was easier than measuring the induration[34]. Histological examination showed that the in vivo reaction to PHA is characterized by cellular infiltration located around the vessels and cutaneous adnexa in the dermis and the upper subcutaneous area of the skin, which is similar to that seen in the delayed hypersensitivity reaction to environmental microbial antigens[5,6,9]. The PHA skin response is distinct from histological findings of the Arthus reaction[6]. Thus, morphologically and chronologically the skin response to PHA appears to represent a delayed hypersensitivity response.

Since PHA causes nonimmune lymphocytes to attack and kill various target cells in vitro, the skin reaction observed may reflect nonspecific lympho-cyte-mediated cytotoxicity in vivo[23].

The first steps in testing the clinical application of the PHA skin test are to study whether it can be applied to various age groups in adults, and whether it can be used repeatedly. Carcinogenesis occurs more frequently in elderly individuals, so it seems important to know accurately the general immunocompetence of host in elderly subjects. Recently, Barnes et al.[4] suggested that anomalies in the immunological reactivities of cancer patients may be due to age differences in the control subjects selected, because the DNCB skin response and in vitro lymphocyte transformation are influenced by age in adults[4,18]. For diagnostic purposes, it seems of great value that skin reactivity to PHA was founded to be very similar in all age groups of adults tested. Burgio et al.[10] also found that the PHA skin response was not influenced by age in adults.

Studies on the antigenicity of mitogenic factors in PHA, Astaldi et al.[3] showed that PHA, when it was injected intravenously into patients with aplastic anemia, caused formation of circulating antibodies capable of neutralizing the blastogenic action of PHA. However, we observed no significant increase or decrease in skin reactivity 24 hr after injection of 5 μg of PHA in successive tests. This difference may be due to the different route of administration, and more particularly to the different dose used. Thus it seems that the skin test with PHA is repeatable when PHA is injected intradermally at a diagnostic dose.

It is known that the skin reactivity to PHA decreases in Hodgkin's disease and increases in chronic lymphocytic leukemia[1,6], but the reactivities of patients with nonlymphomatous cancer have not been studied extensively. Moreover, there are no reports on alterations in skin response to PHA in cases of neoplasmas during anticancer therapy. We found that the skin reactivity to PHA was impaired in many cancer patients, particularly those under anticancer therapy. It is clear from our previous studies that malignant neoplasmas have a definite systemic effect on nonspecific immuno-competence in patients with gastric cancer[34]. We compared the skin response to PHA of patients with the four stages of gastric cancer before therapy, and found that the skin reactivity was decreased in cases with the advanced stages, III and IV of gastric cancer. On the other hand, 75 % of 20 patients with gastric cancer who showed indications of requiring operation for curative resection, showed a positive response to an initial PHA skin test, whereas only 37.5 % of 24 cancer patients without such indications showed a positive reactivity to PHA[35]. Thus the degree of the initial skin response to PHA was correlated with the clinical stages, and the results seemed helpful in evaluating the therapy required. As described above, various degrees of immunosuppression are observed in neoplasmas, due to the disease itself and to the type and dosage of anticancer agents used. Accordingly, the cases with neoplasmas were used in this study to compare the PHA skin test with other in vitro and in vivo tests of cellular immunity. Our results showed significant correlations between responses in the PHA skin test and both in vitro PHA blastogenesis of lymphocytes and the delayed hypersensitivity responses to DNCB and PPD in cancer patients. Responses in the PHA skin test were also correlated, though less significantly, with the number of peripheral T-cells. Discrepancies between in vitro and in vivo responses to PHA were observed in some cancer patients. These discrepancies may have been due to insufficient T-cells, low production of lymphocyte mediators, change in vascular permeability, abnormal macrophage function and the presence of serum inhibitors.

The PHA skin test seems to be less sensitive than the response to DNCB because in our study all patients who showed qualitatively different responses in the two tests showed a positive response to PHA and negative response to DNCB.

Recently, much attention has been paid to enhancement of general immunity in patients with neoplasma. Using various nonspecific immunostimulants,such as BCG, Corynebacterium pavum and levamisole,various combinations of chemotherapy,surgical or radiation therapy with immunotherapy have been devised to obtain good responses[19,22,28,29,31,37]. It is now possible to convert immunoincompetence to immunocompetence in some patients with neoplasmas during therapy, if the disease can be controlled[2,8,16,21]. Therefore, the immunocompetence of the host must be evaluated repeatedly during therapy of cases of malignancies. The methods used most widely are measurements of in vitro lymphocyte transformation, peripheral T-cells and delayed hypersensitivity to DNCB[2,8,12,14,16,21,26]. Sequential evaluations of nonspecific immunological reactivity in patients with neoplasmas indicated that alteration in immunological reactivity during and after therapy is more important than the status before therapy[12,21]. Serial studies of in vivo and in vitro measures of cellular immunity correlate with the extent of tumors and the clinical course of cancer patients[13,15,33]. However, in practical terms these tests have several disadvantages, such as that they involve complicated techniques which are only possible in specialized laboratories or that the response to DNCB requires presensitization. Accordingly, we studied the availability of sequential skin tests on reactivity to PHA for use instead of the other methods described above for diagnosis of cellular immunocompetence,because the skin reactivity to PHA does not require prior exposure, and because the test is simple and rapid. Sequential tests showed that in almost all patients with advanced stages of cancer (Fig.2) there was a progressive dcrease in the patient's ability to react to PHA, and that the PHA skin response was markedly depressed within about 35 days of death. Skin reactivity to PHA appears to change in parallell with the progress of the disease. On the other hand, lympho-reticular malignancies directly involve the immune effector system responsible for cellular immunity, and therefore the initial immunological impairment could be reversed if successful control of disease was achieved[2,8,21]. Our observations also suggested that prognosis was good in patients who changed from immunoincompetence to immunocompetence, or maintained immunocompetence during remission induction. Continued suppression of the PHA skin reactivity as a result of therapy was associated with a poor prognosis. The present results showed that there was a good correlation between the skin reactivity to PHA and the response of lymphoreticular malignancies to chemotherapy.

It is also important to determine the effect of chemotherapy on immuno-logical defense mechanism because their suppression impairs the patient's resistance to infection and the antitumor response. Our results showed that several type of chemotherapy can inhibit PHA skin reactivity in man. Of the therapeutic regimens used, DCMP (daunomycin,cytosine arabinoside,6-mercapto-prine and prednisolone) was the most immunosuppressive. The rapid rise in PHA skin reactivity after intensive combination chemotherapy seen in some leukemic patients (Figs.3,4) resembles the rebound of in vitro lymphocyte reactivity to PHA after intensive combination chemotherapy in patients with neoplasmas described by Hersh and Oppenheim[20].

Sequential evaluation of immunocompetence showed that the clinical course correlated better with the skin reactivity to PHA than with results of the in vitro lymphocyte stimulation test. Our results indicated that 1) the skin reactivity to PHA could be used not only qualitatively, but also quantitatively and it was better than other tests for assessing general immunocompetence,including cellular immunocompetence, in patients with neoplasmas during anticancer therapy, and 2) serial PHA skin tests were useful in assessing the course of disease and the effect of therapy.

4. SUMMARY

Skin test with 5 µg of purified phytohemagglutinin (PHA) were performed in 69 normal subjects and 149 patients with nonlymphomatous malignancies. A positive reaction was observed in 67 (97.1%) of 69 normal subjects, 40 (49.4%) of 81 untreated patients with cancer,and 24 (35.3%) of 68 cancer patients under anticancer therapy. The PHA skin reactivities of 301 adults of different age groups without malignancies were very similar. A method for serial evaluation of the PHA skin response was established, and serial PHA skin tests in 17 cancer patients showed that the skin reactivity was correlated with the tumor progression and the prognosis, and the PHA skin responses was markedly depressed within 35 days of death in almost all these patients. On the other hand,in 8 patients with lymphoreticular malignancies during remission induction, change from hyporeactivity to normal reactivity to PHA during therapy was associated with remission, whereas continued depression of the skin reactivity to PHA was associated with a poor response to therapy.
Other in vitro and in vivo tests for assessing cellular immunity were performed simultaneously for comparison with the PHA skin test. Results of the PHA skin test correlated well with those on delayed hypersensitivity to DNCB ($P < 0.01$) in 29 (82.9%) of 35 cancer patients and with results on in vitro lymphocyte transformation ($P < 0.001$) in 87 subjects. Results of the PHA skin test were also significantly correlated with the cutaneous response to PPD ($P < 0.01$) in 177 cases of cancer, and less significantly with the number of peripheral T-cells in 82 subjects.
These results indicate that the skin reactivity to PHA reflects the host's cellular immunocompetence, and that sequential evaluation of PHA skin reactivity can be made in cancer patients of various ages, and is useful in assessing the immunological status and prognosis of the patients and their responses to therapy.

5. ACKNOWLEDGMENT

This work was supported by a Grant-in-Aid for Scientific Research from the Japan Ministry of Education, Science and Culture.

TABLE I. PHA Skin Tests in Various Groups

Group	No. of subjects	No. of positive subjects	positive rate (%)	Positive Diameter of response (mm) ± standard deviation			
				24 hr Erythema	24 hr Induration	48 hr Erythema	48 hr Induration
Normal subjects	69	67	97.1	37.0± 6.4	12.4±3.9	26.9±14.8	7.0±3.5
Patients with cancer	149	64	43.0	23.1±10.4	9.1±4.6	17.8±11.0	6.7±3.8
untreated[a]	81	40	49.4	24.8±10.5	9.2±4.4	19.8±13.0	6.7±4.0
treated[b]	68	24	35.3	21.0±10.0	9.0±4.9	16.0±10.9	6.9±3.5

All subjects were tested by intradermal injection of 5 μg of PHA in 0.1 ml.
a) Untreated: Skin tests were performed before anticancer therapy in 35 cases of gastric cancer, 10 of lung cancer, 14 of breast cancer, 6 of cancer of the colon, 6 of hepatoma, 2 of thyroid cancer, and 8 others.

b) Treated: Skin tests were performed during or after anticancer therapy in 37 cases of lung cancer, 8 of gastric cancer, 7 of cancer of the uterus, 3 of melanoma, 2 of esophageal cancer, 2 of cancer of the tongue, 2 of cancer of the colon, and 7 others.

TABLE II. Skin Reactivity to PHA in Repeated Tests

Response after 24 hr[a]	Weeks after initial skin test[b]			
	0	4	9	12
Erythema	34.7±5.5	34.1±5.4	33.6±4.2	31.5±4.1
Induration	10.0±1.9	10.5±2.0	9.2±1.2	9.5±2.3

a) Diameter of response (mm) ± standard deviation.
b) Skin tests with 5 μg of PHA were repeated 4 times on 21 hospitalized patients without malignancies who showed an initial positive skin response to PHA.

TABLE III. Correlation of PHA and PPD Skin Responses in Cancer Patients

Group	No. tested	PPD skin test[a]		PHA skin test[b] Positive	Negative
Untreated[c]	118	Positive	75 (63.6%)	59	16
		Negative	43 (36.4%)	19	24
				78 (66.1%)	40 (33.9%)
Treated[d]	59	Positive	14 (23.7%)	12	2
		Negative	45 (76.3%)	15	30
				27 (45.8%)	32 (54.2%)

a) Positive PPD skin response: Erythema of 10 mm diameter or more 48 hr after intradermal injection of 0.05 μg of PPD.
b) Positive PHA skin response: Erythema of 25 mm diameter or more 24 hr after intradermal injection of 5 μg of PHA.
c),d) Untreated and under anticancer therapy,respectively.

TABLE IV. Correlation Between PHA Skin Test and Delayed Cutaneous Hypersensitivity to DNCB

Skin response to DNCB	PHA skin test	
	Positive	Negative
Positive	12 (34.3%)	0 (0.0%)
Negative	6 (17.1%)	17 (48.6%)

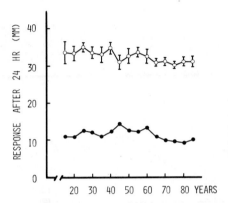

FIG. 1. Skin reactivity to PHA in 301 subjects of various age groups without malignancies or debility. Subjects were treated with 5 µg of PHA. o—o Erythema and ●—● induration are shown as the mean diameters of the skin responses in the various age groups. Bars show standard errors.

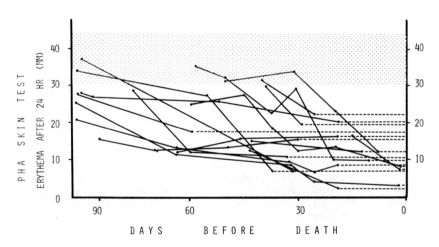

FIG. 2. Serial skin tests with PHA for 3 months before death were performed in 17 cases of nonlymphomatous malignancies during anticancer therapy.

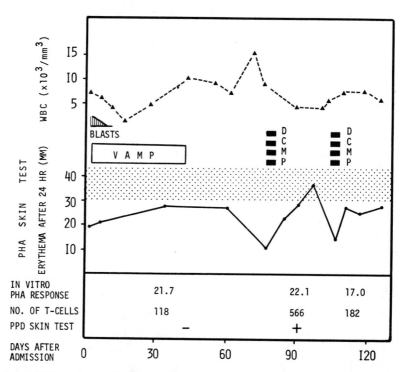

·FIG. 3. Effect of combination chemotherapy on the PHA skin reactivity of a patient with acute leukemia. The patient received the following drugs (in mg/kg body weight): VAMP (vincristine 0.04 mg/week, and methotrexate 0.9 mg daily for 6 weeks), and DCMP (daunomycin 0.4-0.5 mg, cytosine arabinoside 1.4 mg, 6-mercaptoprine 1.8 mg and prednisolone 0.7 mg daily for 4 days) and responded well to the therapy.

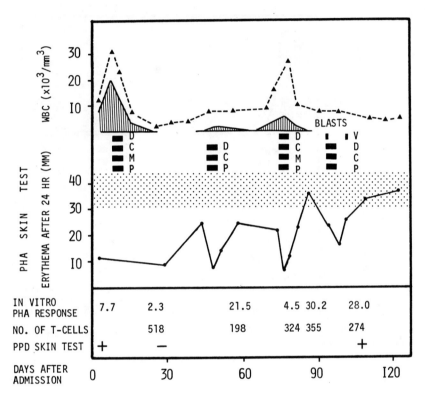

FIG. 4. Effect of intermittent intensive chemotherapy on the PHA skin reactivity of a patient with acute myelogenous leukemia. This patient received the following drugs (in mg/kg body weight per day): DCMP (daunomycin 0.7 mg, cytosine arabinoside (CA) 2.1 mg, 6-mercaptoprine 2.5 mg and prednisolone 1.5 mg daily for 4 days), DCP (daunomycin 0.6 mg, CA 2.2 mg and prednisolone 1.5 mg daily for 4 days), and VDCP (vincristine 0.03 mg twice weekly, and daunomycin 0.7 mg, CA 2.0 mg and prednisolone 1.0 mg daily for 4 days), and showed remission.

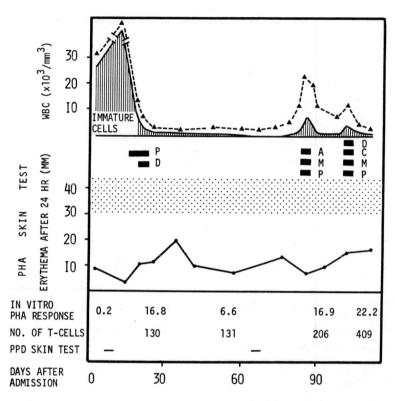

FIG. 5. Effect of intermittent intensive chemotherapy on the PHA skin reactivity of a patient with acute lymphocytic leukemia. The patient received the following drugs (in mg/kg body weight): PD (prednisolone 1.5 mg daily for 11 days and daunomycin 0.9 mg daily for 4 days) and AMP (adriamycin 0.3 mg, 6-mercaptoprine 2.0 mg and prednisolone 1.1 mg daily for 4 aays) and DCMP (daunomycin 0.9 mg, cytosine arabinoside 2.7 mg, 6-mercaptoprine 2.9 mg and prednisolone 1.8 mg daily for 4 days), but did not show remission.

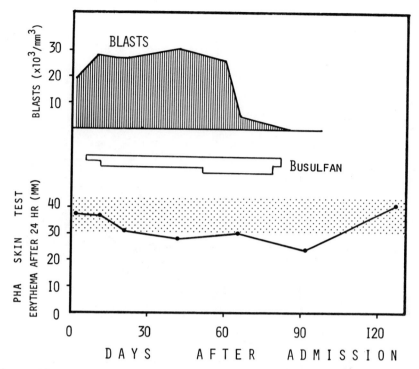

FIG. 6. Effect of chemotherapy on the PHA skin reactivity of a patient
with chronic myelogenous leukemia. The patient received the drug (in mg/kg
body weight per day): Busulfan (0.05 mg for 6 days, 0.07 mg for 28 days,
0.1 mg for 26 days and 0.05 mg for 3 days consecutively by the oral route),
and responded well to the therapy.

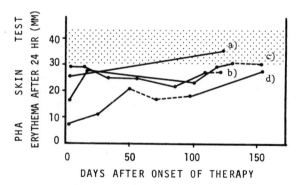

FIG. 7. Follow-ups on patients with reticulum cell sarcoma during remission induction. The staging classification revealed: a); stage II_A,b);
and c); stage III_A,d); stage III_B. All patients received VEMP therapy
●——● : vincristine 0.02 mg per week, cyclophosphamide 0.8-1.4 mg/day,
6-mercaptoprine 0.9-1.4 mg/day, and prednisolone 0.5-0.7 mg/day, and all
cases responded completely to therapy except one case of d) who responded
only partially.

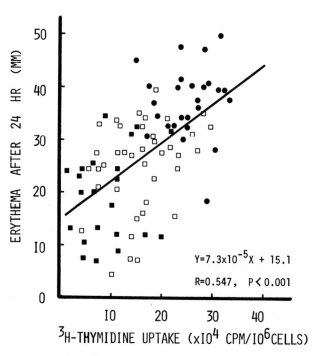

FIG. 8. Correlation of In vivo and in vitro PHA responses. The PHA skin test and in vitro lymphocyte blastogenic response to PHA were measured simultaneously in (●)26 normal subjects, (□)39 cancer patients before anticancer therapy, and (■)22 cancer patients under anticancer therapy.

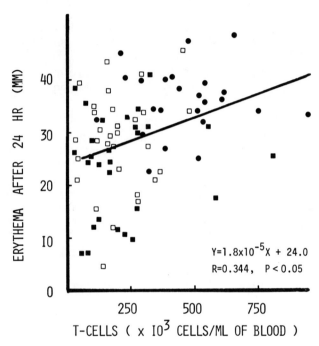

FIG. 9. Correlation between skin reactivity to PHA and number of peripheral T-cells were measured in (●)24 normal subjects, (□)30 cancer patients before anticancer therapy, and (■)28 cancer patients under anticancer therapy.

REFERENCES

1. Airo,R.,Mihailescu,E., Astaldi,G., and Meardi,G. Skin Reactions To Phytohemagglutinin. Lancet., 1:899-900, 1967.

2. Aisenberg,A.C., Studies On Delayed Hypersensitivity In Hodgkin's Disease. J.Clin.Invest., 41:1964-1970, 1962.

3. Astaldi,G., Airo,R., Lisino,T., Paradisi,E.R., and Novelli,E. Antibodies To Phytohemagglutinin. Lancet, 2:502-503, 1966.

4. Barnes,E.W., Farmer,A., Penhale,W.J., Irvine,W.J., Roscoe,P., and Horne, N.W. Phytohemagglutinin-Induced Lymphocyte Transformation In Newly Presenting Patients With Primary Carcinoma Of The Lung. Cancer, 36:187-193, 1975.

5. Blaese,R.M., Weiden,P., Oppenheim,J.J., and Waldman,T.A. Phyto-hemagglutinin As A Skin Test For The Evaluation Of Cellular Immune Competence In Man. J.Lab.Clin.Med. 81:538-548, 1973.

6. Bonforte,R.J., Topilsky,M., Siltzbach,L.E., and Glade,P.R. Phyto-hemagglutinin Skin Test: A Possible In Vivo Measure of Cell-Mediated Immunity. J. Pediatr., 81:775-780, 1972.

7. Bøyum,R. Separation Of White Blood Cells. Nature, 21:793-794, 1964.

8. Brown,R.S., Haynes,H.A., Foley,H.T., Goodwin,H.A., Bernard,C.W., and Carbone,P.P. Hodgkin's Disease - Immunologic, Clinical and Histologic Features Of Fifty Untreated Patients. Ann. Intern. Med, 67:291-302, 1967.

9. Burgio,G.R., Astaldi,G., Genova,R., and Curtoni,E. Cytology Of Skin Reactions To Different Inoculated Substances (Tuberculin, Streptokinase, Lipopolysaccharide Of S.Typhi, Phytohemagglutinin, And Pokeweed Mitogen) Path. Europ., 4:138-151, 1969.

10. Burgio,G.R., Rizzoni,G., and Marni,E. Age And Skin Reactivity. Lancet, 2:411, 1968.

11. Carbone,P.P., Kapalan,H.S., Musshof,K., Smithers,D.W., and Tubiana,M. Report Of The Committe On Hodgkin's Disease Staging Classification. Cancer Res., 31:1860-1861, 1971.

12. Cheema,A.R., and Hersh,E.M. Patient Survival After Chemotherapy And Its Relationship To In Vitro Lymphocyte Blastogenesis. Cancer, 28:851-855, 1971.

13. Chretien,P.B., Crowder,W.L., Gertner,H.R., Sample,W.F., and Catalona, W.J. Correlation Of Preoperative Lymphocyte Reactivity With The Clinical Course of Cancer Patients. Surg. Gynecol. Obstet., 136:380-384, 1973.

14. Dellon,A.L., Potvin,C., and Chretien,P.B. Thymus-Dependent Lymphocyte Levels In Bronchogenic Carcinoma: Correlation With Histology, Clinical Stage And Clinical Course After Surgical Treatment. Cancer, 35:687-694, 1975.

15. Eilber,F.R., and Morton,D.L. Impaired Immunologic Reactivity And Recurrence Following Cancer Surgery. Cancer, 25:362-367, 1970.

16. Eilber,F.R., Nizze,J.A., and Morton,D.L. Sequential Evaluation Of General Immune Competence In Cancer Patients: Correlation With Clinical Course. Cancer, 35:660-665, 1975.

17. Greaves,M.F., Janossy,G., and Doenhoff,M. Activation Of Human T And B Lymphocytes By Polyclonal Mitogens. Nature, 248:698-701, 1974.

18. Gross,L. Immunological Defect In Aged Population And Its Relationship To Cancer. Cancer, 18:201-204, 1965.

19. Gutterman,J.U., McBride,C., Freireich,E.J., Mavligit,G., Frei III,E., and Hersh,E.M. Active Immunotherapy With BCG For Recurrent Malignant Melanoma. Lancet, 1:1208-1212, 1973.

20. Hersh,E.M., and Oppenheim,J.J. Inhibition Of In Vitro Lymphocyte Transformation During Chemotherapy In Man. Cancer Res., 27:98-105, 1967.

21. Hersh,E.M., Whitecar,J.P., McCredie,K.B., Bodey,G.P., and Freireich,E.J. Chemotherapy,Immunocompetence,Immunosuppression And Prognosis In Acute Leukemia. New Engl. J. Med., 285:1211-1216, 1971.

22. Holmes,E.C., Eilber,F.R., and Morton,D.L. Immunotherapy Of Malignancy In Humans: Current Status. JAMA., 232:1052-1055, 1975.

23. Holm,G., and Perlmann,R. Cytotoxic Potential Of Stimulated Human Lymphocytes. J. Exp. Med., 125:721-726, 1967.

24. Krant,M.J., Manskopf,G., Brandrup,C.S., and Madoff,M.A. Immunologic Alterations In Bronchogenic Cancer. Cancer, 21:623-631, 1968.

25. Lawlor,G.J., Stiehm,E.R., Kaplan,M.S., Sengar,E.P.S., and Terasaki,P.I. Phytohemagglutinin (PHA) Skin Test In The Diagnosis Of Cellular Immunodeficiency. J. Allergy Clin. Immunol., 52:31-37, 1973.

26. Lee,Y.N., Sparks,F.C., Eilber,F.R., and Morton,D.L. Delayed Cutaneous Hypersensitivity And Peripheral Lymphocyte Counts In Patients With Advanced Cancer. Cancer, 35:748-755, 1975.

27. Levitt,M., Marsh,J.C., DeConti,R.C., Mitchell,M.S., Skeel,R.T., Farber,L.R., and Bertino,J.R. Combination Sequential Chemotherapy In Advanced Reticulum Cell Sarcoma. Cancer, 29:630-636, 1972.

28. Mathe,G., Amiel,J.L., Schwarzenberg,L., Schneider,M., Gattan,A., Schlumberger,J.R., Hayat,M., and De Vassal,F. Active Immunotherapy For Acute Lymphoblastic Leukemia. Lancet, 1:697-699, 1969.

29. Morton,D.L., Eilber,F.R., Malmgren,R.A., and Wood,W.C. Immunological Factors Which Influence Response To Immunotherapy In Malignant Melanoma. Surgery, 68:158-164, 1970.

30. Oppenheim,J.J., Blaese,R.M., and Waldmann,T.A. Defective Lymphocyte Transformation And Delayed Hypersensitivity In Wiskott-Aldrich Syndrome. J. Immunol., 104:835-844, 1970.

31. Powles,R.L., Crowther,D., Bateman,C.J.T., Beard,M.E.J., McElwain,T.J., Russell,J.,Lister,T.A., Whitehouse,J.M.A., Wrigley,P.F.M., Pike,M., Alexander,P., and Hamilton Fairley,G. Immunotherapy For Acute Myelogenous Leukemia. Brit. J. Cancer, 28:365-376, 1973.

32. Schrek,R., and Stefani,S.S. Lymphocytic And Intradermal Reactions To Phytohemagglutinin. Fed. Proc., 22:428, 1963.

33. Solowey,A.C., and Rapaport,J.T. Immunologic Responses In Cancer Patients. Surg. Gynecol. Obstet., 121:756-760, 1965.

34. Sone,S., Taoka,S., Yata,K., Tsubura,E., Nakano,Y., Taguchi,T., Saijo, N., and Niitani,H. Phytohemagglutinin Skin Test: Diagnostic Value For Showing Immunodeficiency In Patients With Cancer. Gann, 66:641-648, 1975.

35. Sone,S., Taoka,S., Yata,K., Tsubura,E., Nakano,Y., Taguchi,T., Saijo, N., and Niitani,H. Phytohemagglutinin Skin Test: Sequential Evaluation Of Cellular Immunocompetence In Neoplastic Disease. 13th Annual Meeting of the Japan Society for Cancer Therapy. Proceeding of the Japan Society for Cancer Therapy, 185, 1975. (in Japanese)

36. Southam,C.M. The Immunologic Status Of Patients With Nonlymphomatous Cancer. Cancer Res., 28:1433-1440, 1968.

37. Tripodi,D., Parks,L.C., and Brugmans,J. Drug-Induced Restoration Of Cutaneous Delayed Hypersensitivity In Anergic Patients With Cancer. New Engl. J. Med., 289:354-357, 1973.

38. Wybran,J., and Fudenberg,H.H. Thymus-Derived Rosette-Forming Cells In Various Human Disease States: Cancer, Lymphoma, Bacterial And Viral Infection, and Other Diseases. J. Clin. Invest., 52:1026-1032, 1973.

FULMINATING BREAST CANCER:
CLINICAL FEATURES

N. Mourali, M.D.

F. Tabbane, M.D.

M. Djazizi, M.D.

M. Cammoun, M.D.

R. Ben Attia, M.D.

S. Belhassen, M.D.

Institut Salah Azaiz
Tunis, Tunisia

INTRODUCTION

During the course of their evolution a number of breast cancers acquire clinical and radiological traits characterized by a great aggressiveness which indicates a poor prognosis. The different degrees of inflammation are a major factor in the clinical picture and their presence justifies the diagnosis of "poussee evolutive" (PEV) as described by the Institut Gustave Roussy (Villejuif) (5). The search for traits peculiar to the clinical as well as radiological inflammation has been carried out by our Institute since its creation in 1969. The PEV parameter used in association with TNM classification takes into

Editor's Note: References cited in this article are available directly from the author consideration the existence or the non-existence of these signs. We have tried to better define the clinical, radiological and the biological characteristics of this particular form. The advent of PEV is, in fact, a serious event, in the natural history of a breast cancer and its diagnosis requires an adaptation in treatment.

We shall strive, during this presentation, to report the clinical, radiological and biological feature that we have been able to define up to the present date.

PROCEDURES AND MATERIALS

Between January 1969 and December 1973, 504 cases were examined before any treatment at the Institut Salah Azaiz (ISA) in Tunis. The diagnosis of PEV was made after complete and systematic examination where the procedures used were exactly the same for each patient. These consisted of a local, regional and general clinical examination but also included a systematic search for a color modification of the breast skin and cutaneous infiltration by edema. The X-ray examination consisted of mammography and examination of the chest and pelvis. X-ray for other areas were carried out if metastases were suspected.

All this information having been collected, the breast tumor committee classified the patients according to the TNM classification and the PEV parameter was graded from 0 to 3 according to the criteria as follows:

PEV 0 - Total absence of inflammatory signs

PEV 1 - The recent

increase in volume without clinical inflammatory signs. Any tumor having doubled in size in less than six months is included in this group.

PEV 2 - The acute or subacute form of the tumor accompanied by pseudo-inflammatory signs located in the tumor or its vicinity.

PEV 3 - An acute, massive cancer, invading the whole breast. When the diagnosis of PEV was established with young women, non-menopausal or 2 years post-menopausal, we performed an exploratory laparotomy searching for intra-abdominal metastases while carrying out ovariectomy.

The study of host response was initiated in March 1973 and included 96 patients in this series. 24 other women free of cancer, in the same age group, were also tested. This study consisted only of the DNCB test, a measurement of the individual's capacity to develop a delayed hypersensitivity skin reaction. Sensitization was performed with the application of 1/10 ml DNCB (1 mg/1 ml) to forearm skin. Two weeks after sensitization, two dilutions of DNCB (1/20, 1/40) were applied by ring to the opposite forearm. Results of this second application were recorded after 48 hours. No reaction was considered negative, 1+ was recorded if inflammation and warmth were present; 2+ was induration and minor vesiculation; and 3+ was edema with large vesicules and redness.

RESULTS

Clinical Findings

The distribution of the 504 cases in relation to the various levels of PEV is given in Table I. 45% of the cases consisted of PEV 0, the less aggressive tumor, and the PEV group comprised 55%. The high frequency of PEV 3 is striking and represents 42% of the total and 76% of the aggressive tumors. This incidence is the highest that we know of, especially if we compare this series with the data from Villejuif where the same classification is used; less than 20% of their breast cancers are PEV.

For this reason, the TNM classification of the 279 cases expressed in percent, shows the large extent of the tumor (Table II). Table II shows that the tumor is often large - T 3 and T 4 in 90% of the cases; adenopathy is massive - N2 and N3 in 70% of the cases; metastases are found clinically in 37% of the cases and are often large. They are located in the bones, the skin, the pleura, the liver, the axillary and subclavicular cross lateral nodes, etc.

The results of the intra-abdominal exploration carried out systematically during castration have been more striking. This exploration was carried out on 80 women without clinical metastasis; in 28 or 37% of them occult metastases were discovered.

The correlation between the PEV degrees and the existence of these occult intra-abdominal metastases was established and is shown in Table III.

Host Response to DNCB Skin Test

Analysis of the skin tests is shown in Table IV.

The first results differ significantly according to the aggressiveness of the cancer ($0.02 < p < 0.05$). No difference in DNCB reaction was found between the women with slowly growing breast cancer and non-cancerous controls. The difference in skin test results between the two groups of cancer patients does not appear to depend on the existence or absence of metastasis in the patients who were tested ($0.3 < p < 0.05$).

Prognosis

The 175 PEV patients free of clinical metastases were treated with

cobalt 60-therapy with a dose of 4500 rads to the breast and lymph nodes (axillary, supra-clavicular and internal mammary). Irradiation up to 7500 to 9000 rads was carried out on the tumoral and remaining lymph nodes.

Mastectomy was suggested to patients 4 to 6 months after irradiation when the reaction to radiotherapy regressed and subsequent metastases did not appear. The 3 year survival for PEV cases is very low as shown in Table V, 29 patients accepted mastectomy and of this group, 21 had residual tumor. The 3 year survival in PEV 1 (25%) was m less than the 60% five year survival in PEV 0 cases.

DISCUSSION

The purpose of this report is to point out the existence of a particularly aggressive form of breast cancer which in our experience may appear either early or late in the evolution of the tumor. The aggressiveness and the large size are not solely due to delayed diagnosis since we have seen PEV tumors occurring in patients with lesions as small as 2 cm. The inflammation with edema is not dependent on axillary blockage and PEV cases are often seen without lymph node involvement.

As we reported previously (6) this aggressive form is seen in all age groups above 15 years, with the highest relative frequency at 40 and 60 years. It should be noted, however, that all breast cancer observed in young women under the age of 25 showed signs of PEV. PEV is frequently seen in young women who have the constant hormonal stimulation of pregnancy, being found in 70% of our series of 47 pregnant breast cancer patients (6). Because of the poor prognosis and necessary modification of treatment it is very important to recognize the PEV form of breast cancer. The real problem in diagnosis is recognizing PEV 1, as PEV 2 and PEV 3 present no major difficulties.

Recognition of PEV 1 is difficult because it is based upon one subjective factor; namely, the interview. It is obviously underestimated due to the absence of objective criteria.

We are presently trying to define objective criteria in addition to clinical evaluation and mammography.

Thermography may be very useful. Recently Gros, Gautherie et al have measured intra-tumoral temperature and have shown that the higher the level of thermogenesis, the shorter the duration of survival (2). Lloys has confirmed this fact on another series of patients (3). Using the results of dynamic telethermography which makes it possible to obtain quantitative and qualitative data, we are presently gathering information based on cutaneous vascularization, the local thermic elevation gradient, and the extent of the hot spot. Using these criteria Amalric and Al. (Marseille) (1), have defined a PEV 1 TH category characterized by a hyperthermic surface of less than half the breast surface (S1) with a thermic elevation gradient of at least 5°.

A clinical PEV 1 cancer should appear as a hyperthermic PEV. We are currently investigating this possibility, but we cannot as yet draw conclusions from our limited experience.

PEV 2 and PEV 3 are recognized more easily. In PEV 2 the tumor varies in size, usually being quite large. The covering skin is often discreetly inflammatory which requires a comparative study of the two breasts. The skin has a thickened appearance like peau d'orange; the edema covers the tumor area and sometimes extends beyond it.

PEV 3 is the ultimate form. The tumor is always large and often covers the whole breast. The inflammatory aspects are varied. The edema is constant and spreads towards the axilla. The identification of PEV 3 is easy from both the clinical and radiologic point of view.

551

In PEV 2, mammography shows a stellar tumoral or
nodular picture without a clear border occasionally with a
nucleus of micro- calcifications. There is a dense
cutaneous thickening around the tumor which is only seen in
the area of the lesion.

In PEV 3 mammographic interpretation is also very easy.
The homogeneous tumoral density sometimes involves the whole
breast and acquires either a marbled or a spotted aspect.
The tumor gives the impression of having exploded in the
gland taking the shape of multiple tumoral opacities. Skin
thickening is characteristic, covering the whole breast from
4 mm to more than 3 cm. The thickening may be evenly
distributed or it may be predominant in the sloping part of
the breast. The subcutaneous transparency disappears due to
the subcutaneous edema. An umbilication of the nipple with
the thickened areolar plane is often visualized with a
subareolar funnel connecting the tumor to the nipple.

As in PEV 1, thermography also may be useful in PEV 2
and 3. The immunological study is consistent with the
findings of other workers who note a correlation between
DNCB reactivity and prognosis. Larger numbers are needed
before final conclusions can be made, however. We are now
using additional antigens, including tumor-related antigens,
and we are evaluating the hormonal aspects as well.

The 3 year survival indicates the poor prognosis of
these aggressive tumors. Since current methods clearly do
not achieve long term control, treatment now should be
readjusted in the light of recent developments in
chemotherapy.

TABLE I

Distribution of Patients According to the PEV Classification

PEV	Number of Cases	% Total		
0	225	44.6		
1	20	4	279	7.2% PEV
2	46	9.1	55.4%	16.5% PEV
3	213	42.3		76.3% PEV
Total	504	100		

TABLE II

TNM Classification of PEV
(figures express%)

T	N0 MO	N0 M+	N1 MO	N1 M+	N2 MO	N2 M+	N3 MO	N3 M+	Total MO	Total M+
T1	-	-	0.7	-	0.3	-	-	-	1	-
T2	1	-	3.4	0.3	1.7	1	-	2	6.1	3.3
T3	3.1	-	13.9	1.7	12.5	4.1	6.4	4.7	35.9	10.5
T4	0.3	-	3.4	0.3	7.8	5.1	6.1	17.3	17.6	22.7
TX	-	-	1.7	-	0.3	-	-	0.6	2	0.6
Total	4.4	-	23	2.3	22.7	10.1	12.5	24.7	62.7	37.3

TABLE III

Correlation between Degrees of PEV
and Occult Metastases

PEV	Percentage of Cases	Percentage with Metastases
3	82	93
2	13	7
1	5	0
Total	100	100

TABLE IV

Results of DNCB Tests

Patient Group	Patients Free of Cancer		PEV 0		PEV	
DNCB	Number	%	Number	%	Number	%
-	2	8	1	4	19	27
+	1	4	6	24	21	30
++	10	42	12	48	15	21
+++	11	46	6	24	16	23
Total	24	100	25	100	71	100

TABLE V

Patients' Survival According to PEV

Yrs.	PEV 1			PEV 2			PEV 3		
	No.	Living	Survival (%)	No.	Living	Survival (%)	No.	Living	Survival (%)
1	11	9	82	28	22	79	136	83	61
2	8	5	63	24	8	33	88	25	28
3	4	1	25	22	5	23	51	9	18

IMMUNOBIOLOGY OF OPERABLE BREAST CANCER
AN ASSESSMENT OF BIOLOGIC RISK BY IMMUNOPARAMETERS

Harold J. Wanebo, M.D., Paul P. Rosen, M.D., Howard Thaler, Ph.D.
Jerome Urban, M.D. and Herbert Oettgen, M.D.

Memorial Sloan-Kettering Cancer Center
New York, N. Y.

INTRODUCTION

The prognostic determinants in patients with operable breast cancer can be described in terms of tumor factors. Tumor factors are directly related to the biologic aggressiveness of the cancer and can be described in terms of histology and pathologic extent of disease (Table I). Host factors are those that influence tumor resistance and have been demonstrated morphologically as round cell infiltration of the primary tumor, sinus histiocytosis in lymph nodes, and other patterns of lymph node reactivity (Table II). Attempts to measure specific host tumor reactions have included the skin window technique [3], skin testing with breast cancer extracts [1, 33], and measurements of the responses to breast cancer antigens by lymphocytes [4, 14, 15] or humoral antibody [17, 9, 29]. General immune reactivity has been measured by skin testing with common antigens [16, 24, 25, 32] or by measuring the dermal response to de novo sensitization to chemicals such as DNCB [10, 28]. In vitro methods have included measurement of peripheral lymphocyte counts [22, 26] and lymphocyte subpopulations [35] or lymphocyte stimulation studies [12, 36, 42] and have shown great variability in results. Marked depression of PHA response has been reported by some workers [42] whereas minimal or no depression has been reported by others [36].

In this study we have compared detailed measurements of general immune reactivity in malignant and benign breast disease and have correlated these findings with the pathologic stage of disease in the

555

cancer patients. We have attempted to determine which measures of general immune reactivity correlate best with the 'risk of recurrence' as determined by the pathologic extent of disease.

PATHOLOGIC STAGE OF DISEASE - CONCEPT OF 'RISK'
(RETROSPECTIVE FINDINGS)

Pathologic factors that show a major correlation with recurrence and survival rates include histology and size of primary, and number and extent of nodal metastases. In patients with infiltrating cancer but without nodal metastases the 18 month recurrence rate is 6% [13]. In those with one to three nodal metastases 16 to 19% have recurrence and in those with < 4 nodal metastases 45% have recurrence at 18 months [13, 31]. The extent of nodal metastases is important [18]. The prognosis is better in patients with micrometastases (<2 mm) than in those with macrometastases (<2 mm). The eight-year survival was 62% in patients with macrometastases at Level I compared to 94% in those with micrometastases at that level. Patients with macrometastases at Level I had survival (62%) to those with micrometastases at Level III (59%). The survival in patients with macrometastases at Level III was only 29%. Utilizing data from these clinicopathologic studies we have constructed a table of 'risk of recurrence' in which there are three categories based on the pathologic extent of disease (Table I). Because of the strong correlation of the pathologic stage with known recurrence and survival rates, this table provides a good assessment of future prognosis, and as such can serve as a standard for analyzing the multiple variables of immune reactivity that we have measured.

MATERIALS AND METHODS

Skin Tests

Patients were tested for pre-existing delayed hypersensitivity to Dermatophyton-0, mumps skin test antigen, intermediate strength tuberculin and streptokinase/streptodornase as previously reported [21,28]. The antigens were injected intradermally in volumes of 0.1 ml. The tests were read at 48 hours and considered positive when the diameter of induration was 5 mm or more.

Sensitization and challenge with 2,4-dinitrochlorobenzene (DNCB) was carried out according to the method of Eilber and Morton [10]. DNCB 2000 mg dissolved in 0.1 ml of acetone was applied to the inner aspect of the upper arm, within the confines of a plastic ring measuring 2 cm in diameter, and allowed to evaporate. Prior hypersensitivity to DNCB was excluded by control testing with 100μg and 25μg DNCB in 0.1 ml acetone applied simultaneously to the ipsilateral forearm and read at 48 hours. If there were no erythema and induration at the 100 and 25μg sites after two weeks, the patients were re-challenged on the ipsilateral extremity with 100, 50 and 25μg of DNCB. The reaction was considered positive if there was induration of 5 mm or greater at 48 hours at the challenge sites.

In Vitro Tests
Stimulation of Lymphocytes by Mitogens and Antigens

Lymphocyte transformation in vitro was performed using a micro method. Lymphocytes were obtained from heparinized blood on Ficoll-Hypaque ("Lymphoprep") density gradients, and re-suspended in RPMI 1640 with Hepes buffer, glutamine (0.25 mg/cc), penicillin 10 units/cc, streptomycin 10 units/cc, heparin 10 i.u./cc, and 15% pooled normal human serum. Lympho-cyte culture was performed in flat bottom microtiter plates (Falcon #3040) by adding 100,000 lymphocytes in 200λ of media. Transformation of lymphocytes was measured in terms of incorporation of C^{14} thymidine which was added after 72 hours (for mitogens) or 120 hours (for antigens) and then incubated 24 hours. Cultures were performed in triplicate. Dilutions of mitogens or antigens which had been prepared in advance and stored at $-20^{0}C$ were freshly thawed and were added to the cultures in 25 λ volumes. The concentrations of phytohemagglutinin (PHA-P) used were 500, 250, 50, 10 and 5 mcg/ml, conconavalin A (Con A Difco) at 125, 42, 15 and 5 mcg/ml, pokeweed mitogen (PWM Gibco) at 2000, 400 and 80 mcg/ml. The following antigen preparations were used in tenfold dilutions (four dilutions each): candida albicans (Hollister Stier Laboratories) 1:10 dilution, streptokinase/streptodornase (Lederle) 25,000 units in 2 ml, staph aureus 1×10^{9} organisms/ml, heat inactivated, E. coli 1×10^{9} organisms/ml, heat inactivated, mixed bacterial vaccine (MBV) 1:10 dilu-tion, mumps antigen (Lilly mumps skin test antigen) 1:10 dilution.

T Lymphocyte Rosettes (E-R)

T lymphocyte rosettes in the peripheral blood were determined by a modification of the method of Jondal [20]. Equal volumes (0.1 ml) of a lymphocyte suspension $(3 \times 10^9$ cells/ml) and a suspension of washed sheep red cells (SRBC 0.5%) were mixed with 0.1 ml of human AB serum previously absorbed with RBC of the same sheep. The mixture was rotated at 20 rpm in a waterbath at 37^0C for five minutes, then centrifuged at 50μg for 5 minutes, and finally left at 4^0C for 18 hours. A drop of trypan blue was added, the cells were resuspended with a Pasteur pipette, and the rosettes were counted in a hemocytometer. Two hundred viable cells were counted and big (three or more RBC) and small (one or two SRBC) rosettes were recorded. Each test was done in triplicate.

B Lymphocyte Rosettes (EAC-R)

B lymphocytes were determined as C^3 receptor lymphocytes, using a modification of the technique described by Bianco [2]. Human A-1 erythrocytes (E) were sensitized with inactivated rabbit anti-A-1 serum at 37^0C for 30 minutes with frequent shaking. Sensitized cells (EA) were washed with culture medium in the cold and a 5% EA suspension was diluted in 1:10 in C^5-deficient AKR mouse serum, and the mixture (EAC) was incubated for 30 minutes at 37^0C and then washed in the cold. Equal volumes (0.1 ml) of lymphocytes $(3 \times 10^6$ ml) and EAC (0.5%) were mixed and rotated at 20 rpm in a waterbath at 37^0C for 30 minutes. The cells were resuspended, shaken on a vortex shaker and placed in an ice bath, a drop of trypan blue was added, and rosettes were counted within 30 minutes. Ingestion of latex particles was used as a marker for excluding phagocytic monocytes [7]. Two hundred living cells were counted, and large and small rosettes were recorded separately.

Serum Immunoglobulins

The concentration of IgG, IgM and IgA was determined by radial immune diffusion using anti-immunoglobulin plates purchased from the Behring Company (Tri-Partigen plates). Patient sera and prediluted standards are placed in the wells and the diameter of the antigen-antibody precipitate is measured at 24 hours.

B Lymphocytes Bearing Surface Immunoglobulins [27]

Approximately 10^5 lymphocytes in 0.025 ml of phosphate-buffered saline with 3% bovine serum albumin (BSA-PBS) were mixed with 0.025 ml of fluoroscein-conjugated polyvalent Ig-antiserum (purchased from Behring Diagnostics) in the presence of 0.02% sodium azide and kept in an ice bath for 30 minutes. The cells were washed in the cold four times with BSA-PBS containing 0.02% sodium azide. A drop of the cell suspension on a slide, covered with a cover-glass and sealed with nail polish, was examined under a Leitz fluorescence microscope. Phase contrast microscopy for identification of cells and examination under ultraviolet light were carried out on the same preparations. A minimum of 200 lymphocytes was examined on every slide. Cells showing intracellular fluorescence in the form of a dense fluorescein deposit were considered non-viable and were not counted.

Pathology

Surgical specimens were examined microscopically to determine the size of the primary lesion and the presence of nodal metastases. Levels of axillary nodes were designated by the surgeon at the time of the operation. Level I refers to lymph nodes lying lateral to the pectoralis major muscles; Level II encompasses lymph nodes beneath the pectoralis minor muscle; and Level III lymph nodes are those located to the medial border of the pectoralis minor. Histologic examination concentrated on evidence of multicentricity, invasion of inframammary lymphatics and the presence of cellular infiltrates. Lymph nodes were evaluated for micro (less than 2 mm) or macro (greater than 2 mm) metastases and the presence of sinus histiocytosis or follicular hyperplasia.

RESULTS

Patients

One hundred and twenty-seven patients with breast cancer and 63 patients with benign breast lesions were studied. The mean age was 55.9 ± 13 years in the patients with cancer and 45.7 ± 12 years in the group with benign lesions. The median age was 55 years respectively. In the malignant group 27% were premenopausal, and 73% were postmenopausal. In the benign patients these results were 44% vs. 56%. Nine percent had non-infiltrating cancer and the rest had infiltrating cancer, mostly of the ductal type. Patients were classified into the general histologic types of non-infiltrating cancer, and infiltrating cancer, with or without node metastases. Patients were also classified in terms of prognosis according to the extent of disease into three defined risk groups as suggested by Fisher's data [13].

Skin Tests for Delayed Hypersensitivity

The DNCB test was positive in 10 of 11 patients with benign lesions (91%), 8 of 9 patients with non-infiltrating cancer (89%), 23 of 25 patients with infiltrating cancer without nodal metastases (89%) and 55 of 69 patients with infiltrating cancer and axillary metastases (80%). The differences in DNCB responses were not significant, nor were there any significant differences in the responses to common antigens.

Skin test responses to DNCB and intradermal antigens were evaluated in the breast cancer patients according to their pathologic stage (extent of disease) or 'risk category.' There was not a direct correlation of DNCB responsiveness with progressing stage of disease. The frequency of DNCB responsiveness according to the risk category was 91% in the 'low risk,' 77% in 'intermediate risk' and 89% in the 'high risk' group. None of the differences in DNCB responses nor in the intradermal responses was significant.

In Vitro Tests - Benign vs Malignant Breast Disease
Lymphocytes and Lymphocyte Subpopulations

There were no significant differences between the breast cancer patients and those with benign disease in either the absolute lymphocyte counts (2107 $\pm$ 157 cells/mm^3 vs 2213 $\pm$ 152 cells/mm^3), nor in the percent T cell counts (87.1 $\pm$ 0.83 vs 88.2 $\pm$ 0.95). There was no significant difference between the two groups in EAC rosetting cells (11.0 vs 13.2, P=0.073). There was a significant increase in the number of S-Ig bearing cells in the breast cancer group (11.7 $\pm$ 0.8 vs 9.6 $\pm$ 0.7, P< 0.05).

LYMPHOCYTE STIMULATION RESPONSES TO MITOGENS AND ANTIGENS BENIGN VS MALIGNANT BREAST DISEASE

There were no significant differences in the mean maximum lymphocyte response to the mitogens (PHA, PWM, Con A) between the malignant and benign breast groups (Table II). There were differences in the lymphocyte responses to certain antigens of which stimulation with candida albicans and E. coli showed the clearest differences between the cancer and the benign patients. A significantly greater proportion of the cancer patients were in the 'low responder' group, and had CPM less than 2500 in response to both candida albicans and E. coli (P <.05). There were no significant differences between the malignant and benign breast group if one compared only the mean maximum CPM of either candida albicans or E. coli.

Lymphocyte Count and Lymphocyte Subpopulation
in Breast Cancer Subgroups

There were no differences in absolute lymphocyte counts nor in the percentage of T cells, EAC rosettes or B cells bearing surface immuno-globulins when patients with nodal metastases were compared to those without nodal metastases. When the breast cancer patients were classified according to extent of disease (pathologic state), there were slight but not significant decreases in the absolute lymphocyte counts in the patients with high risk lesions compared to those with low risk lesions (Figure 1).

Lymphocyte Stimulation Responses in Breast Cancer Subgroups

The mean PHA response was slightly diminished, whereas Con A and PWM responses were slightly increased in the patients with infiltrating cancer who had nodal metastases compared to the patients with negative nodes (not significant). The lymphocyte responses to common antigens showed a generalized increase in the group with nodal metastases (not significant).

A similar analysis was made of the results in the breast cancer patients when they were classified according to pathologic stage of disease (risk). Lymphocyte stimulation with mitogens showed a linear decrease in response to PHA with increasing stage of disease. There were paradoxically increased responses to Con A and PWM in patients with 'high risk' breast cancer (Stage III) compared to those with 'low risk' lesions. Lymphocyte responses to antigens were generally increased in the patients with 'high risk' cancer except for the responses to candida albicans. The data was best analyzed by constructing a standardized score for all of the parameters tested which would facilitate comparison of results (Figure 2). The Standardized Score was calculated as follows: for each parameter the grand mean of all groups was subtracted from the 'risk' group means and the differences divided by the pooled estimate of the standard deviation. This places all the parameters on a comparative scale and permits comparison of trends. Figure 2 shows the relationships of the standardized scores of lymphocyte stimulation values between patients with 'low risk,' 'intermediate risk' and 'high risk' operable breast cancer. There was a linear decrease in the PHA scores in patients with increasing stage of disease (increasing risk) (P < .05). In contrast, although there was a decrease in the scores of PWM, Con A and the common antigens between the benign group and the patients with low risk cancer, there was a generalized increase in these standardized scores in patients with intermediate and high risk breast cancer. A "V-shaped" pattern existed for the scores of certain tests - PWM, E. coli, staph aureus and MBV - when one plotted the scores of the benign patients, the low risk group and the high risk groups (P <.05 for each score).

Clinical Follow-up of Breast Cancer Subgroups

Preliminary evaluation of patient subgroups who had 18 month follow-up showed that the recurrence rates in each pathologic stage or 'risk' category paralleled the expected rate as predicted from historical data. There were no recurrences in 25 patients with pathologic Stage I (low risk) but the recurrence rate increased in Stage II (6 of 34) and Stage III (15 of 36). The relationship of low PHA to recurrence and survival is not apparent at this time. Thirteen of 70 patients had a preoperative maximum PHA stimulation of < 20,000 (less than the 10th percentile of the control group). (Ten of these patients were in Stage II and III). Thus far, after 18 months of follow-up there have been eight recurrences (three in Stage II, five in Stage III). Only one of these patients with recurrence had a preoperative PHA < 20,000 cpm.

DISCUSSION

Patients with operable breast cancer showed some impairment of cellular immune function as measured by skin tests and *in vitro* immune parameters. DNCB reactivity was almost normal in breast cancer patients without nodal metastases (89%) and was only slightly reduced in patients with infiltrating cancer who had nodal metastases (80%). There was no further depression in patients with Stage III cancer ('high risk' group). The frequency of DNCB responders in breast cancer patients was strikingly higher than what we have observed in patients with operable cancers of the head and neck, lung, and rectum and colon who were tested in similar fashion [39,40]. Breast cancer patients had normal lymphocyte levels, and T cell counts, but had different B cell levels than their benign counterparts. In the cancer patients the numbers of B cells bearing surface immunoglobulins (S-Ig) were increased, whereas the B cells carrying complement receptors were decreased in comparison to the benign group. There were also differences in B cell levels measured by these two techniques within the benign and malignant breast groups. In the benign

562

patients the number of complement receptor lymphocytes (CRL) was significantly higher than the number of lymphocytes bearing surface immunoglobulins (S-Ig). In the cancer patients B cell measurements by both techniques gave similar results. The meaning of the differences in B cell levels between these patient groups is not determined. The increase in lymphocytes bearing S-Ig in the breast patients will require further analysis because in this technique determination of B lymphocytes by anti-surface immunoglobulin fluorescence using whole immunoglobulin reagents has been shown to overestimate the true number of B lymphocytes [43] and may be detecting a third lymphocyte population termed K cells.

Lymphocyte stimulation studies with mitogens and a battery of antigens showed selected differences between the benign and breast cancer groups. The breast cancer patients showed significant impairment in their response to certain antigens, candida albicans and E. coli. There were no significant differences in the mitogen responses (PHA, PWM, Con A) when the benign patients were compared to the total breast cancer group. When the breast cancer patients were segregated into groups according to the pathologic extent of the disease ('risk') there were significant differences in the lymphocyte responses to certain mitogens and antigens. The analysis of these results was greatly facilitated by converting lymphocyte stimulation values to a standardized score which allowed simultaneous comparison of 10 variables of lymphocyte function within three cancer subgroups. Only lymphocyte stimulation with PHA showed a linear decrease with increasing stage of disease. Certain lymphocyte responses actually gave a "V-shaped" pattern and showed maximum depression in patients with Stage I cancer and then a paradoxical increase in patients with Stage II and III cancer. These findings occurred with the mitogens PWM and Con A, and with the antigens staph aureus, E. coli and MBV. These findings suggest that in breast cancer patients nodal metastases and more extensive local disease may be associated with stimulation of certain lymphocyte responses. Indeed, Whitehead et al. have reported that a significant depression of T cell levels exists in Stage I and II breast cancer whereas in Stage III patients the values have returned to the normal range [41]. Although we did not observe these differences in our measurements of T cell levels, these results mimic our findings with lymphocyte stimulation studies (most antigens and mitogens gave a paradoxical stimulation in Stage III). Fisher et al. have found that in lymphocyte stimulation studies with diluted PHA, lymphocytes from

563

the lowest axillary nodes (closest to the tumor) had much higher stimulation responses than found in lymphocytes from high axillary nodes (further removed from the tumor), or in peripheral blood lymphocytes [12]. Lymphocytes from the high axillary nodes gave stimulation values similar to peripheral blood lymphocytes. Similar findings have been reported by Ellis et al. who tested lymphocytes in the peripheral blood and regional nodes of breast cancer patients using a breast cancer extract and a macrophage inhibition test and found greater activity in peripheral node lymphocytes than in the peripheral blood [11]. These studies suggest that a regional node lymphocytes adjacent to primary breast cancer may be in a state of chronic stimulation. There may also be increased stimulation of peripheral blood lymphocytes in patients with locally advanced breast cancer. In our study peripheral blood lymphocytes cultured with the majority of antigens and mitogens did show a paradoxical increase in stimulation values in patient with the greatest tumor burden ('high risk' group). The apparent general increase in lymphocyte function as shown by lymphocyte stimulation studies in patients with locally advanced (Stage III) breast cancer is reversed in patients who developed visceral metastases. These patients often show profound depression of lymphocyte function (unpublished observation) [40]. There seems to be a fine balance in the host-tumor relationship in breast cancer patients in whom up to a point increasing tumor burden is associated with general lymphocyte stimulation, whereupon further increase in tumor burden is associated with depression.

The most striking feature in our study has been the demonstration that only lymphocyte stimulation studies with PHA showed a linear decreased response in the patients with increasing stage of disease or 'risk' category. The lymphocyte population affected by PHA may be uniquely sensitive to increasing tumor burden. A major question now is whether this test has any prognostic value beyond its being a general reflector of tumor burden. Preliminary follow-up results show that the 'risk' categories as defined pathologically do reflect the recurrence rates predicted from previous historical data. At this point in follow-up, eight patients (of 70 with PHA values) have developed recurrence, and the majority are in Stage III ('high risk' category). Only one had low PHA values (PHA <20,000 CPM) as previously defined. Conversely, in the overall group of 13 patients who had low PHA values preoperatively (mainly in Stage II and III) only this single patient has developed early recurrence. These results are preliminary but suggest that although the PHA lymphocyte stimulation test is a reasonable indicator of tumor burden and extent of disease in a population of patients with breast cancer, it is not of necessity an indication of individual prognosis.

SUMMARY

The concept of whether immune function was related to risk of recurrence was examined in patients with operable breast cancer in whom careful clinical and pathologic staging had been performed.

Immune reactivity was assessed by skin tests, by measurement of absolute lymphocyte count, T and B cells, lymphocyte stimulation by mitogens and a battery of common antigens, serum immunoglobulins and complement levels. There were 127 patients with operable breast cancer and 62 patients with benign breast lesions. The breast cancer patients showed minimal or no impairment of DNCB skin tests. Only patients with nodal metastases showed a slight but not significant impairment of DNCB responses (80% were DNCB positive compared to 90% in the controls).

The lymphocyte responses to mitogens were normal in the breast cancer patients, but there was a significant depression of lymphocyte responses to certain recall antigens such as candida albicans and E. coli.

The absolute lymphocyte count and the T cell counts were normal, but B cells bearing complement receptors were decreased and B cells bearing surface immunoglobulins were increased in the breast cancer patients.

Immune function was also analyzed according to the pathologic stage of disease 'risk of recurrence' categories. There was no correlation with skin tests nor lymphocyte levels. A striking and paradoxical finding was the demonstration that patients with 'low risk' cancer overall had markedly lower responses to the battery of stimulating mitogens and antigens than found in patients with 'high risk' or 'intermediate risk' disease. Only the lymphocyte response to PHA showed a significant linear correlation with increasing pathologic stage or 'risk of recur-rence.' Current evidence from this study suggests that PHA response is markedly influenced by the primary tumor burden and thus indirectly reflects the risk of recurrence.

ACKNOWLEDGMENT

Supported by Cancer Research Institute, Inc., New York, N. Y.

Table I
BREAST CANCER
TUMOR FACTORS - CONCEPT OF "RISK" *

Pathologic Extent of Disease - "Risk"	Pts. Rate	Recurrence 18 Mo.	Survival 5 Yr.	NED 10 Yr.
I. "Low Risk" (minimal breast Ca) Infil. cancer < 3 cm, neg. nodes Non-infiltrating cancer	158	6%	80%	73%
II. "Intermediate Risk" 1 - 3 nodal metastases Macrometastases level I [†]	72	19%	70%	50% < 62%
III. "High Risk" > 4 nodal metastases Macrometastases level II or III [†]	61	45%	37%	22%

* Constructed from data of Rosen, Urban, Miké 1975
[†] Huvos 1971

Table II
OPERABLE BREAST CANCER
LYMPHOCYTE RESPONSE TO SELECTED
MITOGENS AND ANTIGENS*

	Benign	Malignant	P value
Mitogens			
PHA	27.6 ± .72	25.6 ± .88	NS
CON A	26.0 ± .78	24.1 ± .83	N.S.
PWM	17.8 ± .74	17.1 ± .69	N.S.
Antigens			
Candida albicans	6.1 ± 1.2	4.8 ± 1.0	NS
Non-responder [†]	12 (23%)	31 (43%)	< 0.05
E. coli	3.1 ± .31	2.6 ± .30	NS
Non-responder	22 (42%)	48 (66%)	< 0.05

* stimulation values = CPM × 1000

[†] stimulation values = < 2.5 CPM × 1000

No. of pts. 57 benign, 71 malignant

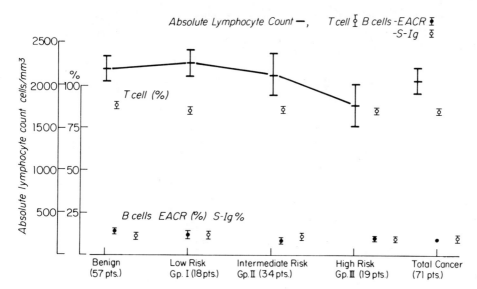

LYMPHOCYTES AND LYMPHOCYTE SUBPOPULATIONS
ACCORDING TO EXTENT OF DISEASE "RISK"

FIG. 1. There was a moderate but not statistically significant decrease in the absolute lymphocyte count in the high risk patients. There were no differences in the percentages of T cells nor B cells as measured by EAC rosettes and surface immunoglobulins.

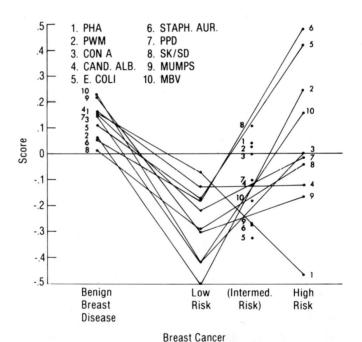

IMMUNE REACTIVITY IN OPERABLE BREAST CANCER

STANDARDIZED SCORES FOR LYMPHOCYTE STIMULATION VALUES
ACCORDING TO RISK CATEGORY

FIG. 2. Comparison of standardized scores of lymphocyte stimulation values between patients with benign breast lesions and breast cancer patients who were categorized according to risk. Only the response to PHA showed a decrease associated with increasing extent of disease (risk). There was a paradoxical increase in the lymphocyte stimulation scores of the other mitogens and antigens with increase in risk of disease.

REFERENCES

1. Alford, T. C., Hollinshead, A., Herberman, R. B.: Delayed cutaneous hypersensitivity reactions to extracts of malignant and normal human breast cells. Ann. Surg. 178:20, 1973.

2. Bianco, C., Patrick, R. and Nussenzweig, V.: A population of lymphocytes bearing a membrane receptor for antigen-antibody-complement complexes. J. Exp. Med. 132:702, 1970.

3. Black, M. M. and Lois, N. P. Jr.: Cellular response to autologous breast cancer tissue: correlation with stage and lymphoreticular reactivity. Cancer 28: 268-73, 1971.

4. Black, M. M., Lois, H. P, Shore, B. and Zachran, R. E.: Cellular hypersensitivity to breast cancer: assessment by a leukocyte migration procedure. Cancer 33:952-958, 1974.

5. Black, M. D.: Immunology of breast cancer: clinical implications. 1975 Progress in Clinical Cancer (Ed. I. Ariel).

6. Catalona, W. J., Sample, W. F. and Chretien, P. B.: Lymphocyte reactivity in cancer patients, correlation with tumor histology and clinical stage. Cancer 31:65-71, 1973.

7. Cline, M. J. and Lehrer, R. I.: Phagocytosis by human monocytes. Blood 32:423, 1968.

8. Dellon, A., Potvin, C., Chretien, P. B.: T cell levels in bronchogenic carcinoma: correlations with tumor stage and clinical course. Cancer, in press.

9. Edynak, E. M.. Hirshaut, Y., Bernhard, M. and Trempe, G.: Fluorescent antibody studies of human breast cancer. J. Natl. Cancer Inst. 48:1137, 1972.

10. Eilber, F. R., and Morton, D. L.: Impaired immunologic reactivity and recurrence following cancer surgery. Cancer 25:362-367, 1970.

11. Ellis, R. J., Werneck, G., Zabriske, J. B.and Goldman, L. J.: Immunologic competence of regional lymph nodes in patients with breast cancer. Cancer 35:655-659, 1975.

12. a. Fisher, B., Saffer, T. A. and Fisher, E. R.: Studies concerning the regional lymph node in cancer. III. Response of regional lymph node cells from breast and colon cancer patients to PHA stimulation. Cancer 30:1202-15, 1972.
    b. VII. Thymidine uptake cells from nodes of breast cancer patients relative to axillary locations and histopathologic discriminants. Cancer 33: 271-279, 1974.

13. Fisher, B., Slack, N.H., Bross, I. D. J.: Cancer of the breast: size of neoplasm abd prognosis. Cancer 24:1071-1080, 1960.

14. Fossati, G., Canevan, S., Della Porte, G., Balzarini, G. P. and Veronisi, V.: Cellular immunity to human breast carcinoma: Int. J. Cancer 10: 391-396, 1972.

15. Hellstrom, I, Hellstrom, K. E., Sjogren, H. O. and Warner, G. A.: Demonstration of cell-mediated immunity to human neoplasms of various histological types. Int. J. Cancer 7:1-10, 1971.

16. Hughes, L. E. and Mackay, W. D.: Suppression of the tuberculin response in malignant disease. Brit. Med. J. 2:1346-1348, 1965.

17. Humphrey, L. J., Estes, N. C., Norse, P. A., Jewell, W. R., Boudet, R. A. and Hudscn, M.J . K.: Serum antiboty in patients with mammary disease. Cancer 34:1516-1520, 1974.

18. Huvos, A. G., Hutter, R. V. P. and Berg, J.: Significance of axillary macrometastases and micrometastases in mammary cancer. Ann.Surg. 173: 44-46, 1971.

19. Johnston, R. N., Ritchie, R. T. and Murray, I. H. F.: Declining tuberculin sensitivity with advancing age. Brit. Med. J. 2:720-724, 1963.

20. Jondal, M., Holm, G. and Wigzell, H.: Surface markers on human T and B lymphocytes. A large population of lymphocytes forming non-immune rosettes with sheep red blood cells. J. Exp. Med. 136:207, 1972.

21. Lundy, J., Wanebo, H. J., Pinsky, C., Strong, E. and Oettgen, H.: Delayed hypersensitivity reactions in patients with squamous cell cancer of the head and neck. Am. J. Surg. 128:530-533, 1974.

22. McCredie, J. A., Inch, W. R., Sutherland, R. M.: Peripheral blood lymphocytes and breast cancer.. Arch. Surg. 107:162-165, 1973.

23. Magnus, K. and Horowitz, O. Tuberculin allergy and cancer risk. J. Chronic Dis. 24:635-641, 1971.

24. Mitchell, R. J.: The delayed hypersensitivity response in primary breast carcinoma as an index of host resistance. Brit. J. Surg. 59:505-506, 1972.

25. Nelson, H. S.: Delayed hypersensitivity in cancer patients. Cutaneous and in vitro lymphocyte response to specific antigens. J. Nat. Cancer Inst. 42:705-770, 1969.

26. Papatestas, A. E., Lesnick, G. J., Genkins, G and Aufses, A. H.: The prognostic significance of peripheral lymphocyte counts in patients with breast cancer. Cancer 37:164-168, 1976.

27. Pernis, B., Ferrarini, M., Forni, L. and Amante, L.: Immunoglobulins on lymphocyte membranes. In Amos, B. (Ed.): Progress in Immunology, New York, Academic Press, 1971.

28. Pinsky, C. M., El Domieri, A., Caron, A. S., Knapper, W. H. and Oettgen, H. F.: Delayed hypersensitivity reactions in patients with cancer. In: Recent Results in Cancer Research. (G. Mathe and F. Weiner, Eds.) Springer-Verlag, New York, 1974.

29. Priori, E . A., Anderson, D. E., Williams, W. C. and Dinochowski, L.: Immunological studies on human breast cancer and mouse mammary tumor. J. Natl. Cancer Inst. 48:1134, 1972.

30. Renaud, M.: La cuti-reaction a la tuberculine chez cancereux. Bull. Soc. Med. Paris 50:1441-1442, 1926.

31. Rosen, P. P., Urban, J. A. and Mike, V.: Breast cancer study, Memorial Sloan-Kettering Cancer Center, 1964. Preliminary results.

32. Roberts, M. M. and Jones-Williams, W.: The delayed hypersensitivity reaction in breast cancer. Brit. J. Surg. 61:549-552, 1974.

33. Sample, W. F., Gertner, H. R. and Chretien, P. R.: Inhibition of phytohemagglutinin-induced in vitro lymphocyte transformation by serum from patients with carcinoma. J. Natl. Cancer Inst. 46:1291-1297, 197-

34. Stewart, T. H. and Orizago, M.: The presence of delayed hypersensitivity reactions in patients toward cellular extracts of their malignant tumors. The frequency, duration and cross reactivity of the phenomenon in patients with breast cancer and its correlation with survival. Cancer 28:1472-1478, 1971.

35. Stjernsward, J. et al: Lymphopenia and change in distribution of human B and T lymphocytes in peripheral blood induced by irradiation for mammary carcinoma. Lancet 1:1352-1356, 1972.

36. Sutherland, R. M., Inch, W. R., McRedie, J. A.: Phytohemagglutinin (PH-A)-induced transformation of lymphocytes from patients with cancer. Cancer 75:574-578, 1971.

37. Urban, J. A.: Changing patterns of breast cancer. Cancer 37: 111, 1976.

38. Wanebo, H. J., Huvos, A. G. and Urban, J. A.: Treatment of minimal breast cancer. Cancer 33:349-356, 1974.

39. Wanebo, H. J., Moo Young Jun, Strong, E. and Oettgen, H.: T cell deficiency in patients with squamous cell cancer of the head and neck. Am. J. Surg. 130:445-451, 1975.

40. Wanebo, H. J.: Personal observation

41. Whitehead, R. H., Thatcher, J., Teasdale, C., Roberts, G. P. and Hughes, L. E.: T and B lymphocyte depression by enzyme treatment in vitro. Lancet 1:330-332, 1976.

42. Whittaker, M. E., Rees, K. and Clark, G. C.: Reduced lymphocyte transformation in breast cancer. Lancet 1:892-893, 1971.

43. Winchester, R. J., Fu, S. M., Hoffman, T and Kunkel, H. G.: IgG on lymphocyte surfaces, technical problems and the significance of a third cell population. J. Immun. 114:1210-1212, 1975.

INDUCTION OF CUTANEOUS DHR TO IRRADIATED AUTOLOGOUS TUMOR CELLS IN INOPERABLE BREAST CANCER

Aliza Adler, Joseph A. Stein and Bernard Czernobilsky *

Institute of Oncology and Radioisotopes, Hadassah Hospital, Tel-Aviv
University Sackler Medical School, Balfour Street, Tel-Aviv, Israel
and * Institute of Pathology, Kaplan Hospital, Rehovot, Israel.

It is the object of this study to test the feasibility of active specific
anti-tumor immunization as a regularly applicable procedure in breast
cancer patients and to look for possible beneficial clinical effects resulting from immunotherapy. For the exploratory phases of such a study
patients with inoperable breast cancer are suitable since they were shown
to an adequate level of general immunocompetence (1), rendering them
potentially capable for active immunization toward a specific tumor
associated antigen. Spontaneous skin DHR toward autologous tumor extract
was reportedly elicited in 26% of operable breast cancer patients (2).
We found such a reaction in only 2 of 23 patients with inoperable breast
cancer. Reported methods of active immunization with BCG - tumor cell
mixtures (3,4,5) were adopted and modified to devise a procedure leading
to regular induction of skin DHR toward autologous irradiated tumor cells
in inoperable breast cancer patients.

Patient Material and Method of Evaluation

23 breast cancer patients, 5 pre- and 17 post menopausal females and one
male, aged 42-70, are described in this report. 17 of these patients had
locally advanced inoperable tumors but had no demonstrable distant metastases and 6 patients had manifest metastatic dissemination. Excisional
biopsy was performed on each patient for diagnosis and in order to obtain
tumor tissue for immunization. When the yield of recoverable tumor cells
from the primary source was insufficient, tumor cells were sometimes obtained from excised lymph nodes involved with tumor.

Each patient had a thorough physical examination, laboratory tests, X-
ray survey of the skeleton, liver scan and evaluation of her general immunocompetence by skin testing with PPD and DNCB, lymphocyte stimulation
by PHA and PPD, total peripheral blood lymphocyte number and E-rosette
formation. Initially PPD negative patients had repeated BCG inoculations
until converted to full PPD positivity.

Immunization Procedure

Autologous irradiated tumor cells (T) are prepared from the freshly received, sterile surgical biopsy specimen. Macroscopic tumor is dissected

from the surrounding tissue and a small sample is taken from every piece
for histological confirmation. Normal tissue is collected whenever possible. Tissues are finely cut, manually teased and the spilled cells are
collected in saline. Cells are washed in saline, counted and resuspended
at a concentration of 1×10^7 cells/ml saline. A smear of the suspension
is examined in the microscope. The cell suspension is then irradiated in
plastic containers to a dose of 6000 rad with telecobalt, output appr.
200 rad / minute. The cell suspension is then subdivided into vials,
each containing the dose required for one immunization and is stored at
minus 70°C. A sample of (T) taken before freezing is tested for sterility under aerobic and anaerobic conditions. Non sterile material is discarded. (T) is also tested for viability by trypan blue exclusion test
before use. Normal tissues for control studies are treated in exactly
the same way.

BCG freeze - dried intradermal vaccine (Glaxo) containing approximately
10×10^6 viable organisms / ampoule as specified for each batch was employed. The highest dilution of BCG in saline which would still evoke a
palpable skin granuloma of 10 to 15 mm diameter - but is just short of
causing necrosis - was determined for each individual patient prior to
immunization. BCG had to be further diluted with progressive immunization as patients' reactivity to it increases.

The mixture (M) of BCG and (T) is prepared by adding 0.3 ml of the
thawed (T) to 0.3 ml of BCG in double strength of the required dilution.
This sample contains 3×10^6 tumor cells. The mixture (M) is injected
intradermally in a rosette - like arrangement at six sites, each site
receiving 5×10^5 tumor cells in 0.1 ml. At the center of the rosette a
test inoculum of (T) containing 1×10^6 cells in 0.1 ml is injected.
Another control inoculum of (T) is placed ten cm outside the rosette to
show the response to tumor cells at a distance from BCG. Rosettes were
placed on the patients' body in proximity to main sites of draining
lymph nodes. When a positive response to (T) is well established, normal
autologous tissue is injected as control. Patients' skin reactivity toward (T) is checked every month and if a decreased reaction is found additional boosters of (M) are administered. A 6 mm diameter punch biopsy
was performed on all positive skin responses to (T) and on some to (M).
Specimens were fixed in 10% neutral formalin, stained with hematoxyline
and eosine and were examined histologically.

RESULTS

In Vivo Observations

A positive response toward irradiated autologous tumor cells (T), as
evident by a strong and progressive cutaneous reaction at the site of
(T) inoculation, has been elicited in 19 of 23 patients who were given
repeated weekly inoculations of (M). When it appeared, the response to
(T) was indistinguishable from that to (M). (Fig. 1, 2). Positive skin
response to (T) was observed between the second and sixth week of the
immunizing procedure, appearing as a reddish elevated infiltration in
the skin of palpable thickness and of a 10 - 25 mm diameter. When established, the positive response to (T) is sometimes found already 12
hours after inoculation reaching its maximal dimensions at 24 hours.
Early (T) responses usually fade after two days but as inoculations are
carried on the skin response to (T) becomes more pronounced in size and

574

bulk, reaching diameters of 20 - 25 mm and persisting up to four days, with central necrosis appearing on the second or third day. Inoculi of (M) remain in a state of activity for 3 to 4 weeks due to the presence of the BCG component. It was found that positive response toward tumor cells - though apparent after 2 to 6 weekly inoculations of (M) rosettes - attained its greatest dimensions after the sixth to ninth (M) rosette procedure.

In each of the 17 inoperable patients the attempted immunization procedure resulted in the induction of a positive strong response to (T) and it was also elicited in two of the six patients with metastatic disease. However, these two patients did not attain maximal levels of positive response even though they had nine repeated trials each.

In two inoperable patients the "flare up" phenomenon was observed, simultaneously with the first evidence of immunization toward (T). These patients had received (M) rosettes with central (T) test inoculi for three consecutive weeks without result. After the fourth (M) rosette administration a positive response to (T) appeared in the center, together with identical central responses inside the three previous (M) rosettes. These spontaneous "flare up" responses lasted for 11 and 14 days respectively and proceeded to central necrosis (Fig. 3).

Response to (T) Relative to Dose

Skin response relative to dose of injected tumor cells was examined in four patients with vigorous reactivity to (T). Four concentrations of (T) were employed: $1x10^6$, $1x10^5$, $1x10^4$ and $1x10^3$ cells / 0.1 ml. The smallest dose of tumor cells evoked a relatively weak but positive response with erythema and induration of 6 - 8 mm across; the larger doses of tumor cells produced infiltrative lesions of proportional bulk, with the highest dose measuring 20-25 mm across with occasional central necrosis (Fig. 4). It is thus evident that the degree of skin response to (T) is dose related.

Maintenance of Response to (T)

Patients were observed for maintenance of positive response to (T) during periods ranging from 2 - 8 months. Response to (T), retested every month, was steadily elicited in all but two patients who required additional booster with mixture (M).

Response to Normal Autologous Tissue

Suspensions of normal autologous skin tissue and of peripheral leukocytes were irradiated, stored like the tumor tissue and were employed to test the possibility of non specific auto-immune response to normal cell components. In no case was a reaction toward inoculi of skin tissue observed; three patients showed a transient response toward their own leukocyte inoculum.

Response to Non-Irradiated Autologous Tumor Cells

Six immunized patients were examined for response toward non-irradiated autologous tumor cells which were otherwise prepared and stored in the same way as (T). A positive skin response to these inoculi was observed similar to that toward irradiated tumor cells. It is not known - and we are reluctant to try - whether patients can be immunized by means of non-irradiated cells. However, the above finding indicates that irradiation does not alter the antigenic properties of tumor cells under our experimental conditions.

Individual BCG Dilution

Using "personalised" BCG doses for each patient enabled us to proceed through at least nine repeated immunizations without causing such side effects in highly sensitized patients as usually accompany massive BCG inoculations. None of the patients treated by repeated immunizations developed severe necrotising lesions in the skin nor systemic reactions of malaise, fever or BCG induced visceral granulomas. The majority of patients had slight reactive regional lymphadenitis. All patients treated with dilute BCG mixed with tumor cells have also shown stimulation of general immunocompetence by known parameters of cell mediated immunity.

Histopathological Findings

Skin biopsy specimens of (T) excised at the peak of response showed prominent perivascular lymphocyte "cuffing" and diffuse infiltration of the upper dermal layer with lymphocytes, histiocytes, eosinophils and neutrophils, with some edema. (Fig. 6, 7). The microscopic appearancs is rather uniform in all patients examined and is consistent with delayed hypersensitivity cellular reaction. Skin biopsy specimens of (M) showed a pattern of cellular reaction similar to that of (T) (Fig. 5) with the additional feature of characteristic granulomas composed of histiocytes, lymphocytes and Langhans type giant cells appearing three to four days following injection. Histological reaction to (M) is in effect quite comparable to that toward BCG alone.

In sequential biopsies of (T) inoculi the microscopic picture in the skin after 12 - 24 hours is characterised by the prominence of the neutrophils in the early phases of the response, with subsequent predominance of lymphocytes, histiocytes and eosinophil cells in later phases, after 48 - 72 hours. In one instance, (S.V.) an 11 days old (T) lesion showed - in addition to the above features - progress to acute epidermal inflammatory reaction with bullous formation containing massive neutrophils and with the appearance of a single granuloma in the upper portion of the dermis, composed of histiocytes and lymphocytes.

The effect of inoculation with increasing doses of tumor cells is recognisable by the degree of pleomorphism of the inflammatory infiltrate developing in response to the larger inoculi of (T). A dose of 10^{3-4} tumor cells produced a predominantly lymphocytic response in the dermis whereas higher doses of (T), 10^{5-6} tumor cells, showed in addition a rich assembly of neutrophils, histiocytes and eosinophils as well foci of dermal necrosis and focal necrotising vasculitis in small subcutaneous arteries. Though carefully searched for, none of the injected tumor cells could be detected even in biopsies taken 12 hours after (T) inoculation.

Case Report (Patients S.V.)

Manifestation of spontaneous systemic immunological host - tumor interaction may take considerable time following immunization. Relative to this point is the report of one of our first immunized patients, 62 years old. She presented with auto-amputation of the right breast by a massive ulcerating tumor extending over the entire right chest wall, with peau d'orange and deep masses palpable in the left breast and with bilateral coarse lymphnodes involved with tumor in the axillae. Although aware of her disease for three years the patient had sought no treatment. Still, no evidence of metastatic disease dissemination was found on thorough clinical examination. The patient was actively immunized eight months ago with the mixture of BCG and her own tumor cells. When she was seen with her first positive skin response to (T) after the fourth weekly inoculation of rosettes she showed a simultaneous "flare up" of the (T) inoculi at the center of the three previously injected rosettes. (Fig. 3). After the induction of a strong positive skin DHR to (T) the right and left breasts were treated by tangential irradiation with telecobalt to a uniform dose of 3000 rad in three weeks. The bulk of the tumor regressed soon after this relatively small dose of radiation. The BCG - (T) mixture was once again inoculated following radiotherapy and since then the patient was given a test dose of (T) every month and her response is steadily positive.

During the past four months this patient has presented with a clinical syndrome of bouts of fever, malaise and chills recurring every 3 to 4 weeks. These bouts are accompanied by a hot, red, angry inflammation suffusing a clinically tumor free margin of the chest regions on all sides. Inside the inflamed skin belt, small satellite like lesions appear which on multiple biopsies were proven to be microscopic foci of nests of anaplastic carcinoma in the subcutaneous tissue; above these a dense cellular infiltrate and perivascular lymphocyte cuffing were found histologically characteristic of DHR. (Fig. 8, 9, 10). The local and systemic manifestations subside after 2 - 3 days. The described syndrome is suggestive of the patient's acquisition of self-activated, systemic hypersensitivity reaction toward actively growing tumor microfoci, appearing in the wake of specific immunotherapeutic intervention. Whether this acquired reactivity toward viable tumor will be effective in the further control of tumor foci in the patient's body - remains to be seen.

COMMENT

Though this series of patients with locally advanced breast cancer is as yet relatively small for evaluation the results indicate that the induction of cutaneous DHR toward autologous tumor associated antigen is going to be feasible in a large proportion of such patients. It is hoped that evidence of spontaneous host - tumor interaction at sites of tumor deposits such as described in the case report will be forthcoming and observable in further instances among the patients who are immunized. Notably, in the patient described, the spontaneous reaction around the tumor did not occur at the site of the main tumor residue in the breast region but was directed against tiny foci of tumor cells dispersed throughout the adjacent deep dermal layers. This finding may well serve as a reflection of the relative forces operating between the tumor and the immune system - tipping the balance in favour of the latter only when the former is of microscopic dimensions. This is probably the reason why we have not been able to observe signs of clinical tumor regression among this series of patients who are harboring relatively large volumes of tumor tissue in the breast region. It is conceivable that in another host-tumor setting, such as the early post-mastectomy patient, induced acquisition of anti-tumor immunity might be effective in the arrest or the elimination of occult dispersed micrometastatic deposits which are the cause of eventual clinical disease recurrence.

SUMMARY

Cuteneous delayed hypersensitivity reaction (DHR) toward autologous irradiated tumor cells was induced in 17 successive patients with locally advanced, inoperable breast cancer and in 2 of 6 patients with disseminated metastatic disease. Positive DHR appeared after 3 to 6 weekly inoculations with a mixture of BCG and irradiated tumor cells (M), injected in a circular, rosette - like formation, with a single tumor cell inoculum (T) in the center. The rosettes were placed in proximity to axillary, supraclavicular and inguinal lymph nodes. Maximal response to (T) was observed after the 6th to 9th weekly inoculation, appearing as a bulky infiltration of 20 - 25 mm diameter, with central necrosis. This response was detectable after 12 hours and persisted for 2 - 4 days. Degree of skin response to (T) was found proportional to dose of tumor cells injected. Individual patient response to dilutions of BCG (Glaxo) just short of necrosis was determined for preparation of the immunising mixture of BCG and tumor cells. The histological appearance of foci of positive skin response to (T) is characteristic of the delayed hypersensitivity reaction, showing perivascular "cuffing" by lymphocytes with a rich cellular infiltrate in the dermis. This is initially mainly composed of neutrophils with subsequent predominance of lymphocytes, histiocytes and eosinophils. Necrotizing vasculitis of small arteries as well as a granulomatous reaction to (T) were found.

Patients are receiving periodically booster inoculations of (T), according to immunological monitoring by skin tests and in vitro correlates of cell mediated immunity and close clinical follow up observations are recorded.

Clinical and histological findings are presented in detail on one treated patient who has subsequently shown evidence of spontaneous DHR toward subcutaneous foci of carcinoma.

Acknowledgments

The cooperation and help of Drs. R. Rozin and Z. Teva, Chiefs of Surgical Departments is greatly appreciated.

This study was supported in part by the Jehudit Segal Cancer Research Foundation and the Frida Sharfhartz Cancer Research Fund.

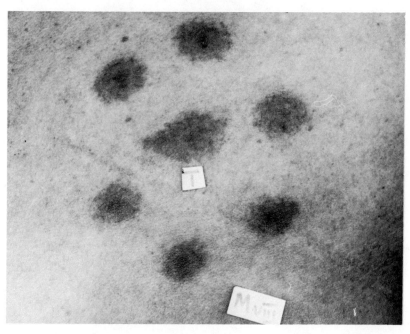

FIG. 1. Pat. H.M., Close up of (M) rosette with positive (T) in center; photographed 24 hours after inoculation of skin.

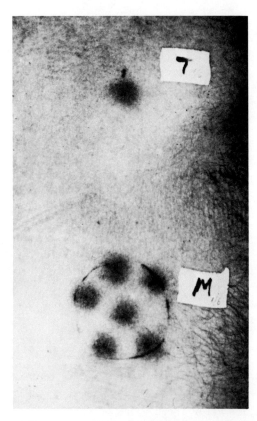

FIG. 2. Pat. S.S., (M) rosette with positive (T) in center and positive reaction to (T) injected 10 cm outside rosette - 24 hours after inoculation.

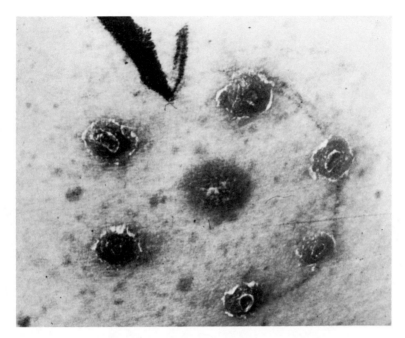

FIG. 3. Pat. S.V., Four weeks old (M) rosette with "flare up" reaction to (T) in the center after patient became immunized toward her own tumor cells. Note the central necrosis in the flaring (T) inoculum.

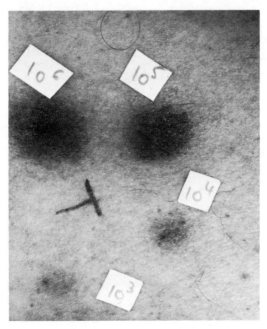

FIG. 4. Pat. S.S., Graded reaction to 5 concentrations of (T) after 24 hours: 10^6, 10^5, 10^4 and 10^3 tumor cells in each resp. inoculum.

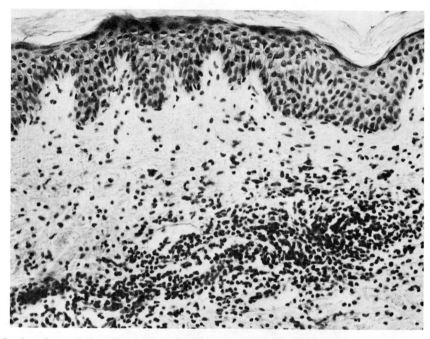

FIG. 5. Pat. H.M., Inoculum of (M) - irradiated tumor cell + BCG mixture;
Punch biopsy of skin taken 36 hours after inoculation. Histological
appearance is same as in Figure 6; heavy perivascular infiltration of
lymphocytes. (H & E x 100).

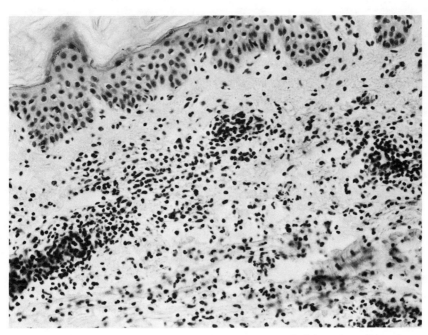

FIG. 6. Same patient as in Figure 5; inoculum of (T) - irradiated tumor
cells, biopsied after 37 hours. The prominent histological feature is
"cuffing", heavy perivascular lymphocyte infiltration in upper dermis.
(H & E x 100).

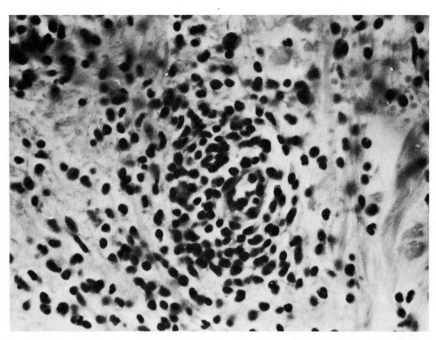

FIG. 7.   Same patient as in Figure 2; skin biopsy taken from (T) inoculum
at 10 cm distance from (M) rosette. Close up of prominent perivascular
lymphocyte "cuffing", same as in (T) in the center of the rosette. (H & E
x 400)

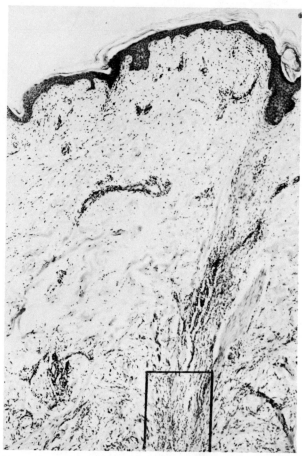

FIG. 8. Pat. S.V., Low power view of biopsy from inflamed skin, taken from region adjacent to breast tumor. There is diffuse and perivascular infiltration in the upper dermis above strands of anaplastic tumor cells in the lower portion of the dermis (inset at bottom of the figure). (H & E x 40)

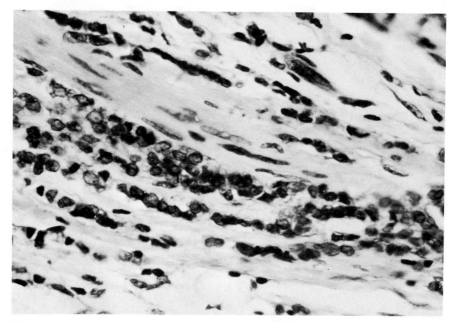

FIG. 9. Same patient as in Figure 8; high power view of inset. Strands of anaplastic tumor cells infiltrating into the depth of the dermis. (H & E x 400)

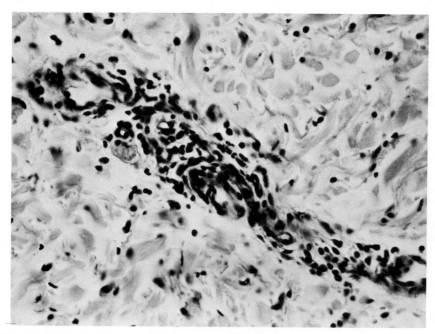

FIG. 10. Same patient as in Figure 8; high power view of region above the inset. Perivascular cuffing with mononuclear cells in upper dermis. (H & E x 350)

REFERENCES

1. Adler, A., Stein J.A., Ben Efraim, S. and Maor, M. A close study of delayed hypersensitivity skin reaction and PHA lymphocyte stimulation in 220 breast cancer patients; relation to stage and activity of disease and to radiation treatment. XI Internatl. Cancer Congress, Florence, Abstracts 2: 113, 1974.

2. Stewart, T.H.M. The presence of delayed hypersensitivity reactions in patients toward cellular extracts of their malignant tumors. I. The role of tissue antigen, non specific reactions of nuclear material and bacterial antigen as a source for this phenomenon. Cancer, 23: 1368 - 1379, 1969.

3. Bartlett, L.G. and Zbar, B. Tumor specific vaccine containing Mycobacterium bovis and tumore cells; safety and efficacy. J. Natl. Cancer Inst., 48: 1709 - 1726, 1972.

4. Morton, D.L., Eibler, F.R., Joseph, W.L., Wood, W.C., Trahan, E. and Ketcham, A.S. Immunological factors in human sarcomas and melanomas; a rational basis for immunotherapy. Ann. Intern. Medicine, 74: 587 - 604, 1971.

5. Currie, G.A. and Mc Elwain, T.G. Active immunotherapy in the treatment of disseminated malignant melanoma. A pilot study. Brit. J. Cancer, 31: 143 - 156, 1974. `

IMMUNOTHERAPY OF CANCER BY BACTERIAL VACCINES

Helen C. Nauts

Executive Director
Cancer Research Institute, Inc.*

The treatment of cancer by bacterial vaccines is based on observations over the past 200 years of dramatic cancer regressions, following acute bacterial infections, principally streptococcal and staphylococcal (1).

Approximately 430 histories of cancer patients in whom an infection developed spontaneously, or by inoculation, have been analyzed (1). Of these, 222 had histologic confirmation of diagnosis, and 106 of these determinate cases were apparent cures, traced 5 to 54 years later (Fig. 1). Of the 116 failures, 21 survived far longer than expected (5 to 30 years) (2). We have also analyzed 894 determinate cases of cancer treated by mixed toxins of Streptococcus pyogenes and Serratia marcescens (Coley Toxins). Of these, 426 were followed from 5 to 79 years after onset of their neoplasm. In the majority of patients who developed concurrent infections or who received toxin therapy, the condition was inoperable when toxins were begun.

The highest percentage of successes in the toxin-treated cases occurred in sarcoma of soft tissues (6), and malignant lymphomas, including reticulum cell sarcoma of both bone and soft tissues (3,7). Complete or partial regressions were also obtained in inoperable or metastatic carcinomas of the breast (8), colon (9), head and neck (2), uterus (2), ovary (2), renal (11) and testicular (12) cancer, malignant melanoma (13), neuroblastoma (14), and various bone tumors (3,4,5,23). Other beneficial effects included marked decrease or cessation of pain, improved appetite and weight gain (up to 50 pounds), reduction or disappearance of lymphedema, ascites or pleural effusion and remarkable regeneration of bone (2-5,14,17, 19,23,24) Significant palliation, (symptom-free up to five years) and one apparently permanent result occurred in multiple myeloma (24) (Table I) Fig. 2).

Most of the osteogenic sarcoma cases involved the long bones, and received toxin therapy as an adjuvant to surgery (5). Coley was the first to try saving the limb as well as the life in patients with sarcoma or giant cell tumor of the extremities (6-13). A few other surgeons followed his example. Of the 128 cases in which amputation was not performed, 73 (57%) were permanent successes, as compared to 32% of the 166 cases in which amputation was performed. The highest percentage of success with conservative surgery occurred in giant cell tumor (96%) and in operable sarcoma of soft tissues (80%). The poorest occurred in Ewing's sarcoma of

*Name changed to Cancer Research Institute, Inc., in 1973.

bone, as most of these young patients received excessive immunosuppresive radiation therapy prior to toxin therapy (13). Sykes found that bone marrow may be permanently aplastic following radiation (25) (Tables I and II).

Of the 891 toxin treated cases, 86 died of their original cancers more than 5 years after onset, and 60 subsequently developed an entirely different type of neoplasm up to 63 years after recovery from the first. Of these, 30 occurred in tissues irradiated prior to toxin therapy, consisting principally of basal cell carcinomas in the irradiated skin and 6 osteogenic sarcomas in irradiated bone. Of these 60 second primaries, 43 proved fatal. One patient developed a second reticulum cell sarcoma (tibia), 9 years after the first (femur) (3). Another patient developed a second giant cell tumor in the contralateral femur 7 years after the first (4).

In addition to these second primary solid tumors, 4 patients developed fatal acute myelogenous leukemia 23 to 57 years after onset of their primary neoplasm. Two had received massive radittion therapy to the chest "to prevent lung metastases" from their osteogenic sarcomas (5). Another had received radiation for a second primary. The fourth had had prolonged x-ray monitoring of the pelvis over a 23 year period.

Gershon reported that immunologic defense against metastases in tumor bearing hamsters is impaired <u>if the tumor is removed before full development of immunity</u>. In such cases, metastases occur far more frequently than if the tumor is not removed too soon (25a). The clinical findings seem to bear this out, especially in osteogenic sarcoma and reticulum cell sarcoma of bone. Patients treated very soon after onset did less well than those treated 6 to 9 months after onset (3,4,5). Timing is therefore crucial.

The studies of a great many investigators, both in the laboratory and clinic, including Old and Klein, have stressed the vital importance of the immunological system in our defense against cancer (6,14-24,34-37,54). Thus, any agent which suppresses its function can be deleterious while those which stimulate, such as infections and microbial products, including Coley Toxins, Staphage Lysate, BCG and C. parvum, can be beneficial.

Discussion

Only recently have modern oncologists and hematologists recognized that concurrent infections and vaccines may increase the survival rate of cancer or leukemia patients. Huth(1953) was the first to do so with leukemia(38-40). Nauts (1958) discussed the remarkable remissions occurring in leukemia, principally after pyogenic infections but also in 7 patients in whom malaria developed or was induced, and in 2 patients treated by Coley Toxins (41). Clarkson et al.(1975) analyzed the factors affecting prognosis in acute leukemia in adults and noted that the cases receiving Pseudominas aeruginosa vaccine maintained drug induced remissions longer than controls treated only with chemotherapy (42,43).

Several thoracic surgeons have reported a significantly higher survival of their lung cancer patients who developed empyema (44-49). Takita,
at Roswell Park, observed that 54% of his bronchogenic cancer cases with
postoperative infection survived five years. Staphylococcus and Pseudomonas aeruginosa were the two most frequently isolated organisms (49).
Orton used a streptococcal vaccine prior to removing the lesion. This
patient developed a lung abscess and remained well 15 years later (5).
Spontaneous regression of an inoperable bronchogenic cancer has been reported following concurrent infection (51).

Since empyema is a serious complication which one cannot induce
therapeutically, one may achieve the same immunostimulation by administering bacterial vaccines such as Staphage Lysate, SPL (Delmont Laboratories)
or BAC (Hoffmann Laboratories) or Pseudomonas aeruginosa vaccine by aerosol and by intracutaneous injections before, as well as after lung surgery. These agents are non-toxic and can be continued on an ambulatory
basis. McKneally, et al. have used intrapleural BCG (a single postoperative injection in 40 patients). BCG increased survival significantly in
patients with a limited tumor burden: no recurrance or deaths in 17 Stage
I cases as compared to 9 of 22 controls (50).

Meyer and Benjafield have postulated that a contributory factor to
the increase in cancer may be the widespread use of antibiotics since
1940: "The antibiotics may absolve the body of the need to bring the normal immunological mechanism into use - a mechanism that has been acquired
and perfected through millions of years of evolution" (54). The incidence of lung cancer began to increase very rapidly in just the period in
which tuberculosis had been controlled so successfully. Of course,
cigarette smoking has played a role in this increase.

The beneficial effect of fever, heat and inflammation has also been
studied, not only on existing cancer but on cancer incidence (56). In
Japan, the daily use of the hot, full bath (42°-48°C.) may destroy incipient cancers before they are apparent. This practice may be one reason
why the incidence of cancers of the breast, penis, testis and skin is
much lower in Japan than elsewhere (57).

The most dramatic of the so-called spontaneous regressions of cancer
reported in the past 200 years occurred following an acute febrile bacterial infection (55).* Duration of such infections played a significant
role in survival. A brief attack of erysipelas produced the largest number of initial complete or partial regressions, but the largest number of
permanent results occurred after the more prolonged suppurative types of
infections such as the staphylococcal or mixed pyogenic infections (1).

In this connection, it was found that in the treatment of cancer by
Coley Toxins the duration of this form of immunotherapy was of critical
importance. Fourteen of 17 osteogenic sarcoma patients treated for 4
months or more were permanent successes. The 3 who died survived 4-13
years after onset. These tumors treated by amputation alone usually died
of pulmonary metastases within 10 to 12 months (58).(Fig. 5)

 * Patients receiving Coley Toxins had a higher percentage of permanent
results if febrile reactions averaged over 38.5°C, especially in the inoperable cases. (Fig. 4)

Extensive inoperable vascular tumors involving the soft tissues or pelvic girdle should not be destroyed so rapidly with bacterial vaccines that the excretory, reticuloendothelial and lymphoid tissues are overwhelmed and toxemia develops (2, 4, 5, 14). To avoid this problem, some of the necrotic tumor may be evacuated, or drainage established. Streptococcal enzymes may also be used (59, 60). Through their catalytic and enzymatic properties they facilitate the elimination of necrotic debris, permit more effective use of drugs, and aid in healing and regeneration of tissues destroyed by the tumor.

Thornes has made extensive studies since 1961 of the role of proteolytic enzymes in the treatment of cancer and leukemia (61). Immunotherapy of cancer requires an active immune system. Prognosis is poor in patients with anergy (inactive or blocked T lymphocytes) (61). By using streptokinase or Protease I (Brinase) from Aspergillus oryzae, he was able to induce fibrinolysis for long periods. The first controlled study involved carcinoma of the colon and rectum following resection (62). A single dose of streptokinase increased 5 year survival in the treated group to 76% as compared to 42% in the controls. It is believed that, in addition to its fibrinolytic effect, streptokinase stimulates the immune mechanism: it decreases postoperative fall in lymphocytes (32% as compared to 50% in the controls) (63).

In order to convert anergic patients with Brinase therapy it is necessary to use 100 mg. by intravenous infusion over one hour and to make the intradermal antigen injections within 4 hours after Brinase infusion. Weekly infusion of Brinase and vaccination with BCG resulted in conversion of 4 patients from anergy to allergy. Leukocyte migration is also much stimulated immediately after an infusion of Brinase (64). Thornes stated: "No patient previously anergic, but treated with Brinase or streptokinase with a minimum tumor load following successful surgery, has reverted to a state of anergy since we started in 1972" (62). The lysosomal activity of patients' leukocytes is markedly increased following induction of fibrinolysis: approximately 300% as compared to a 50% increase after Levamisole therapy.

Thornes observed that "many immunosuppressed cancer patients do not give any history of infectious disease" (65). Ungar also reported a much lower incidence of infectious diseases and allergies in a large number of cancer patients as compared to the non-cancerous over a period of years in Basel. He cited similar observations by other physicians (66). In cancer patients who are anergic to a spectrum of agents that induce delayed hypersensitivity, Brinase aids the return of immunologic competence (67, 68).

Possibly much of the benefit observed following streptococcal infections may be due to streptokinase activity. Since such enzymes are thermolabile, the heat-killed preparations of Coley Toxins did not contain them. At the present time the possible benefit of combining Brinase or streptokinase with bacterial vaccine therapy of cancer should be widely explored.

Wolf and Ransberger have used proteolytic enzymes for many years in the treatment of a large number of cancer patients (69).

In recent years a number of clinical studies of various microbial products have been undertaken here and abroad, including BCG (70-75),

Corynebacterium parvum (76-78), and to a lesser extent, Glucan (79-81) and Staphage Lysate (LPS) (82-85), and Streptokinase (63, 67, 68). These last three agents deserve more widespread use.

Since bacterial vaccines greatly increase the nonspecific resistance of cancer patients to infections, provided they are administered prior to the terminal stage, and since they promote wound healing, regeneration of bone, potentiation of response to radiation or chemotherapy, oncologists should now consider using them routinely before surgery, radiation or chemotherapy of solid tumors or leukemia (2-5, 14, 17, 19, 23, 24, 31, 33, 57).

It is hoped that our study of results obtained with Coley Toxins, which parallel those seen with other immunotherapeutic microbial products, may encourage wider use of such agents at the present time, not merely as a last resort when the immune status of cancer patients is seriously compromised, but prior to, during and after the conventional modalities.

Conclusions

The end result studies cited above revealed the following significant findings which affected prognosis with this method, and which were not readily apparent until these studies were made (2-5, 14-24, 57).

1. The variability of the 16 preparations of Coley Toxins.

2. The lack of recognition of the critical importance of the site of injection, dose level and frequency, and especially of the duration of toxin therapy.

3. The stage of the disease: far advanced or terminal cancers in elderly patients, or in those whose immune responses had been destroyed or weakened by prior immunosuppressive therapy, produced few permanent successes, although in many such cases significant palliation occurred.

4. The importance of timing in combination therapies: the best results occurred when injections were begun prior to surgery, irradiation, or chemotherapy.

5. With inoperable cases, partial removal, by reducing the tumor burden, may increase the percentage of permanent results.

6. In the operable cases, when used as an adjuvant to surgery, injections should be started prior to excision or amputation, making some injections into the tumor or its immediate periphery to increase the inflammatory and immunological reactions in the tumor site.

7. Proteolytic enzymes such as streptokinase or Brinase should now be evaluated in conjunction with BCG and bacterial vaccine therapy.

8. The several mechanisms of action whereby microbial vaccines and enzymes exert their effects in destroying tumors must receive much further

study on an international cooperative scale, so that modern oncologists can use these agents to greatest advantage in the overall treatment of neoplastic diseases.

Acknowledgment

The author wishes to express her deepest appreciation to Drs. Alexander Brunschwig, George A. Fowler, Norman L. Higinbotham, Theodore R. Miller, Louis Pelner, Gregory Schwartzman, Walker E. Swift, and most especially, to Dr. Lloyd J. Old, for their invaluable guidance and encouragement over the years; to Lilian Delmonte, Ph.D. for her invaluable help in preparing the graphs and tables, and to Carol Landrey for typing the manuscript.

TABLE I. 5-Year Survival of 894 Patients with Various Types of Tumors Treated with Coley's Toxins

| Type of Tumor | Total No. of Cases | 5-Year Survival | | | |
| | | Inoperable | | Operable | |
		No.	%	No.	%
Bone Tumors					
Ewing's Sarcoma	114	11/52	21	18/62	29
Osteogenic Sarcoma	162	3/23	13	43/139	31
Retic. Cell Sarcoma	72	9/49	18	13/23	57
Multiple Myeloma	12	4/ 8	50	2/ 4	50
Giant Cell Tumor	57	15/19	79	33/38	87
Soft Tissue Sarcomas					
Lymphosarcoma	86	42/86	49	-	-
Hodgkin's Disease	15	10/15	67	-	-
Other Soft Tissue Sarcomas	186	77/137	56	35/49	72
Gynecological Tumors					
Breast Cancer	33	13/20	65	13/13	100
Ovarian Cancer	16	10/15	67	1/1	(100)
Cervical Carcinoma	3	2/ 3	67	-	-
Uterine Sarcoma	11	8/11	73	-	-
Other Tumors					
Testicular Cancer*	64	14/43*	34	15/21	71
Malignant Melanoma	31	10/17	60	10/14	71
Colorectal Cancer	13	5/11	46	2/ 2	(100)
Renal Cancer (adult)	8	3/ 7	43	1/ 1	(100)
Renal Cancer (Wilms' Tumor)	3	-	-	1/ 3	33
Neuroblastoma	9	1/ 6	17	2/ 3	67
TOTAL	894	237/522	45	189/373	51

*including 16 terminal cases

TABLE II. Immunotherapy (Coley's Toxins) Combined with Conservation Surgery or Amputation

Type of Tumor	Total No. of Cases	Permanent Successes*			
		Conservative Surgery		Amputation	
		No. of Cases	%	No. of Cases	%
Retic. Cell Sarcoma	29	16/ 26	62	1/ 3	33
Soft Tissue Sarcomas					
Inoperable	21	6/ 17	35	0/ 4	0
Operable	22	8/ 10	80	6/ 12	50
Osteogenic Sarcoma	126	9/ 15	60	36/111	33
Giant Cell Tumor	43	24/ 25	96	4/ 18	22
Ewing's Tumor	53	10/ 35	29	6/ 18	30
TOTAL	294	73/128	57	53/166	32

* Traced 5-58 Years

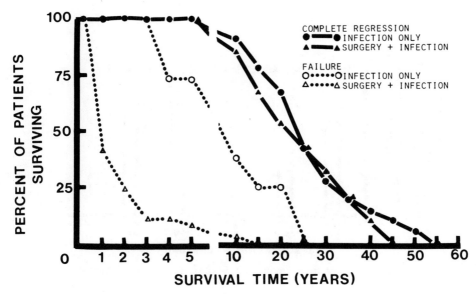

FIG. 1. Clinical Course of 222 patients with cancer, after acute bacterial infection.

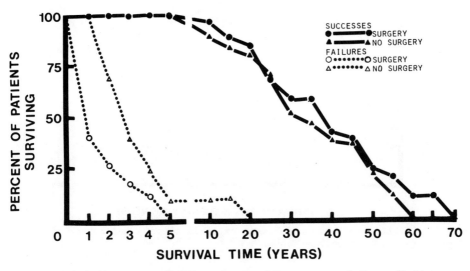

FIG. 2. Clinical course of 180 patients with sarcoma of the soft tissues (non-lymphomatous) treated with toxins.

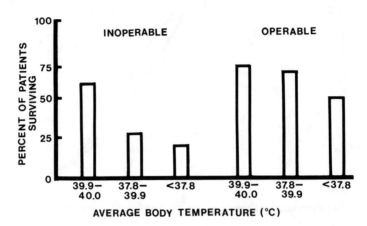

FIG. 3. Correlation between fever and 5-year survival of patients with cancer.

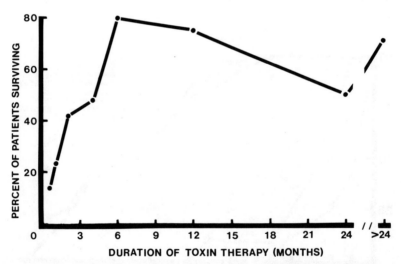

FIG. 4. Correlation between duration of toxin therapy and 5-year survival of patients with inoperable cancer.

References

1. Nauts, H. C. The Apparently Beneficial Effects of Bacterial Infections On Host Resistance To Cancer: End Results In 435 Cases. New York Cancer Research Institute* Monogr. (N.Y.) 8: 1-829, 1969. (969 References)

2. Nauts, H. C., Fowler, G. A., Bogatko, F. H. A Review Of The Influence Of Bacterial Infection And Of Bacterial Products (Coley's Toxins) On Malignant Tumors In Man. Acta Med. Scand. 45, Suppl. 276: 1-103, April, 1953.

3. Miller, T. N., Nicholson, J. T. End Results In Reticulum Cell Sarcoma Of Bone Treated By Toxin Therapy Alone Or Combined With Surgery And/Or Radiation (47 Cases) Or With Concurrent Infection (5 Cases). Cancer 27: 524-548, 1971.

4. Nauts, H. C. Giant Cell Tumor Of Bone: End Results Following Immunotherapy (Coley Toxins) Alone Or Combined With Surgery And/Or Radiation (66 Cases), Or With Concurrent Infection (4 Cases). Cancer Research Institute Monogr. (N.Y.) 4: 1976.

5. Nauts, H. C. Osteogenic Sarcoma: End Results Following Immunotherapy (Bacterial Vaccines) 165 Cases, Or Concurrent Infections, Inflammation Or Fever, 41 Cases. Cancer Research Institute Monogr. (N.Y.) 15:1-120, 1975.

6. Coley, W. B. A Plea For More Conservative Treatment Of Sarcoma Of the Long Bones. J.A.M.A. 54: 333-343, 1910.

7. Coley, W. B. Central Sarcoma Of The Lower End Of The Femur With Extensive Involvement Of The Knee Joint Successfully Treated With The Mixed Toxins Of Erysipelas And Bacillus Prodigiosus. Ann. Surg. 65:370-373, 1917.

8. Coley, W. B. Central Sarcoma Of The Radius. Clinical And X-Ray Diagnosis, Inoperable Without Sacrifice Of The Arm. Ann.Surg. 69:551-553, 1919.

9. Coley, W. B. Very Large Inoperable Sarcoma Of The Upper Portion Of The Femur, Following A Recent Fracture; Disappearance Under Combined Toxins And Radium Treatment. Ann. Surg. 69: 553-554, 1919.

10. Coley, W. B. Periosteal Spindle-celled Sarcoma Of the Tibia, With Metastases In The Inguinal And Femoral Glands; Disappearance Under Toxin And Radium Treatment; Well At Present Nearly Two Years. Ann. Surg. 69: 654-657, 1919.

11. Coley, W. B. Further Observations On The Conservative Treatment Of Sarcoma Of The Long Bones. Ann. Surg. 70: 633-660, 1919.

12. Coley, W. B. The Value Of Conservative Treatment In Sarcoma Of The Long Bones. Ann. Surg. 74: 655-661, 1921.

13. Coley, W. B. Endothelial Myeloma Or Ewing's Sarcoma. Radiology 16: 627-656, 1931.

14. Nauts, H. C. Beneficial Effects Of Immunotherapy (Bacterial Toxins) On Sarcoma Of The Soft Tissues, Other Than Lymphosarcoma. Cancer Research Institute Monogr. (N.Y.) 16: 1-219, 1975.

15. Nauts, H. C., Fowler, G. A. End Results In Lymphosarcoma Treated By Toxin Therapy Alone Or Combined With Surgery And/Or Radiation. New York Cancer Research Institute* Monogr. (N.Y.) 6: 1-119, 1969.

16. Nauts, H. C. Immunological Factors Affecting Incidence, Prognosis And Survival In Breast Cancer. Part 1: The Immunopotentiating Effects Of Concurrent Infections, Inflammation Or Fever. Part II: Immunotherapy, Effects Of Bacterial Vaccines. Cancer Research Institute Monogr.(N.Y.) 17: To Be Published.

17. Fowler, G. A. Beneficial Effects Of Acute Bacterial Infections Or Bacterial Toxin Therapy On Cancer Of The Colon Or Rectum. New York Cancer Research Institute* Monogr. (N.Y.) 10: 1-57, 1969.

18. Cancer Research Institute Records, Data Not Yet Published.

19. Nauts, H. C. Enhancement Of Natural Resistance To Renal Cancer: Beneficial Effects Of Concurrent Infections And Immunotherapy With Bacterial Vaccines. New York Cancer Research Institute* Monogr. (N.Y.) 12: 1-96, 1973.

20. Fowler, G. A. Testicular Cancer Treated By Bacterial Toxin Therapy As A Means Of Enhancing Host Resistance. End Results In 63 Determinate Cases. New York Cancer Research Institute* Monogr. (N.Y.) 7: 1-38, 1968.

21. Fowler, G. A. Enhancement Of Natural Resistance To Malignant Melanoma With Special Reference To The Beneficial Effects Of Concurrent Infections And Bacterial Toxin Therapy. New York Cancer Research Institute* Monogr. (N.Y.) 9: 1-85, 1969.

22. Fowler, G. A., Nauts, H. C. The Apparently Beneficial Effects of Concurrent Infections, Inflammation Or Fever, And Of Bacterial Toxin Therapy, On Neuroblastoma. New York Cancer Research Institute* Monogr. (N.Y.) 11: 1-82, 1970.

23. Nauts, H. C. Ewing's Sarcoma Of Bone: End Results Following Immunotherapy (Bacterial Toxins) Combined With Surgery And/Or Radiation. Cancer Research Institute Monogr. (N.Y.) 14: 1-108, 1974.

24. Nauts, H. C. Multiple Myeloma: Beneficial Effects Of Acute Infections Or Immunotherapy (Bacterial Vaccines). Cancer Research Institute Monogr. (N.Y.) 12: 1-96, 1975.

25. Sykes, M. P., Chu, F., Case, T. S., McKenzie, S. Follow-up On The Long Term Effects Of Therapeutic Irradiation On Bone Marrow. Radiology 113: 179-180, 1974.

25a. Gershon, R. K., Carter, R. L. Factors Controlling Concomitant Immunity In Tumor Bearing Hamster. The Effects Of Prior Splenectomy And Of Tumor Removal. J. Natl. Cancer Inst. 43:533-543, 1969.

26. Coley, W. B. Treatment Of Inoperable Malignant Tumors With Toxins Of Erysipelas And The Bacillus Prodigiosus. Trans. Amer. Surg. Assn. 12: 183-212, 1894.

27. Coley, W. B. Further Observations Upon The Treatment Of Malignant Tumors With The Mixed Toxins Of Erysipelas And Bacillus Prodigiosus With A Report Of 160 Cases. Bull. Johns Hopkins Hosp. 65:157-162,1896. (Abst. J.A.M.A. 27: 1001, 1896; Canada Pract. 21: 737-750, 1896; Canada Lancet 29: 67-77, 1896.)

28. Coley, W. B. The Treatment Of Inoperable Sarcoma By Bacterial Toxins (The Mixed Toxins Of The Streptococcus Of Erysipelas And The Baccillus Prodigiosus). Practitioner (London) 83: 589-613, 1909.(Also in Proc. Royal Soc. Med., Surg., Sect. 3: 1-48, 1909-1910; Abst. Brit. M.J. 2: 144-145, 1909)

29. Coley, W. B. The Treatment Of Malignant Inoperable Tumors With The Mixed Toxins Of Erysipelas And Bacillus Prodigiosus, With A Brief Report of 80 Cases Successfully Treated With the Toxins From 1893-1914. M. Weissenbruch, Brussels, p.172, 1914.

30. Ainsworth, E. J., Forbes, P. D. The Effect Of Pseudomonas Pyrogen On Survival Of Irradiated Mice. Radiation Research 14: 767-774, 1961.

31. Hollcraft, J. W., Smith, W. W. Endotoxin Treatment And X-Irradiation In Mice Bearing Transplanted Tumors. J. Nat. Cancer Inst. 21:311-330, 1958.

32. Smith, W. W., Alderman, I. M., Gillespie, R. E. Increased Survival In Irradiated Animals Treated With Bacterial Endotoxins. Amer.J.Physiol. 191: 124-130, 1957.

33. Smith, W. W., Alderman, I. M., Gillespie, R. E. Hematopoietic Recovery Induced By Bacterial Endotoxin In Irradiated Mice. Amer.J. Physiol. 192: 549-556, 1958.

34. Old, L. J., Benacerraf, B., Clarke, D. A., Carswell, E. A., Stockert, E. The Role Of the Reticuloendothelial System In The Host Reaction To Neoplasia. Cancer Research 21: 1281-1300, 1961.

35. Old, L. J., Boyse, E. A. Current Enigmas In Cancer Research. The Harvey Lectures, Series 67: 273-315, 1973.

36. Klein, G. Immunological Surveillance Against Neoplasia. The Harvey Lectures, Series 69: 71-102, 1975.

37. Nauts, H. C. Host Resistance to Cancer. Review Of The Early And Recent Literature.New York Cancer Research Inst.*Mongr.(N.Y.) 5: 1-403, 1970.

38. Huth, E. Die Bedeutung Der Sogenannten Spontanheilungen Und Remissionen Für Die Therapie Und Pathogenese Der Leukosen Und Malignen Tumoren. Zeitschr. F. Krebsf. 58: 524-575, 1952.

39. Huth, E. Leukamie Und Infektion. Kinderarzliche Praxis 25: 448-456, 1957.

40. Huth, E. Die Rolle Der Bakteriellen Infektionen Bei Der Spontanremiss-ion Maligner Tumoren Und Leukosen. In: Körpereigene Abwehr Und Bö-ŝartige Geschwülste. Tumorbeeinglussung Durch Hyperthermie Under Hyper amie. Lambert, H., Selawry, O., eds. Ulm, 1957.

41. Nauts, H. C., Fowler, G. A., Pelner, L. Effects Of Concurrent Infect-ions And Their Toxins On The Course Of Leukemia. Acta Med. Scand. 162: Supple. 338, 1958.

42. Clarkson, B., Dowling, M. D., Gee, T. S., Cunningham, I., Burchenal, J. H. Treatment Of Acute Leukemia In Adults. Cancer 36: 775-795, 1975.

43. Young, L. S., Meyer, R. D., Armstrong, D. Pseudomonas Acruginosa Vaccine In Cancer Patients. Ann. Intern. Med. 79: 518-527, 1973.

44. LeRoux, B. T. Empyema Thoracis. Brit. J. Surg. 52: 89-99,1965.

45. Moore, G. E. Iatrogenic Immunotherapy Of Lung Cancer. New Eng. J. Med. 287: 1041-1043, 1972.

46. Ruckdeschel, J. C., Codish, S. D., Stranahan, A., McKneally, M. F. Post-Operative Empyema Improves Survival In Lung Cancer. Documentation And Analysis Of A Natural Experiment. New Eng. J. Med. 267: 1013-1017, 1972.

47. Cady, B., Cliffton, E. E. Empyema And Survival Following Surgery For Bronchogenic Carcinoma. J. Thorac. and Cardio. Surg. 53: 102-108, 1967.

48. Sensenig, D. M., Rossi, N. P., Ehrenhaft, J. L. Results Of Surgical Treatment Of Bronchiogenic Carcinoma. Surg. Gyn. and Obst. 116: 279-284, 1963.

49. Takita, H. Effect Of Postoperative Empyema On Survival of Patients With Bronchogenic Carcinoma. J. Thoracic Cardiovascular Surg. 59: 642-644, 1970.

50. McKneally, M. F., Maver, C., Kausel, H. W. Regional Immunotherapy Of Lung Cancer With Intrapleural BCG. Lancet 1: 377-379, 1976.

51. Blades, B., McCorkle, R. C., Jr. A Case Of Spontaneous Regression Of An Untreated Bronchiogenic Carcinoma. J. Thoracic Surg. 27: 415-419, 1954.

52. Shayegani, M., DeCourcy, S. J., Jr., Mudd, S. Cell-Mediated Immunity In Mice Infected With S. Aureus And Elicited With Specific Bacterial Antigens. J. Reticuloendothelial Soc. 14: 44-51, 1973.

53. Editorial: Postoperative Immunosuppression. Lancet 2: 817-818, 1975.

54. Meyer, B. A., Benjafield, J. D. Carcinoma And Antibiotics. Med. Press 234: 206-208, 1955.

55. Nauts, H. C. Pyrogen Therapy Of Cancer: An Historical Overview And Current Activities. Read At The International Symposium On Cancer Therapy By Hyperthermia And Radiation, Washington, D.C., April, 1975. (In Press)

56. Glynn, L. E., Holborrow, J. The Production Of Complete Antigens From Polysaccharide Haptenes By Streptococci And Other Organisms. J. Path. And Bact. 64: 775-783, 1952.

57. Nauts, H. C. Immunotherapy Of Cancer By Microbial Products. In: Host Defense Against Cancer And Its Potentiation. Mizuno, D., et al, eds. University Of Tokyo Press, Tokyo., Univ. Park Press, Baltimore, pp. 337-351, 1975.

58. Kuehn, P. G., Tamoney, H. J., Gossling, H. R. Iliac Vein Occlusion Prior To Amputation For Sarcoma. Cancer 26: 536-546, 1970.

59. Johnson, A. J. Cytological Studies In Association With Local Injections Of Streptokinase-streptodornase In Patients. J. Clin. Invest. 29: 1376-1386, 1950.

60. Tillett, W. S., Sherry, S., Christensen, L. R., Johnson, A. J. Hazelhurst, G. Streptococcal Enzymatic Debridement. Ann. Surg. 131: 12-22, 1950.

61. Thornes, R. D., Kee, J. L., Devlin, J. G., MacDonell, J. D. Complement Dependent Cytotoxic Autoantibodies In Patients With Acute Leukaemia Following Fibrinolytic Therapy By Protease I Of Aspergillus Oryzae. Irish J. Med. Sc. 3: 107-114, 1970.

62. Thornes, R. D. Adjuvant Therapy Of Cancer Via Cellular Immune Mechanism Or Fibrin By Induced Fibrinolysis And Oral Anticoagulants. Cancer 35: 91-97, 1975.

63. Clery, A. P., Hogan, B. L., Holland, P. D. L., Widdness, J. D. H., Ryan, M., Doyle, S. J., Burke, G. J., Thornes, R. D. Early Experience In A Controlled Clinical Trial Using Streptokinase Induced Fibrinolysis During Resections For Colon And Rectal Carcinomas In An Attempt To Prevent Haematogenous Metastasis. J. Irish Coll. Phys. & Surg. 1: 91-94, 1972.

64. Holland, P. D. J., Browne, O., Thornes, R. D. The Enhancing Influence Of Proteolysis On E Rosette Forming Lymphocytes (T Cells) In Vivo And In Vitro. Br. J. Cancer 31: 164-169, 1975.

65. Thornes, R. D. Immunological Control Of Cancer. Lancet 1: 626, 1975.

66. Ungar, F. H. Problems Of Allergy And Malignant Tumors. Acta Unio. Intern. Contra Cancrum. 9: 213-216, 1953.

67. Thornes, R. D., Smyth, H., Browne, O., O'Gorman, M., Reen, D. J., Holland, P. D. J. The Effects Of Proteolysis On The Human Immune Mechanism; A Preliminary Communication. J. Med. 5: 92-97, 1974.

68. Thornes, R. D. Fibrinolytic Therapy In Leukaemia. J. Royal Coll. Surg. Ireland 6: 123-128, 1971.

69. Wolf, M., Ransberger, K. Enzyme Therapy. Vantage Press, New York, pp. 1-240, 1972.

70. Nathanson, L. Use Of BCG In The Treatment Of Human Neoplasms:A Review. Seminars In Oncol. 1: 337-350, 1974.

71. Mastrangelo, M. J., Bellet, R. E., Berkelhammer, J., Clark, W. H., Jr. Regression Of Pulmonary Metastatic Disease Associated With Intralesional BCG Therapy Of Intracutaneous Melanoma Metastases. Cancer 36: 1305-1308, 1975.

72. Morton, D. L., Eilber, F. R., Holmes, E. C., Hunt, J. S., Ketcham, A. S., Silverstein, M. J., Sparks, F. C. BCG Immunotherapy Of Malignant Melanoma. Summary Of A Seven Year Experience. Ann. Surg. 180: 635-643, 1974.

73. Maviglit, G. M., Gutterman, J. U., Burgess, M. A., Khankhanian, N., Seibert, G. B., Speer, J. F., Reed, R. C., Jubert, A. V., Margin,R.C., McBride, C. M., Copeland, E. M., Gehan, E. A., Hersh, E. M. Prolongation Of Postoperative Disease-free Interval And Survival By Administration Of Bacillus Calmette-Guerin (BCG) vs. BCG Plus 5-Fluorouracil In Human Colo-rectal Cancer Of The Duke's Classification. (In Press)

74. Eilber, F. R., Morton, D. L., Holmes,K. P., Sparks, F. C., Ramming, K. P. Adjuvant Immunotherapy With BCG In Treatment Of Regional Lymph Node Metastases From Malignant Melanoma. New Eng. J. Med. 294:237-240,1976.

75. Cardenas, J. O., Gutterman, J. U., Hersh, E. M., Maviglit, G. M., Blumenschein, G. R., Livingston, R. B., Freirich, E. J., Gottlieb,J.A. Chemoimmunotherapy Of Disseminated Breast Cancer:Prolongation Of Remission And Survival With BCG. (In Press)

76. Halpern, B., Fray, A., Crepin, Y., Platica, O., Lorinet, L., Isac, R. Corynebacterium Parvum, A Potent Immunostimulant In Experimental Infections And In Malignancies. In: Immunopotentiation. Ciba Foundation Symposium 18 (new series) ASP Elsevier, Excerpta Medica, North Holland, Amsterdam, 1973.

77. Israel, L. Report On 414 Cases Of Human Tumors Treated With Corynebacteria. In: Corynebacterium Parvum, Applications In Experimental And Clinical Oncology. Halpern, B. N., ed., Plenum Press, New York, pp. 389-401, 1975.

78. Israel, L., Edelstein, R., Depierre, A., Dimitrov, N. Daily Intravenous Injections Of Corynebacterium Parvum in 20 Patients With Disseminated Cancer; A Preliminary Report And Biological findings. J. Nat. Cancer Inst. 55: 29-33, 1974.

79. Mansell, P. W. A., Ichinose, H., Reed, R. J., Krementz, E. T.,McNamee, R., Di Luzio, N. R. Macrophage Mediated Destruction Of Human Malignant Cells In Vivo. J. Nat. Cancer Inst. 54: 571-580, 1975.

80. Di Luzio, N. R., Pisano, J. C., Saba, T. M. Evaluation Of The Mechanism Of Glucan-Induced Stimulation Of The Reticuloendothelial System. J. Reticuloendothelial Soc. 7: 731-742, 1970.

81. Di Luzio, N. R., McNamee, R., Jones, E., Lasoff, S., Sear, W., Hoffman, E. O. Inhibition Of Growth Of Shay Myelogenous Leukemia Tumor In Rats By Glucan And Activated Macrophages. In: Proc. VII. International Congress Of The Reticuloendothelial Society. Plenum Press, N. Y., 1975.

82. Mudd, S. Resistance Against Staphylococcus Aureus. J.A.M.A. 218: 1671-1673, 1971.

83. Dean, H. J., Silva, J. S., McCoy, J. L., Chan, S. P. Baker, J. J., Leonard, C., Herberman, R. B. In Vitro Human Reactivity To Staphylococcal Phage Lysate. J. Immun. 115: 1060-1064, 1975.

84. Dean, J. H. Silva, J. S., McCoy, J. L., Leonard, C. M., Cannon, G. B., Herberman, R. B. Functional Activities Of Rosette Separated Human Peripheral Blood Lymphocytes. J. Immun. 115: 1449-1455, 1975.

85. Mudd, S., Baker, A. G. Nonspecific Cell Mediated Immunity In The Treatment of Recurrent Herpes Virus And Aphthous Ulcers. In: Proc. First Intersectional Congress Of IAMS, Hasegawa, T., ed., Science Council of Japan, 4: 459-470, 1975.

Chapter 5

ENDOCRINOLOGY

USE OF HORMONES AND HUMAN TUMORIGENESIS

Edward F. Lewison, M.D.

Johns Hopkins Hospital
Baltimore, Maryland

Among the many aphorisms of Osler perhaps one of the most famous is the maxim that "medicine is a science of uncertainty and an art of probability" (4). However, today with our more modern epidemiologic methods, our micro-hormonal immuno-assays and the cornucopia of the computer, our clinical science is becoming more precise and our clinical dilemmas are being successfully solved. Certainly this seems true regarding the causal relationship of the use of hormones to the development of certain kinds of human tumors both benign and malignant.

In the present discussion I will limit my remarks to four specific types of human tumors all of which appear to show some correlation with the use of hormones. These tumors are (1) breast, (2) endometrium, (3) vagina and (4) liver. The long-term use of exogenous hormones has been implicated as a possible etiologic agent in each of these human tumors. Whether these remarkable hormonal agents will prove to the miracles of our modern age or the malice and mischief-makers of our materia medica remains to be seen. The triumphs and the thorns of our everyday clinical experience will determine the ultimate role in our clinical practice of these so-called "wonder-drugs".

Breast

There is ample experimental evidence (animal models) to indicate that the breast is a hormone sensitive end-organ. Doisey and Allen (10) in 1923 demonstrated that crude ovarian extracts were remarkably potent growth stimulants for the epithelium of the female genital tract. Human breast development in the female begins at puberty with the onset of hormonal activity. The importance of ovarian activity in the development of breast cancer is indicated by the fact that this malignant disease never occurs prior to the dawn of estrogenic awakening. However, during the reproductive years there is a marked exponential increase in its incidence. Cyclic menstrual changes in the breast are in part related to periodic hormonal changes and certainly the hypertrophy and enlargement of the breast which occurs with pregnancy is primarily a hormonal response.

The notable discovery of the existence of estrogen receptors and other steroid hormone receptors in breast cancer

and breast cell cytoplasm has led to the development of estrogen receptor assays and prolactin and other steroid hormone
assays which can be of immense value in the clinical treatment
of this disease. About one-third of all breast cancer patients
have a high level of positive estrogen receptor in their cytoplasm. Also, of great importance in implicating estrogens in
the etiology of breast cancer is the fact that more tha 99 per
cent of the patients are female and less than one per cent of
patients are male.

Gynecomastia can be caused by hormonal stimulation in men
receiving estrogens for cancer of the prostate or other medical
reasons. Enlargement of the male breast has been observed in
stilbestrol factory workers, as well as in men with estrogen
producing tumors. Therefore, it seems quite obvious that both
endogenous and exogenous hormones --- particularly estrogens --
can affect the breast and thus may be important in the etiology
of breast cancer.

Almost a hundred years ago Schinziger (20) suggested
surgical castration for patients with advanced breast cancer.
Shortly thereafter Beatson (5) of Glasgow first reported a
series of women some of whom were successfully treated by
ovariectomy. "Eight months after castration all vestiges of
(breast) cancer had disappeared."

More modern studies have shown that bilateral oophorec-
tomy performed in premenopausal women for pelvic disease unrelated to the breast resulted in a lowered incidence of breast
cancer. Feinleib (13) of Boston has shown that women who
undergo an artificial menopause early in life by the removal
of their ovaries have a reduced risk of developing breast
cancer by about 75 per cent. MacMahon et al (17) has reported
that those women with first births after the age of 35 had
three times the risk of breast cancer than those with first
births before the age of 18. Statistical studies both here
and abroad have noted a definite break or "hook" in the
incidence of breast cancer during the age-range of the menopause. This has been attributed to hormonal changes within
the body occurring at this time of life. As a "mastiatrist"
and surgeon treating breast disease I have frequently observed
that the signs and symptoms of chronic cystic mastitis have a
tendency to subside after the menopause. Many large series
·the world over have uniformly indicated that in premenopausal
women with advanced breast cancer therapeutic castration
produces a clinical improvement and objective regression of the
disease in about 35 per cent of these relatively young and
hormone responsive patients.

Although it is well recognized that small doses of
exogenous estrogens have a stimulating effect upon a pre-
existing breast cancer, yet how ominous is the threat of
long-term low-dose estrogen therapy or oral contraceptives
in high-risk, premalignant or carcinoma-in-situ breast lesions?
Whereas, some women take estrogens to remain feminine forever--
in the illusion of being "a thing of beauty and a joy forever"
--there are other women who may require estrogens for medically sound and sensible reasons. Yet, what is the risk-benefit
ratio regarding the use of these hormones and the development
of human cancer?

Estrogens have been clearly shown by Lyons, Li and Johnson (16) to act directly on normal breast tissue cells to
promote their growth and differentiation. Estrogen also
stimulates the release of pituitary prolactic which in turn
also effects the breast cells. As Boyland (8) has noted more
than a hundred different species of plants contain estrogenic
substances some of which we eat in our daily diet and become
a rarely recognized source of exogenous hormone ingestion.
Other plant estrogens are eaten by domestic farm animals
which we ultimately consume as meat. The biologic in vivo
activity of these estrogenic food-stuffs is, of course,
dependent upon many factors most important of which is the
activity of our liver and digestive tract.

Breast cancer is "easy to see, but hard to foresee". In
my opinion prudence requires that women with a "high-risk"
predisposition for breast cancer, as well as for cancer of
other sites, should avoid the long-term stimulation of estrogen therapy to prevent the possibility of tumor progression
or tumor development. In the case of breast cancer clinical
experience bears sad witness to the fact that the co-existence
of pregnancy, with its markedly elevated level of estrogens,
and the onset of breast cancer carries with it a most ominous
kind of prognosis. A recent report by Symmers (22) in the
British Medical Journal describes the tragedy of two male
transvestites both of whom developed and died of breast cancer
after long-term estrogen therapy. A young female child taking
her mother's birth control pills by mistake has been reported
to have developed breast cancer. However, all of these wisps
of evidence are merely straws in a wistful wind.

There have been, however, several important epidemiologic
studies which have explored the relationship between breast
cancer, estrogens and the pill. These include our own study
at the Johns Hopkins Hospital (1), as well as the Boston
Drug Survey (7), the retrospective study of Vessey, Doll and
Sutton (23), the reports of Black and Leis (6), and Burch,
Byrd and Vaugh (9), as well as the comprehensive report of the
Royal College of General Practitioners (19) and the most recent
case-control study of Fasal and Paffenbarger (11). These
investigations surveyed 1770 San Francisco women, including
452 with breast cancer and 446 with benign breast disease and
872 controls. This extensive study, however, included only
oral contraceptives and did not include estrogenic hormones
taken for other purposes. "Although the relative risk of
developing breast cancer among the 'ever-users' of the pill
was only 1.1, the risk among women using the pill for from
2 to 4 years was significantly increased to 1.9 and this risk
increased to 2.5 for these 2 to 4 year users who were on the
pill when interviewed." Moreover, a prior operation for benign breast disease increased the cancer risk among long-term
users of the pill by as much as 11-fold. However, in our
Johns Hopkins Hospital study (2) of more than 1332 women
with breast tumors (1048 benign and 284 malignant) and 1085
controls there appeared to be no convincing evidence of a
causal association between breast cancer and the prior use of
either estrogens or the pill. Perhaps we will need a much
larger number of subjects and a much longer period of time

between the drug and the disease to delineate this important and serious relationship.

A new and rather unexpected association between the drug Rauwolfia (Reserpine therapy) and breast cancer has been recently confirmed by three separate international studies. All reveal a three to four fold increase of breast cancer in women taking Reserpine. Most of these women were postmenopausal and the risk factor correlated well with the dosage and duration of treatment. It is well known that certain pharmacologic agents such as reserpine, chlorpromazine and other phenothiazines block the synthesis or action of prolactin inhibiting-factor leading to an increased secretion of prolactin. Prolactin dependence has been directly demonstrated in animal tumors and in about one-third of all human breast cancer. Therefore, even non-hormonal drugs which increase the secretion of prolactin may be of importance in either initiating or enhancing the growth of breast cancer by their action on the hormonal production of prolactin.

Endometrium

In the most recent FDA Drug Bulletin (Feb.-March 1976)(12) there is a warning that "prolonged use of estrogens by postmenopausal women apparently is associated with a marked increase in risk of cancer of the endometrium". This is the result of strong epidemiologic evidence that has appeared within the last few months. Whereas further scientific confirmation is needed, these findings clearly alter the benefit/risk ratio for menopausal women who are currently taking estrogens.

This new medical evidence is provided by four recent reports of considerable significance. A case-control study by Ziel and Finkle (24) from the Kaiser Permanente Medical Center in Los Angeles compared 94 women with endometrial cancer with 188 matched controls. Analysis of the clinical records revealed a much more frequent use of conjugated estrogens in the cancer patients (57 %) compared to the controls (15 %). The estimated risk ratio for endometrial cancer (i.e. risk in estrogen users compared with risk in non-users) was 7.6 overall and this was related to the duration of hormone use. In a second study by Smith and his associates (21) there were 317 women (all over 48 years of age) with endometrial cancer who were compared with an equal number of matched control patients from the same institution. Nearly one-half of the endometrial cancer patients (152) were estrogen users whereas only about one-sixth of the controls (54) used hormones. This resulted in a significant 4.5 fold increase in risk of endometrial cancer among the estrogen exposed women.

The cancer risk as indicated by these studies is, in public health terms, a highly significant one. The Advisory Committee on Obstetrics and Gynecology of the FDA has concluded that these studies provided strong evidence that postmenopausal estrogen therapy increases the risk of endometrial cancer. The Committee agreed that there was need for further data to clarify the relationship between the risk of endometrial cancer and such factors as drug dosage, duration of treatment and cyclic administration. The Food and Drug Administration believes that these new findings linking post-menopausal estrogen administration to endometrial cancer must be considered carefully by every physician who prescribes these drugs and by every woman who takes them. The FDA is planning to provide full warning on the packaging label and to advise physicians regarding the indications for treatment, as well as recommendations that appear to be less hazardous, such as "cyclic administration of the lowest effective dose for the shortest possible time with appropriate monitoring for endometrial cancer".

Vagina

Cancer of the vagina is a relatively rare disease, accounting for only about 2 per cent of all malignant tumors of the female genital tract. The most common histologic type is the squamous cell carcinoma, which usually occurs in women over the age of 50 years. Clear-cell adenocarcinomas are extremely rare, and prior to 1966 they were almost unknown in young women. However quite unexpectedly between 1966 and 1969 seven cases of clear-cell adenocarcinoma of the vagina were seen and reported by Herbst (14) all in patients between the ages of 14 and 22 years of age. A retrospective case-control epidemiologic study at the Massachusetts General Hospital (15) revealed a highly significant association with the ingestion of Diethylstilbestrol (DES) during pregnancy by the mothers of these young patients.

During the mid 1940's, 1950's and 1960's DES was used by hundreds of thousands of pregnant women to support high-risk pregnancy and thus reduce fetal loss. This was accepted practice. By 1971 the Food and Drug Administration warned physicians that these drugs (non-steroid estrogens) were contraindicated during pregnancy because of the demonstrated association with vaginal and cervical clear-cell adenocarcinoma in the exposed female offspring. This 20 or 30 year time lag is quite characteristic of many human carcinogens and the "time-bomb" of this particular hormone has now assumed ominous importance.

Although more than 250 cases of vaginal or cervical clear-cell carcinoma in young females have been reported to the Registry thus far, yet considering the extremely large number of pregnant women exposed to DES during their pregnancy, the risk of development of this type of cancer still remains exceedingly low at the present time. Asymptomatic patients are now being discovered by careful screening examination and local treatment has been highly successful in controlling these early lesions.

The Federal Drug Administration now requires package inserts for DES and closely related congeners (Benzestrol, Dienestrol, Hexestrol, Promethestrol, etc.) warning of the danges of vaginal adenosis and vaginal adenocarcinoma.

Liver

Primary tumors of the liver which were relatively rare among women in the United States previously, have now begun to occur with increasing frequency. Many recent reports have focused our attention on the possible relationship between the long-term use of oral contraceptives and the development of liver tumors and nodular hyperplasia in young women. Baum and his colleagues (3) in 1973 presented the clinical characteristics of seven patients with benign hepatic tumors five of whom presented with massive intraperitoneal hemorrhage and severe shock. The rarity of liver tumors in young women led Baum to speculate on the possible etiologic relationship between these liver tumors and the pill.

Mays and his Associates (18) have recently reported 13 primary hepatic tumors developing in young women all of whom had been taking contraceptive steroids. Nine of these tumors were benign, and four were malignant. However in six of these young women the tumors ruptured spontaneously and caused life-threatening hemorrhage and shock.

Contraceptive hormones have been associated with liver damage and numerous changes in liver function. Impairment of bile-secretory activity as measured by the bromsulphalein test has been noted in between 10 to 40 per cent of women on the pill. Jaundice, hepatomegaly and alterations in other liver function tests have been frequently reported.

Recent clinical experience indicates a markedly increased incidence of liver hyperplasia, liver adenomas and primary liver tumors both benign and malignant in young women who have been taking the pill. Although the etiologic role of these contraceptive hormones remains unproved, yet an associated and close causal link appears likely. It is of considerable importance to note that long-term use as well as the exact type of synthetic estrogen in the pill may be very important factors in determining the ultimate risk in each individual patient.

During the past few years hepatocellular cancers have been reported in a small number of young men who have been taking androgenic-anabolic hormones for a variety of therapeutic reasons --- but mainly for aplastic anemia. These malignant liver tumors metastasize slowly and in some patients the tumors have been known to completely regress after the hormone was discontinued.

Finally, in this discussion concerning the use of hormones and the development of human cancer, we must consider the corticosteroids which are often used as immunosuppressive agents and which have been suspected of contributing to the high incidence of cancer among the recipients of organ transplants. In a recent follow-up study of over 6000 kidney transplants, the risk of lymphoma in a transplant patient was about 35 times normal --- mainly due to the very high incidence of reticulum cell sarcoma. Although corticosteroids are often used with other immunosuppressive agents, it seems reasonable to speculate that this hormone is involved in some alteration of the host defense mechanism leading to an excess incidence of malignancy.

Summary and Conclusions

Thus, the list of evidence is long regarding the use of hormones and human tumorigenesis, but it is still based upon a rather short clinical experience. Final verification and proof require that "we see today with the eyes of tomorrow." Yet, in our present every-day practice we must recognize the uncertainty but continue to rely upon first-hand clinical judgement and epidemiologic evidence which does not become second-hand when used. Cancer is a monstrously destructive disease and the carcinogenic potential of these hormones in some patients must clearly alter the benefit/risk ratio for many women and some men in the high-risk category. In our "science of uncertainty and art of probability" prudence is a virtue which we owe to all our patients.

References

1. Arthes, F.G., Sartwell, P.E. and Lewison, E.F.: The pill, estrogens and the breast. Epidemiologic aspects. Cancer 28:1391-1394, 1971.

2. Arthes, F.G., Sartwell, P.E., Lewison, E.F. and Tonascia, J.: Breast cancer, estrogens and the pill: Presented at the XI International Cancer Conference, Florence, Italy, Oct. 23, 1974.

3. Baum, J.K., Bookstein, J.J., Holtz, F. et al: Possible association between benign hepatomas and oral contraceptives. Lancet 2:926-929, 1973.

4. Bean, R.B.: Sir William Osler Aphorisms, 2nd printing, Springfield, Ill. Charles C. Thomas, 1961, p. 129.

5. Beatson, G.T.: On the treatment of inoperable cases of carcinoma of the mammae: suggestions for new method of treatment. Lancet 2:104-107, 1896.

6. Black, M.M. and Leis, H.P. Jr.: Mammary carcinogenesis - influence of parity and estrogens. N.Y. St. J. Med. 72: 1601, 1972.

7. Boston Collaborative Drug Surveillance Programme: Oral contraceptives and venous thromboembolic disease, surgically confirmed gall-bladder disease and breast tumors. Lancet 1:1399-1404, 1973.

8. Boyland, E.: Natural oestrogens and the safe level of oestrogen intake. Tumori 53:19, 1967.

9. Burch, J.C., Byrd, B.F. and Vaugh, W.K.: The effects of long-term estrogen on hysterectomized women. Am. J. Obst. Gyn. 118:778, 1974.

10. Doisey, E.A. and Allen, E.: Ovarian hormone; preliminary report on its localisation, extraction and partial purification and action in test animals. JAMA 81:819-821, 1923.

11. Fasal, E. and Paffenbarger, R.S.: Oral contraceptives as related to cancer and benign lesions of the breast. J. Natl. Cancer Inst. 55:767-773, 1975.

12. F.D.A. Drug Bulletin: Estrogens and endometrial cancer. 6:18-20, 1976.

13. Feinleib, M.: Breast cancer and artificial menopause: a cohort study. J. Nat. Cancer Inst. 41:315-329, 1968.

14. Herbst, A.L., Scully, R.E.: Adenocarcinoma of the vagina in adolescence: a report of 7 cases including 6 clear-cell carcinomas (so-called mesonephromas). Cancer 25:745, 1970.

15. Herbst, A.L., Ulfelder, H. and Poskanzer, D.C.: Adeno-carcinoma of the vagina: association of maternal stilbes-trol therapy with tumor appearance in young women. N.Eng. J. Med. 284:878, 1971.

16. Lyons, W.R., Li, C.H., and Johnson, R.E.: Recent Progress Hormone Research 14:219, 1958.

17. MacMahon, B., Cole, P. and Brown, J.: Etiology of human breast cancer: A review. J. Natl. Cancer Inst. 50:21-42, 1973.

18. Mays, E.T., Christopherson, W.M., Mahr, M.M. and Williams, H.C.: Hepatic changes in young women ingesting contra-ceptive steroids. JAMA 236:730-732, 1976.

19. Royal College of General Practitioners: Oral contracep-tives and health: an interim report. Pitman Medical, London, 1974, p. 98.

20. Schinzinger, A.: Verh. Deutsch. Ges. Chir. 18:28, 1889.

21. Smith, D.C., Prentice, R., Thompson, D.J. and Herrmann, W.L.: Association of exogenous estrogen and endometrial carcinoma. N.Eng.J. Med. 293:1164-1167, 1975.

22. Symmers, W.S.: Carcinoma of breast in trans-sexual individuals after surgical and hormonal interference with primary and secondary sex characteristics. Brit. Med. J. 2:82-86, 1968.

23. Vessey, M.P., Doll, R. and Sutton, P.M.: Investigation of the possible relationship between oral contraceptives and benign and malignant breast disease. Cancer: 28:1395-1399, 1971.

24. Ziel, H.K. and Finkle, W.D.: Increased risk of endometrial carcinoma among users of conjugated estrogens. N.Eng.J. Med. 293:1167-1170, 1975.

TUMORAL GROWTH OF HUMAN BREAST CANCER
CELL LINE (MCF-7) IN ATHYMIC MICE*

J. Russo, C. McGrath, I.H. Russo and M.A. Rich

Department of Biology
Michigan Cancer Foundation
110 East Warren Avenue
Detroit, Michigan 48201

MCF-7 is a stable human mammary carcinoma cell line (19). Its cells are morphologically characteristic of breast epithelium (2). Its breast origin is confirmed by its capacity to synthesize the human milk protein alpha lactalbumin (13). The presence of high-affinity estrogen, androgens, progesterone, and glucocorticoid receptors has been demonstrated (3,9). The malignancy of these cells has been assessed *in vitro* by their growth in soft agar and their agglutinability by Concanavalin A (20). Their malignant origin may, in addition, be inferred from their capacity to reproduce the original histopathological pattern when grown in a three dimensional sponge matrix (15).

It has been suggested that an important criterion of malignancy is the ability of transformed cells to grow in an adequate heterotransplantation system (17). Immunologically depressed athymic mice (nu/nu) (5, 7, 12, 16) have the striking capability of discriminating between normal and neoplastic cells. Normal cells do not induce tumors (7), whereas malignant cells do.

The heterotransplantation study described here assesses the malignancy of MCF-7 cells and determines the importance of the hormonal status of the host in the resultant tumor evolution.

MATERIALS AND METHODS

MCF-7 cells, cultured as previously described (15), were removed from the culture vessel by trypsinization following transfers 163 and 164 and were suspended in Eagle's minimum essential medium with Earle's salt solution and antibiotics.

Forty-seven 21-day-old Balb/c (nu/nu) mice[1] received 1×10^7 cells in 0.05 ml inoculated into the mammary gland fat pad which was cleared according to the method of DeOme (4). Inoculated mice were divided into four groups: *Group I*. Male mice inoculated with MCF-7 cells; *Group II*.

*This study was conducted with the support of Contract NO1 CP 33347 within the Virus Cancer Program of the National Cancer Institute, NIH, PHS, and an Institutional Grant from the United Foundation of Greater Detroit.

[1]Nude mice were generously provided by W.M. Farrow through the cooperation of the Office of Resources and Logistics, Virus Cancer Program, National Cancer Institute.

617

Female mice inoculated with MCF-7 cells; *Group III*. Female mice were inoculated with MCF-7 cells. Two pituitaries obtained from syngeneic 60-day-old female mice were grafted into their perirenal fat; *Group IV*. Female mice were inoculated with MCF-7 cells. Two ovaries obtained from 60-day-old syngeneic mice were grafted into their perirenal fat. The animals were inspected every three days; when palpable tumors appeared, the animals were sacrificed and autopsied. Liver, spleen, kidneys, lungs, lymph nodes, and the grafted ovaries and pituitaries were removed and fixed in Bouin's fluid for light microscopy study. The tumors and the contralateral (non-inoculated) mammary gland were divided into two portions: one was fixed in Bouin's fluid for light microscopy and the other was fixed in Karnovsky's fluid (9) for subsequent electron microscopy study. Histological material was dehydrated, embedded in paraffin and sectioned at a thickness of 5μ. Sections were stained with hematoxylin and eosin or Masson's trichrome stain (1). Material fixed for electron microscopy was embedded in plastic, sectioned at a thickness of 1μ, and stained with 1% toluidine blue in 4% borax solution.

RESULTS

Pathology
  Groups I and II: No tumors appeared in either male or female mice inoculated with MCF-7 cells. These two groups were kept under surveillance (two months) until death due to wasting syndrome (11, 18) occurred. The gross examination of the area of cell inoculation and the histological study revealed a complete absence of the inoculated cells; only disorganization of the fat and some fibrosis were observed.
  Group III: Nine of the eleven (82%) inoculated female mice which received pituitary grafts developed palpable tumors within 12-18 days after inoculation. The tumors adhered to the skin and underlying muscle. No macroscopic metastatic growths were observed.
  Group IV: Eight of the thirteen (61.5%) inoculated female mice which received ovary grafts developed palpable tumors within 12-18 days. Tumors were attached to the skin and underlying muscles; no metastatic growths were observed.

Macroscopic examination
  The tumors were small, oblong masses of 1.5-2.5 mm at their largest diameter. They adhered to the dermis of the skin and to the muscle of the abdominal wall. The tumors were firm, of a rubbery consistency, and presented resistance to sectioning. The tumor's vascular bed was well-developed. The area of the tumor was easily distinguished from the scar produced by the cauterization and the incision made during the transplant procedure.

Microscopic examination
  The histological pattern of the 17 tumors studied was identical. The tumors were composed of nests of cells arranged in either clusters or single or double-row strands (Fig. 1). The inoculated epithelial cells were surrounded by a dense stroma formed by collagen fibers and fibroblasts (Figs. 1 and 2). Blood vessels were scarce in the central portion of the tumor and more abundant in the periphery and in areas of invasion.
  The cells presented a considerable degree of pleomorphism and hyperplasia. The nucleus was oval with few indentations. The nucleoplasm was pale, and a thin layer of heterochromatin was observed on the inner side of the nuclear envelope. More than two nucleoli per nucleus were

618

frequently observed (Figs. 2 and 3). Intracellular lumina with cellular detritus within were present in some cells (Fig. 2). When stained with toluidine blue, the cytoplasm of most cells appeared strongly basophilic. A few cells with pale cytoplasm were also observed (Fig. 3). Similar epithelial cells were also observed in the dermis of the skin overlying the inoculation site and among muscular fibers of the abdominal wall (Fig. 3). The intense fibrous reaction observed at the inoculation site (Figs. 1 and 2) and in the dermis was not observed around cells invading skeletal muscle (Fig. 3.). Mitoses were frequently observed in areas of invasion (Fig. 4).

No metastases were found in any of the tissues studied; however, clusters of cells attached to the adventitia of blood vessels (Fig. 4) or adjacent to the perineurium (Fig. 5) were observed in the periphery of the tumor. Invasion of blood vessels or nerves by neoplastic cells was not observed in serial sections. The tumors observed in groups III and IV were indistinguishable.

DISCUSSION

The successful heterotransplantation of human tumors (12, 16) and cultured human malignant cells (5,6) into nude mice has proven to be an excellent model for the study of neoplastic tissue and an effective diagnostic tool for differentiating malignant from benign cells (7). In our experiments, we have used cells derived from a human breast carcinoma (19). The growth of MCF-7 cells as tumors in nude mice might be predicted by the malignant nature of the tumor of origin (22) and by the demonstration of several transformation markers (23). However, MCF-7 cells did not form tumors in all inoculated mice but only in those receiving pituitary or ovarian grafts, thus suggesting a hormone dependency for *in vivo* growth. The fact that more tumors were observed in mice receiving pituitary grafts (82%) than in those receiving ovarian grafts (61.5%) suggested that some pituitary hormone could be involved in the development of these tumors. The mice were sexually immature at the time of inoculation. Further study is needed to determine whether the hypophysis graft acts directly on the tumor or by means of ovarian stimulation.

The inoculation of MCF-7 cells into nude mice induces tumors morphologically similar to the tumor of origin. This property of malignant cells has been described for other cell lines maintained for almost 100 passages *in vitro* (7) and transplanted into nude mice, and for human tumors transplanted into the anterior chamber of the guinea pig eye (8).

MCF-7 cells develop a histological pattern in the nude mice similar to that observed in the tumor of origin. The tumor of origin was an infiltrative ductal carcinoma with productive fibrosis (commonly called scirrhous carcinoma). This same pattern of epithelial cells surrounded by a dense stroma is observed in the mouse, suggesting that it is the neoplastic epithelial cell that elicits a stromal response in the host. This observation was also supported by results obtained in an experimental model developed for the study of scirrhous carcinoma (14).

SUMMARY

MCF-7 is a stable breast cancer cell line which can be stimulated to synthesize an RNA tumor virus-like particle. The expression of malignancy by MCF-7 cells has been assessed by its transplantability into the nude mouse.

Cultured MCF-7 cells were inoculated into the mammary fat pad of 21-day-old Balb/c (nude/nude) mice. Four groups were inoculated: pituitary-grafted females, ovary-grafted females, non-grafted males, and non-grafted female mice. Pituitaries and ovaries from syngeneic mice were implanted into the perirenal fat at the time of cell inoculation. Sixty-one and a half percent of the animals receiving ovary grafts and 82% of the animals receiving pituitary grafts developed tumors of 1.5-2.5 mm diameter within 12-18 days of inoculation. None of the animals that did not receive ovary or pituitary implants developed tumors.

The tumors were infiltrative ductal carcinomas with productive fibrosis, and were invasive to the surrounding dermis and muscle. The morphological features of the neoplastic cells were identical to those observed in both MCF-7 cells in culture and in the primary tumor from which MCF-7 cells were originally derived.

The absence of tumors in untreated animals could be explained by an inadequate hormonal milieu for the growth of MCF-7 cells. The fact that the original tumor from which MCF-7 cells were derived was responsive to hormones and that MCF-7 cells still retain specific high-affinity estradiol and progesterone receptors after 160 passages in culture, supports this hypothesis.

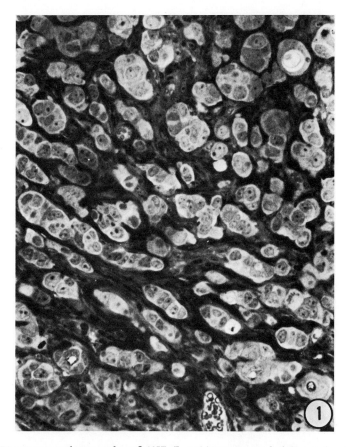

FIG. 1. Clusters and strands of MCF-7 cells surrounded by a dense stromal
reaction in a nude mouse tumor. X80. 1 μ sections of plastic embedded
material stained with toluidine blue.

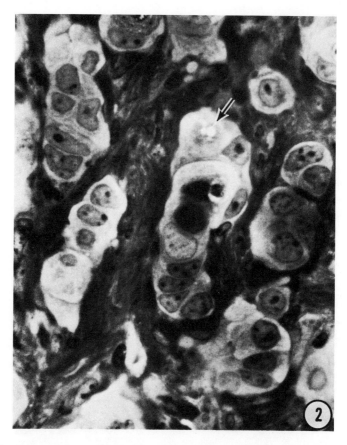

FIG. 2. Striking pleomorphism in cell strands among dense collagen fibers. Intracytoplasmic lumen (arrow). X240. 1 μ sections of plastic embedded material stained with toluidine blue.

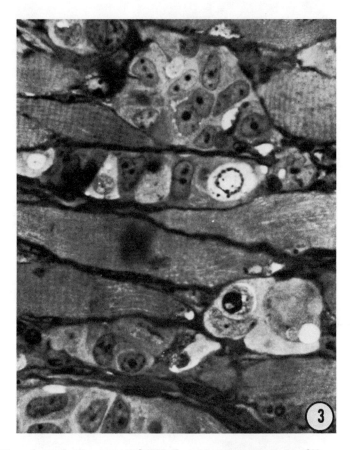

FIG. 3. Strands and clusters of MCF-7 cells among muscle fibers. X240.
1 µ sections of plastic embedded material stained with toluidine blue.

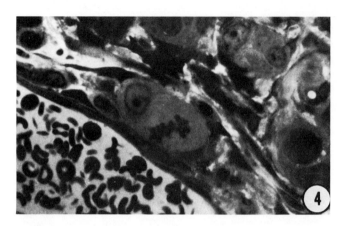

FIG. 4. Two MCF-7 cells, one of them in mitosis, apposed to the adventitia
of a blood vessel. X240. 1 μ sections of plastic embedded material
stained with toluidine blue.

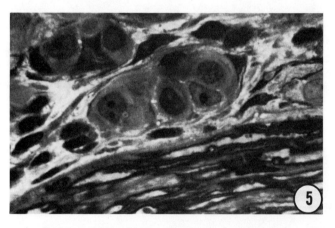

FIG. 5. Cluster of MCF-7 cells apposed to the perineurium. X240. 1 μ
sections of plastic embedded material stained with toluidine blue.

REFERENCES

1. Armed Forces Institute of Pathology. 1957. Manual of Histologic and Special Staining Techniques. Washington, D.C.

2. Arnold, W.J., Soule, H.D., and Russo, J. Fine Structure of a Human Mammary Carcinoma Cell Line, MCF-7. In Vitro, 10: 356, 1975.

3. Brooks, S.C., Locke, B.R., and Soule, H.D. Estrogen Receptor in a Human Cell Line (MCF-7) from Breast Carcinoma. J. Biol. Chem., 243: 6251-6253, 1973.

4. DeOme, K.B., Faulkin, J.R. Jr., Bern, H.A., and Blair, P.B. Development of Mammary Tumors from Hyperplastic Alveolar Nodules Transplanted into Gland-Free Mammary Fat Pads of Female C3H Mice. Cancer Res., 19: 350-359, 1959.

5. Giovanella, B.C., Stehlin, J.S., and Williams, L.J. Jr. Development of Invasive Tumors in the "Nude" Mouse after Injection of Cultured Human Melanoma Cells. J. Natl. Cancer Inst., 48: 1531-1533, 1972.

6. Giovanella, B.C., Stehlin, J.S. Heterotransplantation of Human Malignant Tumors in "Nude" Thymusless Mice. I. Breeding and Maintenance of "Nude" Mice. J. Natl. Cancer Inst., 51: 615-619, 1973.

7. Giovanella, B.C., Stehlin, J.S., and Williams, L.J. Jr. Heterotransplantation of Human Malignant Tumors in "Nude" Thymusless Mice. II. Malignant Tumors Induced by Injection of Cell Cultures Derived from Human Solid Tumors. J. Natl. Cancer Inst., 52: 921-930, 1974.

8. Greene, H.S.N. The Significance of the Heterologous Transplantability of Human Cancer. Cancer, 5: 24-44, 1952.

9. Horwitz, K.B., Costlow, M.E. and McGuire, W.L. MCF-7: A Human Breast Cancer Cell Line with Estrogen, Androgen, Progesterone, and Glucocorticoid Receptors. Steroids, 26: 785-795, 1975.

10. Karnovsky, M.J. A Formaldehyde-Glutaraldehyde Fixative of High Osmolarity for Use in Electron Microscopy. J. Cell Biol., 27: 137A, 1965.

11. Outzen, H.C., Custer, R.P., Eaton, G.J., and Prehn, R.T. Spontaneous and Induced Tumor Incidence in Germfree "Nude" Mice. J. Reticuloendothelial Soc., 17: 1-9, 1975.

12. Povlsen, C.O., Fialkow, P.J., Klein, E. Growth and Antigenic Properties of a Biopsy-Derived Burkitt's Lymphoma in Thymusless (Nude) Mice. Intl. J. Cancer, 11: 30-39, 1973.

13. Rose, H.N. and McGrath, C.M. α-Lactalbumin production in Human Mammary Carcinoma. Science, 190: 673-675, 1975.

14. Russo, J., and McGrath, C.M. Scirrhous Carcinoma in the Mouse: A Model for Human Mammary Carcinoma. Excerpta Medica, Amsterdam, 488, 1975.

15. Russo, J., Soule, H.D., McGrath, C.M., and Rich, M.A. Re-Expression of the Original tumor Pattern by a Human breast Carcinoma Cell Line (MCF-7) in Sponge Culture. J. Natl. Cancer Inst., 56: 279-282, 1976.

16. Rygaard, J., Povlsen, C.O. Heterotransplantation of a Human Malignant Tumor to "Nude" Mice. Acta Pathol. Microbiol. Scand., 77: 758-760, 1969.

17. Sanford, K.K. Biologic Manifestation of Oncogenesis In Vitro: A critique. J. Natl. Cancer Inst., 53: 1481-1485, 1974.

18. Sebesteny, A., and Hill, A.C. Hepatitis and Brain Lesions Due to Mouse Hepatitis Virus Accompanied by Wasting in Nude Mice. Lab Animal., 8: 317-325, 1974.

19. Soule, H.D., Vazquez, J., Long, A., Albert, S., and Brennan, M. A Human Cell Line from a Pleural Effusion derived from a Breast Carcinoma. J. Natl. Cancer Inst., 51: 1409-1416, 1973.

20. Voyles, B.A., Soule, H.D. and McGrath, C.M. Normal and Neoplastic Mammary Epithelium: Concanavalin A Mediated Hemadsorption and Growth in Agar Suspension. In Vitro, 10: 389a, 1975.

HUMAN BREAST CANCER: STUDIES ON URINARY EXCRETION OF ENDOGENOUS OESTROGENS AND ITS CHANGES AFTER HORMONE TREATMENT

Giuseppe Paparopoli [*]
Adele Traina [*]
Biagio Agostara [*]

Luigi Castagnetta [Ø*]
Giancarlo Brucoli [Ø]

Cancer Hospital Center [*]
Via del Vespro Palermo
Italy

Department of Biochemistry [Ø]
Facoltà di Medicina Policlinico
Palermo Italy

Experimental research work on urinary excretion patterns of oestrogens in patients with various kinds of tumours has been carried out by number of authors: several data concerning blood rates and urinary excretion rates of oestrogens in female patients with breast cancer are thus available (1-5). On the contrary, data concerning male patients with breast cancer are quite scarce, due to the low incidence of this kind of tumour (6-7). The role of oestrogens in determining or influencing breast cancer, i.e. their mechanism of action, is still unknown (8).

Recent experimental work has been carried out on the effects of synthetic oestrogens in cases with breast cancer (patients in pre-and post-menopausal age) (9).

A few years ago Mac Mahon oberved a higher incidence of breast cancer in American women, than in Asiatic women, and assumed such difference as reflecting lower or higher urinary oestriol excretion (10).

Quite recently Lemon contributed more satisfactory data to this problem and showed how oestriol exerts an exceptionally protective action against 7-12-DMBA induced breast cancer in rats (11). Moreover Schwartz observed a further -though different- protective action of oestradiol in human breast cancer tissue in vitro (12).

627

Bulbrook suggested that breast cancer might be more frequent in women whose urinary excretion of oestrogens and 17-ketosteroids is below normal values (13).

The opinion prevails now that oestrogens exert an indirect carcinogenic action due to their role in considerably increasing prolactin rates (14-15).

On the other hand Heuson suggests that the oestrogen-like properties of ethinyl-oestradiol and Nafoxidine-which might induce breast cancer regression- are independant of their effect on prolaction secretion (16).

According to a very recent study on male breast cancer by Dao the data available show that in such patients oestrogen metabolism follows an abnormal pathway (17).

Most authors deal almost exclusively with "classical" oestrogen metabolites, i.e. $E_1 + E_2 + E_3$. Our work was focused on the evaluation of some urinary oestrogen metabolites which are usually absent (or are present in very small amounts) in normal urine but are present in male and female patients with breast cancer. We also studied the alterations of those urinary oestrogen excretion patterns after the administration of synthetic oestrogens.

PROCEDURES AND MATERIALS USED

Our investigation was carried out on 9 male patients with breast cancer and 21 selected cases of female patients with post-menopausal, metastasized and advanced breast cancer. The latter group was chosen among patients whose urinary oestrogen excretion pattern was atypical.They were further subdivided into two groups according to the amount of "classical" oestrogens excreted.

30 women of post-menopausal age and I2 men of about the same age as our patients were taken as normal control subjects.

None of the patients admitted to the present study had impaired liver function, either before or during the course of our investigation. Moreover the urine (and blood specimens) belong to patients who had received no treatment,other than hormone treatment, either before or during the course of our study.

Urine specimens were collected for 24 hours without added preservatives and were sometimes frozen (-20° C). In most cases, however, specimens were processed immediately upon arrival at our laboratory.

Urinary steroids were assayed before tratment and then 72 h and 15 days after treatment had been stopped. Further assays were performed at irregular intervals.

Methods : urine specimens were first purified and then hydrolysed (both acid and enzyme hydrolysis). Purification, hydrolysis extraction and thin layer chromatography, preparation of derivatives and gas-liquid chromatography were carried out according to methods already described (18).

Assays were performed on at least two stationary phases for each specimen (18). 17-ketosteroids were assayed using the method described by Kirschner (19).

RESULTS

a. Urinary oestrogen excretion pattern before treatment.

(1) FEMALE BREAST CANCER: GROUP 1 (35% of all cases under study).

In this group findings were: decrease of oestriol ratio; decrease of "classical" oestrogens; marked decrease of oestriol. In these cases metabolites unusual in human urine are present in high amounts and the ratio between "classical" oestrogens and unusual metabolites is absolutely unbalanced. Urinary oestrogen excretion pattern is atypical.Moreover the amount of all urinary oestrogen metabolites is very high as shown in Table.

(2) FEMALE BREAST CANCER: GROUP II (64% of all cases under study).

In this group findings were: marked and significant increase of oestriol rate; increase of "classical" oestrogens; oestriol ratio mostly above normal values. In these cases unusual metabolites are present in large amounts, although less than in group I. Urinary oestrogen excretion pattern is atypical. The total amount of oestrogen metabolites excreted is very high (Table).

(3) MALE BREAST CANCER: GROUP III.

In this group findings were: significant increase of "classical" oestrogens in urine; high amounts of unusual oestrogen metabolites. Urinary oestrogen excretion pattern is very atypical.

629

Fractionated 17-ketosteroids were assayed in all groups and showed significantly lower values than normal in all investigated cases.

b. Clinical conditions after treatment.

In cases with female breast cancer atypical urinary oestrogen excretion patterns were modified after treatment with Hexestrol (HES) and/or Diethylstilboestrol (DES). Such changes were in good agreement with clinical improvement in group I. In group II, however, treatment with HES and/or DES brought about only very slight changes in urinary oestrogen excretion patterns. Clinical conditions were stabilized in some cases and worse in others.

In the cases with male breast cancer, atypical excretion patterns were modified by treatment with DES only, which also caused clinical improvement of patients in group III. The other cases were not treated with DES .

c. Changes in urinary oestrogen excretion patterns after treatment.

(1) GROUP I: Fig.1 shows the changes observed in urinary excretion patterns after treatment which correspond to a complete reversal of patterns found before treatment. Normal conditions were thus restored. Unusual oestrogen metabolites were mostly due to an increase of "classical" oestro-"classical" oestrogens increased. Such increase is reflected in oestrogen ratios. Changes in the ratio between "classical" oestrogen and unusual oestrogen metabolites were mostly due to an increase of "classical" oestrogen metabolites. These latter attained levels much higher than normal. Urinary oestrogen excretion pattern cannot be therefore considered as normalized, at least in the period immediately following withdrawal of treatment.

(2) GROUP II: as shown in Fig.2, urinary excretion patterns of endogenous oestrogens was but slightly affected by treatment. Absolute values and "classical" oestrogen ratios were unchanged after treatment.

The ratio of unusual metabolites (still present in these specimens) was unchanged too, though their excretion rate was lower then before treatment.

(3) GROUP III: treated cases and data are few, but changes in urinary

oestrogen excretion patterns appear to be in good agreement with those obtained from group I.

DISCUSSION

The most important feature in our findings is the presence of some oestrogen metabolites, referred to as "unusual metabolites", attaining ve ry high levels in the urines of cases with breast cancer under study.

Most of these metabolites were already shown to be present, though in small amounts, in the bile and in the urine of pregnant women (20-21).

Their presence may be therefore considered as due to physiological oestrogen hypersecretion. We still ignore the meaning of such phenomenon in cases with human breast cancer.

Our findings, however, allow to establish some relationship between the presence of these unusual metabolites, and their amount, related to rate of "classical" oestrogens, on one hand, and clinical conditions, on the other. We also found a remarkable variability concerning basic values of "classical" oestrogen rates and basic values of oestriol ratios in the three groups of patients under study.

Our data seem thus to confirm previous report of Lemon (22).

Such variability is strongly influenced by the administration of oestrogen metabolites, referred to as "unusual metabolites", attaining ve-the same on our three groups.

According to recent data (11-12), it appears that different metabolites of "classical" oestrogens may exert different, and probably several, biological actions in organism (23).

The distinction between biologically active and non active metabolites may appear thus to be outdated (24).

Our data also show the importance of wide ranging investigation on all oestrogen metabolites, and draw particular attention on the ratio between "classical" and "unusual" metabolites in human urine.

The relationship between the presence of such unusual metabolites and breast cancer deserves further investigation too.

SUMMARY

Gas-chromatographic patterns of urinary excretion of endogenous oestrogens were studied in some cases of histologically proven male and female breast cancer. In our survey levels of total urinary oestrogen were higher (by a factor of 3, 4, or more) than normal control values.

Moreover we found unusual patterns of urinary oestrogen excretion and a particularly remarkable reversal of the ratio between "classical" oestrogens (E_1 + E_2 + E_3) and other metabolites usually present in very low amounts in human urine.

After treatment with hexestrol and/or diethylstilboestrol the ratio between "classical" and unusual metabolites showed a remarkable increase. Infact the normal patterns of urinary oestrogen excretion were restored and characterized by the return to normal (or increased) levels of oestriol ratio and by the increase of the excretion rate of 17-beta-oestradiol, oestriol and oestrone. Clinical improval was in good agreement with changes in urinary excretion patterns in a series of cases, with female,and in treated, with male breast cancer. Our studies show clearly the importance of further investigation concerning all metabolites of urinary oestrogens, with special attention to the ratios between "classical" and unusual metabolites and to the relationship between the presence of unusual metabolites in urine and human breast cancer.

ACKNOWLEDGMENTS

This study was partially supported by a grant from the "Donazione R. and M. Nuccio".

We wish to thank Miss Michelina M.Nuccio for financial support and Prof. L.Boniforti (Istituto Superiore di Sanità, Rome) for presenting us with OV 61 stationary phase.

TABLE I. Urinary Oestrogen Profiles Before and After Treatment in Postmenopausal Patients with Breast Cancer and in Controls

	mean values in µg/24 hr				
	CLASSICAL OESTROGENS	OESTRIOL	OESTRIOL RATIO	UNUSUAL METABOLITES	TOTAL OESTROGENS
GROUP I					
(1)	15.4 ± 4.7 ‡	8.1 ±3.6 †	0.84 ±0.33 **	44.2 ±20.0 **	59.6 ±22.6 **
(2)	27.6 ±10.6 †	19.2 ±8.1 **	2.45 ±0.61 †	5.5 ± 3.6	32.9 ±13.3 **
N.C.	18.3 ± 4.4	12.3 ±5.5	2.10 ±0.45	N.D.	18.3 ± 4.4
GROUP II					
(1)	35.0 ±11.3 **	25.7 ±8.7 **	2.60 ±0.80 †	25.3 ± 8.9 **	60.2 ±18.4 **
(2)	28.2 ± 7.4 **	14.8 ±3.9 ‡	1.20 ±0.68 **	18.6 ± 6.3 **	44.5 ±13.5 **

(1)=Before treatment   N.C.=Normal Controls
(2)=After treatment   N.D.=Not Detectable
** p < 0.001   † < 0.01   ‡ p < 0.05

The total amounts of 16EpiOestriol, 16-αHydroxyOestrone, 11Dehydro-17αOestradiol, 17αOestradiol, 17EpiOestriol, 16-17EpiOestriol, 16-KetoOestrone are referred to as Unusual Metabolites.

    All the data before and after treatment were the averages of, at least three determinations ± S.D.

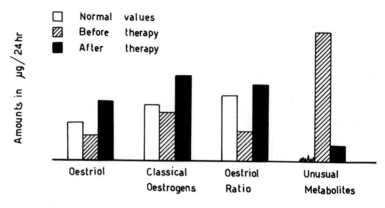

FIG. 1

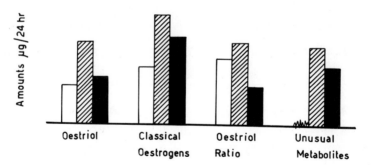

FIG. 2

REFERENCES

(1) Nocke,W. In Vivo Studies on the Endocrine Activity of Normal and Tumo rous Ovaries in Post-menopausal Women. In: Advances in the Bioscien ces, 3. Ed.: Gerard Raspé.Pergamon Press,Berlin, 129-49,1969.

(2) Lemon, H.M. Abnormal Estrogen Metabolism and Tissue Estrogen Receptor Proteins in Breast Cancer. Cancer, 25:423-435,1970.

(3) Dao,T.L., and Libby,P.R. Steroid Sulphate Formation in Human Breast Tumor and Hormone Dependency. In : Estrogen Target Tissues and Neopla sia. Chicago, University of Chicago Press,181-200,1972.

(4) Abraham,G.E. Radioimmunoassay of Plasma Steroids Hormones. In: Modern Methods in Steroids Analysis. Ed. E.Heftman. Academic Press,New York, 451-465,1973.

(5) MacMahon,B.,Cole,P.,and Brown,J. Etiology of Human Breast Cancer. J. Nat.Cancer Inst.,50:21-42,1973.

(6) Treves,N. The Treatment.......of the Male Breast Cancer by Ablative Surgery and Hormone (estrogens and corticosteroids) Therapy........ Cancer,12:820-832,1959.

(7) Donegan,W.L.,and Perez-Mesa,C.M. Carcinoma of the Male Breast. Arch. Surg.,106:273-279,1973.

(8) Jensen,E.V.,and DeSombre,E.R. Mechanism of Action of the Female Sex Hormones.Ann.Rev.Biochem.,41:203-230,1972.

(9) Burch,J.C.,and Byrd,B.F. Effects of Long Term Administration of Estro gen on the Occurrence of Mammary Cancer in Women.Ann.Surg.,174:414-418,1971.

(10) MacMahon,B.,Cole,P.,Brown,J.S.,Aoki,K.,Lin,T.M.,Morgan,R.W. and Woo, N.C. Oestrogen Profiles of Asian and North American Women. Lancet, 2:900-902,1971.

(11) Lemon,H.M. Estriol Prevention of Mammary Carcinoma Induced by 7-12 DMBA and Procarbazine. Cancer Res.,35:1341-53,1975

(12) Schwarz,A.G. The Protective Effect of Estradiol 17 beta against Poly-ciclic Hydrocarb.Cytotoxicity. Cancer Res.,33:2431-36,1973.

(13) Bulbrook,R.D. Hormonal Factors in the Etiology and Treatment of Breast Cancer.Sixth Canadian Cancer Research Conference. Pergamon Press,New York, pp.36-49,1966.

(14) Frantz,A.G.,Kleinberg,D.L.,and Noel,G.L. Studies on Prolactin in Man. Recent Progr.Horm.Res., 28:527-590,1972.

(15) Kwa,H.G., Engelsman, E.,De Jong-Bakker, M.,Cleton, F.G. Plasma Pro-lactionin Human Breast Cancer.Lancet 1,433-434,1974.

(16) L'Heremite, M., Robin C.,Heuson,J.C., and Rozenscweig, M. Breast Cancer Regression under Oestrogen Therapy. Brith.Med.J.,1:390--,1974.

(17) Dao,T.L.,Morreal,C.,and Nemoto,T. Urinary Estrogens Excretion in Man with Breast Cancer. New Engl.J.Med.,289:138-140,1973.

(18) Castagnetta,L.,Brucoli,G.,Bologna,P.,and Paternò,F. 17-alfa Oestra-diol in Human Urine in a Case of Male Breast Carcinoma.Experientia, 1976, in press.

(19) Kirschner, M.A.,and Lipsett,M.B. Gas-liquid Chromatography in the Quantitative Analysis of Urinary 11oxy- 17-Ketosteroids. J. Clin.Invest.,23:255-260,1963.

(20) Adlercreutz, H. Studies on Oestrogen Excretion in Human Bile. Acta Endocr.,Suppl.,72:156-194,1962.

(21) Adlercreutz, H.,and Luukkainen, T. Studies on Estrogen Metabolism in the Adult Human Organism in Vivo. Advances in the Biosciences, 3:53-70,1969.

(22) Lemon,H.M.,Wotiz, H.H., Parsons, L., and Mozden P.J. Reduced Estriol Excretion in Patients with Breast Cancer Prior to Endocrine Therapy. J.Amer.Med.Assoc.,196:1128-1136,1966.

(23) Mueller, G.C., Vonderhaar, B., Kim, U.H.,and Le Mahieu, M. Estrogen Action: An Inroad to Cell Biology. Recent Progr. Horm. Res., 28:1-49,1972.

(24) Emmens, C.W. Estrogens. In : Methods in Hormone Research. Ed.: Ralph I. Dorfman. Vol. II Academic Press. Inc.,New York, pp. 61-120, 1969.

THE VALUE OF URINARY STEROID ANALYSIS
IN CHORIONIC NEOPLASIA

Toshiko Kodama, Mitsuo Kodama and
Ryozo Totani

Aichi Cancer Center
Research Institute and
Nagoya National Hospital
Nagoya, Japan.

I. INTRODUCTION

Chorionic neoplasia is a spectrum disease of 3 sequential entities by
definition. The malignancy increases in the order of hydatidiform mole,
chorioadenoma destruens and choriocarcinoma. The tumor tissue releases
a high amount of human chorionic gonadotropin (HCG) to the periphery.
But the fetus is absent in uterus, and the steroidogenesis of the target
tissue (ovary) under the influence of neoplastic HCG is to be differentiated from that in normal pregnancy.

The purpose of this investigation is to provide more information about
the steroid excretion in chorionic neoplasia so that the distinction
among the 3 entities of chorionic neoplasia and normal pregnancy may
hopefully become feasible by urinary steroid analysis.

II. PROCEDURES AND MATERIALS USED

A 50 ml urine sample was processed by Horning's method to form 0-methyl-
oxime-trimethyl silyl ether derivatives of steroids, and a total of 14
neutral steroids were estimated separately by gas liquid chromatography.
In addition, the whole chromatogram was divided into 3 fractions by
appropriate MU values, and sum of identified and unidentified peaks was
calculated for each fraction. The names of identified steroids in the
3 fractions are listed below together with their abbreviations.
1) Fraction 1: androsterone(A), etiocholanolone(E), dehydroepiandroste-

637

rone(D) and 11-ketoandrosterone(KA). 2) Fraction 2 (menstruation-dependent in excretion): 11-hydroxyandrosterone(HA), 11-hydroxyetiocholanolone
(Het), pregnanediol(Pd) and pregnanetriol(Pt). 3) Fraction 3: tetrahydro-
cortisone(THE), tetrahydrocorticosterone(THB), tetrahydrocortisol(THF),
cortolone(Cn), β-cortolone and β-cortol(β) and cortol(Cl). The details of
steroid analysis and statistical technic are described elsewhere (Kodama
and Kodama, 1975).

This study includes 152 specimens from 20 pregnant women, 23 specimens
from 23 patients with hydatidiform mole, 238 specimens from 9 patients
with chorioadenoma destruens and 6 specimens from 2 patients with choriocarcinoma. In addition, the data with over 200 non-pregnant women served
for setting the normal range of steroid excretion. The figures for non-
pregnant women are also referred to in the preceding paper (Kodama et al.,
1975).

III. RESULTS

The steroid excretions in normal pregnancy and chorionic neoplasia were
first compared with the values of a non-pregnant woman of luteal phase (20
days after the start of the last menstruation). Figure 1 illustrates their
deviations from the non-pregnant control. The normal pregnancy is characterised by a remarkable increase of F_2 steroid excretions and a general
decrease of F_1 and F_3 steroids.   Likewise, the hydatidiform mole is
associated with a decrease of F_1 and F_3 steroid excretions, but the
excretion of F_2 steroids is reduced to the level of luteal phase.   The
level of F_2 steroid excretions drops further in chorioadenoma destruens.
The F_3 steroid excretions are generally decreased in the same group, but
androsterone is rather increased, as compared with the non-pregnant control. To sum up, the general decrease in F_3 steroid excretion is a common
feature among normal pregnancy, hydatidiform mole and chorioadenoma destruens, but the ratio of F_2 to F_1 steroids may serve as a discriminant parameter for these 3 entities.   In choriocarcinoma, the level of F_3 steroids
remains at the level of luteal phase, and some of F_1 and F_2 steroids are
reduced remarkably, a finding to indicate a general devastation of ovarian
steroidogenesis. The discriminant capacity of log F_2/F_1 was tested with
a set of normal pregnancy, hydatitiform mole, chorioadenoma destruens
and non-pregnant controls of luteal and follicular phase. Before the
calculation of mean and standard deviation, logarithmic transformation

was applied to normalize the frequency distribution of that parameter, F_2/F_1. Figure 2 shows that the separation of hydatidiform mole from chorioadenoma destruens is much better than from normal pregnancy. Actually, a remarkable drop of log F_2/F_1 was observed in 6 cases of chorionic neoplasia tested during the clinical transition from hydatidiform mole to chorioadenoma destruens. Figure 3 shows that the level of log F_2/F_1 in chorioadenoma destruens remains no less higher than that of a non-pregnant woman of follicular phase, unless the titer of HCG is reduced to a normal level by chemotherapy. It is clear that the neoplastic tissue exerts a depressant effect on the production of luteal hormone by the ovary. In the absence of tumor HCG, the pituitary gonadotropin restores the menstrual cycle in the ovary.

IV. DISCUSSION

The mean value of log F_2/F_1 increases in the order of a) follicular phase, b) luteal phase and c) normal pregnancy (Fig. 2). It is indicated that the above parameter reflects the activity of the ovarian corpus luteum. During pregnancy, the ovary produces a high amount of progesterone under the influence of placental HCG. Stepwise reductions of log F_2/F_1 were observed in the series of normal pregnancy, hydatidiform mole and chorioadenoma destruens. These findings suggest that the steroidal deviations in chorionic neoplasia, as compared with normal pregnancy, are related to the deficient activity of the ovarian corpus luteum, and that the HCG from chorionic tissues is depleted of luteotropic action in spite of high antigenic activity. A remarkable drop of this parameter took place in the course of clinical transition from hydatidiform mole to chorioadenoma destruens for six cases tested, and the separation between hydatidiform mole and chorioadenoma destruens groups with log F_2/F_1 was good enough for clinical differentiation. In other combinations of comparison, the log F_2/F_1 alone was not effective for distinction, even if the difference was found statistically significant. The differential incidence of chorionic neoplasia between Asia and the West has been well established (Joint Project,1959). Fox and Tow (1966) found that the level of urinary HCG in Chinese women with normal pregnancy was reduced as compared with that of Caucasian women. They tentatively related their findings to the preference of chorionic neoplasia for the Asian

women. So far, there is no evidence that the steroidal changes in
chorionic neoplasia are implicated in the genesis of this desease.

V. SUMMARY

The urinary excretion of steroids in chorionic neoplasia was compared
with that of pregnant and non-pregnant healthy control by use of gas
liquid chromatography. Hydatidiform mole, as compared with the normal
pregnancy, was characterized by the reduction of menstruation-dependent
steroids (F_2). The reduction of F_2 steroids proceeds further through
the clinical transition to chorioadenoma destruens, and the ratio of F_2
to F_1 steroids (11-deoxy-17-ketosteroids) was found useful in differentiating chorioadenoma destruens from the benign mole. In choriocarcinoma,
deficient excretion was observed in both F_1 and F_2 steroids. It is
indicated that the above finding is relevant to the activity of ovary
under the influence of deficient HCG from tumors.

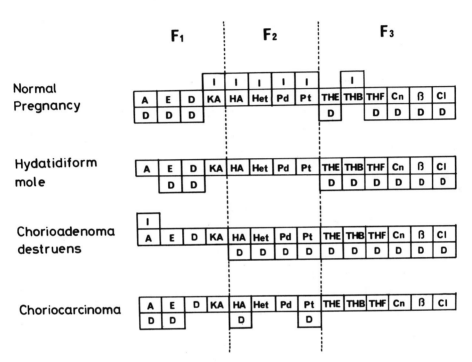

FIG. 1. Steroidal deviations of urine of normal pregnancy and chorionic neoplasia from the non-pregnant healthy control (luteal phase). Abbreviations used: Fraction 1 (F_1), Fraction 2 (F_2), Fraction 3 (F_3), Androsterona (A), Etiocholanolone (E), Dehydroepiandrosterone (D), 11-keto-androsterone (KA), 11-hydroxyandrosterone (HA), 11-hydroxyetiocholanolone (Het), Pregnanediol (Pd), Pregnanetriol (pt), Tetrahydrocortisone (THE), Tetrahydrocorticosterone (THB), Tetrahydrocortisol (THF), Cortolone (Cn), ß-cortolone and ß-cortol (ß), Cortol (Cl), Increase (I), and Decrease (D).

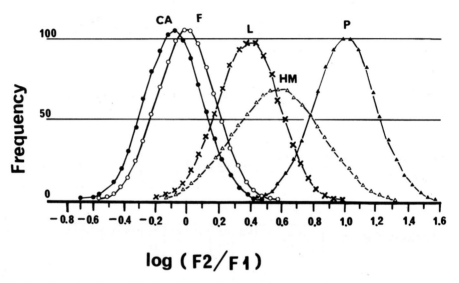

FIG. 2. Distinction of hydatidiform mole and chorioadenoma destruens from normal pregnancy with log F_2/F_1. Abbreviations used: Normal pregnancy (P), Hydatidiform mole (HM), Chorioadenoma destruens (CA), Luteal phase (L), and Follicular phase (F).

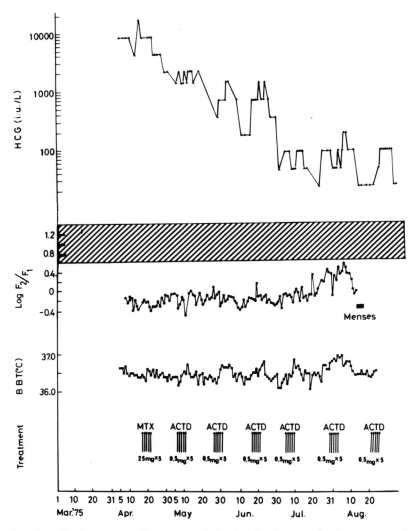

FIG. 3. Clinical course of a case with chorioadenoma destruens. Abbreviations used: Human chorionic gonadotropin (HCG), Basal body temperature (BBT), Methotrexate (MTX), and Actinomycin D (ACTD). The shadowy zone in the middle indicates the range of normal pregnancy for log F_2/F_1.

REFERENCES

1. Fox, F.J., and Tow, W.S.H. Immunologically determined chorionic gonadotropin titers in Singapore women with hydatidiform mole, choriocarcinoma, and normal intrauterine pregnancy. A preliminaty report. Am. J. Obstet. & Gynec., 95:239-248,1966.
2. Joint project for study of choriocarcinoma and hydatidiform mole in Asia. Ann. New York Acad. Sc., 80:176-196,1959.
3. Kodama, M., and Kodama, T. Hormonal status of breast cancer. I. Theoretical basis for the analysis of steroid profile. J. nat. Cancer Inst., 54:1023-1029,1975.
4. Kodama, M., Kodama, T., Yoshida, M., Totani, R., and Aoki, K. Hormonal status of breast cancer. II. Abnormal urinary steroid excretion. J. nat. Cancer Inst., 54:1275-1282,1975.

HEIGHTENED ANDROGEN AFFINITY OF HUMAN PROSTATIC CANCER

Wells E. Farnsworth and James R. Brown

Department of Biochemistry
State University of New York at Buffalo
and
Veterans Administration Hospital
Buffalo, New York

INTRODUCTION

Most would agree that aberrant hormone levels do not account for malignant transformation of the human prostate. They would hasten to add that the differentiated adenocarcinoma is androgen-dependent and never arises in the atrophic gland of a castrate. The long-recognized need of this gland for testosterone (T) (or biologically related steroids) underlies the diverse and extensive efforts of the past 35 years to attenuate prostatic cancer by removing or inactivating testicular and 19-carbon adrenal secretions. Although there has been a flurry of antiandrogen work, there has been relatively little consideration of how the cancerous gland may differ from the normal in its response to its hormonal milieu, and how its capability may be affected by circulating, nonsteroidal factors. Infusion and perfusion studies also abound, but they suffer from the inability to either duplicate the mix of hormones and plasma proteins that bathe the prostate in vivo, or to account for the effects of pools of endogenous hormones within the tissue.

Our current study represents the first attempt to discern the steady state relationships of the diseased prostate to its environment.

In order to know what to look for in our work, we had to think about what variables should be interacting to determine how much of what hormone(s) would be incorporated into the gland. We concluded that we must consider the following:

A. Androgen secretion. For example, we know (1) that the level of testicular androgens is lower in unstressed subjects with benign prostatic hypertrophy (BPH) (Table I) than in younger individuals. Though an increase in dihydrotestosterone (DHT) offsets in part the fall in testosterone, the net androgen concentration is over 20% less in the elderly than in the young. Probably the increase in conversion of T to DHT occurs in the prostate for we have seen as much as 70% conversion of T to DHT by prostate slices in vitro and Mahoudeau et al (2) found the concentration of DHT in prostatic vein blood to be well above that in the peripheral circulation.

B.   Androgen availability. Vermeulen has shown (3) that it is not
enough to know how much androgen is in the blood. For much of the testosterone is bound to sex hormone binding globulin (SHBG) and is unavailable
for metabolism or to exert a biological effect. In the aged man (4,5),
not only is the total testosterone decreased, but less is free (Table II).
This is true because,

C.   The level of circulating estrogens is higher and this induces
synthesis of more SHBG. Both the testes and the adrenals contribute this
estrogen. There is more FSH and LH being secreted (6) by a hypersensitive
pituitary (Table III). We know from the effect of chorionic gonadotrophin
(HCG) and ACTH that both glands can contribute. Table IV shows that if
the testicular source is inhibited by estrogen or eliminated by orchiectomy, the adrenal compensates by producing more testosterone and androstenedione for peripheral aromatization (7,8). A decline in sulfurylation
of the estrogen also contributes (9) by lessening renal clearance as
estrogen sulfates. Still further increasing the ratio of estrogen to
androgen is the fact that the affinity of SHBG for T is greater than for
estradiol (10,11). Therefore, as more SHBG becomes available, it selectively binds the T and leaves the estrogen free.

D.   As a consequence of having more free estrogen, there is inhibition of the hypothalamic release of LHRF, FSHRF and PIF. This decreases
pituitary output of LH and FSH but permits a rise in prolactin secretion.
We (12) and others (13) have found that prolactin increases the affinity
of the prostate cell for androgen. In fact, we have seen that binding
of testosterone to prostatic microsomes increases in parallel with increased binding of lactogen. Meites' group (14) has seen that testosterone increases binding of lactogen to prostatic plasma membranes. In
our hands, this is a biologically effective association for lactogen
seems to amplify the ability of testosterone to increase prostatic acid
phosphatase. Also, immunological depletion of endogenous lactogen undoes
this synergistic effect.

E.   Besides the lactogen-mediated actions of the estrogens are
others of a more direct nature. The uptake of androgen is influenced
by the nature of the entering steroid and by the capacity of the cell to
bind it. Presumably, uptake of testosterone can only occur down a concentration gradient. This gradient is maintained by the rapid intracellular reduction of the entering T to DHT by the enzyme, 5 alpha-
reductase, and then binding of the DHT to a cytosolic receptor protein.
The superfusion studies of Giorgi's group (15) show that estrogen, as
well as cyproterone and its acetate, directly increases the entry and
uptake of T and DHT into the prostate cell. On the other hand, Shimazaki
(16) and we (17) have shown that estrogens inhibit the 5 alpha-reductase
and Fraser (18) has now reported that they also inhibit binding of DHT
to the receptor protein. Perhaps this inhibition of binding is due to
competition for the steroid by another protein in the cytosol of the
benign hypertrophic prostate which is distinguishable only with much
difficulty from plasma SHBG. It is suggested that steroid bound to the
SHBG-like protein may be unavailable for either transmission to the
nucleus to activate transcription of the genome or for export to the
blood stream. Whether or not this SHBG-like protein of the BPH cell is
induced by estrogen, as is its circulating analogue, has not been investigated.

PROCEDURES AND METHODS USED

Our study was conducted on 13 patients with BPH and 6 with advanced carcinoma of the prostate from whom we obtained blood and prostate tissue samples at the time of prostatectomy. Both plasma T and tissue T, DHT and 5 alpha-androstane-3 alpha,17 beta-diol, extracted with Delsal's reagent, were quantitated by competitive protein binding after careful chromatographic separation of these tissue steroids. Details are being published elsewhere (19).

RESULTS AND DISCUSSION

In our study (Fig. 1) we found that the plasma testosterone concentration in the BPH patients was equal to that in those with carcinoma but was about 30% less than in 10 normal young subjects assayed by the same method. Harper et al (20) (Table V) have just confirmed that the levels of testosterone, androstenedione and estradiol are the same in the two elderly groups.

We found that the concentration of androgen within both the BPH and cancerous glands was nearly 4-fold that in the blood. In spite of almost equal plasma concentrations of testosterone, the cancer tissue accumulated a nearly 30% greater level of testosterone and its metabolites than did the BPH tissue. An examination of the proportional distribution of the steroids revealed that in both cancer and BPH tissues about 70% was DHT, 12% DIOL and 18% unmetabolized T.

Logically, the greater androgen uptake of the cancer tissue could be due to either more capability to extract steroid from the plasma pool or to a more accessible form of steroid in the pool. It was remembered that not all of the circulating testosterone is free, that the greater part of the circulating androgen is bound to the sex hormone binding globulin. The apparent free testosterone concentration (AFTC) is a better index of androgenicity. To test this possibility, the ^{3}H-DHT-labelled plasma of our study patients was fractionated by $(NH_4)_2SO_4$ precipitation of the SHBG-bound steroid. After correction for the albumin-bound fraction, the AFTC was determined. Contrary to expectations, we found that, due to a 21% higher SHBG binding capacity in the blood of the cancer patients, the AFTC was not higher, but lower than that of the BPH subjects. Therefore, it appears that the cancer tissue does not acquire its richer store of androgen because more is freely available in the blood but through either an enhanced intrinsic androphilia or the action of some extraprostatic agent which imparts this affinity to it.

From what has been discussed earlier, it is natural to suspect that the cancer tissue is being subjected to a richer effective estrogen environment. This would account for the higher SHBG binding capacity. We have mentioned that with more androgen bound, more estrogen is set free from the globulin.

As mentioned before, Harper et al (20) saw no difference in the total estrogens of BPH and cancer patients' blood. This does not tell us that the amount of unbound estrogen is the same in the two groups. Argu-ing that it may not be the same as the report of Kaul et al (21) of a decline in urinary estrogen excretion in patients with carcinoma of the prostate. This may very well mean that less of the estrogen is con-jugated as sulfate; that more is free. With more free estrogen, androgen uptake could be expedited by the estrogen directly (cf. Giorgi, 15) and/or by the mediation of an estrogen-evoked, increase in prolactin secretion. Harper et al (20) (Table VI) found that the level of serum prolactin in their prostate cancer patients was more than twice that in their BPH patients. The difference was highly significant. This was not surprizing for Asano (22) long ago showed that the level of urinary prolactin excre-tion is directly correlated with the stage of prostate cancer.

What are the biological implications or consequences of these differences in prostatic androgen?

Although there is 30% more androgenic steroid in the cancer than in the BPH tissue, the percent distribution is identical. This suggests that we are observing an equilibrium mixture of T and its metabolites in which some 80% of the penetrating T is reduced to DHT. The action of 3 alpha-OH-steroid dehydrogenase then further reduces about 15% of the DHT to the androstanediol. Horst et al (23) achieved a similar distribu-tion in BPH tissue after infusing 5 alpha-androstane-3 alpha,17 beta-diol. Perhaps one can conclude that the difference between BPH and cancer tissue is only the intensity (concentration) and not the qualitative nature of steroid action. This is an important observation for Schmidt et al (24) have shown that DHT is a more potent stimulus of proliferation than is T but that the two steroids effect about equal stimulation of metabolic processes and attendant biosynthetic activities.

But we should also know the role of the androstanediol. From the studies of steroid metabolism just described, the DIOL appears as a reserve supply of DHT. It is hard to discern the effect of this steroid in systems where it can be readily metabolized to DHT. Several workers have observed that 5 alpha-androstane-3 beta,17 beta-diol is not mitogenic but is a more potent agent for maintenance of epithelial cell height and stimulation of secretion. We wonder if its peculiar effect is due to its limited conversion to DHT. Would both epimers have this metabolic effect if they were equally preserved, i.e. not converted to DHT? This is a difficult question to answer by bioassay. Data from Dorfman and Shipley (25) (Table VII) show what different effects one obtains from systemic treatment of the seminal vesicle as compared to local inunction of the chick comb. Reduction of the 3 ketone of DHT to a 3 alpha alcohol (5 alpha-androstane-3 alpha,17 beta-diol) diminishes the effect on the seminal vesicle to 1/6th and, if to the 3 beta-ol, to 1/12th that of DHT. In contrast, stimulation of comb growth is equally good with the 3 alpha, 17 beta-diol as with DHT. Identical relationships are seen upon 3 alpha- and 3 beta-reduction of the far less potent (1/10th DHT) 5 alpha-andro-stane-3,17-dione. It is evident that the 3 beta epimer is less effective than the 3 alpha compound in both test systems.

The shift to molecular parameters has obviated the problem. We can study action of hormones on prostate enzymes directly- Griffiths et al (26) have found that the DNA polymerase of dog prostate is stimulated by testosterone and 5 alpha-androstane-3 alpha,17 beta-diol but not by DHT or the 3 beta-epimer of the DIOL. Incidentally, Jean Wilson (27) has succeeded in inducing BPH in canine prostate by chronic treatment with the 3 alpha,17 beta-diol. Neither T nor DHT is effective. This is peculiar to this species, we suspect, for both T and DHT are excellent stimuli of DNA polymerase in human BPH. The nuclear RNA polymerase of the canine prostate (28) is responsive to DHT but only slightly to the 3 beta,17 beta-diol, whereas the enzyme from rat prostate is equally stimulated by both DIOL epimers and especially by DHT.

These data provide an answer to part of our question. They tell us that, subject to species differences, both epimers of the 17 beta-diol are effective agents. They do not tell if the DIOL action in only mitogenic or also metabolic.

An important facet of metabolic and biosynthetic activity is active transport with its component $(Na^+ + K^+)$-dependent ATPase. Studies in our laboratory have shown that active transport of the nonmetabolizable amino acid, alpha-aminoisobutyric acid, into human prostate slices is stimulated by the presence of $10^{-9}M$ testosterone in the incubation medium. Since this indicates that the androgen affects the Na^+ pump we (29) have assessed the influence of DHT and the 3 alpha,17 beta-diol on the ATPase. Fifteen minute pretreatment of human prostate microsomes with these steroids at a concentration of $10^{-12}M$ was found to increase the $(Na^+ + K^+)$-dependent ATPase activity an average of 28% with the DIOL and 38% with DHT. This suggests that the 3 alpha,17 beta-DIOL has both proliferative and metabolic properties. The 3 beta epimer is inactive (30).

SUMMARY

From our study of 13 BPH and 6 cancer patients, we find that the prostate of the aged human male has the capacity to accumulate androgenic steroids against a formidable concentration gradient and from a plasma pool of testosterone which is not only less concentrated than that in the younger individual but made less accessible by an increased per cent of binding to sex hormone binding globulin. A higher concentration of estrogen, derived from both testis and adrenal, probably accounts for the high SHBG capacity, the decreased T secretion and some increase in circulating prolactin. It may, in addition, directly increase androgen uptake. The interaction of these several factors is such that the cancerous prostate achieves a 30% greater androgen concentration than does the benign hypertrophic gland, despite an even smaller pool of free T available to the cancer tissue. Although it is evident that the steroids sequestered in the glands have different biological actions, their per cent distribution in BPH and CA is identical. We can only conclude that the cancerous gland is subjected to more intense stimulation by its enriched internal milieu.

ACKNOWLEDGMENTS

This work was supported by Veterans Administration Hospital, Buffalo, New York Project Number 2746-01. The author's wish to express their gratitude for the cooperation of area Urologists, the VA Hospital's Department of Medical Illustration and especially the invaluable help of Mrs. Pamela Snyder.

TABLE I. Effects of Age on Blood Androgens (ng/100 ml)

Age (yrs.)	No.	T	DHT	T + DHT	T/DHT
60 - 90	41	466	89	555	5.2
20 - 39	16	660	49	709	13.5

From: Horton, R., et al (1)

TABLE II. Hormone Levels in Man

	Age (yrs.)	
	22 - 61	67 - 90
	n = 50	n = 34
Testosterone (ng/100 ml)	545	459
Estradiol-17 beta (ng/100 ml)	1.66	2.56
Estrone (ng/100 ml)	2.81	3.41
SHBG capacity (ug T/100 ml)	1.44	2.05

From: Pirke, K.M., and Doerr, P. (4)
       Doerr, P. (5)

TABLE III. Age on Gonadotrophin Secretion
(Effect 200 µg LHRH, i.v.)

	Young Men (<50 yrs.)	Elderly Men (>65 yrs.)
LH		
Basal	13.0	22.5
After 40' treatment	69.1	78.3
FSH		
Basal	6.6	15.0
After 40' treatment	11.1	19.8

FROM: Rubens et al (6)

TABLE IV. ACTH on Plasma Androgens in Prostate
Cancer (Plasma Steroid, ng/100 ml)

Patients No.	Testosterone		Androstenedione	
	Control	ACTH	Control	ACTH
Untreated 14	488	386	74	152
Honvan 7	34	67	52	167
DES 3	43	73	53	238
Castrate 1	0	6.5	20	85
Castrate +				
Hovan 1	23	120	108	380

From: Cowley et al (8)

TABLE V.   Plasma Steroids in Prostatic Disease

Patients	Testosterone (ng/ml)	Androstenedione (ng/ml)	Estradiol (pg/ml)
Without disease	6.4 (35)	0.56 (32)	40 (34)
BPH	5.9 (41)	0.59 (27)	41.7 (41)
CA	5.45 (33)	0.70 (23)	38.5 (30)

From: Harper et al (20)

TABLE VI.   Plasma Gonadotrophins in Prostatic Disease

Patients	LH (mIU/ml)	FSH (mIU/ml)	Prolactin (mamp/ml)
Without disease	7.0 (35)	14.0 (31)	16.4 (35)
BPH	11.1 (41)	6.6 (37)	9.5 (41)[*]
CA	8.2 (33)	6.9 (31)	19.0 (32) [*]

[*]BPH vs CA: $P \ll 0.01$

From: Harper et al (20)

TABLE VII.   Relative Biological Activities of 5 alpha-Androstane Derivatives on Seminal Vesicles of Immature Rats and Capon's Comb (Testosterone = 100%)

Derivative	Seminal Vesicle	Capon Comb
17 beta-ol, 3-one (DHT)	200	75
17 beta-ol, 3 alpha-ol	33	75
17 beta-ol, 3 beta-ol	14	3
17 keto, 3-one	20	12
17 keto, 3 alpha-ol	10	10
17 keto, 3 beta-ol	3	2

From: Dorfman and Shipley (25)

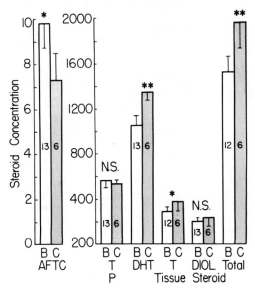

FIG. 1

REFERENCES

1. Horton, R., Hsieh, P., Barberia, J., Pages, L., and Cosgrove, M. Altered Blood Androgens In Elderly Men With Prostate Hyperplasia. J. Clin. Endocrinol. Metab., 41:793-796, 1975.
2. Mahoudeau, J., Dallasalle,A., and Bricaire, R. Secretion Of Dihydrotestosterone By Human Prostate In Benign Prostatic Hypertrophy. Acta Endocrinologica, 77:401-407, 1974.
3. Vermeulen, A., Stoica, T., and Verdonck, L. The Apparent Free Testosterone Concentration, An Index of Androgenicity. J. Clin. Endocrinol. Metab., 33:759-767, 1971.
4. Pirke, K.M., and Doerr, P. Age Related Changes and Interrelationships Between Plasma Testosterone, Oestradiol and Testosterone-Binding Globulin In Normal Adult Males. Acta Endocrinol., 74:792-800, 1973.
5. Doerr, P. Radioimmunoassay Of Oestrone In Plasma. Acta Endocrinol., 81:655-667, 1976.
6. Rubens, R., Dhont, M., and Vermeulen, A. Further Studies On Leydig Cell Function In Old Age. J. Clin. Endocrinol. Metab., 39:40-45, 1974.
7. Kley, H.K., Nieschlag, E., and Kruskemper, H.L. Age Dependence Of Plasma Oestrogen Response to HCG and ACTH In Men. Acta Endocrinologica, 79:95-101, 1975.
8. Cowley, T.H., Brownsey, B.G., Harper, M.E., Peeling, W.B., and Griffiths,K. The Effect Of ACTH On Plasma Testosterone And Androstenedione Concentrations In Patients With Prostatic Carcinoma. Acta Endocrinologica, 8:310-320, 1976.
9. Sköldefors, H., Carlström, K., and Furuhjelm, M. Aging And Urinary Oestrogen Excretion In The Male. Acta Obstet. Gynec. Scand., 54:89-90, 1975.
10. Hemsell, D.L., Grodin, J.M., Brenner, P.F., Siiteri, P.K., and MacDonald, P.C. Plasma Precursors Of Estrogen. II. Correlation Of The Extent Of Conversion Of Plasma Androstenedione To Estrone With Age. J. Clin. Endocrinol. Metab., 38:476-479, 1974.
11. Burke, C.W., and Anderson, D.C. Sex-Hormone-Binding Globulin Is An Oestrogen Amplifier. Nature, 240:38-40, 1972.
12. Farnsworth, W.E. Role Of Lactogen In Prostatic Physiology. Urological Res., 3:129-132, 1975.
13. Lloyd, J.W., Thomas, J.A., and Mawhinney, M.G. A Difference In The In Vitro Accumulation And Metabolism Of Testosterone-1,2-^{3}H By The Rat Prostate Gland Following Incubation With Ovine Or Bovine Prolactin. Steroids, 22:473-483, 1973.
14. Kledzik, G.S., Marshall, S., Campbell, G.A., Helato, M., and Meites, J. Effects Of Castration, Testosterone, Estradiol And Prolactin On Specific Prolactin-Binding Activity In Ventral Prostate Of Male Rats. Endocrinol., 98:373-379, 1976.
15. Giorgi, E.P., Moses, T.F., Grant, J.K., Scott, R., and Sinclair, J. In Vitro Studies Of The Regulation Of Androgen-Tissue Relationship In Normal Canine And Hyperplastic Human Prostate. Mol. Cell. Endocrinol., 1:271-284, 1974.
16. Shimazaki, J., Kurihara, H., Ito, Y., and Shida, K. Testosterone Metabolism In Prostate; Formation Of Androstan-17 beta-ol-3-one And Androst-4-ene-3,17-dione And The Inhibitory Effect Of Natural And Synthetic Estrogens. Gunma J. Med. Sci., 14:313-325, 1965.
17. Farnsworth, W.E. A Direct Effect Of Estrogens On Prostatic Metabolism Of Testosterone. Invest. Urol., 6:423-427, 1969.

18. Fraser, H.M., Mitchell, A.J.H., Anderson, C.K., and Oakey, R.E. The Interaction Of Dihydrotestosterone On Oestradiol-17 beta With Macromolecules In Human Hyperplastic Prostate Tissue. Acta Endocrinologica, 76:773-782, 1974.

19. Farnsworth, W.E., and Brown, J.R. Androgens Of The Human Prostate. Endocrine Research Communications, 3 - in press.

20. Harper, M.E., Peeling, W.B., Cowley, T., Brownsey, B.G., Phillips, M.E.A., Groom, G., Fahmy, D.R., and Griffiths, K. Plasma Steroid And Protein Hormone Concentrations In Patients With Prostatic Carcinoma, Before And During Oestrogen Therapy. Acta Endocrinologica, 81:409-425, 1976.

21. Kaul, P., Prasad, G.C., Gupta, R.C., and Udupa, K.N. A Comparative Study of Urinary Oestrogens In The Cancer Of The Breast And Prostate. Indian J. Cancer, 11:162-167, 1974.

22. Asano, M. Studies On Urinary Prolactin With Special Reference To Carcinoma Of The Prostate. Jap. J. Urol., 53:901-918, 1962.

23. Horst, H.-J., Dennis, M., Kaufmann, J., and Voigt, K.D. In Vivo Uptake And Metabolism Of ^{3}H-5 alpha-Androstane-3 alpha,17 beta-diol And Of ^{3}H 5 alpha-Androstane-3 beta,17 beta-diol By Human Prostatic Hypertrophy. Acta Endocrinologica, 79:394-402, 1975.

24. Schmidt, H., Noack, I., and Voight, K.D. Metabolism And Mode Of Action Of Androgens In Target Tissues Of Male Rats. II. Mode Of Action Of Testosterone And 5 alpha-Dihydrotestosterone At A Cellular Level On Seminal Vesicles And Prostates Of Rats. Acta Endocrinologica, 69:165-173, 1972.

25. Dorfman, R.I., and Shipley, R.A. Androgens, Biochemistry, Physiology and Clinical Significance. John Wiley, New York, p. 118, 1956.

26. Griffiths, K., Harper, M.E., Groom, M.A., Pike, A.W., Fahmy, A.R., and Pierrepoint, C.G. Testosterone Metabolism in the Dog Prostate with Regard to its Growth and Function. In: Some Aspects of the Aetiology and Biochemistry of Prostatic Cancer. Eds: Griffiths, K., Pierrepoint, C.G. Alpha Omega Alpha Publishing Co., Cardiff, pp. 88-94, 1970.

27. Wilson, J. Presented at Workshop on BPH at NIH, February, 1975.

28. Davies, P., Fahmy, A.R., Pierrepoint, C.G., and Griffiths, K. Hormonal Effects In Vitro On Prostatic Ribunucleic Acid Polymerase. Biochem. J., 129:1167-1169, 1972.

29. Farnsworth, W.E. The Role Of The Steroid-Sensitive Cation-Dependent ATPase In Human Prostatic Tissue. J. Endocr., 54:375-385, 1972.

30. Farnsworth, W.E. Androgen Stimulation of Prostatic Cation-Dependent ATPase. In: The Biochemistry of Steroid Hormone Action. Ed.: Smellie, R.M.S., London, Academic Press, Inc., London, pp. 129-132, 1971.

Chapter 6

NUTRITION

FOOD: A CARCINOGENIC HAZARD ?

Robert Kroes

Laboratory of Pathology
National Institute of Public Health
P.O.Box 1, Bilthoven, The Netherlands

INTRODUCTION

For many thousand years man has consumed foods, selected on his own experience. This selection was made on the basis of appreciation of the product,
and on the basis of absence of acute toxicity signs. Many food intems have
become in use and their consumption is so common and universal that, even
today, nobody cares for their possible delayed toxicity. One may state
that a great number of food items is eaten because they have been eaten
for centuries and not because they have been evaluated toxicologically for
their safety. In this paper an attempt will be made to discuss the possible carcinogenic hazard of food in a philosophical way. Not only "known"
factors will be considered but also "unknown" factors which may contribute
directly or indirectly to the possible carcinogenic hazard of food.

Chemicals in Foods

Chemicals in foods may be present as natural or as man-made chemicals.
Many of the latter are essential in that they either preserve or stabilize
foods; others, though not essential, are used on large scale for food-
colouring or flavouring.

Natural Chemicals in Food

Natural chemicals in food may be present as natural components of food
products or as natural contaminants of food products. In considering natural components of food products legislation in most countries will prohibit the introduction of new components which will bear suspicion for
carcinogenicity. Many components however, have been consumed for centuries
and are therefore considered to be safe. This might be a false assumption:
although a major threat should have been detected, a minor one can still
be present since so many factors are involved in cancercausation of man,
that decent epidemiological studies may not detect such a minor threat.
For example, the consumption of spinach, leek or purslaine has not been
under suspicion until recently. The presence of nitrate in these foods and
its subsequent reduction to nitrite in saliva, might create a problem

since nitrite may react with secondary or tertiary amines, present in the food or taken as a drug to form carcinogenic nitrosamines. In addition as yet unknown factors may be present, which may directly or indirectly lead to cancer. Important in this respect is the current believe that nutrition may affect the incidence of a large number of the human cancers (Wynder, 1975). Experimentally it has been shown that food restriction inhibits tumor formation in several tissues. In addition, changes in the level of fat and protein may effect tumor formation as well, merely by altering the metabolism of carcinogens or their modifying factors (Clayson, 1975, Carroll and Khor, 1975, Reddy et al, 1976).

When natural contaminants in food are considered, the natural carcinogens are of primary interest. Compounds as aflatoxin, cycasin, safrole, sterigmatocystine, penicillic acid, patulin, luteoskyrin, cyclochlorotine, and pyrolizidine alkaloids have been shown to be present in man's diet (Purchase, 1974). Some of these compounds belong to the most potent carcinogens identified to date, in particular aflatoxins. In nuts levels range from 5-260 μg/kg, in prepared foods from 2-100 μg/kg (Preussmann, 1975). Elimination of these compounds from the food is of great importance. Complete elimination might however be impossible since these products may enter the human food via several routes. For example, aflatoxin B_1 usually present at low levels in animal feed is partially metabolized and excreted in cows milk as aflatoxin M_1, the 4-hydroxy derivative of aflatoxin B_1. Recent surveys in the Netherlands and Western Germany indicate that the majority of milk samples are contaminated at low levels (Schuller et al, 1976). These levels do not decrease in technological procedures, such as pasteurization and sterilization and even increase proportionally to its initial content in the preparation of cheese (Stoloff and Trucksess, 1974, Verhülsdonk et al, 1976). In addition to the natural carcinogens other natural toxins may indirectly influence the cancer causation.

Man-made Chemicals in Food

Man-made chemicals may be present in food as additives, as chemicals derived from packaging materials, as residues of agricultural chemicals and as contaminants. In addition man-made chemicals may enter or develop in food processing.

In most countries legislation is directed towards a prohibition of the use of new food additives which are known to be carcinogenic. Thus the introduction of new carcinogenic compounds in food as an additive seems less likely. In the past however, several additives have been permitted for use, but were withdrawn on the basis of new findings, indicating their possible carcinogenicity (butter jellow, ponceaux SX, ponceaux 3R, guinea green, fuchsin, amaranth furfurylfuramide (AF-2), dulcin).

Another cause for concern give chemicals which enter the food through migration from packaging materials. Especially the finding that the monomer vinylchloride is carcinogenic to man and animals (Creech and Johnson, 1974, Viola, 1971, Maltoni, 1974) has prompted many governmental agencies into action to reduce or to prohibit the use of this compound in packaging materials. Although the migrating quantities are usually small, though levels of 20 mg/kg have been found (IARC, 1974), they do add to the total carcinogenic burden. In addition other migrating components as yet unknown may give the same problem. The presence of agricultural chemicals as residues in food is another route in which carcinogenic compounds may reach the food. Although in general no carcinogens are utilized as pesticides or fertilizers, some are known to be used even in the western world, and

may, especially when inaccurately handled, enter the food. Carcinogenic
compounds or compounds suspected for carcinogenicity still employed in many
countries are a.o. dibromoethane, dibromochloropropane, aramite, chlorde-
cone, lindane (BHC), DDT, Aldrin and Dieldrin. Evidence of the danger of
nitrogen fertilizers was recently given by Armyo and Coulson (1975) who
noticed a high correlation between stomach cancer death rates in man in
Chile and cumulative per capita exposure to nitrogenfertilizers. Nitrogenfertilizers are considered to be the precursors for the in vivo nitrosation
of secondary or tertiary amines into nitrosamines, a process most presumable occuring in the stomach (Sander et al, 1968).
Possibly the most important is the variety of carcinogenic compounds reaching
food as a result of environmental pollution, or as a contamination during
storage or transport. The use of carcinogenic compounds or compounds suspected for carcinogenicity for many purposes, such as desinfection, growth
promotion, insectcontrol, weedcontrol and the use of carcinogenic compounds
in chemical synthesis, will in most instances sooner or later result in
the introduction of these compounds in the food, especially if they are
persistant. Although the quantities as a rule may be small, the diversity
of the compounds used, will certainly have an influence on the total carcinogenic burden in food. An example may be the use of coccidiostatic
agents and growth promotors in animal husbandry. In the Netherlands the
use of such agents in pig husbandry amounts 25.000 kg a year. Several of
these compounds have been shown to be carcinogenic or are suspected for
carcinogenicity and even though they will not lead to residues in the animal products, they will pollute and will reach human food as long as they
are stable and difficultly biodegradated. The animal manure heavily contaminated with such compounds will be used as fertilizer and thus the compound may enter the agricultural products.
Another good example was given by Engst and Fritz (1975). They investigated
the extent and sources of environmental pollution and the contamination
of foodstuffs by measuring the content of carcinogenic polycyclic aromatic
hydrocarbons in vegetables, fruits and oils. They concluded that the degree of contamination parralled the degree of contamination in the soil.
Fritz (1971) estimated the total amount of Benz(a)pyrene ingested per man
per year at about 0.35-1.2 mg, the most important sources being vegetables,
grain and fruits.
The last possible source of carcinogens in food is the possible development of such agents in the course of processing of food. There are no indications that irradiation of food bears a carcinogenic hazard. The carcinogenicity studies carried out as yet do not indicate that irradiation of
food may lead to the development of carcinogens. Smoke-curing of food however, as is practisized with some types of fish, meat and cheeses, has
demonstrated to be a source of newly formed carcinogens, especially the
polycyclic aromatic hydrocarbons. These compounds develop in every system
where organic material is burned or smoulded. In such products levels of
0.02-14.6 microgram/kg Benz(a)pyrene can be found, whereas in special
home-made products even levels of 23-107 microgram/kg have been found
(Preussmann, 1975). Polycyclic aromatic hydrocarbons do also develop on
charcoalfires, due to pyrolysis of fat burned in the fire. The use of
fungi in the processing of certain cheeses and other products may lead to
the formation of mycotoxins. Cheeses checked for the presence of aflatoxin
in our Institute have fortunately always been negative.
Finally the curing of fish and meat by nitrite and nitrate must be emphasized. No better example can be given to demonstrate the development of
strong carcinogens during processing. In this respect several types of
nitrosamines have been identified: nitrosodimethylamine, nitrosodiethyl-

amine, nitrosopyrrolidine and nitrosopiperidine. Meatproducts, especially
bacon, but also other products such as salami, smoked meat and some types
of hams, have been shown to contain N-nitrosamines in the order of µg/kg
(Preussmann, 1975, Stephany et al, 1976). Since detection of nitrosamines
is extremely difficult it may well be that other as yet unknown N-nitrosamines, will be found in the future, especially since the introduction of
the so-called thermal energy analysis (TEA) detector (Fine et al, 1975)
has made the detection considerable easier than before.

DISCUSSION

It has been shown that carcinogens may be present in food in a great variety. Usually the levels found are extremely low. This does however not imply that there is no danger. Although no definite proof exists at the moment, there is a general agreement that the majority of cancers in man are
chemically induced (W.H.O. TRS 276, 1964, Boyland, 1969, Clayson, 1967,
Higginson, 1968, and Higginson and Muir, 1976). If this is true, a considerable part of these carcinogenic chemicals must reach man via food and
drinking water. It is of the utmost importance to reduce and eliminate at
least the known carcinogens as far as possible from food and drinking water.
This will not be an easy task since only 3000 of the existing 2 million
chemical compounds have been adequately tested for carcinogenic properies
(Anon. 1976). But prevention should not only consist of elimination of
known carcinogens from the food but should also be reflected in the approach of public health officials towards the use of carcinogens for other
purposes. In addition attempts should be made to change habits such as
colouring food, curing and smoking food, or change these processes in such
a way that the risk is reduced.
Finally, a better insight is needed on the importance of dietary factors
and especially of the impact of modifying factors on cancer causation. It
is hoped that the ultimate goal: the reduction of carcinogenic compounds
in man's food and environment to the best possible minimum will be reached
as soon as possible through the shared efforts of scientists, politicians
and public health officials.

SUMMARY

In food known as well as unknown, intentional as well as non-intentional
food contaminants may endanger health. A great number of food items has
become in use and their consumption is so common and universal that nobody cares for their possible delayed toxicity. For example natural food
components such as spinach have not been under suspicion until recently,
due to the presence of nitrate which is a precursor of nitrosamine. Many
known carcinogenic natural contaminants may be present in food at low quan-
taties. Man-made chemicals may be present in food as additives, as chemicals derived from packaging materials, as residues of agricultural chemicals and as contaminants. Although intentional food additives are expected to be thoroughly investigated before introduction, some have been shown
to be carcinogenic after they had permitted for use. Migration of chemicals into the food of packaging materials raises another problem, especially since vinylchloride has been shown to be carcinogenic. The use of some
pesticides which are carcinogenic may be another possibility to enter the

food via residues or contaminants. Possibly the most important variety of carcinogenic compounds reaches food as a contaminant from environmental pollution. A further possible source of carcinogens in food is their development in food processing (smoking, grilling, curing). Since there are reasons to believe that a majority of cancers is chemically induced, it must be assumed that at least a considerable part of these chemicals is present in food and drinking water. The only feasible solution to this problem is prevention. Prevention should not only consist of elimination of known carcinogenic elements from the food but should also be directed to the elimination of such compounds for other purposes. It cannot be emphasized enough that the production and use of carcinogens for whatever purpose will inevitably lead to the introduction of the compounds in the food as a contaminant. Prevention should also include the attempt to change certain habits such as colouring, curing and smoking of food, as long as such processes may give rise to a greater risk. Prevention should mean the promotion of studies performed to investigate the importance of the composition of the food: the protein carbonhydrate, fat and raw matter contents and their influence on tumorproduction and tumor prevention. Last but not least prevention should mean the development of better methods to detect the carcinogenic action of compounds and to predict the impact of modifying factors in order to be able to eliminate the burden of compounds which endanger man's health.

REFERENCES

1. Anonymus. Control Of Toxic Substances: An Idea Whose Time Has Nearly Come. Science, 191: 541, 1976.
2. Armyo, R., and Coulson, A.H. Epidemiology Of Stomach Cancer In Chile: The Role Of Nitrogen Fertilizers. Int.J.Epid., 4: 301-309, 1975.
3. Boyland, E. The Correlation Of Experimental Carcinogenesis And Cancer In Man. Prog.Exp.Tumor Res., 11: 222-234, 1969.
4. Carroll, K.K., and Kohr, H.T. Dietary Fat In Relation To Tumorigenesis. Progr.Biochem.Pharmacol., 10: 308-353, 1975.
5. Clayson, D.B. Chemicals And Environmental Carcinogenisis In Man. Europ.J.Cancer, 3: 405-416, 1967.
6. Clayson, D.B. Nutrition And Experimental Carcinogenesis: A Review. Cancer Res., 35: 3292-3300, 1975.
7. Creech, J.L., and Johnson, M.N. Angiosarcoma Of Liver In The Manufacture Of Polyvinyl Chloride. J.Occ.Med., 16: 150-151, 1974.
8. Engst, R., and Fritz, W. Environment Pollution Of Foodstuffs By Carcinogenic Hydrocarbons. ROC ZN PZH, 26(1): 113-118, 1975.
9. Fine, D.H., and Rounbehler, D.P. Trace-analysis Of Volatile N-nitroso-compounds By Combined Gaschromatography And Thermal Energy Analysis (TEA). J.Chrom., 109: 271-279, 1975.
10. Fritz, W. Umfang Und Quellen Der Kontamination Von Lebensmitteln Mit Krebserzeugenden Kohlen-wasserstoffen. Ernährungsforschung, 16: 547-557, 1971.
11. Higginson, J. Present Trends In Cancer Epidemiology. Proc.8th Canad. Cancer Conference, Pergamon, Toronto, p. 40-75, 1968.
12. Higginson, J., and Muir, C.S. The Role Of Epidemiology In Elucidating The Importance Of Environmental Factors In Human Cancer. Cancer Prevention and Detection. International Symposium Journal, no.1, April 1976.
13. IARC. IARC Monographs On The Evaluation Of Carcinogenic Risk Of Chem-

icals To Man, 7, Some Anti-thyroid And Related Substances, Nitrofurans And Industrial Chemicals, p. 291-305, 1974.

14. Maltoni, C., and Lefemine, G. Carcinogenicity Bio-assays Of Vinylchloride. Environm.Res., $\underline{7}$: 387-405, 1974.

15. Preussmann, R. Chemische Carcinogene In Der Menschlichen Umwelt. Handbuch Der Allgemeinen Pathologie. Springer Verlag, Berlin, $\underline{6}$: 421-594, 1975.

16. Purchase, I.F.H. Mycotoxins. Elseviers Scientific Publishing Company, Amsterdam - Oxford - New York, p. 1-428, 1974.

17. Reddy, B.S., Narisawa, T., Vukisch, D., Weisburger, J.H., and Wynder, E.L. Effect Of Quality And Quantity Of Dietary Fat And Dimethylhydrazine In Colon Carcinogenesis In Rats. Proc.Soc.Exp.Biol.and Med., $\underline{151}$: 237-239, 1976.

18. Sander, J., Schweinsberg, F., and Menz, H.P. Untersuchungen Uber Die Entstehung Cancerogener Nitrosamine Im Magen. Z.Physiol.Chem., $\underline{349}$: 1691-1695, 1968.

19. Schuller, P.L., Verhülsdonk, C.A.H., and Paulsch, W.E. Aflatoxin M_1 In Liquid And Powdered Milk. Second Int.Symp.On Mycotoxins In Food, 1974, IUPAC PAN, Pulawy, Poland in press, 1976.

20. Stephany, R.W., Freudenthal, J., and Schuller, P.L. Quantitative And Qualitative Determination Of Some Volatile N-nitrosamines In Various Meat Products. IARC scient.publication, No.13 in press, 1976.

21. Stoloff, L., and Trucksess, M. Studies On Stability Of Aflatoxin M_1 In Milk. Manuscript FDA, Bureau Of Foods, Washington, 1974.

22. Verhülsdonk, C.A.H., Egmond, H.van, Leussink, A.B., and Paulsch, W.E. De Invloed Van Een Aantal Technologische Processen Op Het Gehalte Aan Aflatoxine M_1 In Melk En Melkproducten. Report Nat.Inst.Publ.Health, The Netherlands, no.51, 1976.

23. Viola, P.L., Bigotti, A., and Caputo, A. Oncogenic Response Of Rat Skin, Lungs And Bones To Vinylchloride. Cancer Res., $\underline{31}$: 516-522, 1971.

24. WHO. WHO Technical Report Series No.276 Prevention Of Cancer, Geneva, 1964.

25. Wynder, E.L. Introductory Remarks On The Symposium Nutrition In The Causation Of Cancer. Cancer Res., $\underline{35}$: 3238-3239, 1975.

NUTRITIONAL MODULATION OF CARCINOGENESIS

Paul M. Newberne, Adrianne E. Rogers and Robert L. Gross

Department of Nutrition and Food Science
Massachusetts Institute of Technology
Cambridge, Massachusetts

I. INTRODUCTION.

The concept that diet, nutrition and some forms of cancer are inter-related is relatively recent. Only in recent years have epidemiologists begun to point the way for biologists and analytical chemists to follow toward the resolution of some questions about the food we eat and certain undesirable consequences, including cancer.

Evidence clearly points out a relationship in the United States between nutrition and cancer of five major target organs. Table I lists statistics for 1975 in which cancer of five organ sites comprise about 200,000 new cases, roughly one-third of all new cancer cases for the year. Further evidence, on the international level, is shown in Table II. It is particularly interesting that there is an inverse relationship between stomach and colon cancer; when one is high the other is low, and con-versely.

The following pages will describe examples where epidemiologic studies and experimental data coincide to support or deny an hypothesis for nutritional modification of carcinogenesis.

II. PROCEDURES AND RESULTS.

The wide variation in incidence of some types of cancer in various populations of ethnic groups living in different geographic locations as shown in Table II and the change in risk of migrant populations as they relocate and assume dietary habits and nutritive status of low or high risk groups, strongly support a role for nutrition in resistance or sus-ceptibility to cancer. Other dietary factors which may be related to differences in cancer incidence are carcinogens (or their precursors) found as contaminants in foods. Some of these are mycotoxins, nitrosa-mines, pesticides, and synthetic hormones. Other chemicals such as food additives used to improve texture, flavor, color, or nutritive value are also suspect in some cases.

The effects of nutrition on carcinogenesis in experimental animals are sometimes conspicuous and easily recognized; more often, however, they are subtle and may be expressed only as changes in induction time or in the type or distribution of tumors. Nutritive status relevant to human cancer is probably in the nature of a marginal deficit or imbalance rather than a severely abnormal situation which makes the job of identifying the important nutritional factors very difficult; but at the same time impor-tant opportunities and challenges to the nutritionist in our continuing search for cancer cause and prevention are provided.

A. Esophageal Carcinoma.

There is a varied geographic distribution of esophageal cancer with a high incidence in Puerto Rico, Chile and in selected areas of Japan, France and South and East Africa; a low incidence has been reported in Norway, and the disease is practically unknown in West Africa (1). Other reports indicate high rates of esophageal cancer in parts of the Soviet Union. The high frequency in some areas appears to be a development of the past 30-40 years. In New York City, patients with esophageal cancer tend to be heavy smokers and often consume large quantities of alcohol with decreased consumption of milk, eggs and green leafy vegetables. On the island of Curacao and in several counties of South Carolina a high incidence of esophageal cancer has been associated with use of local plants for beverages and medicinal purposes but nutrient deficiencies have not been ruled out. Dietary factors have been associated with eso-phageal cancer in each of the areas of high incidence (2-7).

In Puerto Rico where less fresh fruits and vegetables, meat, eggs and milk are consumed, the diet is high in carbohydrates; foods and beverages and alcohol from uncontrolled fermentation have been associated with esophageal cancer but this is an unknown quantity. Similar studies in Africa have suggested that contamination of beer by mycotoxins and nitrosamines found in maize, is a factor in esophageal cancer (8,9).

In the United States significant correlations between esophageal cancer, percent of the population living in urban communities, cigarette and alcohol sales have been demonstrated. A geographic correlation between mortality rates from esophageal cancer and per capita consumption of spirits and beer has also been shown. Alcoholics may exhibit deficiencies of vitamins or of some of the trace elements, all of which may contribute in some way to tumor development (10-13).

An association of low intake of vitamins A, C and riboflavin, animal protein, and fresh fruit and vegetables and an increased incidence of esophageal cancer has been established in Iran (14). Further, these studies have also demonstrated a relationship between this form of cancer and wheat-eating, as opposed to rice-eating populations. In China the high incidence areas also are areas of wheat-eating populations rather than rice-eating peoples and nitrosamines have been identified in the local environment; a high incidence of esophageal cancer in chickens as well as people has been reported from well defined areas of the People's Republic of China (15). In the geographical areas of very high incidence, the predominance of esophageal cancer in males decreases and women have an equal or even slightly greater incidence. In these areas of high incidence, as in Iran, the association with tobacco and alcohol is less strong. There may be other environmental carcinogens to which women may be more susceptible than men along with other factors such as deficiency concomitant to childbearing and poor intake of nutrients resulting from poverty. All of these conditions are coexistant in many of these population groups (16).

Animal studies in our laboratories have provided data which suggest that deficiencies and dietary contamination may interact in esophageal carcinogenesis. We have examined the effects of feeding N-nitrosodiethylamine (DEN) to lipotrope-deficient rats and have found a significant enhancement of esophageal carcinogenesis (Table III) (17). The tumors induced in these investigations were invasive squamous cell carcinomas, morphologically identical to those in man. However, it must be pointed out that in this study the diet was also high in fat. Currently, in collaboration with Dr. W.C. Chan and Dr. Lin in Hong Kong and with Dr. Natth Bhamarapravati in Thailand, we are exploring nutrition and esophageal cancer. In these areas food contaminants, malnutrition and a high incidence of esophgeal cancer coexist.

Both epidemiologic and experimental data point to a role for nutritional deficiencies in esophageal cancer, perhaps acting in concert with other unidentified environmental interactants to modify the individual exposed to carcinogens.

B. Gastric Cancer

Cancer of the stomach has a remarkable variability in incidence according to geographic location. Populations in Japan, Chile, Columbia, Austria, Iceland and Finland exhibit a high incidence while a low incidence is recorded in the United States and Canada (1). A number of dietary factors have been implicated in its etiology but studies about food habits in gastric cancer patients have yielded few if any significant differences in intake of specific nutrients when compared to control groups (18-20). The high incidence of gastric cancer in Iceland has been associated with a large intake of smoked food but this hypothesis has not been substantiated (21). Talc, most of which contains asbestos, has been assigned a role in stomach cancer in Japan (22), but epidemiologic data and experimental work is largely yet to be developed.

There has been a progressive decrease in mortality from gastric cancer in the United States during the past four decades. There is a gradient of increasing frequency with decreasing socioeconomic status in gastric cancer; the lowest socioeconomic groups are reported to have three times the incidence of upper social groups (23). Stomach cancer in Japanese migrants to Hawaii is about equal in incidence to their native Japanese cohorts in high risk areas even though the immigrants eat western type diets; however, their offspring have lower risks. In a United States study (24) it was revealed that gastric cancer patients ate raw vegetables less often than controls but there was no relation between fried foods, meats, or alcohol consumption and the disease.

An inverse relationship exists between cancer of the stomach and cancer of the colon according to epidemiologic surveys. Migration from a high risk area for stomach cancer in Japan to a relatively low risk area of California resulted in a decreasing incidence of gastric cancer and increasing incidence of colon cancer (25), the incidence of both types similar to the area to which they migrated (Table IV)(26).

Although there is convincing evidence from epidemiologic data that nutritional factors are important to the etiology of gastric carcinoma, experimental evidence is equivocal. Tatematsu et al. (27) have shown that sodium chloride increased the incidence of gastric carcinoma with either N-methyl-N-Nitroso-N'-nitroguanidine (MNNG) or N-nitrosoquinoline (NQO) but the manner in which salt was administered clearly influenced the results. Single weekly doses of saturated NaCl were more effective in enhancing gastric cancer than continuous administration of salt either in water or diet. Sodium chloride alone under these conditions enhanced the effects of the two carcinogens. These authors suggest that salt may have modified the mucopolysaccharides and mucosal barrier rendering the stomach lining more permeable to the carcinogen.

In our own laboratories at M.I.T., we have found that increased intakes of vitamin A reduced the number of papillomas of the forestomach in hamsters given carcinogenic doses of benzo(a)pyrene intratracheally although the increased vitamin A had no influence on cancer of the respiratory tree (28); others have confirmed this (29). Other studies in our laboratory revealed that a diet marginal in lipotropes and high in fat had no effect on the incidence of gastric squamous carcinoma. Other investigators have shown that antioxidant food additives can reduce gastric tumor incidence in mice (30,31).

It thus appears that although there is highly suggestive evidence that nutrition is related to gastric cancer in some human populations, specific agents are yet to be identified and, in the case of animal experiments, the evidence is variable and sometimes conflicting.

C. Colon Cancer.

There is a strong negative correlation between gastric and colon cancer; where one is relatively common, the other is often rare. Cancer of the colon is associated with environmental factors and a number of studies have suggested a role for nutrition in the etiology of this type of malignancy. The mortality from colon cancer is high in Scotland, Canada and the United States and low in Japan and Chile (1).

Epidemiological studies have implicated a high fat diet in the etiology of colon cancer; however, these same populations usually consume considerable protein because most of the dietary fat is consumed along with animal protein (beef) (32). In Japan where the incidence of colon cancer is low, fat intake accounts for about 12% of calories and the fat is primarily unsaturated. In the U.S. 40-44% of calories derive from fat, including the diet eaten by immigrants to the United States from Japan (32, 33). In contrast (Table IV) to gastric cancer, colon cancer incidence rises in the immigrants, and their children have a much higher incidence of colon cancer than those born in Japan. Adoption of a Western style diet and a higher standard of living may account for this difference.

669

It is interesting to note that the incidence of colon cancer in the United States does not vary appreciably with race or ethnic group or with socio-economic status (33,34). Mortality from colon cancer in migrants from Poland and Norway to the U.S. has shifted upward to United States levels. Bjelke (35) has reported no correlation between blood-cholesterol level and mortality from colon cancer in Norway but a particularly high risk of colon cancer in people consuming an excess of processed meats; the data of Rose et al. (36) are in agreement.

It has been observed that populations in areas with a high incidence of colon cancer consume diets high in refined foods and low in fiber. Refined foods result in small stools and long intestinal transit time while high fiber diets are associated with large stools, rapid transit time (37-40) and differences in the bacterial flora (41). There are higher anaerobic bacteria counts and lower counts of aerobic bacteria; higher levels of total neutral steroids and more degraded cholesterol and bile acids in feces of individuals from areas of high risk for colon cancer. It has been postulated that certain metabolites of bile salts may be carcinogenic. There is disagreement on the relative amounts of fecal bile salts in groups consuming vegetarian diets (42). Thus, as more recent observations illustrate (43), the relation of a number of dietary habits and constituents to colon cancer is a complex one and require many more epidemiologic studies followed by in-depth analytical studies designed to identify etiologic agents or conditions in areas of high risk.

Cancer of the colon occurs rarely as a spontaneous disease in laboratory animals; it can be induced readily however by a number of chemical carcinogens. Bracken fern, cycasin or MAM (44,45), dimethylhydrazine (DMH) (46), and aflatoxin (47,48) are all associated with colon cancer in laboratory animals. Investigations in our laboratory as well as others have shown that diet can modify the incidence of the tumor induced by chemical agents (45-49).

Diet may modify the induction of colon cancer through its influence on the intestinal microflora (50), by changing the sensitivity of the colon mucosa to carcinogens or perhaps by liberating an active metabolite or supplying promotors or accelerators to act on the colon mucosa. Rats fed a diet high in fat excreted more bile acids and steroid metabolites and were more susceptible to DMH-induced colon cancer than rats fed a diet low in fat (51).

Our own studies (52) have shown that a diet high in fat and marginal in lipotropes increased the incidence of colon carcinoma induced by DMH (Table V). Chronic dietary deficiency of vitamin A only slightly increased the incidence of DMH-induced colon tumors and slightly decreased induction time. A high level of vitamin A in the diet had no affect on tumor incidence but decreased the number of tumors per rat (Table VI) (51).

Aflatoxin B[1] (49), normally considered a liver carcinogen in laboratory animals, induced a significant number of colon tumors in rats fed diets low or marginal in vitamin A; an indication that there was a change in target organ from liver to colon (Table VII). This suggests a change in sensitivity of the colon or a change in metabolite(s) associated with vitamin A deficiency and a plethora of factors or mechanisms may be involved; if mediated through a change in gut microflora, a change in drug metabolizing enzymes, altered quantity or quality of the secretion of colon glycopeptides which are vitamin A-dependent (53) or a combination of these. High dietary vitamin A had no appreciable effect on liver or colon tumor incidence.

Recent studies (54,55) have clearly shown that intestinal aryl hydrocarbon hydroxylase (AHH) can be modified by diet; this in turn can modify chemical carcinogenesis. The activity of AHH in the intestine of the rat can be changed by exogenous inducers in foods including Brussels sprouts, turnips, cabbage, alfalfa and other dietary components, suggesting an important role for natural dietary ingredients in modulation of carcinogenesis through enzyme systems. These observations have important implications for human cancer.

D. Liver Cancer.

In some population groups of Africa, South China, Hawaii, Thailand, Mozambique, and other areas, primary liver cancer is a major problem, particularly in males (2,3,4,56-58). Liver cancer is the commonest of all forms of cancer south of the Sahara in Africa representing from 10 to 30% of all tumors in men in that part of the world. In the Bantu of Mozambique it accounts for two-thirds of cancer in men, a rate 500 times that of the same age group in the United States. The U.S. rate is about 2.4 per 100,000.

Reports of Shank et al., in Thailand, (57) and observations from East and South Africa clearly implicate carcinogenic dietary contaminants

in the etiology of liver cancer (58). These contaminants appear to interact with nutritional deficits or imbalances in some manner to enhance carcinogenesis. The tumors are mainly of the hepatocellular type. It has
been suggested that the high frequency in Africa and Asia results from an
increased incidence of cirrhosis which enhances susceptibility to tumor
development. Cirrhosis may be induced by malnutrition or it may be the
result of dietary contaminants, infectious disease, or of a combination
of these and other factors. A role for nutrition is indicated, but the
complex problem is probably a result of many different interactions. In
the United States, hepatocarcinoma is associated with alcoholic cirrhosis,
another disease resulting from complex interactions of diet, toxins and
possibly viral liver disease.

Dietary effects on chemical induction of hepatocarcinoma in experimental animals have been studied extensively in our laboratory. Increased dietary lipid, particularly the unsaturated types, are associated
with increased tumor incidence (60). If the diet is both high in fat and
deficient in the lipotropes choline, methionine and folic acid, induction of liver tumors by carcinogens of several chemical classes is markedly enhanced (Table VIII). Aflatoxin B_1, nitrosamines, and N-2-
fluorenylacetamide (AAF) all induced liver tumors earlier or in higher
incidence in deficient rats, compared to rats fed adequate, balanced
lipotropes (17,30). Trends for the influence of vitamin A on chemical
carcinogenesis in experimental animals is shown in Table IX; it is interesting that the effects of lipotropes and of vitamin A do not coincide
(compare Tables VIII and IX).

The most likely mechanism by which the lipotrope deficiency, high
fat diet influences carcinogenesis is through alteration of the metabolism of carcinogens by the tissues. Deficient rats had decreased basal
(resting) levels of hepatic microsomal oxidases (Table X) which could be
induced by phenobarbital and, in some cases, by AAF but not by AFB_1
(61,62). Deficient rats cleared diethylnitrosamine (DEN), an hepato-
carcinogen for the rat, from their blood slightly but significantly less
rapidly than normal rats (Table XII); this correlated with tumor incidence.

Studies in progress on AAF metabolism in collaboration with Poirier
and Grantham at the National Cancer Institute, Bethesda, indicate that
urinary excretion of N-hydroxy AAF, an intermediate on the pathway of

activation of AAF, may be increased in deficient rats following prolonged feeding. S-adenosyl-methionine (SAM) content in the liver of deficient rats, a direct biochemical measure of lipotrope deficiency, was decreased in deficient rats. It diminished in both deficient and adequately-fed rats when AAF was fed which may indicate its participation in some aspect of AAF metabolism. Hepatic content of reduced glutathione, which reacts with many exogenous toxic chemicals to detoxify them, was normal in deficient rats and was not affected by AAF.

In collaboration with Suit and Luria at M.I.T., we are using the in vitro mutagenesis assay and specific bacterial strains developed by Ames (63) to determine whether the observed dietary effects on chemical carcinogenesis operate through alteration of hepatic activation of carcinogens. In agreement with the data on microsomal oxidases, liver preparations from deficient rats converted only about one-third to one-half as much AFB_1 to a bacterial mutagen as preparations from adequately fed rats; conversion of AAF also was decreased. Treatment of rats with carcinogen modified the capacity of the liver preparations to convert the carcinogen to a mutagen. Preliminary studies have indicated that after AAF treatment of rats, liver preparations from lipotrope-deficient rats are as effective as preparations from normal rats in conversion of AAF to a mutagen. AFB_1 treatment either decreased the capacity of liver preparations from adequately-fed rats to convert AFB_1 to a mutagen without affecting conversion by preparations from deficient rats, or enhanced the conversion by both groups depending on time and dose. More extensive studies are required for confirmation of these results and these are now in progress. Results of these studies agree with our other studies of microsomal oxidases and demonstrate a diet-induced difference in hepatic carcinogen activation, insofar as it is indicated by mutagen production. They do not, however, fully explain the enhancement of carcinogenesis in deficient rats.

In addition to its effect on hepatic enzymes, the lipotrope-deficient high fat diet induces and maintains increased DNA synthesis and mitosis in hepatocytes; presumably this is the result of increased cell turnover although significant necrosis is not evident histologically. Studies in collaboration with Leffert at the Salk Institute, La Jolla, have demonstrated that there is a significant drop in serum very low density lipoproteins (VLDL) in the marginally deficient animals although it is not as marked as in severely deficient ones (Table XII). Serum VLDL inhibit the initiation of hepatocyte DNA synthesis both in vitro and in vivo and may, in conjunction with several hormones, control cell division in the liver (64). Therefore the dietary effect on VLDL may interfere with normal regulatory growth controls and render the hepatocytes more susceptible to chemical carcinogens.

Other nutrients which influence tumor induction in the liver include protein, riboflavin and vitamin B_{12}. Protein deficiency sufficient to decrease hepatic microsomal oxidases blocked induction of hepatic tumors by DMN and enhanced induction of renal tumors, presumably because DMN was cleared from the blood less rapidly in deficient rats (65). Diets either marginally deficient or excessive in protein have variable effects on induction of liver and other tumors, most notably bladder tumors which may be increased by increased urinary levels of tryptophan metabolites (66).

Riboflavin specifically decreases hepatic tumor induction by the aminoazobenzes since it is a co-factor for the enzyme which metabolizes those compounds.

High concentrations of vitamin B_{12} is reported to be cocarcinogenic for the induction of liver tumors by DAB and DEN (67). No mechanism for the effect has been proposed; it may be related to an abnormality in one carbon metabolism, as we have found in lipotrope deficient, high fat diets, but has a different end result.

E. Breast Cancer.

Breast cancer incidence is correlated with socioeconomic status and therefore, it is assumed with differences in nutritive status. It is not common in women in developing societies nor in Japanese women but the incidence increases in these population groups when they migrate to the United States (68). Breast cancer is increasing in young women in the United States; this increase may be associated with a higher fat consumption; however, there is insufficient evidence at this time to incriminate fat per se in breast cancer. As noted earlier, increased fat intake in the United States is almost always accompanied by increased protein intake and protein levels per se have not been examined in this regard. Breast cancer patients have been reported to be obese compared to control groups but recent studies have indicated that the difference is more closely related to body mass, i.e., influence by both height and weight (69). A

674

possible mechanism for increased breast cancer in the obese is increased synthesis of estrone from stored fat, thus exposing the individual to continued, excessive levels of this estrogen.

An interesting possible mechanism for increased breast cancer associated with fat is related to the intestinal flora; people consuming a western, high-fat diet have a higher proportion of strictly anaerobic microflora in the intestine. These organisms can produce estrogens from biliary steroids which also are increased in subjects consuming high fat diets (51).

A number of other dietary factors which may modify individuals have been associated with breast cancer in epidemiologic studies, including iodine deficiency (70), the cadmium content of the water (71), and high rate of beer consumption (72). These suggestions are speculative, however, and require more extensive epidemiologic and experimental support.

In experimental studies, diets high in corn oil enhanced mammary tumor induction in rats by 7,12-dimethylbenz(a)anthracene (DMBA) but the tumors were inhibited by the synthetic antioxidants BHA, BHT, and ethoxyquin (54) and by sulfur-containing compounds benzylthiocyanate, disulfuram and dimethyldithiocarbamate (73). In mice, dietary restriction (74), riboflavin deficiency (75), and phenylalanine deficiency (76) inhibited the formation of mammary gland tumors.

Experiments in our laboratory using a diet marginal in lipotropes and high in fat have modified the induction of breast cancer in two strains of female rats by AAF or DMBA. Dietary AAF induced fewer mammary tumors in Sprauge-Dawley rats fed the low lipotrope, high-fat diet than in rats fed an adequate diet (Table XIII). Tumor incidence was lower in the marginally lipotrope deficient rats and death from mammary tumors was slowed by 4-6 weeks, compared to the controls. In Fischer rats, which are resistant to AAF induction of mammary tumors, hepatic carcinomas developed in a significantly greater incidence in the deficient rats, a result in accord with findings in male rats discussed above.

In Sprague-Dawley rats fed the marginal lipotrope, high-fat diet, mammary tumor incidence induced by DMBA also was reduced similar to the result with AAF.

The alteration of mammary tumor incidence in rats fed the high fat diet is particularly important because it is opposed to previous results in experimental animals which have shown an enhancement of mammary

675

carcinogenesis by high fat diets. The marginal lipotrope status of the
rats may account for the observed difference in tumor induction. It should
be noted, however, that the marginal deficiency of lipotropes was not of
such severity as to significantly depress growth or caloric intake.

III. DISCUSSION.

Recognition that nutritional factors can have a profound influence on
the susceptibility of individuals to carcinogenesis is a first step toward
utilizing these mechanisms to protect populations from unidentified carcinogens or from those that are known and for various reasons cannot be
eliminated from the environment. Epidemiologic studies and animal experimentation have clearly indicated that dietary factors and nutrients may
be important in altering the response of individuals to environmental carcinogens. There is a critical need to learn more about what these factors
are and how they modify people's responses so that they can be used in the
prevention of cancer.

Cancers of five different organ sites associated in some manner with
nutrition account for about one-third of the mortality from all cancer in
the United States which makes these types of neoplasia prime targets for
epidemiologic and experimental studies designed to examine interactions
between nutritive status and other environmental factors in tumor induction in specific populations. Nitrosamines now known to be environmental
contaminants and to develop in vivo from dietary nitrites and amines,
cause esophageal cancer in experimental animals. Esophageal cancer in the
United States is highest in alcoholics, who are as a group notorious for
nutritional deficiencies. Critical studies in alcoholics may yield valuable insight into mechanisms of esophageal cancer induction. Trace elements, particularly zinc, as well as vitamin A, both associated with maintenance of esophageal integrity should form the basis for intriguing
investigations. Heavy smokers among alcoholics would be particularly
interesting since tobacco smoke contains nitrosamines. Study of interactions among nutrients, contaminants, and esophageal cancer may produce
data important in prevention of the disease.

Although stomach cancer occurs in the United States in a relatively
low incidence compared to tumors of certain other organs and compared to
the incidence in other countries, it merits intense study. If a relationship to diet and nutrition could be found to explain why the incidence
is high in Japan but low and declining in the United States, it might
conceivably illuminate other etiologic interrelationships. It is

interesting that epidemiolgoic evidence just now in hand indicates that gastric cancer in Japan is declining and that this correlates well with increased consumption of milk, dairy products and eggs.

Colon cancer has been associated with a number of dietary factors, most notably quantity and quality of fat and type and amount of fiber. That some environmental factor(s) are involved in cancer of the colon can no longer be doubted, based on both epidemiologic and animal experimental studies. In the association between fat intake and colon cancer, mechanisms such as bile salt metabolism with production of carcinogens, cholesterol degradation by microflora, decreased bulk and longer intestinal transit time allowing for longer periods of microbial action and contact of a potential carcinogen with mucosa, or combinations of these have been suggested. Evidence from experimental animals in recent studies does not strongly support an anticarcinogenic effect of fiber but only a few studies have been reported. Our studies favor a relationship between dietary fat and colon cancer in an experimental animal model. The relationship is not simply to the amount of fat but includes also a factor of abnormal fat metabolism.

The influence of vitamin A on colon tumors associated with aflatoxin B_1 opens an exciting new dimension in studies of colon cancer. A number of possible explanations exist including modification of carcinogen metabolism by microsomal enzymes or change in sensitivity of colonic mucosa to chemical carcinogenesis.

The geographical distribution of liver cancer strongly implies an environmental etiology which is probably an interaction of dietary contamination and nutritional imbalance. In some areas of the world (South Africa, Southeast Asia), where liver cancer incidence is highest, malnutrition is common as is dietary contamination with a number of hepatotoxins and carcinogens (mycotoxins, nitrosamines). If animal data can be accepted as indicative of human response, this epidemiologic data can be related to experimental evidence that nutritional imbalances such as are induced by marginal lipotrope and high fat intake can significantly enhance carcinogenesis, most likely through modification of the liver microsomal enzyme systems. In areas such as South Africa, Mozambique and in Southeast Asia, the lipid content of the diet is significantly lower than that of United States, yet many if not most of the victims of liver cancer have some degree of fatty liver and cirrhosis. This suggests that hepatic damage by some nutritional imbalance enhances hepatic tumor development

677

although the imbalance may not be induced by dietary fat as it is in the animal model.

Protein, riboflavin and vitamin B_{12} appear, from animal studies also to influence liver tumor induction. The data on these are fragmentary and require further investigation.

Breast cancer has been positively correlated by epidemiologists with socioeconomic status. This seems to imply that at least ample and possibly overnourishment (obesity) may be involved. Further, saturated fats appear to be related in some way to increased breast cancer in women in many widely dispersed geographic locations. In considering animal fat, it is usually the case that a relatively high level of protein is taken in along with fat since those countries where breast cancer (and fat consumption) is highest derive much of their protein from beef and to a lesser extent, pork.

Obesity may have a detectible influence on breast cancer; it has been postulated that this may be via increased synthesis of estrone in fat cells which increases exposure to this hormone which is carcinogenic in experimental animals. It appears, however, that body mass, that is both height and weight, has a greater influence than obesity alone. Clearly, much remains to be done in this area of research into the human disease. In the case of animal experiments, in some cases dietary fat has been shown to promote mammary tumors; our studies have shown an effect by fat opposite to that; these observations, where increased fat resulted in fewer breast tumors, are very provocative and are being further investigated.

Nutritional modification of individuals offers one of the most exciting means for changing the course of cancer morbidity and mortality. There can be no doubt that in many population groups dietary habits are central to the incidence of some forms of cancer and through astute observations and experimentations we can learn to use nutrition as a major modifier in our efforts toward cancer prevention.

IV. SUMMARY.

Compelling evidence is now available to indicate that nutrition is associated with resistance to the development of cancer in man and other animals. The convincing nature of epidemiologic studies which clearly show a change in incidence of some forms of cancer, when populations move from one geographic location to another and change food habits, is further supported in some cases by animal studies. Of the more than three-hundred thousand new cases of cancer reported in the United States during the past year, about one-third could be associated with nutritional factors in one way or another. The primary sites include the esophagus, stomach, colon, liver and breast. Although a number of factors have been related to tumors at each site in people or experimental animals, the following positive associations are best established: 1) esophagus: heavy consumption of cigarettes and alcohol, wheat bread and tea consumption; 2) stomach: low socioeconomic status, consumption of salted, smoked, or fermented foods and decreased consumption of raw vegetables; 3) colon: increased consumption of meat, saturated fats, and highly refined carbohydrates with low dietary fiber and decreased vitamin A; 4) liver: decreased dietary lipotropes and increased fat, consumption of toxins such as alcohol and mycotoxins and modified microsomal oxidases; 5) breast: higher, socioeconomic status with increased consumption of animal fat, obesity or increased height or both, potential increases in estrogen synthesis.

From these preliminary observations there must be development of vigorous programs in epidemiology which include in-depth and precise analyses of diets and nutritional status of people and in animal experimentation. Properly utilized these integrated efforts can hasten the time when nutrition, which touches everyone everyday, can be used in the prevention or alleviation of cancer development.

TABLE I. Morbidity and Mortality in U.S. from Cancers During One Year Which May be Related to Diet

Organ Site	Estimated Statistics for 1975	
	New Cases	Deaths
Esophagus	7,400	6,500
Stomach	22,900	14,400
Colon	69,000	38,600
Breast	88,700	32,900
Liver (and Bile Ducts)	11,500	9,800
Total	199,500	102,200
All Cancer	665,000	365,000

TABLE II. Age Adjusted Death Rate/100,000 Population - 1968-1969

Country	Primary Cancer Site				Breast
	Stomach		Colon and Rectum		
	Male	Female	Male	Female	Female
U.S.A.	9	4	19	16	22
Japan	66	34	9	7	4
Scotland	23	12	25	21	26
Germany (F.R.)	33	18	21	17	19
Netherlands	26	13	18	17	26
Chile	59	36	7	7	11

(Compiled from data in References 1-4)

TABLE III. Tumor Incidence in Rats Fed N-Nitrosodiethylamine

Diet	Number of Rats	N-Nitroso-diethylamine Intake (total mg/rat)	Body Wt. (g)[a]	% of Rats with Tumor in Esophagus
Control (1)	23	179	657	35
Marginal Lipotrope (2)	34	176	702	44

[a] Average weight at end of N-nitrosodiethylamine treatment.

TABLE IV. Mortality from Cancer of Stomach and Colon for Japanese in Japan and Japanese and Caucasians in California

	Japan= (Japanese)		California Foreign-Born		U.S.-Born		Caucasian	
	Men	Women	Men	Women	Men	Women	Men	Women
Stomach (151)	58.4	30.9	29.9	13.0	11.7	11.3	8.0	4.0
Colon (153)	1.9	2.1	6.1	7.0	6.3	10.4	7.9	8.3
TOTAL	60.3	33.0	36.0	20.0	18.0	21.7	15.9	12.3

(From Ackerman, 1972, abridged.)

TABLE V. Tumor Induction by Dimethylhydrazine in Rats Fed Control or Marginal Lipotrope, High Fat Diets

Diet	Total DMH (mg kg^{-1})	% Mortality[a]	% Rats Dead with Carcinoma of Colon[b]
Control	300	100	86
High Fat	300	100	100
Control	150	80	56
High Fat	150	68	85

[a] 40 weeks after initial dose of DMH.

[b] Adenocarcinoma with varying degrees of differentiation and mucus production.

TABLE VI. Colon Tumors in Rats Given DMH and Vitamin A

Treatment	Amount of DMH (mg/kg body weight)	Rats with Colon Carcinoma (%)
Control	420	60
10 ug/g vitamin A	275	56
Deficient	420	100
0-1 ug/g vitamin A	275	77
Excess	420	60
165 ug/g vitamin A	275	60

(From Reference 24)

TABLE VII. Incidence of Liver and Colon Tumors in Rats Fed Aflatoxin B_1 and Diets Low or Normal in Vitamin A Content

	Animal Nos.	Sex	Liver	Colon	Percentage of Tumors Liver Only	Colon Only	Both
Control							
3.0 ug/g RA	1-24	M	0/24	0/24	0	0	0
3.0 ug/g RA	25-51	F	0/26	0/26	0	0	0
3.0 ug/g RA + AFB₁	52-76	M	21/24	1/24	83	0	4
3.0 ug/g RA + AFB₁	77-101	F	19/24	2/24	70	0	8
Low Vitamin A							
0.3 ug/g RA	102-111	M	0/10	0/10	0	0	0
0.3 ug/g RA	112-123	F	0/12	0/12	0	0	0
0.3 ug/g RA + AFB₁	124-190	M	59/66	19/66	62	3	26
0.3 ug/g RA + AFB₁	191-232	F	32/42	12/42	64	16	11

TABLE VIII. Summation of Effects of Marginal Lipotrope, High Fat Diet on Chemical Carcinogenesis in Rats

| Carcinogen | Tumor Induction | | |
	Enhanced in:	Depressed in:	Not Affected in:
	Males		
AFB$_1$	Liver	--	--
DEN	Liver, Esophagus	--	--
DBN	Liver	--	Esophagus, Lung, Bladder
DMN	--	--	Liver, Kidney
AAF	Liver	--	Zymbal's Gland
DMH	Colon	Zymbal's Gland	Small Intestine
MNNG	--	--	Forestomach
FANFT	--	--	Bladder
	Females		
AAF (Sprague-Dawley)	--	Mammary Gland	Zymbal's Gland
AAF (Fischer)	Liver	--	--
DMBA	--	Mammary Gland	--

TABLE IX. Effect of Vitamin A on Chemical Carcinogenesis

| Carcinogen | Species | Dietary Vitamin A | Tumor Induction | | |
			Enhanced in:	Depressed in:	Not Affected in:
BP	Hamster	Increased	--	Esophagus, Forestomach	Respiratory Tract
BP	Hamster	Decreased	Respiratory Tract	--	--
AFB$_1$	Rat	Decreased	Colon	Liver	--
AFB$_1$	Rat	Increased	--	--	Liver
DMH	Rat	Decreased	Colon	--	Small Intestine
DMH	Rat	Increased	--	--	Colon, Small Intestine
FANFT	Rat	Increased	Bladder	--	--

(Taken from Reference 27 and 60)

TABLE X. Liver Enzymes, AAF and Diet, Female Rats

Diet	PNA ug P-Nitrophenol g/liver	BPOH Quinine Units g/liver
Control	142 + 16	8 + 4
Control + AAF	187 + 14	13 + 6
Marginal Lipotrope, High Fat	105 + 14	7 + 3
Marginal Lipotrope, High Fat + AAF	147 + 20	5 + 3

TABLE XI. Blood Content of DEN at Intervals After Intraperitoneal Injection[a]

Time After DEN Injection (min)	DEN in Blood (ug/ml + S.E.)	
	Control	Deficient
4	36.1 + 2.0	31.2 + 3.1
20	19.8 + 2.6	19.0 + 1.6
40	13.9 + 3.0	15.0 + 4.4
60	11.2 + 3.0	12.1 + 1.4
120	3.1 + 1.5	5.5 + 0.9
210	None Detectable[b]	0.6 + 0.2

[a] Rats were given 25 mg/kg DEN; 4-5 rats/diet were studied at each time period.

[b] 0.05 ug/ml would have been easily detected under the experimental conditions.

(Taken from Reference 62)

TABLE XII. Effect of Lipotrope Deficiency on Hepatocyte DNA Synthesis and Serum VLDL in Weanling Rats

Diet	DNA Synthesis[a]	Serum VLDL[a]
Control	0.5 - 4	75
Marginal Lipotrope	1 - 9	50
Low Lipotrope	5 - 20	25

[a] Expressed in arbitrary units as an index of DNA synthesis and concentration of very low density lipoprotein (VLDL).

TABLE XIII. Mammary Tumor Induction by AAF in Female Rats Fed Control or Marginal Lipotrope, High Fat Diets

Diet	Rat Strain	No. Rats	Mammary Tumors (%)		
			Carcinoma	Adenoma	Total
Control	SD	31	65	3	68
Marginal Lipotrope, High Fat	SD	32	41	9	50
Control	Fischer	25	0	12	12
Marginal Lipotrope, High Fat	Fischer	25	8	0	8

V. REFERENCES.

1. Levin, D.L., Devesa, S.S., Godwin, J.D., and Silverman, D.T. Cancer Rates and Risks. D.H.E.W. Publication #75-691, 1974. National Institutes of Health, Washington D.C.

2. Doll, R. Worldwide Distribution of Gastrointestinal Cancer. Nat. Cancer Inst. Monograph 25: 173-190, 1967.

3. Bailer, J.C. Distribution of Carcinoma of Esophagus, Stomach and Large Bowel. In: Carcinoma of the Alimentary Tract. Ed.: W.J. Burdette. University of Utah Press, Salt Lake City, pp. 3-14, 1965.

4. Cook, P., and Burkitt, D. Cancer in Africa. Brit. Med. Bull. 27: 14-20, 1971.

5. Wynder, E.L., and Bross, I.J. A Study of Etiological Factors in Cancer of the Esophagus. Cancer 14: 389-413, 1961

6. O'Gara, R.W., Lee, C.W., Morton, J.E., Kapadia, G.J., and Dunham, L.J. Sarcoma Induced in Rats by Extracts of Plants and by Fractionated Extract of Krameria ixina. J. Nat. Cancer Inst. 52: 445-448, 1974.

7. Jussawalla, D.J. Report of the International Seminar on Epidemiology of Oesophageal Cancer. Internat. J. Cancer 10: 436-441, 1972.

8. Martinez, I. Factors Associated with Cancer of the Esophagus, Mouth and Pharnyx in Puerto Rico. J. Nat. Cancer Inst. 42: 1069-1094, 1969.

9. Cook, P. Cancer of the Oesophagus in Africa. Brit. J. Cancer 25: 853-880, 1971.

10. Schoenberg, B.S., Bailar, J.C., and Fraumeni, J.F. Certain Mortality Patterns of Esophageal Cancer in the United States 1930-1967. J. Nat. Cancer Inst. 46: 63-73, 1971.

11. Breslow, N.E., and Enstrom, J.E. Geographic Correlations Between Cancer Mortality and Alcohol-Tobacco Consumption in the United States. J. Nat. Cancer Inst. 53: 631-639, 1974.

12. Leevy, C.M. Liver Disease of the Alcoholic. Viewpoints on Digestive Diseases 3: 104, 1971.

13. Halstead, J.A., Smith, J.C., Jr., and Irwin, M.I. A Conspectus of Research on Zinc Requirements of Man. J. Nutr. 104: 345-378, 1974.

14. Hormozdiari, H., Day, N.E., Aramesh, B., and Mahbonbi, E. Dietary Factors and Esophageal Cancer in the Caspian Littoral of Iran. Cancer Res. 35: 3493-3498, 1975.

15. The Coordinating Group for the Research of Esophageal Carcinoma. Chinese Acad. of Medical Sciences, A Report, 1974.

16. Day, N.E. Some Aspects of the Epidemiology of Esophageal Cancer. Cancer Res. 35: 3304-3307, 1975.

17. Rogers, A.E., Sanchez, O., Feinsod, F.M., and Newberne, P.M. Dietary Enhancement of Nitrosamine Carcinogenesis. Cancer Res. 34: 96-99, 1974.

18. Graham, S., Lilienfeld, A.M., and Tidings, J.E. Dietary and Purgation Factors in the Epidemiology of Gastric Cancer. Cancer 20: 2224, 1967.

19. Acheson, E.D., and Doll, R. Dietary Factors in Carcinoma of the Stomach: A Study of 100 Cases and 200 Controls. Gut 5: 126-131, 1964.

20. Higginson, J. Etiological Factors in Gastrointestinal Cancer in Man. J. Nat. Cancer Inst. 37: 527-545, 1966.

21. Dungal, N., and Sigurjonsson, J. Gastric Cancer and Diet. A Pilot Study on Dietary Habits in Two Districts Differing Markedly in Respect of Mortality from Gastric Cancer. Brit. J. Cancer 21: 270-276, 1967.

22. Merliss, R.R. Talc-Treated Rice and Japanese Stomach Cancer. Science 173: 1141-1142, 1971.

23. Lilienfeld, A. Epidemiology of Gastric Cancer. New Eng. J. Med. 286: 316-317, 1972.

24. Haenszel, W., Kurihara, M., Mitsuo, S., and Lee, R.K. Stomach Cancer Among Japanese in Hawaii. J. Nat. Cancer Inst. 49: 969-983, 1972.

25. Graham, S., Schotz, W., and Martino, P. Alimentary Factors in the Epidemiology of Gastric Cancer. Cancer 30: 927-938, 1972.

26. Ackerman, L.V. Some Thoughts on Food and Cancer. Nutr. Today, pp. 2-9, Jan./Feb., 1972.

27. Tatematsu, M., Takahashi, M., Fukushima, S., Hananouchi, M., and Shirai, T. Effects in Rats of Sodium Chloride on Experimental Gastric Cancers Induced by N-methyl-N'-Nitro-N-nitrosoguanidine or 4-Nitro-quinoline-1-oxide. J. Nat. Cancer Inst. 55: 101-106, 1975.

28. Smith, D.M., Rogers, A.E., and Newberne, P.M. Vitamin A and Benzo(a)-pyrene Carcinogenesis in the Respiratory Tract of Hamsters Fed a Semisynthetic Diet. Cancer Res. 35: 1485-1488, 1975.

29. Chu, E.W., and Malmgren, R.A. An Inhibitory Effect of Vitamin A on the Induction of Tumors of Forestomach and Cervix in the Syrian Hamster by Carcinogenic Polycyclic Hydrocarbons. Cancer Res. 25: 884-895, 1965.

30. Rogers, A.E. Variable Effects of a Lipotrope-Deficient, High Fat Diet on Chemical Carcinogenesis in Rats. Cancer Res. 35: 2469-2474, 1975.

31. Wattenberg, L.W. Inhibition of Carcinogenic and Toxic Effects of Poly-cyclic Hydrocarbons by Phenolic Antioxidants and Ethoxyquin. J. Nat. Cancer Inst. 48: 1425-1430, 1972.

32. Wynder, E.L., and Shigematsu, T. Environmental Factors of Cancer of the Colon and Rectum. Cancer 20: 1520-1561, 1967.

33. Haenszel, W.M., and Kurihari, M. Studies of Japanese Migrants. I. Mortality from Cancer and Other Diseases Among Japanese in the United States. J. Nat. Cancer Inst. 40: 43-51, 1968.

34. Haenszel, N., Berg, J.W., Segi, M., Jurihari, M., and Locke, F.B. Large Bowel Cancer in Hawaiian Japanese. J. Nat. Cancer Inst. 51: 1765-1779, 1973.

35. Bjelke, E. Colon Cancer and Blood Cholesterol. The Lancet (June 1), pp. 1116-1117, 1974.

36. Rose, G., Blackburn, H., Keys, A., Taylor, H., Kamel, W., Reid, P.O., and Stamler, J. Colon Cancer and Blood Cholesterol. Lancet 1: 181-183, 1974.

37. Oettle, A.G. Primary Neoplasms of the Alimentary Canal of White and Bantu of the Transvoal 1949-1953. A Histopathological Series. Nat. Cancer Inst. Monograph 25: 97-109, 1967.

38. Burkitt, D.P., Walker, A.R., and Painter, N.S. Effect of Dietary Fiber of Stools and Transit Time and Its Role in Causation of Disease. Lancet ii: 1408-1412, 1972.

39. Walker, A., Walker, B., and Richardson, B.D. Bowel Transit Times in Bantu Populations. Brit. Med. J. 3: 48-49, 1970.

40. Walker, A.R.P. Effect of High Crude Fiber Intake on Transit Time and the Absorption of Nutrients in South African Negro School Children. Am. J. Clin. Nutr. 28: 1161-1169, 1975.

41. Hill, M.J., Drasar, B.S., Aries, V., Crowther, J.S., Hawksworth, G., and Williams, R.E.O. Bacteria and Etiology of Cancer of the Large Bowel. Lancet 1: 95-102, 1971.

42. Walker, A. Diet and Cancer of the Colon. Lancet 1: 593-594, 1971.

43. Wynder, E.L., and Reddy, B.S. Studies of Large Bowel Cancer: Human Leads to Experimental Application. J. Nat. Cancer Inst. 50: 1099-1106, 1973.

44. Hirono, I., Fushimi, H., Mori, T., Miwa, T., and Haga, M. Comparative Study of Carcinogenic Activity of Each Part of Bracken. J. Nat. Cancer Inst. 50: 1367-1371, 1973.

45. Newberne, P.M. Biologic Effects of Plant Toxins and Aflatoxins in Rats. J. Nat. Cancer Inst. 56: 551-555, 1976.

46. Newberne, P.M., and Rogers, A.E. Adenocarcinoma of the Colon: An Animal Model for Human Disease. Am. J. Path. 72: 541-544, 1973.

47. Rogers, A.E., and Newberne, P.M. Dietary Enhancement of Intestinal Carcinogenesis by Dimethylhydrazine in Rats. Nature 246: 491-492, 1973.

48. Newberne, P.M., and Rogers, A.E. Primary Hepatocellular Carcinoma: An Animal Model for Human Disease. Am. J. Path. 72: 137-140, 1973.

49. Newberne, P.M., and Rogers, A.E. Rat Colon Carcinomas Associated with Aflatoxin and Marginal Vitamin A. J. Nat. Cancer Inst. 50: 439-448, 1973.

50. Reddy, B., Weisburger, J.H., Narisawa, T., and Wynder, E.L. Colon Carcinogenesis in Germ-Free Rats with 1,2-Dimethylhydrazine and N-methyl-N'-nitro-N-nitrosoguanidine. Cancer Res. 34: 2368-2372, 1974.

51. Reddy, B., Weisburger, J.H., and Wynder, E.L. Effect of Dietary Fat Levels and Dimethylhydrazine on Fecal Acid and Neutral Sterol Excretion and Colon Carcinogenesis in Rats. J. Nat. Cancer Inst. 52: 507-511, 1974.

52. Rogers, A.E., Herndon, B.J., and Newberne, P.M. Influence of Vitamin A on Dimethylhydrazine-Induced Colon Carcinoma in Rats. Cancer Res. 33: 1003-1009, 1973.

53. Deluca, L., Schumacher, M., Wolf, F., and Newberne, P.M. Biosynthesis of a Fucose-Containing Glycopeptide from Rat Small Intestine in Normal and Vitamin A-Deficient Conditions. J. Biol. Chem. 245: 4551-4558, 1970.

54. Wattenberg, L. Studies of Polycyclic Hydrocarbon Hydroxylases of the Intestine Possibly Related to Cancer. Effect of Diet on Benzpyrene Hydroxylase Activity. Cancer 28: 99-110, 1971.

55. Wattenberg, L. Dietary Modification of Intestinal and Pulmonary Aryl Hydrocarbon Hydroxylase Activity. Toxicol. Appl. Pharmacol. 23: 741-748, 1972.

56. Higginson, J. The Geographical Pathology of Liver Disease in Man. Gastroenterology 57: 587-598, 1969.

57. Shank, R.C., Bhamarapravati, N., Gordon, J.E., and Wogan, G.N. Dietary Aflatoxins and Human Liver Cancer. Incidence of Primary Liver Cancer in Two Municipal Populations of Thailand. Fd. Cosmet. Toxicol. 10: 171-179, 1972.

58. Tuyns, A.J. I.A.R.C. Working Conference on the Role of Aflatoxin in Human Disease. Lyon, France, October 28-30, 1968.

59. van Rensburg, S.J., van der Watt, J.J., Purchase, I.F.H., Pereira Coutenho, L., and Markham, R. Primary Liver Cancer Rate and Aflatoxin Intake in a High Cancer Area. South African Med. J. 48: 2508a-2508d, 1974.

60. Rogers, A.E., and Newberne, P.M. Diet and Aflatoxin B1 Toxicity in Rats. Toxicol. Appl. Pharmacol. 20: 113-121, 1971.

61. Kula, N. Dietary Effects on Induced Sleeping Time and Aflatoxin Response in Rats. Abstr. Fed. Proc. 33: 669, 1974.

62. Rogers, A.E., Wishnok, J.S., and Archer, M.C. Effect of Diet on DEN Clearance and Carcinogenesis in Rats. Brit. J. Cancer 31: 693-695, 1975.

63. Ames, B.N. Am Improved Bacterial Test System for the Detection and Classification of Mutagens and Carcinogens. Proc. Nat. Acad. Sci. 70: 782-786, 1973.

64. Leffert, H.L., and Weinstein, D.B. Growth Control of Fetal Rat Hepatocytes in Primary Monolayer Culture. IX. Specific Inhibition of DNA Synthesis by the Very Low Density Lipoprotein Fraction of Rat Serum and Its Possible Significance to the Problem of Liver Regeneration. In: Rat Liver Pathology - A Workshop. Eds.: Paul M. Newberne and William H. Butler. Elsevier, Amsterdam (in press, 1976).

65. McLean, A.E.M., and Magee, P.N. Increased Renal Carcinogenesis by Dimethylnitrosamine in Protein-Deficient Rats. Brit. J. Exptl. Path. 51: 587-590, 1970.

66. Clayson, D.B. Nutrition and Experimental Carcinogenesis. Cancer Res. 35: 3292-3300, 1975.

67. Poirier, L.A. Hepatocarcinogenesis by Diethylnitrosamine in Rats Fed High Dietary Levels of Lipotropes. J. Nat. Cancer Inst. 54: 137-140, 1975.

68. Buell, P. Changing Incidence of Breast Cancer in Japanese and American Women. J. Nat. Cancer Inst. 51: 1479-1483, 1973.

69. de Waard, F. Breast Cancer Incidence and Nutritional Status with Particular Reference to Body Weight and Height. Cancer Res. 35: 3351-3356, 1975.

70. Eskin, B.A., Parker, J.A., Bassett, J.G., and George, D.L. Human Breast Uptake of Radioactive Iodine. Obst. Gyn. 44: 398-402, 1974.

71. Berg, J.W., and Burbank, F. Correlations Between Carcinogenic Tract Metals in Water Supplies and Cancer Mortality. Ann. N.Y. Acad. Sci. 199: 249-264, 1972.

72. Breslow, N.E., and Enstrom, J.E. Geographic Correlation Between Cancer Mortality Rates and Alcohol-Tobacco Consumption in the United States. J. Nat. Cancer Inst. 53: 631-639, 1974.

73. Wattenerg, L.W. Inhibition of Carcinogenic and Toxic Effects of Polycyclic Hydrocarbons by Several Sulfur-Containing Compounds. J. Nat. Cancer Inst. 52: 1583-1587, 1974.

74. Rowlatt, L.M., Franks, M., and Sheriff, M.U. Mammary Tumor and Hepatoma Suppression by Dietary Restriction in C_3H A^{vy} Mice. Brit. J. Cancer 28: 83, 1973.

75. Morris, H.P. Effects of the Genesis and Growth of Tumors Associated with Vitamin Intake. Ann. N.Y. Acad. Sci. 49: 119-140, 1947.

76. Hui, Y.H., Deome, K.B., and Briggs, G.M. The Developmental Noduligenic and Tumorigenic Potentials of Transplanted Mammary Gland and Primary Ducts from C_3H Mice Previously Fed a Phenylalanine-Deficient Diet. Cancer Res. 32: 57-60, 1972.

EFFECT OF A HIGH BEEF DIET ON BACTERIAL FLORA AND CHEMICAL COMPONENTS OF HUMAN FECES: A SUMMARY OF RESULTS

David J. Hentges, Glenna C. Burton, Margaret A. Flynn,
John M. Franz, Charles W. Gehrke, Klaus O. Gerhardt,
Bruce R. Maier, Robert K. Tsutakawa, and Robert L. Wixom
The University of Missouri - Columbia
Columbia, Missouri

Introduction

Several observations suggest that the incidence of cancer of the colon in a population may be related to diet. Epidemiological studies of areas with populations at high risk for colon cancer and areas with populations at low risk have shown that the most striking difference in those populations is the food they eat. The incidence of colon cancer is much higher in industrialized countries, in northwest Europe and North America, where a great deal of animal fat and protein and refined carbohydrates are consumed, than in the developing countries of Africa, and South America and in rural India and Japan where much less meat is consumed and the diet is high in vegetable fiber (5).

These variations in incidence do not appear to be related to geographical or genetic differences. Migrant groups tend to assume colon cancer incidence rates of their adopted countries (7). In Japan, for example, the death rate for large bowel cancer is relatively low. In a 1968 study of mortality among U.S. Japanese, the migrants to the U.S. showed an increased incidence approaching that of the U.S. population (4). The migrant Japanese retained their low incidence status, provided they did not change their eating habits. The process of "westernization", either in California or Japan, appeared to be associated with a high incidence of colon cancer.

High incidence has been attributed to the nature of the intestinal flora which synthesize carcinogenic agents from the food and intestinal secretions, such as bile acids (3). Diet not only influences the composition of the intestinal flora, but also the quantity of substrates available for the production of carcinogens.

With this in mind, Hill and others (10) examined the fecal flora of individuals from different parts of the world. Fecal samples were obtained from individuals from six areas -- England, Scotland and the United States, with a high incidence of colon cancer and Uganda, India, Japan with a low incidence of colon cancer. The same broad groups of bacteria were found in feces from all the populations studied. However, substantial differences in relative numbers for several of the bacterial groups were observed. The British and American subjects yielded many more gram-negative anaerobes (Bacteroides spp.) than did the Ugandans, Indians, or Japanese. Conversely, the Ugandans, Indians and Japanese had many more aerobic bacteria (streptococci and enterobacteria). Thus, the ratio of anaerobes to aerobes was much higher in the people living on a western diet than in those on the largely vegetarian diets.

In addition, the concentrations of acid and neutral steroids in the feces differed significantly between individuals on high meat and meat-less diets. Feces collected from British and Americans on high meat diets contained much higher concentrations of steroids than feces of Ugandans, Indians, and Japanese whose diets contained little or no animal fats and proteins. The neutral steroid concentration was very low in the feces of Ugandans and Indians, intermediate in the feces of Japanese, and high in the feces of British and Americans. The microbial degradation products of cholesterol, coprostanol and coprostanone, constituted a much smaller proportion of the total neutral steroids in the feces of the Ugandans, Indians, and Japanese than in the feces of the western group. Even more striking differences were noted in the fecal concentration of acid steroids. The acid steroid concentrations were approximately eleven times greater in the feces of British and Americans than in the feces of Ugandans and Indians and approximately seven times greater than in the feces of Japanese. Moreover, the extent of degradation of the acid steroids was higher in the British and Americans than in the other groups.

Similar observations were made by Reddy and Wynder (14) who showed that the daily fecal excretion of cholesterol metabolites was higher in Americans consuming a diet containing meat than in Americans consuming a meatless diet. In a recent study with human volunteers, Reddy, Weisburger and Wynder (13) found that the anaerobic microflora count was significantly greater during high meat consumption than during consumption of a diet containing no meat. Although total fecal bile acid excretion was the same during the two dietary periods, the concentration of steroid metabolites in the feces was greater during high meat consumption.

As a result of all of these observations it was concluded that the typical high meat diet of western peoples supports a microbial flora that is capable of converting fecal steroids into carcinogenic or cocarcinogenic agents. A systematic study was therefore proposed to examine the effect of a diet high in beef on the bacterial and chemical composition of the feces of humans. The data from this study, the subject of this paper, show that there were changes in fecal composition that occurred as a result of high beef consumption, but these changes were different from those previously reported.

Procedures and Materials Used

Ten male graduate and medical student volunteers were placed on a four month diet series consisting of a control diet, a meatless diet, a high meat diet, and again a control diet, each of one month duration. The diets were carefully formulated to standardize calories, proteins, fat, carbohydrates, cholesterol, fiber, minerals, and vitamins. The fat and fiber contents were held constant in all four diets. Total protein was the same in the control and meatless diets, but was doubled during the high meat diet. Meals were prepared and served exclusively in the metabolic kitchen in the University of Missouri Medical Center. Chemical analyses for each of the diets were prepared on composite food samples collected during a one day period. Analyses were made of proximates, minerals, fatty acids, and total individual amino acids, polyamines, creatine, and creatinine.

During the fourth week of each diet, three fecal samples were collected from each of the volunteers. Samples were collected in Gas-Pak jars set into a specially designed commode (11). The commode was constructed so that a mild stream of nitrogen gas purged the collection jar during fecal passage thereby excluding oxygen and protecting oxygen sensitive organisms in the feces.

At the bacteriology laboratories, the anaerobic jars containing the specimens were placed into clear plastic oxygen-free glovebox isolators for processing anaerobic bacteria (1). Moisture determinations were made on all specimens and serial 10-fold dilutions of the specimens were prepared and plated on pre-reduced media (11). The colonies were counted and approximately 35-40 different representative colonies were picked from the anaerobic plates and identified. The facultative laboratory received the 10-fold dilution series from the anaerobe laboratory. These dilutions were plated and approximately 35 colonies were picked and identified. From each stool specimen, a total of approximately 70 colonies were identified. Recovery, expressed as per cent of total microscopic counts, was between 60% and 70%.

After a one gram portion of the specimen was processed by the bacteriology laboratories, the remainder of the specimen was weighed, anaerobically sealed, and frozen for later delivery to the chemists. Three specimens collected from an individual during the last week on each diet were pooled and homogenized in 2 volumes of water under nitrogen. The homogenate was then distributed to the various chemistry laboratories. The feces were analyzed for the major classes of compounds listed in Table I. Details of the procedures used for chemical analyses will be published in separate papers now in preparation.

Results

It is difficult to adequately summarize all the data. An approach is to examine the statistically significant changes that occurred among the variables after the volunteers' diet had changed from a meatless one to one containing a large quantity of meat. If, first of all, the two diets are compared, it is apparent that they differ significantly in several respects. Table II shows that in addition to protein and amino acids, values for total calories, cholesterol, magnesium, creatine and creatinine were greater in the high meat than the meatless diets. Carbohydrate and calcium values, on the other hand, were greater in the meatless diet.

Table III provides a list of results obtained from chemical analysis of feces of the volunteers. When one examines the variables listed in each of the categories, a pattern resulting from high meat consumption does not emerge. The significant increase in the magnesium and spermine contents of the feces and significant decrease in the calcium content corresponds with the higher magnesium and spermine contents and lower calcium content in the high meat diet as compared with the meatless diet.

The high meat diet also contained more C 16:1 fatty acid and cholesterol than the meatless diet. Surprisingly, however, significantly less of the acid and cholesterol and its derivatives, cholestanol and coprostanone were excreted by the volunteers during the high meat regimen than during the meatless regimen. The question arises concerning the fate, in particular, of the cholesterol ingested during the high meat diet. In examining the cholesterol content of the feces of the ten volunteers, it was observed that two of the volunteers excreted considerably more cholesterol than the eight other volunteers, irrespective of diet. The content of the degradation products of cholesterol, cholestanol and coprostanone, were slightly lower in the feces of these two volunteers than in the feces of the other volunteers. Thus, the ratio of cholesterol to degradation products was unusually high in two of the ten volunteers. The B-sitosterol and campesterol levels were also higher in the stools of these two individuals as compared with the other volunteers.

Data from analysis of the acid steroids indicate that diet does not appreciably affect the concentrations of these acids in the feces. Lithocholic and deoxycholic acids were present in the feces in relatively high concentrations under all dietary conditions, and cholic and chenodeoxycholic acids were present in relatively low concentrations.

Dietary change did affect the composition of the microbial flora of the feces of volunteers, but not as anticipated. All of the facultative or aerobic organisms and anaerobic bacteria isolated from the feces were identified to the species level. Total numbers of these two major categories of organisms, isolated from the volunteers, were determined. Figure 1 illustrates the influence of diet on the total numbers of facultative organisms isolated from each volunteer. It is clear that there were great variations in counts obtained from the different individuals. There was no significant difference in the mean counts from the volunteers on high meat or meatless diets. Similar results were obtained when total anaerobic counts were analyzed. The influence of diet on the numbers of anaerobic organisms isolated from each of the volunteers is illustrated in Figure 2. Again, there was no significant difference in mean counts obtained when the volunteers were on high meat and meatless diets. There was, however, a gradual increase in the mean anaerobic count as the volunteers progressed through the dietary series. Thus, the mean count obtained during the final control diet was significantly higher than the count obtained during the initial control diet. This pattern was observed twice when the diets were administered at different times to two groups of five volunteers. There is no explanation for it. It may simply represent a response to a regulated, institutional type of diet. The ratio of total anaerobes to total facultative or aerobic organisms was approximately 24 to 1 during the meatless diet and 86 to 1 during the high meat diet.

Discussion

What conclusions can be drawn about the role of meat in colon cancer on the basis of the data obtained with this study? Our results were not entirely consistent with those reported by Hill and Aries (9), Hill and others (10), and Reddy, Weisburger, and Wynder (13). There were no significant differences in the total numbers of anaerobic, facultative or aerobic organisms isolated from the feces of volunteers between the high meat and meatless diets. Nor was there a significant difference in the counts of the individual genera and species of organisms encountered. Some increase in the ratio of anaerobic bacteria to facultative and aerobic organisms was observed during the high meat diet as compared with the meatless diet, but not of the magnitude reported by Hill and others (10). There was no increase in the concentrations of acid or neutral steroids or their metabolites in the feces of the volunteers during the high meat diet. On the contrary, the concentrations of cholesterol metabolites in the feces was significantly lower during the high meat diet as compared to the meatless diet. Hill and Aries (9), Hill and others (10) and Reddy and Wynder (14) reported significantly higher levels of these compounds in the feces of individuals on high risk as compared with low risk diets.

It may be argued that our studies represent short term experiments and theirs, long term. However, Aries and others (2) reported that there are no differences in numbers and species of organisms in the feces of individuals consuming a mixed diet and in the feces of individuals that consume no animal products at all. Finegold and others (6) found no striking differences in the composition of the flora of Japanese-Americans on a high risk, western type diet and those on a low risk, Japanese type diet. Similar results were obtained by Moore and Holdeman (12) in their studies of three population groups on high risk, moderately high risk, and low risk diets. Although individuals of the low risk group tended to maintain higher concentrations of a few species of bacteria in their feces than the high risk groups, there were no consistent differences in the types of bacteria found among the different populations. In addition to these observations, the degree of neutral steroid conversion in the intestine appears to differ among individuals despite the composition of the diet. Wilkins and Hackman (15), in a study of the neutral steroid composition of the feces of 31 Americans on a normal diet, reported that in approximately one-quarter of the subjects the rate of conversion of cholesterol or plant steroids into degradation products was very low. The feces of these individuals contained higher concentrations of cholesterol and lower concentrations of degradation products than the feces of high converters. We obtained similar results in our studies. Thus, both these long term experiments and our short term experiments failed to confirm the differences in flora composition and steroid concentration that were previously observed between high risk and low risk populations.

It should be emphasized, however, that we examined only the effect of high meat protein consumption on the composition of the feces of humans. The fat content in all of our diets was held constant. There is some evidence that animal fat consumption influences the concentration of steroids in the feces. Hill (8) showed that the acid steroid concentration in the feces of volunteers declined greatly and the neutral steroid concentration declined slightly when fat meat in the diet was replaced by lean meat. High fecal acid steroid concentration and large bowel cancer risk in a population appear to be related (10, 14). Hill and others (10) and Reddy and Wynder (14) have speculated that high fat intake not only changes the composition of fecal steroids but also modifies the bowel flora, which in turn may produce carcinogenic substances from the steroids. Clearly, carefully controlled studies are needed to examine the effects of high animal fat consumption on the composition of the bowel flora and the concentration of steroids in the feces of humans.

Summary

Ten volunteers completed a four month diet series consisting of a control diet, a meatless diet, a high meat diet, and a second control diet, each of one month duration. Fat and fiber contents were essentially the same in all four diets, but protein content was doubled during the high meat diet. During the fourth week on each diet, three stool specimens collected from each volunteer were analyzed for aerobic and anaerobic bacteria, proximates and minerals, individual amino acids, creatine and creatinine, tryptophan metabolites, polyamines, fatty acids, and neutral and acid steroids.

A number of changes in fecal composition occurred as a result of high meat consumption. There was some increase in the proportion of anaerobic to aerobic bacteria in the feces during the high meat diet as compared with the meatless diet. There was no increase in the concentrations of either neutral or acid steroids. Although the high meat diet contained more cholesterol than the meatless diet, less cholesterol and cholesterol metabolites were excreted during high meat consumption. Two of the volunteers excreted significantly greater quantities of cholesterol than the other eight volunteers, irrespective of diet.

ACKNOWLEDGMENT

This research was performed under Contract No. N01 CP 33335 from the Division of Cancer Cause and Prevention, National Cancer Institute. We thank the Clinical Research Center of the University of Missouri-Columbia School of Medicine for providing food used in these studies and assistance in administering the diets.

TABLE I. Chemical Composition of Feces Classes of Compounds Analyzed

1.	Proximates and minerals
2.	Total, total-soluble, and free-soluble amino acid nitrogen
3.	Total, total-soluble, and free-soluble individual amino acids
4.	Creatine and creatinine
5.	Tryptophan metabolites
6.	Polyamines
7.	Total and free fatty acids
8.	Neutral steroids
9.	Acid steroids

TABLE II. Food Composition

Values significantly greater in high-meat than meatless diet	Values significantly greater in meatless than high-meat diet
Calories	Carbohydrates
Protein and Amino Acids	Calcium
Cholesterol	
Magnesium	
Spermine	
Creatine	
Creatinine	
C 16:1 (total)	

TABLE III. Effect of Diet on Chemical Components in Feces

Values significantly greater* during high-meat than meatless diet	Values significantly smaller* during high-meat than meatless diet
Magnesium	Calcium
Phosphorus	C 16:1 (total
Creatine	Cholesterol
Spermine	Cholestanol
C 16:0 (free)	Coprostanone
C 18:0 (free and total)	Campesterol
C 18:2 (free)	Stigmasterol
Cystathionine (total soluble)	Cystine (total soluble)
Ornithine (total soluble)	O-Phosphoserine (free soluble)
Alanine (total soluble)	Threonine (free soluble)
Proline (total)	Glutamine (free soluble)
Glycine (total)	Serine (total)
	Glutamic acid (total
	Methionine (total)
	Histidine (total)
	Arginine (total)
	1-Methylhistidine (total)

*The Wilcoxon test was used to evaluate the data statistically.

TOTAL FACULTATIVE AND AEROBIC ORGANISMS DURING DIFFERENT DIETS

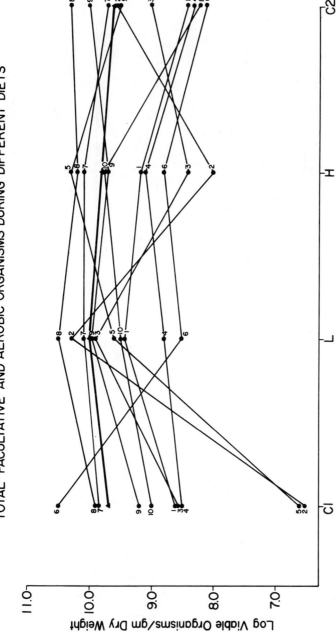

FIG. 1. Influence of diet on the total numbers of facultative and aerobic organisms isolated from the feces of volunteers. C1 signifies control diet 1; L, meatless diet; H, high meat diet; and C2, control diet 2. Numbers on the lines in the graph identify the volunteers. The heavy line connects the plots of the mean values for each diet.

TOTAL ANAEROBIC ORGANISMS DURING DIFFERENT DIETS

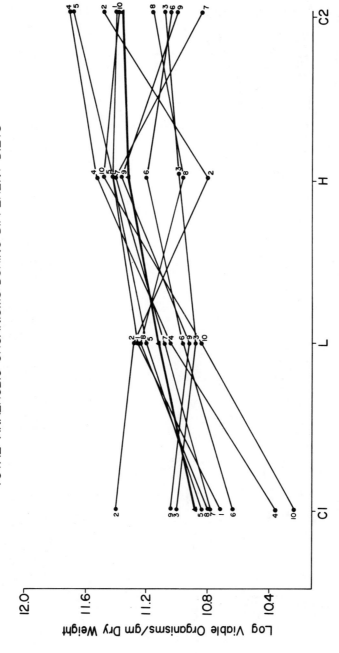

FIG. 2. Influence of diet on the total numbers of anaerobic bacteria isolated from the feces of volunteers. C1 signifies control diet 1; L, meatless diet; H, high meat diet; and C2, control diet 2. Numbers on the lines in the graph identify volunteers. The heavy line connects the plots of the mean values for each diet.

REFERENCES

1. Aranki, A., Syed, S.A., Kenny, E.B. and Freter, R. Isolation Of Anaerobic Bacteria From Human Gingiva And Mouse Cecum By Means Of A Simplified Glove Box Procedure. Appl. Microbiol. 17:568-276, 1969.

2. Aries, V.C., Crowther, J.S., Drasar, B.S., Hill, M.J., and Ellis, F.R. The Effect Of A Strict Vegetarian Diet On The Faecal Flora And Faecal Steroid Concentration. J. Pathol., 103:54-56, 1971.

3. Aries, V.C., Crowther, J.S., Drasar, B.S., Hill, M.J., and Williams, R.E.O. Bacteria And The Aetiology Of Cancer Of The Large Bowel. Gut, 10:334-336, 1969.

4. Buell, P. and Dunn, J. Cancer Mortality Among Japanese Issei And Nisei Of California. Cancer, 18:656-664, 1965.

5. Doll, R. The Geographical Distribution Of Cancer. Brit. J. Cancer, 23:1-8, 1969.

6. Finegold, S.M., Attebery, H.R., and Sutter, V.L. Effect Of Diet On Human Fecal Flora: Comparison Of Japanese And American Diets. Am. J. Clin. Nutr., 27:1456-1469, 1974.

7. Haenszel, W., and Kurihara, M. Studies Of Japanese Migrants. I. Mortality From Cancer And Other Diseases Among Japanese In The United States. J. Natl. Cancer Inst., 40:43-68, 1968.

8. Hill, M.J. The Effect Of Some Factors On The Faecal Concentration of Acid Steroids, Neutral Steroids And Urobilins. J. Pathol., 104:239-245, 1971.

9. Hill, M.J., and Aries, V.C. Faecal Steroid Composition And Its Relationship To Cancer Of The Large Bowel. J. Pathol., 104:129-139, 1971.

10. Hill, M.J., Drasar, B.S., Aries, V.C., Crowther, J.A., Hawksworth, G.M., and Williams, R.E.O. Bacteria And Aetiology Of Cancer Of Large Bowel. Lancet, 1:95-100, 1971.

11. Maier, B.R., Flynn, M.A., Burton, G.C., Tsutakawa, R.K., and Hentges, D.J. Effects Of A High-Beef Diet On Bowel Flora: A Preliminary Report. Am. J. Clin. Nutr., 27:1470-1474, 1974.

12. Moore, W.E.C., and Holdeman, L.V. Discussion Of Current Bacteriological Investigations Of The Relationships Between Intestinal Flora, Diet, And Colon Cancer. Cancer Research, 35:3418-3420, 1975.

13. Reddy, B.S., Weisburger, J.H., and Wynder, E.L. Effect Of High Risk And Low Risk Diets For Colon Carbinogenesis On Fecal Microflora And Steroids In Man. J. Nutr., 105:878-885, 1975.

14. Reddy, B.S., and Wynder, E.L. Large Bowel Carcinogenesis: Fecal Constituents Of Populations With Diverse Incidence Rates Of Colon Cancer. J. Natl. Cancer Inst., 50:1437-1442, 1973.

15. Wilkins, T.D., and Hackman, A.S. Two Patterns Of Neutral Steroid Conversion In The Feces Of Normal North Americans. Cancer Research, 34:2250-2254, 1974.

NEOPLASTIC POTENTIAL IN STRATIFIED
EPITHELIAL GRADIENTS FOLLOWING
METAPLASIA INDUCED BY NUTRITIONAL
DEFICIENCY OF VITAMIN A: AN INTERPRETATION

John H. Van Dyke

Department of Anatomy
Hahnemann Medical College
Philadelphia, Pennsylvania

(1) SPONTANEOUS THYROID METAPLASIA. Utilizing metaplastic foci
(cysts lined by stratified squamous epithelium), induced during chronic
vitamin A deficiency, in the thyroid and thymus of rats, the following experimental studies were designed to define the fate of two distinct strata
of cells (basal vs suprabasal) following co-tumorigenic stimuli. Earlier
studies had identified "new-growths" resembling neogenesis of thyroid
tissue developing spontaneously from basal cells in metaplastic lesions
in many yearling sheep (Van Dyke, '45), and frank cystadenomata from presumably viable, persisting, thin-walled suprabasal cell cysts in thyroids
of old albino rats (Van Dyke, '44).
Since metaplasia and tumor formations never occurred in the isthmus
of these thyroids, we were quite assured that the metaplasia involved in
tumorigenesis was probably a product of a specific portion of the thyroid,
- namely the ultimobranchial tissue component which we have since found,
experimentally, is especially vulnerable to metaplasia. This tissue, as
well as the cytoreticulum of the thymus, has proven ideal for experimental
studies relative to metaplasia, neogenesis and/or tumorigenesis; as well
as the fate of metaplastic lesions during and subsequent to tumor formation. In the rat, much like man, this tissue, after incorporation within
the thyroid, usually becomes induced by its intimate proximity to typical
thyroid parenchyma to transform into thyroid-like cells and vesicles
during embryonic development; and thus ordinarily becomes quite indistinguishable, morphologically, from normal thyroid tissue (Rogers, '27).
Originally thought to function as thyroid tissue by some, it has now been
purported to produce parafollicular or ("C) cells which secrete the new
hormone thyrocalcitonin known to help regulate blood calcium by preventing
osteolysis and thus lower serum calcium.
Initial studies in sheep indicated that ultimobranchial bodies are
represented by large, multiple, bilateral cysts lined by stratified
squamous epithelium. They have been regarded as arising congenitally due
to failure to fuse intimately with thyroid tissue during ontogenesis.
The epithelium of these cysts frequently produced cords or clumps of gland-
like cells that invaded neighboring thyroid tissue in a manner that often
suggested growth of glandular neoplasms. Depending presumably upon state
of activity of the thyroid, these cysts can be the source of at least two
peculiar outgrowths. These may resemble typical thyroid-like tissue

707

(neogenesis ?), or adenoma-like nodules which may be solid and relatively undifferentiated, or densely staining cystic structures composed of columnar epithelium (similar to cystadenomata), and they originate from basal (germinative), and/or suprabasal (degenerating) cell layers, respectively, in these primary cysts during periods of thyroid activity. Ultimobranchial cysts were found in all sheep studied.

In rats, metaplastic ultimobranchial cysts sometimes develop spontaneously, - presumably. They are most often seen in atrophic glands, females, and in older thyroids. As in sheep, basal cells in these squamous cysts can also produce gland-like cells. Following either basal cell outgrowths or delamination of basal cell aggregates from these multilayered cysts, thin-walled cystic remnants persist for long periods. Such remnants are largely only the more superficial, or suprabasal cell layers of original cysts which had been undergoing keratinization. Densely staining, thin-walled cysts characterize thyroids of senile rats. Although some cells were undergoing degeneration, certain other cells apparently remained temporarily viable. These cysts, observed to some degree in all age groups, except newborn, were often contiguous to developing cystadenomata; and the origin of these neoplasms were assigned to certain re-vitalized cells in such degenerating cystic masses in the past. Of ten very old animals, with a total of nine tumors (1 bilateral; all cystadenomata), one tumor was observed directly continuous by a cellular bridge with such a suprabasal cell cyst. One hundred rats (male and female) were studied. It was questionable whether they could all be considered normal.

(a) Experimental tumorigenesis in rat thyroids. Prolonged administration of a goitrogen (propylthiouracil in stock diet) will induce ultimobranchial tissue to undergo neoplasia in a large number of rats, but adjacent areas of thyroid tissue may also be involved. There may even be multiple nodules. Bilateral, incipient neoplasias, largely cystadenomata (some papillary) were readily demonstrated; located centrally in each lateral lobe, - the site typically occupied by ultimobranchial tissue in rats. However, they were not always observed intimately related to metaplastic lesions. Of eighty four female rats, 42% contained cystadenomata; 8% solid, anaplastic undifferentiated tumors. Cystadenomata, also characteristic of senility, occured precociously and in a higher percentage of individuals in old rats than in the young. Controls showed no comparable manifestations (Van Dyke, '53).

(b) Induced metaplastic lesions - thyroid. Thyroids in vitamin A deficient rats invariably show sites of growing, keratinizing cystic metaplasias. These lesions are usually in the center of each lobe, - the precise local occupied by ultimobranchial bodies, and they are predictable. Although these changes are reversible following vitamin A therapy, certain residual, viable (suprabasal) cells or proliferations from these cystic remnants may persist indefinitely after periods of repair and subsequently become tumorigenic. Controls showed few comparable manifestations. For metaplastic lesions resulting from vitamin A deficiency and reparative changes involved subsequent to vitamin A therapy see (Van Dyke, '55 - figures). Chronic A deficiency will induce these lesions in rats of all ages (especially the young), and this has been the basis for many experiments designed to determine the role of epithelial metaplasias in the evolution of particular neoplasms in the thyroid and thymus. Use of a goitrogen plus a carcinogen (during vitamin A deficiency) can demonstrate two distinctly different kinds of tumor in the thyroid that seem clearly derived from basal or suprabasal cells in induced squamous cell cysts and will be reported. Cystadenomata seemingly derived

708

exclusively from persisting suprabasal cells, under the influence of goitrogen alone (during recurring periods of A deficiency) will also be reported here.

Squamous cell metaplasia in the thyroid, similar to that resulting from vitamin A deficiency, has also been associated with repeated injections of estrogenic hormones, but it is not certain whether these hormones induce these lesions or augment pre-existing metaplastic sites. Squamous cell cysts induced by A deficient diet can be markedly augmented by estrogens in thyroids during early vitamin A therapy. This is especially notable in the thymus associated with incipient spindle cell neoplasia during lesion reparation and will be subsequently discussed.

(c) Metaplasia in the thymus. Apparently vitamin A deficiency will induce metaplastic changes in thymus tissue, but this has not been clearly indicated in past literature. Wolbach and Howe ('25a), and Wolbach ('37), in their classical research, included the thymus in their list of structures that showed keratinizing metaplasia during vitamin A deficiency. However, some investigators considered such metaplastic lesions as merely enlarged Hassall's corpuscles and not an effect of vitamin A deficiency. Since the literature suggested that both vitamin A and estrogenic hormones, alone, can induce metaplasia in the adult thymus (notably also in other organs), a combination of these factors might produce epithelial manifestations of some significance; especially during a formative period of postnatal development. Simulating a prenatal environment, as this procedure does, somewhat comparable to that in the fetus (Byrne and Eastman ('43); Williamson('47) might prove advantageous in clarifying not only the character of entodermal cytoreticulum but also the Hassall corpuscle and its relation, if any, to certain metaplasias and possibly neoplasias. Except for occasional diminutive foci, cysts rarely occur in the thyroids and thymus of rats, normally. Normally active thyroids; especially those stimulated by TSH or cold environment show none (Unpublished data). In order to study epithelial metaplasias in thyroids and thymus more precisely and their relation to tumorigenesis; cell types possibly involved and their origin, the following experiments were conducted.

PROCEDURES AND MATERIALS

(1) GOITROGEN/CARCINOGEN DURING A DEFICIENCY - THYROID. Sixty six, primarily Wistar rats (females - grouped as young, adult; old - ave. age 3-16 mos.) were maintained continuously on vitamin A deficienct diet (Nutritional Biochemicals) for periods of time varying from three to fourteen months to induce and/or augment existing foci of squamous cell metaplasia. Concurrently, thyroids in different age groups were mitoticly stimulated by dietary use of 2 mg of the goitrogen allylthiourea plus 2 mg of the carcinogen 2-acetylaminofluorene daily in A deficient diet.

(a) Estrogen during chronic A deficient diet - thymus. In other experiments, the cytoreticulum of the thymus in twenty four young rats (male and female) was simply stimulated by twice weekly injections of estradiol diproprionate (Schering - 0.25 cc. in 0.1% Sesame oil) for only two to six weeks during chronic A deficiency (vitamin A deficient diet - two weeks, followed by A deficient diet plus estrogen injection for two and four weeks).

(2) GOITROGEN/ESTROGEN - ALTERNATING PERIODS OF A DEFICIENCY. In aditional, separate experiments, thyroids and thymus of rats, presumably containing induced metaplastic lesions, were similarly stimulated during

periods of re-acquisition of vitamin A contained in normal ground Purina rat chow (when basal cells separate from suprabasal cells during re-establishment of typical organ epithelia - Classical Repair). Normal diet contained 12 IU/gm of vitamin A and 6.5 ppm of carotene.

(a) Goitrogen - Thyroids. Thyroids of twelve adult female rats were stimulated by thiourea alone (0.2% in water - ad libitum) during recurring periods of vitamin A deficiency. After an initial twenty one days on deficient diet, rats were alternately fed a normal (reparative) diet containing presumably adequate vitamin A for seven days followed by another period of A deficient diet for twenty one days. This alternation of diets was continued for six to eight months, during which time they continuously received thiourea.

(b) Estrogen - Thymus. Thymus glands of sixteen young rats (male and female) were subjected to vitamin A deficient diet for four weeks with estrogen injections. They were then maintained on normal diet for only two weeks during continuous estradiol diproprionate stimulation.

Significant percentages of metaplasia, and specific neoplasias, each related to a particular cell layer gradient, occurred in all experiments; especially after stimulation during lesion repair associated with re-acquisition of vitamin A. Controls, in all experiments, showed very few comparable manifestations. With the exception of fig. 9, all sections (serial) were stained with Hematoxylin and Eosin. Sections were cut at 6-8 microns.

RESULTS

(1) GOITROGEN/CARCINOGEN DURING A DEFICIENCY - THYROID. Feeding rats allylthiourea and 2-acetylaminofluorene, simultaneously, during chronic A deficiency, resulted in the production of two common but distinctly different neoplasias (Figs. 2 and 5). These tumors also occur in the human thyroid. They can occur in each lateral lobe (bilateral), may be multiple, and can be attributed to ultimobranchial bodies following metaplasia. Both types may develop in the same gland. Both types of experimental tumor, in their incipient stages, can be traced back to their cell layer source in cysts lined by stratified squamous epithelium. The solid, anaplastic or undifferentiated nodule is related to the basal or germinative cell layer (s); the cystadenoma to degenerating, but still viable suprabasal cells in cysts. Fig. 1 shows an ultimobranchial cyst proliferating solid clusters of cells (circled by arrows) which are products of basal cells at two points (a; a'). In their origin, such "new-growths" are temporarily quite distinct. Ultimately they produce tumors such as that in figure 2. In their early stages of formation they resemble typical thyroid-like tissue. Rat-eight months old- maintained on allylthiourea and 2-acetylaminofluorene during chronic vitamin A deficiency - six months. Some cysts before becoming tumorigenic (after considerable hyperplasia in situ) can become relatively enormous before undergoing neoplasia (Fig. 3). Presumably these would have ultimately resulted, in time, in solid tumor masses. Adult female rat kept on same experimental diet for eight months. Typically they lie in the plane of section which includes the parathyroid gland; and relatively near center of each thyroid lobe. In older animals, these tumors develop precociously and apparantly become malignant (medullary type). During their inceptive period, they are not unlike basal cell carcinomas in skin.

Another type of tumor (cystadenomata; like incipient tumors - Figs. 5 and 7) may become papillary and carcinomatous. They are related in

710

origin to so-called suprabasal cell components in persisting epithelial lesions (cysts) following loss of proliferating basal cells, in time, to adjacent thyroid parenchyma. Such cystic remnants are therefore thin-walled but contain some viable cells ("differentiating intermitotics"). Figure 4 illustrates one such mitoticly active cyst which is referred to as a "tornado" cyst because of its proliferative capacity; especially notable at both ends (arrows). Such tumors arise from densely staining cells which become re-vitalized while undergoing degeneration in walls of squamous cell, cystic remnants. In one young group of eighteen rats (age 3-8 mos.) kept on this experiment for five-six months, six showed incipient or moderately advanced solid, undifferentiated tumors (33% - all bilateral). In addition, two rats contained unilateral cystic types of tumor. In one old group (age 16 mos.) similarly treated for five months, showed marked solid tumor types in twelve rats (80% - all bilateral). Again, two of these rats also exhibited unilateral cystadenomata in different stages of development.

(a) Estrogen during chronic A deficiency - thymus. Studies using the hormone estradiol diproprionate, in conjunction with vitamin A deficiency, have resulted in marked, localized epithelial metaplasias (cysts) initially restricted peripherally in the cortex near or in the capsule and septa of thymic lobules in young rats. Rats weaned and maintained on vitamin A deficient diet for two to six weeks (associated with estrogen injections during the last 2-4 weeks) demonstrated precociously developing, highly vascularized multiple metaplasias originating in newly induced, aberrant (by position) thymic corpuscles, initially, identical to those of Hassall. Figure 8 demonstrates three such developing aberrant corpuscles at junction of cortex and stroma (arrows). Note absence of such corpuscles in medulla (a). This rat received estrogen for four weeks during chronic vitamin A deficiency. Such induced corpuscles progressively enlarged as multiple cysts lined by hyperplastic stratified squamous epithelium; but usually of the non-keratinizing (mucous) type, - similar to that in the esophagus (Fig. 9 - arrows). Medulla (a) lacked similar manifestations. Rat kept on vitamin A deficient diet four weeks plus estrogen during the last two weeks (Giemsa stain). Cortical areas become largely replaced by these growing epithelial cysts stimulated by estrogen. Some cysts grew so large and became so numerous that they tended to obliterate medullary areas. Original Hassall's corpuscles in the medulla showed no reaction when they could be identified in animals sacrificed at less than maximal periods of experimental time. Aberrant corpuscles and cysts, varying in size and number, to the extreme, were identified in 100% of rats examined.

(2) GOITROGEN DURING RECURRING A DEFICIENCY - THYROID. Thyroid tumors induced by goitogen alone are usually of the cystadenomatous type but are not always intimately or convincingly associated with squamous cell metaplasias. Consequently, in order to attempt to illustrate foci of incipient tumor formation (cystadenomata) which may be related in origin to such metaplastic lesions, adult rats were subjected to thiourea continuously during recurring periods of vitamin A deficiency. In doing so, it was hoped that basal cells in these cysts would be stripped from cysts during periodic repair due to re-acquisition of vitamin A, or proliferate into adjacent thyroid parenchyma during periods of A deficiency due to the stimulatory action of thiourea; and thus more readily expose suprabasal cells to the tumorigenic action of the goitrogen. Rats thus subjected to recurring periods of A deficiency did frequently exhibit developing neoplasms (cystadenomata) clearly contiguous with persisting cystic remnants of metaplastic tissue. During this periodic

711

epithelial repair process, or due to the action of the goitrogen on whole cysts during A deficiency, basal cells separated away from cyst epithelium and apparently contributed to thyroid parenchyma; presumably as parafollicular or ("C) cell elements. All twelve rats showed persisting thin-walled, suprabasal cell cysts; and in nine rats closely associated with cystic tumors. In four rats, these cystic tumors could be traced directly (in serial sections) as strands of neoplastic tissue to cysts some distance removed but nevertheless connected by long, tortuous cellular bridges or pedicles to the remains of partially degenerated, yet still proliferating suprabasal cell cysts (Figs. 6 and 7). Figure 6 exhibits point of origin of tumor from thin-walled cyst (arrow), and figure 7 shows the same neoplasm some distance away in an incipient stage of vesicular formations. Ultimately these vesicles will coalesce and form typical cystadenomata. Controls showed no comparable conditions, although some had cysts.

(3) ESTROGEN - DEFICIENT DIET FOLLOWED BY NORMAL DIET - THYMUS. Epithelial metaplasias (cysts) induced in the thymus of young rats by chronic vitamin A deficiency (augmented by simultaneous injections of estrogen) can be further stimulated to produce rapidly growing, multiple cystic masses containing "new-growths" that can usurp the entire organ, - when estrogen is given during periods of lesion repair (re-acquisition of vitamin A). Figure 10 illustrates this neoplastic devastation of the thymus. Substitution of normal diet (with adequate carotene and vitamin A) initiates a restorative process in these metaplasias in an attempt to re-establish typical organ cytoreticulum, but here the thymus is also under the influence of estrogen; and for only two weeks. Lumina of these multiple cysts contain not only dead, desquamated squamous cells in their centers, but also viable, proliferating suprabasal cells attached to cyst walls at various points on the periphery of the lumina (Figs. 10 and 12). Note points of spindle cell proliferations (arrows), and desquamated products obliterating lumina in figure 10. Figure 11 is of considerable interest because it shows a cyst with normal products of desquamation in the center and two loci of degenerating or growing suprabasal cell aggregates "budding" into the lumen; thus initiating two separate spindle cell "new-growths" (a). Calcium deposites at (b). Remainder of cyst wall (c) is still composed of viable suprabasal cells. Figure 12, under high power, shows one of many proliferation sites in a cyst rapidly sprouting into the cyst lumen (b), but still connected by a pedical (a) to the cyst wall. These new growths eventually coalesce and obliterate the cyst. Since cysts are multiple many such spindle cell masses occur. Figure 13, in a drawing, shows the characteristic detail of spindle cells and their capacity for proliferation (mitosis at (a); remnant of metaplastic lesion (b). These have been identified as spindle cell-like neoplasias derived from re-vitalized suprabasal cells during desquamation in cyst walls under the stimulus of estrogenic hormone. Various degrees of spindle cell neoplasias were observed in 100% of the rats studied. No differences were noted between males and females.

DISCUSSION

(1) THYROID AND THYMUS. Although morphological events in development of epithelial tumors differ frequently, depending upon epithelial surfaces (epidermis differing from glandular and other organs), it is well known that metaplasias are implicated as pre-neoplastic lesions in certain epithelial tumors (Steiner, '53). Metaplasias can also determine

712

the appearance of certain tumors which are peculiar to the organ or region concerned (Karsner, '55). Few investigators have experimentally analysed morphological precursors for epithelial neoplasms; thus too little attention has been devoted to their significance, - origin, manner of development and fate during tumorigenesis. Maugh ('74) has alluded to this in his recent article when he recalls three distinct phases (initiation, preneoplasia, and transformation) which are related to onset of tumors. Additional studies dealing with initiation and fate of metaplasias during experimental tumorigenesis - cell types or strata of cells involved, changes relative to their repair during and/or subsequent to periods of stimulation could be generally rewarding. Such studies are especially important because events occurring or recurring during early life may have considerable significance in determining tumorigenesis in later life. Tumor inducing stimuli may be more effective in the young following metaplasia, or in the old after inception of persisting viable suprabasal cell cysts.

How much vitamin A is required in the human being to prevent preneoplastic metaplasias is not known. Many factors can cause deficiency of vitamin A in addition to minimal intake in foods (liver damage, poor absorption or assimilation; hyperthyroidism, etc.). Since vitamin A is highly toxic in large doses, some substitute, retinol derivatives or synthetic analogs of retinol, perhaps associated with other systemic therapy, is needed to prevent metaplastic lesions and the stimuli concerned in epithelial tumorigenesis. Maintaining proper differentiation of epithelial cells in their respective specialized tissues (i.e., exocrine glands) is a prerequisite in preventing metaplastic lesions; and the occurrence of such indifferent tissue and the stimuli involved (hormonal or otherwise) should have great priority in investigative efforts. Epithelial tumors comprise well over 75% of all human malignancies (Cairns, '75). Prevention against a recurrence of such lesions is also very important because metaplasias may not always undergo proper repair after vitamin A therapy and may not always return to normal function. As latent, potentially malignant cells, some may lie dormant, perhaps for years, until a proper stimulus for malignancy is furnished. Recently, the role of vitamin A deficiency and metaplasia in epithelial tumorigenesis has been questioned; especially in certain organs (colon - Weisburger et al, '76).

In rats, ultimobranchial tissue and thymic cytoreticulum are "labile". Potentially epithelial, they are highly susceptible to metaplasia (squamous or secretory type) under certain conditions. Metaplastic changes, associated with loss of differentiation, can result in particular kinds of neoplasia in thyroids and thymus of rats, under experimental conditions, and concepts presented here may be applicable to neoplastic disease in other organs. Squamous metaplasias, regarded as relatively indifferent tissue, may be subject to demands of induction by parent tissue. It is not inconceivable that some neoplasias represent an aberrant attempt at regeneration in postnatal individuals following tissue degeneration caused by subtle trauma.

In adult baboon, ectopic, cystic ultimobranchial tissue (associated with thymus IV) can apparently give rise to accessory thyroid-like lobules, morphologically identical to thyroid tissue, after birth (Van Dyke, '52). This spontaneous, thyroid-like tissue originated from basal cells in the walls of cysts lined by stratified squamous epithelium, - a manifestation of ultimobranchial tissue not incorporated within the thyroid, and, therefore, could not have been induced by intimate proximity to thyroid parenchyma (neogenesis ?). Such a "new-growth", even

713

development of a tumor from ultimobranchial tissue may well lie dormant until a proper stimulus is provided (perhaps increased endocrine demand, or other factors ?). Other epithelial metaplasias may be subject to neoplasia on the same principle.

Experimental data also supports the concept that ultimobranchial tissue and thymic cytoreticulum (after squamous metaplasia) represents "more or less" indifferent tissue which may be stimulated to produce compensatory "new-growths"; resembling parent tissue; or foreign nodules. Thymic adenomata, resembling thyroid tissue, have been reported in rats subjected to prolonged use of thiourea (Van Dyke, '53). Similar thyroid-like vesicles, non-tumorous in character but receptive to radioactive iodine, develop in thymus tissue of rats after extirpation of the thyroid gland, and this also suggests that thymus tissue (following secretory metaplasia) may be a source of ectopic thyroid hormone (Van Dyke, '54).

Having determined that squamous metaplasias can occur during chronic vitamin A deficiency in rats (invariably), the next objective was to determine, experimentally, the role this vitamin deficiency might play in producing metaplasias that might demonstrate incipient tumorigenesis under certain conditions. We hoped to learn more about mechanisms and perhaps an analysis of cell types involved. Initially, as in young sheep, basal cells seem capable of induction into normal appearing, compensatory thyroid tissue, and, occurring spontaneously (?), may be involved in normal regeneration of "C" cells under influence of a normal milieu (hormonal or otherwise). Under abnormal conditions, and following metaplasia due to A deficiency in rats, they can produce undifferentiated, solid types of neoplasia. Basal cell proliferations are more precocious in development, and may require the action of a carcinogen for malignancy (medullary type). Basal cell proliferations from cyst walls, in time, leave viable suprabasal cell remnants which can persist and ultimately produce cystadenomata.

Suprabasal cells, differentiating toward keratinization and degeneration, retain some viable cells ("differentiating intermitotics") which may revert, re-vitalize during degeneration and subsequently develop in an aberrant manner; possibly the only source of cystadenomata in the thyroid. They seem not capable of "normal" induction characteristic of the organ site. They require more time to develop and differentiate, - especially in the young. They may have a prolonged period of dormancy before onset of carcinogenesis. They develop more readily in older rats. They are more prevelent after prolonged stimulation by a goitrogen alone. Spontaneously, they characterize thyroids of old and senile rats. Here, arising from ultimobranchial tissue metaplasias, suprabasal cells form cystadenomata under the influence of thyrotropin caused primarily by the goitrogen but seem enhanced by the carcinogen.

Thyroids containing cystadenomata induced by a goitrogen, or goitrogen and carcinogen during chronic vitamin A deficiency may show little or no evidence of metaplasia. If squamous cysts had been present, initially, this lack of metaplasia relative to origin of these tumors, could suggest that, in "morphologically activated" glands due to a goitrogen, such neoplasias in advanced stages of growth are usually incompatible with "vestiges" of origin. Cysts can become exhausted, depleted of viable cells and disappear. However, during incipient stages of development, cysts could be identified contiguous to tumors; and this was especially noticeable during periods of recurring vitamin A deficiency, when, after loss of basal cells to the parenchyma, suprabasal cells were apparently more vulnerable to effects of goitrogen, and cystadenomata could be traced directly to their cyst of origin.

714

In the thymus of young rats, using estrogen during periods of vitamin A deficiency, reticular cells produced aberrant thymic corpuscles at the periphery of the cortex. This suggests not only that we stimulated latent reticular cells (probably the earliest formed) which, following centrifugal growth, had reached the periphery of the cortex but cells that can become re-vitalized to produce corpuscles after birth. It recalls fetal conditions of excess estrogen and relative deficiency of vitamin A which may have induced the original Hassall corpuscles before birth.

Spindle cell neoplasias, derived from suprabasal cells in cysts (usually non-keratinizing and with more layers of viable cells), formed very precociously. They were initiated during periods of reparation under the stimulus of estrogenic hormone (when basal cells separate from cyst epithelium and contribute as small vesicles to cytoreticulum). Hence, some suprabasal cells, still viable, are more readily available for stimulation by estrogen. Partially differentiated toward degenerating surface cells, they too may revert, re-vitalize, and proliferate in an abnormal manner. Spindle cell aggregates, here, appear identical to spindle cell thymoma earlier described by Castleman ('55) in patients with myasthenia gravis. They also seem to resemble perithelioma mentioned by Pope and Osgood ('53) as arising from connective tissue elements around blood vessels (sarcomas). It is possible that we are dealing with two different tumors as far as origin is concerned. Despite the pleomorphism of some thymic tumors, thymic cytoreticulum is potentially epithelial. Our studies would substantiate the origin of certain spindle cell-like neoplasias from persisting, viable suprabasal cells induced by estrogen, which are derived from the walls of multiple, reorganizing epithelial cysts following re-acquistion of vitamin A.

Many kinds of glands possess capabilities of regeneration after tissue damage. In doing so, they resume an embryonic-like plasticity or potency for diverse differentiation, including metaplasia (Willis, '58). Duct epithelia, presumably with low thresholds for metaplasia, typically produce these "new-growths" during "normal" regeneration; notably in certain glands (i.e., pancreas). Stimuli for some neoplastic organ tissue may depend on inadequacy of vitamin A resulting in squamous metaplasias, certain incident and latent reactive cells derived therefrom, functional "demand" of organ involved, time; other factors (?). Also, "spontaneous" epidermoid metaplasia, widespread in glandular tissue, may be due to only a relative, or local deficiency of vitamin A instigated by many and varied circumstances; perhaps even resulting from chronic inflammation. Contrary to some prior opinion, some animals (rats) can be maintained for long periods in a partially deficient state, - "stabilized" with minimal liver stores and no vitamin A intake (Parnell and Sherman, '62). Experimentally separated, basal and suprabasal cells from squamous metaplasias can proliferate two distinctly different tumors (Van Dyke, '59; '75 -Preliminary reports) - Thyroids - solid, anaplastic (basal cells); cystadenomata (suprabasal cells). Thymus - spindle cell type (suprabasal cells). Relative organ dysfunction during deprivation of vitamin A followed by up-surge of function subsequent to re-acquisition of vitamin A; and other conditions, may incite "cell nests" seeded during (perhaps recurring) reparative periods. Epithelial transformations occurring during and subsequent to chronic A deficiency in rats can produce outgrowths re-sembling parent tissue (neogenesis ?), or frank neoplasias following appropriate stimulation. Basal cells less differentiated, initially, can be induced to form more benign, compensatory growths (ultimately malignant). Nests of occult suprabasal cells ("differentiating intermitotics"), however, deeply implanted within a propitious organ environment are

715

potentially active. When released from intact stratified squamous epithelium (cysts), during tissue re-organization involving repair of metaplasia, these cells, improperly induced, may be a prime source of epithelial, glandular malignancies.

SUMMARY

Utilizing induced metaplastic foci (cysts lined by stratified squamous epithelium) in thyroids and thymus of rats, studies were designed to define, during incipient stages of tumorigenesis, the fate of two distinct strata of cells (basal vs suprabasal). Thyroids in rats, maintained on vitamin A deficient diets to induce and/or augment existing loci of squamous cell metaplasias, were concurrently mitoticly stimulated by dietary use of goitrogen and carcinogen; thymi of deficient rats by simple intraperitoneal injections of estrogen.

Induced metaplastic lesions were similarly stimulated (thyroids by goitrogen; thymi by estrogen) during periods of re-acquisition of vitamin A (when basal cells separate from suprabasal cells during re-establishment of typical organ epithelia - repair). Specific neoplasms resulted; each related to particular cell layer gradients.

Basal cells from thyroid cysts formed typical thyroid-like tissue; or, in time, undifferentiated, solid carcinomatous masses. Cytoreticulum of thymus produced extramedullary, aberrant thymic corpuscles which ultimately formed multiple cysts. Basal cells in thymic cysts contributed to cytoreticulum. Suprabasal cells from these metaplastic lesions, in both organs, produced highly differentiated "new-growths" (Thyroid - cystadenomata; Thymus - multiple, "spindle cell-like" masses).

Metaplasias due to vitamin A deficiency are very vulnerable to neoplasia. Tumorigenesis may derive from two separate cell layers and may wholly deplete the metaplastic epithelium of origin; ultimately leaving little or no trace. Hence, metaplasias are seldom identified in advanced carcinogenesis. Relative organ dysfunction during deprivation of vitamin A followed by upsurge of function subsequent to re-acquisition of vitamin A (other conditions ?), may incite "cell nests" seeded during (perhaps recurring) reparative periods. Basal cells, initially, produce relatively benign, compensatory growths following induction by adjacent mitoticly active thyroid parenchyma, but they may ultimately become malignant. Suprabasal cells have considerable import. Some cells, still viable ("differentiating intermitotics") but partially differentiated toward degenerating, surface cells may apparently revert, re-vitalize, and yield the more aberrant malignant lesions (thyroid cystadenomata). Spindle cell neoplasias in the thymus, also derived from suprabasal cells, are extremely precocious. Nests of occult suprabasal cells (potentially active), deeply implanted within a propitious organ environment, are most suspect in malignant disease. When released from intact stratified squamous epithelium (cysts), during tissue re-organization involving repair of metaplasia, these cells, improperly induced, may be a prime source of epithelial, glandular malignancies.

Since some neoplasias may represent an aberrant attempt at regeneration of organ epithelia following subtle trauma, comparable studies may help clarify neoplastic phenomena in other epithelial glands with similar low thresholds for metaplasia and should have high priority in investigative efforts.

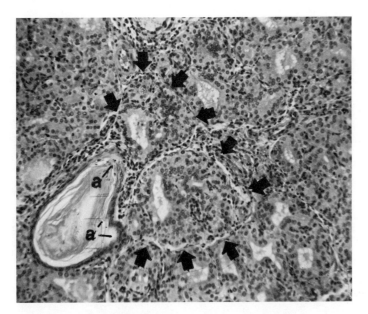

FIG. 1. Hyperplastic squamous cyst proliferating clusters of cells
(arrows) from basal cells at two points (a; a'). They produce tumors
illustrated in Fig. 2. Adult rat kept on goitrogen and carcinogen in
vitamin A deficient diet six months. X 80.

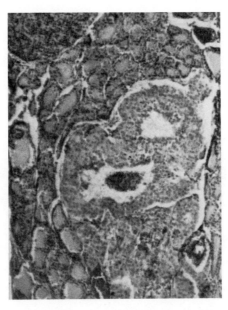

FIG. 2. Highly vascular, centrally located, solid type of tumor (potentially malignant; medullary type) derived from cyst like Fig. 1. Note
parathyroid on left. Experiment similar to Fig. 1. X 50.

717

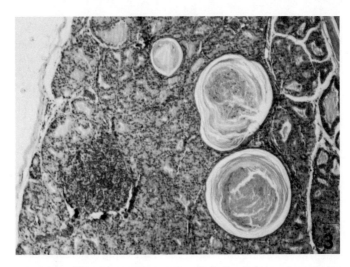

FIG. 3. Enlarged ultimobranchial cysts (intrinsically hyperplastic) which ultimately might have resulted in solid tumor masses. Parathyroid left. Rat kept eight months on same experimental diet. X 80.

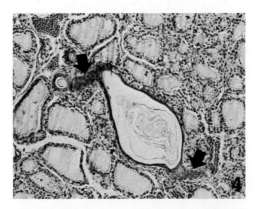

FIG. 4. Persisting, thin-walled suprabasal cell ("tornado") cyst proliferating; especially at both ends (arrows). Some cystadenomata such as in Fig. 5 originate from re-vitalized suprabasal cells during normal degeneration. Age and experiment like that in Fig. 5. 1 to 3. X 100.

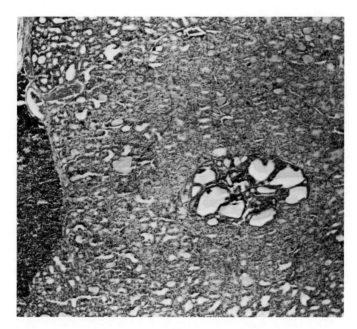

FIG. 5. Incipient cystadenoma like those occurring during A deficiency using goitrogen and carcinogen. Note parathyroid. One cystadenoma formed in opposite lobe. One month old rat fed propylthiouracil for fourteen months. X 60.

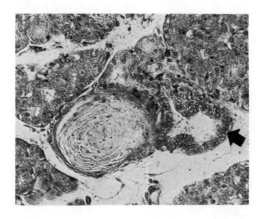

FIG. 6. Small suprabasal cell cyst with attached neoplastic tissue (arrow) that could be traced (serial sections) to incipient, tumor producing cystic vesicles in Fig. 7. Adult rat kept on thiourea during recurring periods of A deficiency for eight months. X 60.

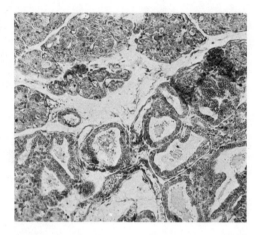

FIG. 7.   Incipient tumor producing cystic vesicles directly traceable to suprabasal cell cyst remnant in Fig. 6.   X 60.

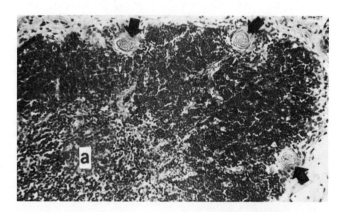

FIG. 8.   Developing, aberrant thymic corpuscles at junction of cortex and stroma (arrows).   Note absence of corpuscles in medulla (a).   Rat received estrogen four weeks during same period of A deficiency.   X 160.

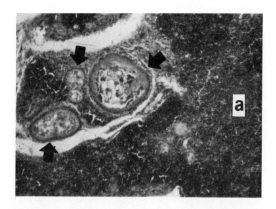

FIG. 9. Apex of thymic lobule showing cluster of enlarged, aberrant corpuscles (cystic) composed of hyperplastic stratified squamous epithelium (arrows). Medulla lacked cysts (a). Rat on A deficient diet four weeks plus estrogen during last two weeks. Giemsa stain. X 60.

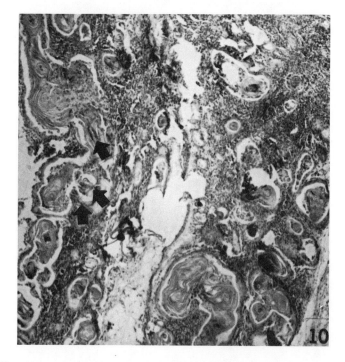

FIG. 10. Extreme cystic metaplasias in two thymic lobes. Points of spindle cell proliferation (arrows) and desquamated products obliterate lumina. Rat on estrogen four weeks during chronic A deficiency; subsequently fed normal diet plus estrogen for two additional final weeks. X 50.

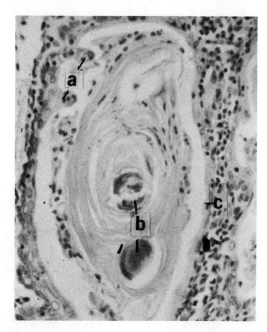

FIG. 11. Same experiment as Fig. 10. Note two discrete points where degenerating suprabasal cells slough off (or proliferate) "buds" of cells contributing to cyst contents (a); calcium deposits (b). Remainder of cyst wall (c), composed of some still viable suprabasal cells which under influence of estrogen, can produce spindle cell masses. X 180.

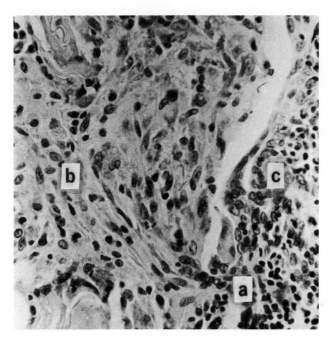

FIG. 12. Same experiment as Fig. 10. One proliferative site within wall
of a cyst (a). These grow into cyst lumina following continuous estrogen
stimulation during repair stages of metaplasia. Because cysts are multiple, and proliferative sites multiple in any one cyst, such spindle cell
masses (b) can be profuse. They apparently derive from intermediate
viable suprabasal cells. Basal cells tend to form vesicles or cords of
cells that mingle with adjacent cytoreticulum (c). X 180.

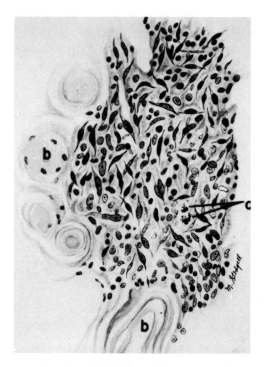

FIG. 13.   Spindle cells from metaplastic epithelium recovering from deficiency of vitamin A under estrogen influence.   Drawing to show detail;
character and proliferative capacity of one incipient spindle cell neoplasm derived from re-vitalized suprabasal cells in a multitude of such
cysts.   Mitosis at (a); remnant of metaplastic lesion (b).   X 200.

REFERENCES

Van Dyke, J. H. Behavior of ultimobranchial tissue in the postnatal thyroid gland: Epithelial cysts, their relation to thyroid parenchyma and to "New-growths" in the thyroid gland of young sheep. Am. J. Anat., 76: 201-251, 1945.

Van Dyke, J. H. Behavior of ultimobranchial tissue in the postnatal thyroid gland: The origin of thyroid cystadenomata in the rat. Anat. Rec., 88: 369-391, 1944.

Rogers, W. M. The fate of the ultimobranchial body in the white rat (Mus norvegicus albinus). Am. J. Anat., 38: 349-377, 1927.

Van Dyke, J. H. Experimental thyroid tumorigenesis in rats. Predominance of neoplasm type and influence of age. A.M.A. Archieves of Pathology, 56: 613-628, 1953.

Van Dyke, J. H. Experimental thyroid metaplasia in the rat. Preliminary report. A.M.A. Archieves of Pathology., 59: 73-81, 1955.

Wolbach, S. B., and Howe, P. R. Tissue changes following deprivation of fat-soluble A vitamin. J. Exper. Med., 42: 753-777, 1925a.

Wolbach, S. B. The pathological changes resulting from vitamin A deficiency. J.A.M.A., 108: 7-13, 1937.

Byrne, J. N., and Eastman, N. J. Vitamin A levels in maternal and fetal blood plasma. Bull. Johns Hopkins Hosp., 73: 132-137, 1943.

Williamson, M. B. Effect of estrogens on plasma vitamin A of normal and thyroidectomized rabbits. Proc. Soc. Exp. Biol. and Med., 66: 621-623, 1947.

Steiner, P. E. Human significance of experimental carcinogenesis. A.M.A. Archives of Pathology., 55: 227-244, 1953.

Maugh II, T. H. Vitamin A: Potential protection from carcinogens. Science., 186: 1198, 1974.

Cairns, J. Mutation selection and natural history of cancer. Nature., 255: 197-200, 1975.

Narisawa, T., Reddy, B. S., Wong, C-Q, and Weisburger, J. H. Effect of vitamin A deficiency on rat colon carcinogenesis by N-Methyl-N' - nitro - N - nitrosoguanidine. Cancer Research., 36: 1379-1383, 1976.

Van Dyke, J. H. Origin of Accessory Thyroid Tissue from Thymus IV in adult baboon. A.M.A. Archives of Pathology., 54: 248-258, 1952.

Van Dyke, J. H. Experimental Aberrant Mediastinal Goiters (Thymic) in the rat. A.M.A. Archives of Pathology., 55: 412-422, 1953.

Pope, R. H., and Osgood, R. Reticular perithelioma of thymus tissue. Am. J. Path., 29: 85-103, 1953.

Karsner, H. T. Human Pathology. J. B. Lippincott Co., Philadelphia, Ed. 8: p. 358, 1955.

Willis, R. A. The Borderland of Embryology and Pathology. Butterworth and Co., London, p. 502, 1958.

Van Dyke, J. H. The Ultimobranchial Bodies. In: Comparative Endocrinology. John Wiley and Sons, Inc., New York, Ed: 1: 320-339, 1959.

Castleman, B. Tumors of the thymus gland. Armed Forces Institute of Pathology., Washington, D. C., pp. 1-82, 1955.

Parnell, J. P. and Sherman, B. S. Effect of Vitamin A on Keratinization in A - Deficient Rat. In: Fundamentals of Keratinization. Am. Assoc. for Advancement of Science, Washington, D. C., pp. 113-131, 1962.

Van Dyke, J. H., Foster, W. C., and Wase, A. W. The thymus as an extrathyroidal source of thyroid hormone. Uptake of radioactive iodine by thymus tissue following thyroidectomy in adult rats. Anat. Rec., 118: 363-364, 1954.

Van Dyke, J. H. An Interpretation; On the origin of glandular neoplasias. Anat. Rec., 191: 542, 1975.

VITAMIN A ACID (RETINOIC ACID) AS AN ADJUVANT TO INCREASE ADRIAMYCIN CYTOTOXICITY IN HUMAN BREAST CANCER CELLS IN VITRO

D. Richard Ishmael
Robert E. Nordquist
Richard H. Bottomley
Jan Zieren

Oklahoma Medical Research Foundation
University of Oklahoma Health Sciences Center
and the Veterans Administration Hospital
Oklahoma City, Oklahoma

I. INTRODUCTION

Adriamycin is a cancer chemotherapeutic antibiotic having activity against a wide variety of human tumors, including solid tumors, lymphomas and leukemias.[1] The usefulness of adriamycin is limited because of cardiotoxicity.[2] This toxicity is related to the total dose of the drug given, is poorly amenable to treatment and is sometimes irreversible.[3] Adriamycin affects human myocardial cells (Girardi Heart Cell line) adversely in tissue culture as much or more than other human tumor cell lines.[4] It seems to be very effective when used in combination with other chemotherapeutic agents.[5] Some of these agents may be acting synergistically rather than additively with adriamycin.[6] The site of action for cell destruction by adriamycin is thought to be through binding to DNA.[7,8] It is possible that resistance to its action is related to differences in membrane permeability to the drug.[9]

Certain agents, including vitamin A and other fat soluble vitamins, are known to affect plasma membranes and make them more permeable.[10] This increased permeability allows certain drugs to pass into the cell more freely. Vitamin A has been shown to increase the activity of certain chemotherapeutic agents, especially the alkylating agents, and therefore act as an adjuvant with these agents.[11] The mechanism is

727

not known, although it has been postulated that vitamin A allows more of the alkylating agents to enter the cell. The specificity of this adjuvant effect for increased killing of cancer cells without a concomitant increase in damage to normal tissue unfortunately is slight.[12] However, the normal nondividing, nonmetabolizing tissues may be less affected by the adjuvant than normal rapidly dividing cells or cancer cells. If an adjuvant could be found to add greater sensitivity to the tumor tissue than to the normal nondividing tissue or the myocardium, then the use of adriamycin could be extended. The first step in looking for an adjuvant would be the development of a rapid cell culture screening technique to look for agents with possible adjuvant activity with adriamycin.

II. METHODS

To look for agents which might have activity as adjuvants, a rapid cell culture screening technique was chosen using a malignant human breast tumor cell line (BOT-2), previously reported.[13] This tumor cell line was derived from an infiltrating duct carcinoma surgically removed from a thirty-one year old patient who had no previous treatment.

A. Tissue Culture

Human breast tumor cells (BOT-2) and Girardi heart cells were each grown in Falcon tissue culture plates in 0.1 ml of Minimum Essential Medium (MEM) in each of the 96 wells. Serial dilutions of adriamycin, adjuvant, or combinations of adriamycin with the adjuvant were added to each well in 50 λ increments. Wells used as controls contained 0.1 ml phosphate buffered saline (PBS). Any wells containing a single agent had 50 λ of PBS added to ensure equal dilution in all wells. All wells contained a total of 0.2 ml of solution.

B. Vitamin A Study

Retinoic acid (vitamin A acid), dissolved in 0.2 N potassium hydroxide, was studied for possible adjuvant activity. The pH was adjusted to 7.5 using 20% potassium acetate (pH 5.0), then the retinoic acid was diluted to various concentrations using PBS. The cells were allowed to incubate for 24 hours before any drugs were added. The plates were then observed at 24 and 48 hours post treatment for growth inhibition or dead cells. Live cells were easily distinguished from dead cells when viewed with an inverted phase microscope. Percentages of live cells were estimated and growth determined by cloning in each well. Actual cell counts were done after the 48 hour reading, using trypan blue to confirm the previous readings. All vitamin A work was done in the dark with safelights.

III. RESULTS

A. BOT-2 Tumor Cells with Adriamycin and Vitamin A

Figures 1, 2 and 3 illustrate the cells as they appeared after 24 hours of treatment with a high concentration of adriamycin, a low concentration of adriamycin, and no adriamycin added. The cells that were called nonviable were nonproliferative, rounded and did not exclude trypan blue (Figure 1). The viable cells in Figure 3 were proliferating, attached to substrate and excluded trypan blue. In Figure 4 are shown the results of adding various concentrations of vitamin A and adriamycin to the cell cultures. These data show that vitamin A does act as an adjuvant to adriamycin at 48 hours, demonstrating increased killing of the cells at vitamin A concentrations of 200, 100 and 10 μg/ml. The adriamycin concentration needed for 100% kill is lowered from 10 μg, when used alone, to 5 μg when combined with 100 μg/ml of vitamin A, thereby halving the dose of adriamycin required.

B. BOT-2 Tumor Cells with Adriamycin and Bleomycin

Figure 5 shows the effect of various concentrations of bleomycin and adriamycin on BOT-2 cells at 48 hours. Bleomycin alone did not kill cells at 48 hours at these concentrations. When bleomycin and adriamycin were combined there was no increased effect observed. An adriamycin and 5-fluorouracil combination did not show a synergistic effect at 24 or 48 hours.

C. Girardi Heart Cells with Vitamin A and Adriamycin

The Girardi heart cell line is a cell line derived from human atria apparently transformed to a malignant state. Figure 6 demonstrates that these cells were exquisitely sensitive to adriamycin. Vitamin A with adriamycin demonstrated no adjuvant effect on the cell line.

IV. DISCUSSION

Adriamycin is an active drug for the treatment of various human malignancies. However, the total dose that can be used is limited by its cardiotoxicity. It would be important to find agents that might prolong the effective use of adriamycin. The initial results of this in vitro study of adriamycin with vitamin A indicate that vitamin A may enhance the activity of adriamycin against a human breast tumor cell line. Two chemotherapeutic agents, bleomycin and 5-fluorouracil, did not enhance the activity of adriamycin against the BOT-2 cell line. There was no enhanced toxicity of the adriamycin-vitamin A combination against the heart cell line. Animal studies are underway to see if a similar adjuvant effect of vitamin A with adriamycin is seen against the L1210 tumor cell line in mice. Cardiotoxicity studies are underway to see if vitamin A also enhances the activity of adriamycin against myocardial tissue.

V. SUMMARY

Vitamin A is known to have adjuvant activity in increasing the killing effect of certain chemotherapeutic agents in certain animal tumor systems. Most of the chemotherapeutic agents previously studied were alkylating agents. Vitamin A is known to increase the permeability of cell membranes to certain substances. We studied the effect of vitamin A acid to see if its presence would increase the killing effect of adriamycin. Adriamycin is a potent antitumor antibiotic, with a dose-limiting cardiotoxicity. This study was undertaken to see if vitamin A could extend the effective use of adriamycin by increasing its toxicity to tumor cells without a concomitant increase in the cardiotoxicity. The first phase of the study does indeed show that vitamin A acid increases the cytotoxicity of adriamycin to cultured human breast cancer cells.

730

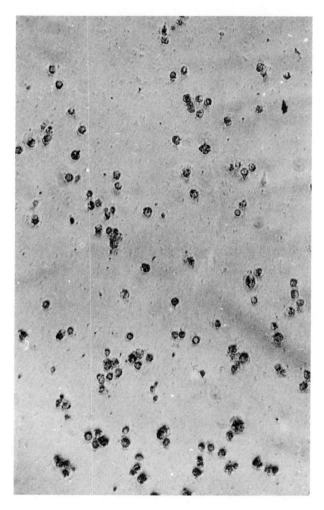

FIG. 1. BOT cells treated with high dose adriamycin.

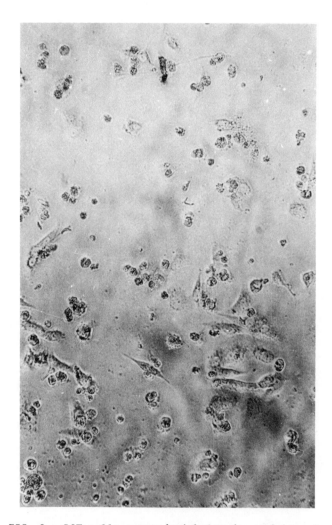

FIG. 2. BOT cells treated with low dose adriamycin.

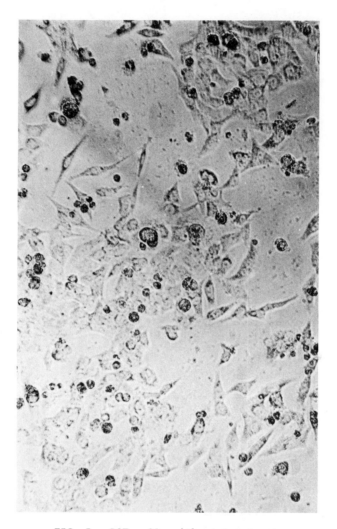

FIG. 3. BOT cells without treatment.

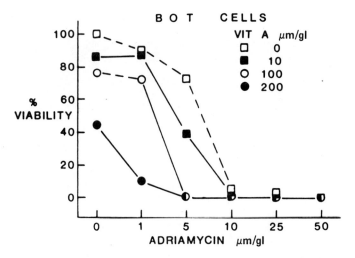

FIG. 4. BOT cells treated with various concentrations of adriamycin and vitamin A.

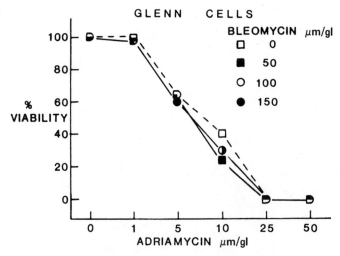

FIG. 5. BOT cells treated with various concentrations of adriamycin and bleomycin.

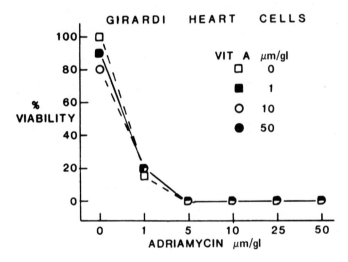

FIG. 6. Girardi Heart Cells treated with various concentrations of adriamycin and vitamin A.

REFERENCES

1. Blum, R.H., and Carter, S.K. Adriamycin: A new anticancer drug with significant clinical activity. Ann. Int. Med., 80:249-259, 1974

2. Cortes, E.P., Lutman, G., Wanka, J., et al. Adriamycin cardio-toxicity in adults with cancer. Clin. Res., 21:412, 1973

3. Lefrak, E., et al. A clinicopathologic analysis of adriamycin cardiotoxicity. Cancer, 32:302-314, 1973

4. Haskell, C.M., and Sullivan, A. Comparative survival in tissue culture of normal and neoplastic human cells exposed to adriamycin. Cancer Res., 34:2991-2994, 1974

5. Gottlieb, J.A., Bakeil, H., Quagliana, J.M., et al. Chemotherapy of sarcomas with a combination of adriamycin and dimethyl triazeno imidazole carboxamide. Cancer, 31:1632-1638, 1972

6. Data of Drug Evaluation Branch, National Cancer Institute.

7. Calendi, E., DiMarco, A., Regiani, M., et al. On physicochemical interactions between daunomycin and nucleic acids. Biochem Biophys Acta, 103:25-49, 1965

8. Lembertenghi-Deliliers, G. Ultrastructural alterations induced in hepatic cell-nucleoli by adriamycin. In: International Symposium on Adriamycin. Springer-Verlag, New York, pp.26-34, 1972

9. Kessel, D., Botteril, U., and Wodinsky, I. Uptake and retention of daunomycin by mouse leukemic cells as factors in drugs response. Cancer Res., 28:938, 1968

10. Lucy, J.A., and Dingle, J.T. Fat-soluble vitamins and biological membranes. Nature, 204:156-160, 1964

11. Cohen, M.H., and Carbone, P. Enhancement of antitumor effect of alkylating agents by Vitamin A. Proc., Amer. Assoc. for Cancer Res., pg. 14, Abst. No. 54, 1969

12. Nathanson, L., Maddock, C.L., and Hall, T.C. Exploratory studies of Vitamin A and cyclophosphamide in tumor-bearing mice. J. Clin. Pharm., 9:359-373, 1969

13. Nordquist, R.E., Ishmael, D.R., Lovig, C.A., Hyder, D.M., and Hoge, A.F. Tissue culture and morphology of human breast tumor cell line BOT-2. Cancer Res., 35:3100-3105, 1975

Chapter 7

SMOKING

SOCIAL AND PSYCHOLOGIC ASPECTS OF STARTING SMOKING

Daniel Horn

National Clearinghouse for Smoking and Health
Center for Disease Control
Atlanta, Georgia

Over a period of years in which we have been responsible for
carrying out both a research programme and a control programme to deal
with the harmful effects of cigarette smoking, we have developed a number
of formulations that were meant to help structure the work. In 1965 (4)
we presented a model that was designed to form a framework for analyzing
whether or not adult smokers would try to give up smoking, and, if they
tried, what were the factors that determined various levels of success.
This same model later became the basis of a self-testing "insight development" instrument (8) for encouraging and improving the success of behavior
change in smoking.

At the same time it was clear that the initiation and the early
formation of the smoking habit which takes place largely among teenagers
involves many quite different elements than does the maintenance of the
smoking habit by an adult in the face of the anti-smoking onslaughts
since the mid-1950's (1)(2)(7)(12). We have now completed a project (6)
which has identified a practical system of measurement of a number of
factors which play a role in the development of the smoking habit among
youth, although knowledge on the patterning of these factors is still
lacking. As with the adult cessation model this also has been published
as a self-testing "insight development" procedure for educational use
with adolescents. A wide variety of research, both on adults and teenagers, their smoking habits and changes in their smoking habits has now
provided voluminous data with which to characterize (1) the initiation,
(2) the development, (3) the maintenance and (4) the cessation or other
hazard-reducing modification of smoking behaviour.

The present report which is concerned with the various aspects of
"starting smoking" deals only with the first two of these four processes - (1) the initiation and (2) the establishment of smoking behaviour.

A. Initiation of the behaviour

The initiation of personal choice health behaviour is usually exploratory in nature, usually takes place in rather young people, sometimes in young children, and is largely dependent on, first, the
availability of an opportunity for engaging in the behaviour; second,
on having a fairly high degree of curiosity about the pleasant effects
of the behaviour; and, third, in finding it a way of either expressing
conformity to the behaviour of others, such as parents, older siblings

or age-equals, or as a way of expressing rebellion against what are
seen as unreasonable proscriptions against the behaviour. Characteristically, the greater the availability or the opportunity for expressing
the behaviour, the less is the necessity for a strong commitment either
to conformity with the behaviour of others or to rebellion against
proscriptions by others. We know that smoking, for example, is much
more common in children of parents who are themselves regular smokers
(2)(10)(11) and this is partly because of the ready availability of cigarettes to children when there is already a smoker in the household and
partly because use of cigarettes by older members of the family sets an
example of acceptable behaviour and stimulates curiosity about what makes
the cigarette so attractive. When smoking first begins to be widespread
in a culture, it tends to be taken up with increasing frequency by
successive waves of young people. Nevertheless substantial numbers of
older people may turn to it, especially if it can serve as a convenient
substitute for previously well-established behaviour, as was the case with
cigarettes replacing cigar and pipe smoking in many male populations between 1910 and 1950.

B. Establishment of the behaviour

The establishment of personal choice health behaviour can be influenced by at least three groups of factors. In the case of cigarette
smoking developing as a continuing habit in adolescents, these are,
first, the costs/benefits evaluation of the behaviour; second, common
stereotypes that characterize perception of the behaviour; and third,
psychological factors characterizing both personal structure and per-
sonality integration factors, particularly as they reflect the relationship of the individual and his needs to society and its demands.

The costs that go into the evaluation of the costs/benefits balance
may include the harmful effects on health (both physical and mental),
economic cost, and the harmful effects on society, such as economic or
as a form of pollution. The benefits may include positive effects on
health (both physical and mental), economic advantages, social utility
(especially in terms of the facilitation of personal interactions),
psychological utility (both in terms of the increase of positive effect
or the reduction of negative effect) and benefits to society. There may
also be quite separate evaluations of a costs/benefits analysis for the
individual and a costs/benefits analysis for society, since for some
individuals, one of these may be more persuasive than the other in producing attempts to change behaviour. For political leaders, the costs/
benefits for society usually takes precedence over the costs/benefits
analysis for the individual. When the behaviour which appears to be
most logical on the basis of a costs/benefits balance and the actual
behaviour of the individual are quite different, another set of factors
consisting of rationalisations or some other set of beliefs may come
into play to reduce the dissonance between the "logical" behaviour and
the actual behaviour. In the case of cigarette smoking, the costs for
the past twenty or so years have largely reflected the increasing evidence of the harmful effects of smoking on health, but in addition to
that such concerns as aesthetic values, and the contribution of smoking
to various forms of pollution, or economic values as reflected by the
financial cost either to the individual or to society, have come
into play. The benefits are wide, ranging from the facilitation of
social interaction, which is perceived or appears as one of the most

valuable benefits of taking up smoking, to the reduction of tension and to the enhancement of states of pleasure which tend to be a later development in the appreciation of benefits. Such common remarks as "I can always give up smoking before it hurts me", or "I don't really smoke enough for it to do any damage" or "The kind of cigarette I smoke (or the way I smoke it) is not very likely to hurt anyone" are characteristic of beliefs of the individual whose perception of potential costs is higher than the perceived benefits and yet who continues to smoke.

Perceptual stereotypes tend to develop as a kind of mythology about what smoking is like, what smokers are like, and why people smoke. These tend to be superficial and frequently inaccurate systems of beliefs and are likely to be derived either from the exaggerations of advertising on the one hand or the exaggerations of counter-advertising by anti-smoking groups on the other. In general, the greater the role played by superficial and inaccurate beliefs about the behaviour, whether positive or negative, the more difficult it is to develop a sound decision-making process on the part of the individual or society as a whole.

A variety of patterns of psychological forces may enter into the determination of personal choice health behaviour, in particular, those that reflect the conflict engendered in individuals by the demands of society or his own inner demands. In the case of smoking behaviour and health, we have identified two such factors. One depends on the strength of the conflict perceived by the individual between the satisfaction of his own needs and the demands imposed on him by society or by its authority figures. The second factor is a reflection of the urgency to the individual of maintaining control over his own behaviour and over his own destiny as opposed to being subject either to the control of others or to the vagaries of chance as represented by "good luck" or by "bad luck".

DISCUSSION:

The utility of a model depends on how much it contributes to improved research designs and the extent to which it suggests new control programmes. In a sense, what has been presented in this paper is a framework for a model rather than the model itself. Figure 1 presents in diagrammatic form both the elements and the processes that have been used in this framework, and Figure 2 elaborates on the factors in the establishment of the behaviour. The processes are illustrated by arrows showing the direction in which change usually takes place and the elements that influence these processes are shown by solid lines. The studies on the epidemiology of lung cancer and coronary heart disease that identified smoking as an important factor in each did much to help develop techniques in the epidemiology of chronic disease. Perhaps the wide range of behavioural research that has been stimulated by the recognition that the reduction of smoking would lead to great improvements in health may serve as well in breaking the ground for better behavioural research into ways of dealing with personal choice health behaviour.

In addition to cigarette smoking, the model appears to be applicable to such well-known problems as those posed by drug abuse, sex behaviour, eating habits, alcohol use, and physical-risk taking such as hazardous sports. It may also be useful in studying such problems as medical care seeking, medical regimen compliance, family planning and other such complex issues. In general, one may define this class of behaviour as comprising normal, socially-acceptable ways of increasing the enjoyment of life or providing mechanisms for coping with the problems of life. They can be useful, and are sometimes necessary, concommitants of life. They share the characteristic that when carried beyond a certain point or when they occur at inappropriate times, that is when they are "abused", they create problems, either health problems or social problems for the individual, the people around him, or the society at large.

At one point in time (3), I have referred to these behaviours as "risk-taking" and later as "gratification" behaviour (5). In the former expression, the emphasis is on the harmful effects of the behaviour, that is the cost. In the latter expression, the emphasis is on the rewarding effect of the behaviour, that is the benefit. The real issue and the matter that involves personal choice is decision-making on the basis of an understanding of the cost/benefits balance. Therefore the term "personal choice health behaviour" or PCHB seems most appropriately descriptive of this area of our concern. In a sense, the role of public health practitioners and especially public health educators, is to develop in people a capability of understanding these behaviours and their effects: to get people to ask "what does it do for me?", "what does it do to me?", and on balance "what do I want to do about this and how do I accomplish it?"

For some reason there seems to have developed a conflict between those who feel that the cigarette problem should be solved by health education directed towards the individual and the other approach supported by those who feel that change should be directed at the cigarette itself and at the way it is promoted and distributed. The same kind of argument exists between those who propose controlling heart disease by regulating the nutritional substances available to the public and those who wish to educate people to make changes in their own diet. Another example is the diminution of death and disability from road accidents by education for safer driving as opposed to changes in car design, road design and driving regulations that would diminish the likelihood of accidents and injury. The recent history of the smoking problem shows that these two approaches need not be alternatives. Not only can they exist side by side, they could be used to reinforce each other. During the past year or two in the United States there has been a rash of legislative and regulatory actions taken to reduce smoking in public places. Such action would have been inconceivable just five years earlier. It was not until the general public and the legislators who represent them became convinced of the serious ill-health that results from smoking that they were willing to support actions for the common good which previously had been viewed as infringements on individual liberty. Since these convictions developed from exposure to health education that was designed to encourage the individual smokers to change his personal smoking habits, it is clear that the same message contributed to a climate in which a new kind of community action became acceptable.

In this paper I have dealt only with those factors concerned with the initiation and establishment of smoking in young people but this is meant in no way to imply that this part of the problem is either more important or less important than the factors which govern the maintenance and the cessation or other modification of smoking in the adult smoker. As further research identifies how the factors I have described above are inter-related and patterned we may be in a better position to design more successful ways of reducing the development of smoking behaviour.

On the basis of our present knowledge, it is clear that we can take the following steps right now to achieve this reduction.

1. Reduce the easy availability of cigarettes to young people.

2. Continue to encourage parents and prominent young and adult role-models important to youth to set the example of not smoking.

3. Reduce the intensity of emotionally charged proscriptions against smoking which serve to stimulate contrary action.

4. Continue to stress the costs associated with smoking without denying the benefits, but encourage young people to achieve these benefits in less damaging ways.

5. Avoid the pitfall of stereotypes about smoking and smokers that turn young people away from the anti-smoking "do-gooders".

6. Help young people develop insight into their own needs and perceptions which appear to make smoking attractive and encourage them to seek alternative, less-damaging means of satisfying these needs.

The challenge of health education is to identify the means whereby we can help people develop the capability of understanding the issues in personal choice health behaviour and the capacity to make choices both in their own self-interest and in the interest of society at large. If this is our goal we must learn to live with the fact that under these conditions many thoughtful people will still make choices that are different from those that we would recommend. In that case, the best we can do is to "manage" the problem by placing boundaries to the amount of damage to themselves and to others that may result from this choice and then to wish the individual well. If studies of the smoking problem and its control throw light on how to deal with some of the other health problems that result from personal behaviour choices, their contribution to good health through this knowledge may, in the long run, be even more in this way than through the reduction of smoking-related disease.

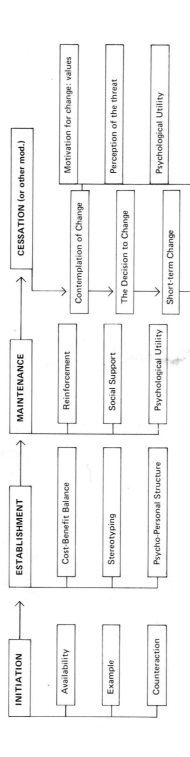

FIG. 1. A schematic outline of a personal choice health behaviour model.
Processes are joined by arrows. Factors, representing critical variables
which determine direction and progression of processes, are joined by
solid lines.

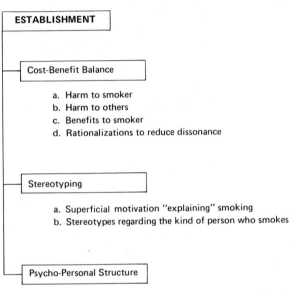

ESTABLISHMENT

Cost-Benefit Balance

    a. Harm to smoker
    b. Harm to others
    c. Benefits to smoker
    d. Rationalizations to reduce dissonance

Stereotyping

    a. Superficial motivation "explaining" smoking
    b. Stereotypes regarding the kind of person who smokes

Psycho-Personal Structure

    a. Perceived conflict between satisfying own needs and meeting demands of
       society and authority figures
    b. Relative importance of controlling one's own destiny as opposed to being
       subject to either "chance" or control by others

FIG. 2. Elaboration of factors governing establishment of the behaviour.

REFERENCES

1. Creswell, W. H., Jr., Huffman, W. J., Stone, D. B., Merki, D. J. & Newman, I. M. University of Illinois anti-smoking education study. Illinois J. Educ., 60, 27 (1969)

2. Horn, D., Courts, F. A., Taylor, R. M. & Solomon, E. S. Cigarette smoking among high school students. Amer. J. publ. Hlth, 49, 1497 (1959)

3. Horn, D. A systematic approach to helping people give up smoking. Southern Medical Bulletin, 54 (2): 23-30 (1966)

4. Horn, D. & Waingrow, S. Some dimensions of a model for smoking behaviour change. Amer. J. publ. Hlth, 56, 21 (1966)

5. Horn, D. Man, cigarettes, and the abuse of gratification. Arch. environm. Hlth, 20, 88 (1970)

6. Milne, A. M. & Colman, J. G. Development of a teenager's self-testing kit (cigarette smoking). Final report. Education and Public Affairs, Washington, D. C. (1973)

7. Salber, E. J. & Abelin, T. Smoking behaviour of Newton school-children - 5-year follow-up. Pediatrics, 40, 363 (1967)

8. US National Clearinghouse for Smoking and Health. Smoker's self-testing kit, U.S.P.H.S. Publication No. 1904 (1969)

9. US National Clearinghouse for Smoking and Health. Teenage self-test: cigarette smoking, US Department of Health, Education and Welfare Publication No. (CDC) 74-8723 (1974)

10. US National Clearinghouse for Smoking and Health. Teenage smoking - national patterns: 1968, 1970, US Department of Health, Education and Welfare Publication No. (HSM) 72-7508 (1972)

11. US National Clearinghouse for Smoking and Health. Teenage smoking - national patterns: 1972, 1974, US Department of Health, Education and Welfare Publication No. (NIH) 76-931 (1976)

12. Williams, T. Summary and implications of review of literature related to adolescent smoking. Education and Public Affairs, Washington, D. C. (1971)

PREVENTION OF SMOKING

Ernst L. Wynder and L.A. Shewchuk
American Health Foundation, New York, N.Y.

Tobacco usage, especially in the form of cigarettes, continues to predominate in the pathogenesis of a variety of human cancers. It represents a major etiological factor for cancers of the lung, oral cavity and larynx in males; 90% of their incidence is attributable to tobacco usage. It also accounts for a significant proportion of the male incidence of cancer of the esophagus, kidney, bladder and pancreas (1-3). Dose responses have been well-established by pro and retrospective studies. We estimate that about 40% of the male cancer deaths in the U.S. are related to tobacco usage (Figure 1). The higher rate of cancer among males, as compared to females, is principally due to differences in smoking habits for those in the cancer age group.

What then has been done or can be done in the future to reduce, if not eliminate, this adverse effect of smoking on human health?

The eradication of any disease entity involves two levels of prevention - primary and secondary. We can think of smoking prevention in the same light. Primary prevention of smoking deals with those who have not yet begun to smoke but who may be at high risk to do so. Secondary prevention is characteristically viewed as early identification and prompt treatment of a disease or disorder. In smoking prevention we deal with the individual who smokes, realizes the risk he is taking by doing so, and who wants to quit smoking.

Research in this paper was supported in part by Contract HSM-21-72-557 of the National Clearinghouse for Smoking and Health, Bureau of Health Education, Center for Disease Control, DHEW; and in part by Grant ACS MG-161 of the American Cancer Society, Inc. and part by Grant CA17867-01 from the National Cancer Institute, DHEW, NIH.

747

HEALTH EDUCATION (PRIMARY PREVENTION)

Our present programs directing children not to smoke have been largely ineffective. As many of our boys smoke today as ten years ago, and the number of girls smoking has drastically increased (Figures 2 and 3). Peer pressure in favor of smoking seems to be much more persuasive to children than rational claims on the future deleterious effects that smoking will have on them.

The American Health Foundation is currently sponsoring KNOW YOUR BODY, a new program for school children which screens them for a variety of risk factors (viz: cholesterol, blood pressure, obesity, the recovery index test for the heart and the history of cigarette smoking). After receiving their results, they then, when necessary, participate in an intervention program aimed collectively and individually at high-risk children.   A case-control study is in progress to determine the success of such an approach. It can already be said, however, that students, teachers and adults involved in ongoing KYB programs have shown an enthusiastic support that has not been experienced with didactic health lectures.

SMOKING CESSATION CLINICS (SECONDARY PREVENTION)

There is a considerable group of smokers who would like to "break" the habit, but they are unable to do so by themselves; they require help. The medical profession and the current hospitable care system is not providing such help on an adequate basis. Instead of merely blaming the tobacco industry for its contribution to the smoking and health issue, we should ask ourselves whether we, as medical professionals, are doing our share to overcome this problem.

Secondary prevention of smoking deals with the individual who smokes but realizes the risk he is taking by doing so. He is the smoker who wants to quit - who may or may not have tried to do so with some measure of success for short periods of time. There is evidence that there are some 20 million such smokers in the U.S.A. today.[4]   Some inroads have therefore been made, especially among educated white adult males, where smoking has gradually decreased. The motivating factor for this decrease seems to be related to the status symbol of the "non-smoker", rather than concern over the health risks involved. Among women the percent of those giving up smoking is less than for males and no educational gradient has been noted (Figure 4).

Most secondary prevention programs focus on the "motivated" smoker and involve them in a variety of rather intense cessation activities. Such attempts have been adequately reviewed by Schwartz.[5]   We at the American Health Foundation do not feel that all smokers need an intensive, time-consuming therapist or smoking specialist-dependent program of activities in order to stop smoking. Shewchuk has reported on the range of smoking cessation activities developed at the AHF.(6)   Essentially we see two basic problems in secondary prevention:

1. to help people stop smoking, and

2. once they have stopped to help them maintain this status.

We have developed four levels of intervention - ranging from complete self-help procedures whereby a smoker is made aware of the personal relevance his smoking has for him and given tips on how to stop smoking on his own to involving smokers in group interaction procedures over many weeks, which capitalizes on group, intra- and inter-personal dynamics.

Figure 5 summarizes the levels of intervention we have studied. At level I, we have responded to surveys showing that the majority of smokers seeking help in stopping smoking are not interested in clinics and group meetings. What they want are effective materials that they can use on their own. One way of filling this demand is with mass communication instructions for the self-directed use of behavior modification techniques. Brengelmann found that his behavior modification smoking program worked almost as well when administered through the mail as when applied on a face-to-face basis.(7) Payment of money and the use of contracts insure adherence to the program. He reported immediate success rates of 65%, although this percentage may be based only on those who adhered to the program. In our data we have learned to expect up to 50% non-compliance.

We have tried similar programs using mail-outs and mass media approaches on TV and radio with relatively good results (i.e., approximately 10-12% immediate or end-of-treatment quit rate which seems to be maintained up to our 1-3 month follow-up points). The difficulty with such programs is attracting and keeping the attention of participants. One other project which we have been working on in conjunction with Dan Horn and The National Clearinghouse for Smoking and Health involves physicians giving stop-smoking messages to patients as they proceed through regular health examinations. The message takes less than two minutes and each participant is given a more detailed message to take home with him to read at his leisure. We have only preliminary results to report at this time, but if the trend continues for all 3,000 participants the implications become very significant.

Table I summarizes the results of two best groups of smokers studied who maintain a 23% success rate six months after being given the physician message. The contrasted group contains other message types as well as "no message" control groups. One feature of the successes in this program indicates that 60% of those who stopped did so by stopping "cold turkey" even though of all the participants who tried to stop smoking there was a 50-50 split in stopping gradually or stopping abruptly. This finding contrasted with that in higher intervention levels where participants generally work at dosage reduction, reach a certain level and then state they quit "cold turkey" tends to confirm what Dan Horn previously suggested [8] that by a gradual dosage reduction program most smokers who want to quit smoking will eventually reach a dosage level whereby quitting will become easier or at best reach a level of markedly reduced risk to tobacco-related diseases. We must, however, bear in mind that the high intervention levels deal with the hard-core smoker and as yet we are not certain if this is the case in the minimal intervention level.

Our Level II programs have been described by Shewchuk. [6] They focus on the utilization of stop smoking materials which are available to smokers through any commercial outlet. Essentially, these techniques are ones which require practice and effort on the part of the smoker, but little in the way of introduction, structure or monitoring by a staff smoking specialist. A number of such techniques are presently on the market in the form of books, tapes and records. Very few, if any, have been systematically and scientifically tested for their effectiveness in helping people stop smoking. Our preliminary data are rather disappointing since half of our population drop out of our studies - reflecting a non-acceptance of the particular aids we chose to study. In spite of the drop outs, overall results show 19% have stopped smoking one month after completing the program. Our efforts in this area will focus on finding more acceptable aids and identifying the characteristics of the smoker who would find this level of intervention most beneficial.

Most of our efforts to date have been directed at Level III intervention programs. Interventions at this level are defined as any smoking cessation technique requiring practice and effort on the part of the smoker and is monitored and structured by some support system such as a group and/or therapist or person specifically trained to deal with issues characterizing the smoking cessation process.

Figure 6 summarizes our results on 2,000 participants taking part in group and individual counseling and hypnosis. These results were achieved without the aid of maintenance procedures and generally confirm other findings of 20-30% success rates at the end of one year. With perfected maintenance programs, we expect to increase our success rates very close to 50%. Our MRFIT program, which involves an elaborate maintenance procedure utilizing weekly telephone calls, periodic clinic visits, support from spouses, etc., achieve one year success rates of approximately 50%. Our maintenance programs are in various stages of development and efforts to date have been described by Shewchuk. [6] We visualize a hierarchy of maintenance programs ranging from self-help techniques to intensive, effort-consuming activities very much parallel to our initial stop smoking interventions. Eventually we hope to be able to identify smoker characteristics which would aid in matching cessation levels (or techniques) to specific smokers to help them stop smoking and then match maintenance levels (or techniques) to specific ex-smokers to help maintain their non-smoking status.

Additional research is being carried out in terms of anti-smoking drugs. Most drugs now on the market seem to have only a placebo effect. We are currently testing the possibility that nicotine aerosol may be useful in helping people overcome smoking habit, with long-term maintenance provided by a prescribed antagonist.

This new means of providing nicotine should prove useful for those persons physiologically dependent on some of the central nervous system and peripheral effects of nicotine. Several earlier studies have shown that substitution of cigarette nicotine by nicotine gum does reduce smoking despite the slow alkaloid release by the chewing gum.[9] Other experiments using cigarettes "spiked" with added nicotine have shown a similar drop in number of cigarettes consumed.[10] These data suggest that many smokers titrate themselves to maintain satisfying blood concentrations of nicotine. Aerosolized nicotine may thus wean "hard core" smokers from the cigarette. With the aid of counseling and the subsequent use of other drugs which block rebound excitability of the nervous system, more "dependent" smokers will be likely to quit. A large scale clinical trial utilizing this methodology is projected in the very near future.

Expansion and improvement of smoking cessation clinics remain a major challenge to the medical and health profession. Further efforts should be directed at exploring "mass media" intervention programs, maintenance programs and the standardization of collecting and reporting results of cessation activities.

PREDICTING THE EX-SMOKER

We have completed some analyses of potential predictors for long-term success in level III programs and have identified nine variables which, in combination, will accurately classify 78% of two extreme groups of quitters and failures. These predictors (of success) include the following:

a) Long previous periods of not smoking.

b) Disagreeing with the statement "I am very aware when not smoking".

c) Never or only occasionally use tranquillizers.

d) Have achieved high educational levels.

e) Have tried to quit on their own in the past.

f)   Having non-smoking family members.

g)   Use automobile shoulder harness.

h)   Have a "bargain hunter" attitude.

i)   Live with a spouse or room-mate but not
     alone or with parents.

At the present time, our cost for group therapy and minimal maintenance contacts is $55 per patient per year. We re-
commend that smoking cessation clinics become an integral part
of every hospital outpatient service. If need be, a third
party carrier could pay for such programs, although there does
appear to be a motivating factor to quit if some fee is paid
by the patient.

LESS HARMFUL CIGARETTES

An additional way of reaching smoke related diseases related to the production of less harmful cigarettes - a
"managerial" aspect of preventive medicine.

The particulate matter of tobacco smoke has been shown to
be largely responsible for the carcinogenic effect of cigarette smoking.[11]   Therefore, a reduction of such condensate can be expected to lead to a reduction of cancer risk
among smokers after a suitable latent period of about ten
years.

Since cigarette "tar" is carcinogenic, as measured experimentally on a gram to gram level, but is lower in amount
than it was 25 years ago (when average "tar" was 40 mg)
(Figure 7) the risk of smokers of modern cigarettes is bound
to be less than for smokers of the cigarettes of 25 years ago,
assuming the number of cigarettes smoked has remained the same.
Even the risk of non-filter smokers should be less than those
of the 1950's, since these cigarettes have also reduced the
"tar" yield. The lower risk of developing cancers of the lung
and larynx for long-term filter smokers is demonstrated in
Figure 8. The differences in risk appear to be particularly
great in ages 40-49, since this group smoked non-filter cigarettes for the least period of time. It should be noted that
all present day filter smokers in the cancer age began their
smoking career with the old non-filter type. The longer low
tar cigarettes have been smoked, the lower the risk should be.
However, we cannot as yet measure the risk of those who have
smoked filter cigarettes exclusively. Females have smoked
filter cigarettes relatively longer than males (Figure 9);
and we thus predict that their risks, though they will be
increasing, will not reach the levels currently reached by
men.

The present data on cigarettes are based on "tar" yields of about 20 mg per cigarette. Since 1968, the percentage of cigarettes with a tar yield of 16 mg or less has been increased and if the present influx takes hold, the future rates of tobacco-related cancers are likely to further decrease. The cigarette of tomorrow is likely to be under 10 mg of particulate matter and will be selectively lower in those smoke components that have been shown to be tumorigenic. Due to our increased knowledge of flavor technology, it will be possible to provide smoking "satisfaction" to smokers of such cigarettes. Such progress in the "managerial area" of preventive medicine will continue to have a major effect on the rate of tobacco-related cancer.

A separate evaluation needs to be made for cardiovascular disease, which requires measuring, in particular, the relative contribution of nicotine and carbon monoxide to its etiology. While nicotine has been reduced, no comparable carbon monoxide reduction has taken place - a reduction which, with the exception of increased ventilation, has proved to be a difficult engineering problem. In terms of chronic obstructive pulmonary disease, the relative roles of particulate matter and gas phase remain to be elucidated. In any case, we must be certain that a less harmful cigarette for cancer does not become a more harmful cigarette for some other tobacco-related disease.

It has been asked, "Why should non-tobacco industry scientists work on less harmful cigarettes?" As long as our society permits smoking, a large percentage of the public will continue to smoke in spite of all efforts and health education, even if such efforts are well-coordinated. It is important for those of us wary of tobacco-related disease to realize that smoking represents an ingrained habit with millions for whom it also provides some satisfaction. The problem will not go away by wishing it away. It requires an organized effort on various fronts in order to make an impact on tobacco-related death rates. Such an impact is beginning to be evident in relation to lung cancer in the younger age groups in the U.S.[12] It is already more visible in England partly because cigarette smoking has a longer history there than in the U.S.[13]

The ultimate triumph for those engaged in the smoking and health area is obviously the reduction of tobacco-related disease. What we now see may be the beginning of the end. With an increased effort on the part of all segments of society we hopefully will, in our lifetime, witness the day when tobacco related diseases will no longer be a scourge of mankind.

TABLE I. Summary of Six Month Success Rate: Physician
Mini-Message Program

MESSAGE CONDITION	N	PERCENT QUIT @ 6 MONTHS
OTHER MESSAGE AND NO MESSAGE GROUPS	529	16
STRUCTURED MESSAGE TO PREVIOUS QUITTERS	80	23
ALL GROUPS	609	17

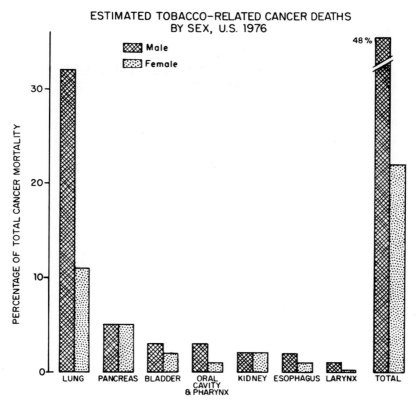

ESTIMATED TOBACCO−RELATED CANCER DEATHS
BY SEX, U.S. 1976

(SOURCE: ACS, FACTS & FIGURES, 1976)

FIG. 1

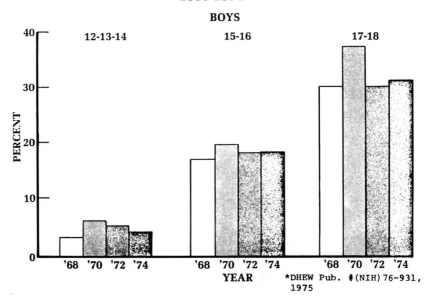

PERCENT
CURRENT REGULAR SMOKERS—TEENAGE,
1968-1974 *

FIG. 2

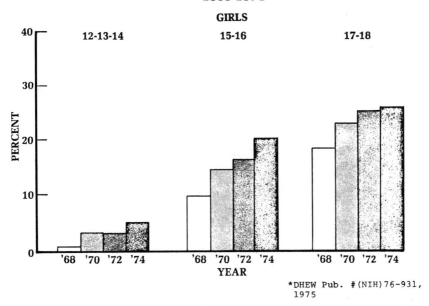

PERCENT
CURRENT REGULAR SMOKERS—TEENAGE,
1968-1974 *

GIRLS

*DHEW Pub. #(NIH)76-931,
1975

FIG. 3

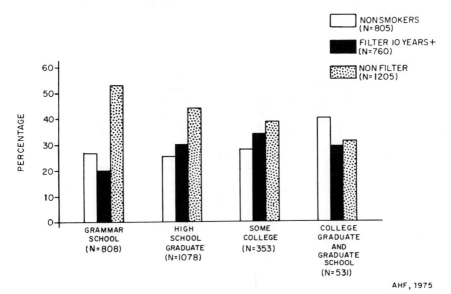

DISTRIBUTION OF SMOKING STATUS AMONG MALE CONTROLS (AGED 40-80) BY
EDUCATIONAL ATTAINMENT.

AHF, 1975

FIG. 4

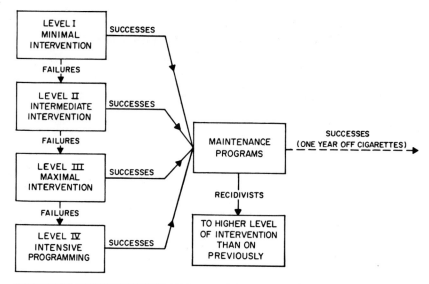

SCHEMATIC REPRESENTATION OF SMOKING CESSATION PROGRAM HIERARCHY:
AMERICAN HEALTH FOUNDATION

FIG. 5

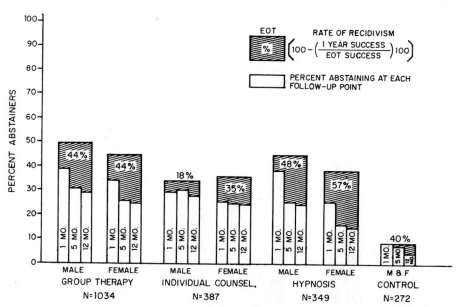

SUMMARY OF END-OF-TREATMENT SUCCESS RATES AND RECIDIVISM RATE FOR
THREE SMOKING CESSATION METHODS (N = 2042)

FIG. 6

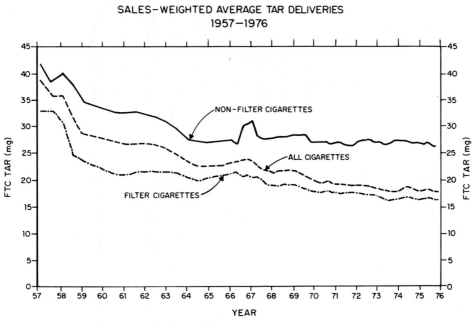

SALES−WEIGHTED AVERAGE TAR DELIVERIES
1957−1976

NON−FILTER CIGARETTES

ALL CIGARETTES

FILTER CIGARETTES

FIG. 7

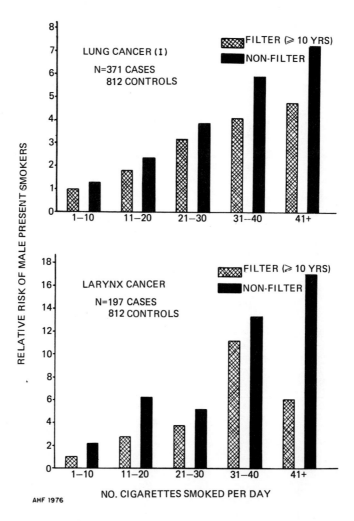

FIG. 8

760

PERCENT OF LIFE−LONG FILTER SMOKERS BY AGE AND SEX

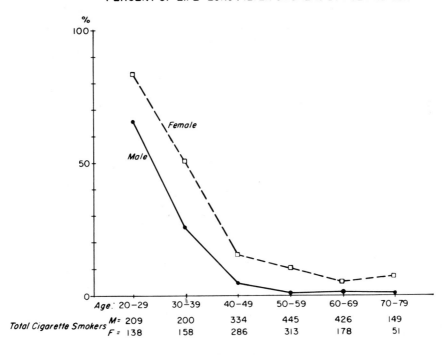

Age:	20−29	30−39	40−49	50−59	60−69	70−79
Total Cigarette Smokers M=	209	200	334	445	426	149
F =	138	158	286	313	178	51

FIG. 9

REFERENCES

1. U.S. Department of Health, Education, and Welfare, Smoking and Health: Report of Advisory Committee to the Surgeon General of the Public Health Service. U.S. Gov. Printing Office, Washington, D.C., 1964.

2. U.S. Department of Health, Education, and Welfare. The Health Consequences of Smoking - 1974. U.S. Gov. Printing Office, Washington, D.C., 1974.

3. World Health Organization, Smoking and Its Effects on Health: Report of a WHO Expert Committee. WHO Technical Report Series 568, Geneva, 1975.

4. McAlister, A. Helping people quit smoking, current progress. In: Applying Behavioral Science to Cardiovascular Risk. Eds.: A.J. Enelow, and Judith Henderson. American Heart Association, 1975.

5. Schwartz, J., and Dubitsky, M. Psychosocial Factors Involved in Cigarette Smoking and Cessation. Smoking Control Research Project, Berkeley, Ca., Sept., 1968.

6. Shewchuk, L.A. Smoking Cessation Programs of the American Health Foundation. Prev. Med., 5: 454-474, 1976.

7. Brengelmann, J. Guidelines for Organizing Smoking Withdrawal Clinics. In: Proceedings of the Third World Conference on Smoking and Health. Eds.: J.L. Steinfeld, W. Griffiths, K.P. Ball, and R.M. Taylor. DHEW Publication, in press.

8. Horn, Daniel. Personal Communication and Discussion, New York, 1973.

9. Brantmark, B., Ohlin, P., and Westling, H. Nicotine containing chewing gum as an anti-smoking aid. Psychopharmacologia, 31: 191-200, 1973.

10. Jarvik, M.E. Further observations on nicotine as the reinforcing agent in smoking. In: Smoking Behavior: Motives and Incentives. Ed.: W.L. Dunn, Jr. Winston and Sons, Washington, D.C., pp.33-49, 1973.

11. Wynder, Ernst L., and Hoffmann, D. Tobacco and Tobacco Smoke. Studies on Experimental Carcinogenesis. Academic Press, New York, p.730, 1967.

12. Wynder, Ernst L. and Gori, G.B. The Current Reduction in Lung Cancer Incidence, in preparation.

13. Wald, Nicholas J. Mortality from lung cancer and coronary heart disease in relation to changes in smoking habits. The Lancet, Jan. 17, 136-138, 1976.

EDUCATIONAL REQUIREMENTS FOR SMOKING AND HEALTH PROGRAMS
THE INTERAGENCY CONCEPT AT NATIONAL, PROVINCIAL AND COMMUNITY LEVELS

Norman C. Delarue
Professor of Surgery
Faculty of Medicine
University of Toronto

The fundamental need for enthusiastic and uncompromising interagency co-operation in all Smoking and Health programs has a very straightforward basis. Thus far we have failed to eradicate the smoking habit and must try to find out why this is so, in order to improve our performance.

In doing this, we must first make certain that we do not forget certain fundamental observations.

CORE ISSUES

In fact, there are only 4 truly core issues.

A. In the first place, at the central core of the problem is the realization that there are only 2 reasons why people do anything.

1. They are forced to do it, - e.g. they have no choice.

2. They want to do it, - e.g. a personal choice is possible.

B. It is with this second reason that we must deal effectively. To be specific there are 3 basic "wants".

1. Personal gratification - e.g. enjoyment of pleasurable experiences.

2. Anticipation of reward.
    This "want" is related to the need for personal security whether
    it be on the emotional or physical plane. There is an ever
    present desire for acceptance and a need to allay anxiety
    concerning future events.

3. The option to pursue "easy" behaviour
    This involves the opportunity to choose the easy way when other
    alternatives are less desirable. Relatively few seek the
    "high road".

Since we must answer these "wants" if we are to secure the attention of continuing smokers we must stress the enjoyable characteristics of the

course we wish people to pursue by indicating the rewards to be anticipated. These may relate to the physical sense of well being, personal
pride in an exemplary leadership role, or self-approbation following rec-
ognised success in any of these areas.

Unfortunately, fear of punishment rarely has an immediate or personal
an impact as have these rewards. Consequently, we should have anticipated the fact that the dreary repetitive recitation of risk alone would
not prove to be as successful as we had hoped.

The "easy" way is made still more attractive when socially acceptable behaviour (as exemplified by the cigarette smoking habit) diverts
people into the acceptable pathway and discourages them from doing what
they know they ought to do to protect their own health.

The fact that smokers now realize the magnitude of the risk of their
habit underscores a conflict we have ourselves forced on the public. The
awareness on the part of smokers that they should not smoke and the realization that they may be unable to give up their habit leads to confusion
and irrational responses which are marked by resentment if they consider
any advice they may be given to represent a direct attack on their personal habit.

C. A Third concept must also be emphasized. Unfortunately, our failure to recognize its importance explains much of our current problem. In
stubborn fashion we have not realized that giving up cigarettes and
consolidating the new non-smoking habit are two completely different matters.

There is abundant evidence that this is true in the reports of the
number of people who have given up at sometime or another only to resume
the habit subsequently. The very high recidivism rate should have al-
armed us long ago.

In dealing with the two very different problems of quitting and
recidivism two different approaches are required.

    1. In providing the motivation to quit "loading dose" therapy is
       appropriate.

    2. In providing the motivation for abstinence a "maintenance"
       program is the only one likely to be successful.

The first objective can be pursued in public, whereas the second
requires more private interaction and is much more difficult to imple-
ment because of the individualization which is required.

Educational efforts have been reasonably successful in the first instance. However, appreciation of risk and dread of disease and death, which are powerful incentives for quitting, are quite impotent in guaranteeing lasting abstinence. This reflects the fact that, for many, the motivation to take another cigarette remains in the long run stronger than the motivation to quit. Indeed, in the smokers who want to quit but don't know how to go about it successfully, a sense of defeatism adds to their frustration and tends to strengthen or buttress their habit.

The motivation to maintain abstinence must, therefore, be continually reinforced. Smokers need this type of support particularly in the privacy of their own world, whether it be in their interpersonal interactions within the community, or amongst their family and friends. This private world can be entered effectively only in highly individualized fashion.

Individualization of this type necessitates an exploration of other "values" which can be used to support the personal resolve. These values, which determine personal interactions, revolve primarily around social needs, such as the herd instinct, family concern, the desire to be liked, admired, or respected, interest in personal appearance, personal beliefs, and active involvement in other interests, such as hobbies and recreational sports activities.

In pursuing these values it is wise to use an oblique rather than a direct approach so that the messages will not be perceived as deliberately educational or forcefully persuasive.

D.   The final concept to be considered as a core issue is the appreciation of the fact that there are 2 broad groups of smokers to be "reached".

1.   Those who are influenced by education alone

2.   Those who remain unaffected by information transfer

The first group represents those who have responded to previous educational efforts. Millions have stopped smoking. Millions have been persuaded not be begin smoking. A significant reduction in tar and nicotine content of cigarettes has also been achieved. Consequently, these established techniques warrant pursuit and information transfer must continue unabated.

However, up to the present time we have not affected those who require additional influences to supplement this type of traditional education. They are aware of the fact that they should stop smoking and

we must now explore the reasons why this "awareness" has not been reflected in positive action.

If we are to improve our position, since we have reached those
amenable to educational persuasion, we must develop new techniques by
which we can "reach" with equal effectiveness those who have as yet remained resistant to our attempts to have them give up their cigarettes.

EXPLANATION OF PAST FAILURE

It is in exploring the reasons why these smokers continue to smoke
when they know they ought to stop that we can build a basic understanding
of the requirements for effective new programs.

They continue smoking for a very simple reason — those influences
which favour persistence of the habit are more relevant for them than
those influences which have been used to discourage it. It is, therefore,
in this context in which we must now concentrate our efforts.

PRESCRIPTION FOR FUTURE SUCCESS

In the first place, in reviewing the fundamental principles which
will govern future actions, attention must be given to all the factors in
the determining facilitation-dissuasion "equation". (Fig. 1). The number
of permutations and combinations of these factors which determine individual smoking patterns are so complex that no single standardized approach can hope to be successful.

1. Facilitating Influences

All facilitating influences must be weakened or eliminated, if
possible. This primarily involves an attempt to change the aura of social
acceptability which is promoted by smoking exemplars and advertising influence.

2. Dissuasive Influences

All dissuasive influences must be strengthened. The risk factor is
a necessary basis for educational programs but it cannot be fruitfully
over-emphasized at the expense of careful attention also to other factors.

The social unacceptability of the habit can be discussed in the
context of the possible risks smoking in enclosed environments poses for
others - and specifically for non-smokers.

The protection required for non-smokers must not encourage their
segregation. They remain in the majority and since they harm no one
there is no need to segregate them. It is the smoker whose habit has the
potential for harming others and who must be segregated. Once segre-

gation is achieved of course it becomes immediately obvious to all that smoking itself can no longer be considered a totally acceptable social habit.

Smoking Withdrawal Assistance Programs must be provided for those who wish help in giving up the cigarette habit. One must not underestimate the effectiveness of these programs since they allow the necessary individualization in approaching smokers whose habits are so very personal.

Large clinics have to be subdivided into small groups since, otherwise, individualization is quite impossible. A large clinic is in essence merely an extension of traditional educational effort and will consequently affect only those already convinced and committed - although admittedly helpful for smokers of this type.

It is important to realize that the success rate for the participants in these programs is a very superficial way of judging their effectiveness in view of the ripples of exemplary influence each successful ex-smoker will take back to the community in which he lives and works. In the process the social acceptability of the non-smoking habit is immeasurably strengthened.

3. Simultaneous Programs of Dissuasion and Elimination of Facilitating Influences

Since a single standardized program is not feasible, all these avenues must be pursued concurrently. Consequently, the entire program becomes too massive an exercise for any single agency to manage, in view of the limited funds available and the limited resource of personnel. A successful approach can only be mounted within an interagency concept.

Some programs are easy and individual agencies may well feel that they can manage them within their own resources with the result that they are comfortable and confident in these programs. However, some programs are much more difficult and expensive and as a result no single agency will attempt to pursue them because their resources are quite inadequate. It is in these areas that pooling of resources is essential so that all necessary programs can be undertaken.

4. Behavioural Approach

It is quite clear now that the problem is primarily a behavioural one, and one which must be approached in the areas of social acceptability. Essentially the conflict lies in the sphere of apposing social influences which determine personal and community behavioural norms.

In this context traditional education alone is no longer adequate, since the objective of creating a fund of knowledge by the passive transfer of information in the expectation that the recipient will then act intelligently on the basis of this knowledge is quite ineffective when behavioural considerations are at stake. Attention must be paid to the entire knowledge-attitude-behaviour triad if success is to be achieved. (Fig. 2). Particular emphasis must be placed on the catalysts required at each stage in the progression through this triad of behavioural change. In order to have knowledge reflected in a change in attitude the information - which created the knowledge must be relevant to the recipient. In order to ensure that the changing attitude is reflected in changing behaviour the attitude must be reinforced by exemplary exposure to acceptable individual and group social customs.

Since we are now becoming involved in matters of social acceptability it is impossible to impose opinions on those we are trying to influence. There are certain "needs" that can be identified if we are to ensure uninterrupted progression through the knowledge-attitude-behaviour sequence. The number and magnitude of the required programs clearly emphasizes the rationale for interagency cooperation.

GENERAL PROPOSALS

Before proceeding to design specific programs it is important to identify the general principles underlying the various program needs.

1. The need for coordination of activities

     To avert public confusion due to multiple programs.

     To avoid unecessary duplication

     To minimize wastage of resources

          a) personnel
          b) financial support

     To eliminate non-productive programs

2. The imperative of total coverage

     a) All factors in the decision to smoke or abstain demand attention.

               Smoking is a unique personal experience

               The habit is determined by the facilitation-dissuasion equation

               The smoker will not be affected by incomplete or isolated programs

b) Total coverage determines the requirements for interagency action

    Programs designed to weaken all facilitating influences

    Programs designed to strengthen all dissuasive influences

    Simultaneous implementation of both types of programs

3. The new educational prerogative

Current programs must be based on the realization that knowledge is no longer the educational end point.

    The new educational objective becomes one of behavioural modification

    This requires emphasis on the catalysts required for progression along the knowledge-attitude-behaviour sequence

        a) provision of relevant information for target groups

        b) continuous reinforcements of changing attitude

SPECIFIC PROGRAM PROPOSALS

One can now proceed from these general principles to the specific program proposals which must represent the basis for interagency cooperation in coordinated activities.

A.   Programs Designed to Strengthen Dissuasive Influences

1. Provision of relevant information for selected target groups
(relevance represents the catalyst for the knowledge-attitude transformation)

    a) disadvantages of smoking — children
       (or advantages of non-smoking)

    b) risks of smoking — adults

    c) expansion of exemplary influence — exemplars of note

2.   Reinforcement Techniques
(the catalyst for attitude-behaviour transformation)

    a) continuing reiteration of relevant information

    b) development of non-smoking behavioural norm

    c) provision of smoking areas

       buses, trains, planes

       restaurants, theatres, meeting places

       offices, factories, retail outlets

3.   Programs for Smokers who Wish Help in Giving Up their Smoking Habit

    a) Smoking Withdrawal Centres — personalized assistance

    b) Kits for personal use — individualized information

B. __Programs Designed to __**Minimize**__ Facilitating Influences__

    1. Lobbying for legislative ban on advertising and promotion

        a) prelegislative influence at the community level

        b) legislative lobby at Provincial and Federal levels

It should be emphasized that the voluntary guidelines undertaken by the industry represent merely subterfuges designed to divert direct governmental intervention.

For example, recent British proposals forbid sexual inferences, signals of masculinity, personal testimonials, youth involvement, or any impression that smoke may be clean and pure.

However, these proposals have no effect on sports sponsorship, coupon schemes, cigar advertising, or other indirect promotions. The incomplete restrictions cannot be expected to prove effective.

    2. __Counter-Advertising Programs__

        a) Programs to stress the social acceptability (advantages)

            of non-smoking

        b) Programs to emphasize the social unacceptability of smoking

            in enclosed spaces (risk to others)

Some of these programs are best implemented at the National level and some at the Community level.

C. __National Programs__

    L - Legislative Lobby

        Control of product advertising and promotion

    I - Information Resource Facility

    F - Financial Distribution Centre

        multi-agency funding for major programs

    T - Technical Support

        cadre of professional specialists

        (advice in research or community activities)

D. __Community Programs__

    1. Prelegislative Lobby

        Prior commitment of elected representatives

    2. Programs designed to expand exemplary influence

        Exemplars of note - personal

                     - institutional

3. Programs designed to enlarge non-smoking behavioural influences

        Establishment of smoking areas

        Involvement of community business interests

4. "SWAP" Programs

        For smokers who seek help in withdrawal.

IMPLEMENTATION

A brief word of warning is in order at this point. Careful thought is required in implementing these programs since any superficial approach will do more harm than good. The health orientated professions have long worked effectively within the traditional educational framework but have little experience in behavioural techniques. Consequently, if these new programs are to affect the smokers who have not been influenced by previous educational efforts, assistance must be sought from the behavioural scientists in designing programs which will deal effectively with this particular problem.

Separate committees will be required for each new program and, despite the almost inexhaustible resource of volunteer energy, committee members must be chosen who are not only dedicated but also knowledgeable and open minded. Enthusisastic support can be anticipated from all professional voluntary agencies since the breadth and scope of the entire program is designed to take advantage of the very special capabilities each agency will bring to the overall program. Agency involvement will, therefore, be recognized without loss of individual agency reputation.

The end result for each program must be appropriate. Care must be taken that the clientele are not "turned-off" or led into other equally unattractive outlets for their frustrations.

Provided care is taken to work within the bounds of the knowledge-attitude-behaviour sequence and emphasis is placed on the required catalysts of relevance and reinforcement it should be possible to accomplish our aims without running these risks.

One can put the knowledge-attitude-behaviour triad in a somewhat different light, if one considers use of the appropriate catalysts to ensure progression through the triad by providing persuasion for the following purposes:

1. Stimulation of interest — by the provision of relevant information
2. The birth of understanding — when relevant information is considered important

3. Encouragement of "involvement" - when the concept of "importance" warrants personal action.

When viewed in this fashion the sequence stresses the importance of communication because persusasion results primarily from a combination of what one sees, hears, or reads - particularly if all one's senses are bombarded simultaneously by influence having the same impact.

In enlisting the cooperation of health professionals acknowledgement can be freely expressed for the experience and judgement which they can bring to programs of this type. These elements of experience and judgement have been fashioned in the fiery crucible of practical involvement and become available with a resource of volunteer personnel which is unmatched in any other field. If interagency cooperation can coordinate all activities in the smoking and health arena the potential dividends to be anticipated with successful pursuit of these further objectives should be motivation for all to join in this great and challenging adventure.

BASIS FOR "ANTI-SMOKING" CAMPAIGNS
THE "FACILITATION-DISSUASION EQUATION"

FACILITATING INFLUENCES   VS   DISSUASIVE INFLUENCES

THE SOCIAL ENVIRONMENT   THE RISK FACTOR

    Social Acceptability   Public Education
    Smoking Exemplars   Governmental Intervention
    Advertising Impact

THE SMOKING ENVIRONMENT   EXEMPLAR INFLUENCE

    Pleasurable Experience   Non-Smoking Exemplars
    Relief From Tension   (Interpersonal Interaction)
    Habituation   Social Unacceptability
    Dependence   Institutional Example

                              GROUP SUPPORT

                               ANTI-SMOKING CLINICS

FIG. 1

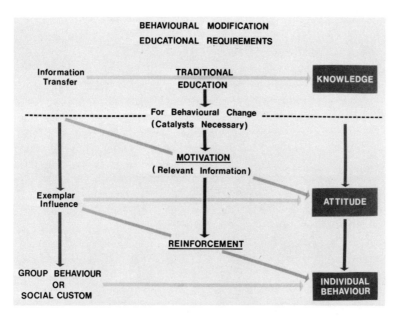

FIG. 2

775

BENEFITS OF STOPPING SMOKING

Lawrence Garfinkel, M.A.

Department of Epidemiology and Statistics
American Cancer Society, Inc.
New York, New York

It is by now well known that cigarette smoking increases the death rate
for coronary heart disease, lung cancer, emphysema and a number of other
diseases, and that the risk increases in proportion to the number of
cigarettes smoked per day. What may perhaps be less well-known are the
benefits of stopping smoking. Stopping cigarette smoking has short term
benefits to many smokers such as an increased taste for food; decreased
coughing, fewer colds, etc. This paper is concerned with the long-range
benefits of stopping; the epidemiologic studies which show the effects
of stopping on the mortality rate and the pathologic studies demonstrating
the effects of stopping cigarette smoking on human tissues.

A number of epidemiologic studies have shown the benefits of stopping. In
Doll and Hill's study of physicians, the death rate from coronary artery
disease for ex-cigarette smokers was 18% less than in physicians who
continued to smoke than in current smokers.

In the Dorn study of smoking and mortality in veterans, ex-smokers, who
stopped for reasons other than doctor's orders, died from coronary heart
disease at a rate 25% less than current smokers.

In the American Cancer Society's prospective study the coronary heart
disease death rate of all ex-cigarette smokers was 39% lower than current
smokers for those who smoked less than 1 pack a day. In those who smoked
1 pack or more a day, the death rate for all ex-cigarette smokers was 50%
less. Furthermore, the death rate decreased according to the number of
years since last smoked. For those who smoked 1 pack or more a day, it
was 37% less for those who gave up smoking less than 1 year; 41% less
in those who gave up smoking 1-4 years; 55% less in those who stopped
5-9 years before the study started; 51% less in those who stopped 10-19
years; and 59% less in those who stopped 20 years.

Ex-cigarette smokers also had lower lung cancer mortality rates than
those who continued to smoke. In the Doll and Hill study, the death
rate from lung cancer was 73% less in ex-smokers than in continuing
smokers. In the Dorn study the death rate was 57% less than for
continuing smokers.

Death rates from lung cancer for ex-smokers in the Doll and Hill study decreased with the length of time they had stopped smoking. It was down 62% for those who quit between one and five years, and 85% for those who quit 20 or more years.

In the American Cancer Society study current cigarette smokers who had smoked less than 1 pack a day had a mortality ratio 7.5 times as high as those who never smoked. Ex-cigarette smokers who formerly had smoked less than 1 pack and had stopped less than 1 year had a rate 7.13 as high as for men who never smoked. It was 3.31 times higher for those who stopped 1-4 years; 1.25 for 5-9 years; and 0.43 for those who stopped 10+ years.

The lung cancer mortality ratio for the 1 pack or more a day smokers was 16.94. It was higher for the ex-cigarette smokers who stopped less than 1 year (17.69); and dropped steadily according to the length of time they had given up smoking. There are 2 major reasons for this higher rate. One reason is that the group who quit smoking less than 1 year before the start of the study is more heavily weighted by those who gave up smoking because of illness than ex-smokers who gave up smoking more than one year.

Another reason for the high death rate in ex-cigarette smokers who recently gave up smoking is that more of them returned to smoking than ex-smokers who had given up smoking more than 1 year before the start of the study. Ex-smokers as classified at any point in time are a heterogenous group containing some who gave up smoking many years ago; some who gave up smoking temporarily and who returned to smoking, and others who gave up smoking because of illness. In the ACS study, 37% of the men who said that they had given up smoking less than 1 year before the study started were smoking cigarettes again 2 years later. Eleven percent who had stopped 1-4 years had resumed smoking; 4% who had stopped 5-9 years resumed smoking; and only 2% who had stopped 10+ years resumed smoking 2 years after the start of the study.

In the ACS study the subjects who smoked 20+ cigarettes a day were classified by whether or not they were in "ill-health" at the start of the study (defined as those who replied that they were "sick at present", or gave a history of heart disease, stroke, high blood pressure, cancer of the lung, buccal cavity, pharynx, larynx or esophagus). They were further classified into 6 sub-groups: never smoked, current smokers; and ex-cigarette smokers classified into 4 groups by time since they had given up smoking.

The "ill-health" group had death rates 2 to 3 times higher than those not in ill-health. In the "ill-health" group, the death rate for the ex-cigarette smokers who had stopped less than 1 year was 9% higher than the death rate for the current smokers. In the "not in ill-health" group, the death rate for the ex-cigarette smokers who stopped less than 1 year was 10% lower than those who continued to smoke. Mortality ratios in the "not in ill-health" group dropped much more rapidly by length of time stopped. Those who had stopped 10 or more years had a death rate only 11% higher than the comparable group who had never smoked.

Another type of evidence of the effect of smoking cessation comes from an autopsy study of bronchial epithelium by Auerbach et al. In a double-blind study, the tracheo-bronchial trees of 72 cigarette smokers were matched for age, residence and occupation (white-collar or blue-collar) with 72 ex-cigarette smokers who formerly smoked the same number of cigarettes per day, and 72 non-smokers. The ex-cigarette smokers were defined as subjects who had smoked for at least 10 years, were primarily cigarette smokers and had given up cigarettes at least 5 years before death. The 216 men were included in a study of 758 persons in which a number of groups who had not died of lung cancer, (urban vs rural, men vs women, young vs old, cigarette smokers vs pipe and cigaresmokers) were being compared for changes in the epithelial lining of the tracheo-bronchial tree.

Fifty-five sections were taken from the tracheo-bronchial tree of each case according to a standard protocol, put in random order, and given a serial number while in that order. For each slide the presence of normal epithelium and pathologic changes such as basal cell hyperplasia, metaplasia, and carcinoma-in-situ were recorded, coded and transfered to punch cards for analysis.

Basal cell hyperplasia was found in 97.8% of slides in smokers; in 57.3% of slides of ex-smokers, and in 12.1% of slides of non-smokers.

Nuclei with atypical cells present in the bronchial epithelium (begining metaplasia) were found in 93% of sections from cigarette smokers; only 6% in ex-cigarette smokers, and 1.2% in non-smokers.

Carcinoma-in-situ (cells that have the cytologic appearance of cancer but have not invaded) was found in 8.0% of the slides in "current" smokers, 0.2% in ex-smokers and 0% in non-smokers.

During the course of the study, a new type of cell was observed, one that had the appearance of a disintegrating cell with a halo around the nucleus. A total of 518 sections with this finding were recorded among the 40,000 slides that were included in this study. All were in ex-smokers. They were present in 15.1% of the 3,436 sections of ex-cigarette smokers. These findings were interpreted as evidence of a healing process in the bronchial epithelium.

Another study by Auerbach et al compared the degree of microscopic evidence of emphysema in autopsied cases in ex-cigarette smokers compared to "current"cigarette smokers and subjects who never smoked. Long-time ex-smokers had less emphysema than those who continued to smoke, but a greater amount of emphysema than non-smokers. There was not much difference in the average degree of emphysema between smokers and ex-smokers who gave up smoking less than 3 years. There was significantly more evidence of emphysema in those who continued cigarette smoking up to the time of death than in matched subjects who had quit 5 or more years before death. These results were interpreted as a halt in damage caused by cigarette smoking upon cessation, and while the damage does not undergo repair, it does not get progressively worse as it does in those who continue to smoke.

Thus there is ample evidence from epidemiologic and pathologic studies that upon cessation of cigarette smoking, the damage to bronchial epithelium and coronary arteries undergo some repair; and that the risk of dying from lung cancer and coronary heart disease decrease in proportion to the length of time stopped. There is a halt in damage in lung parenchyma upon cessation of smoking, but probably no repair of lung parenchymal tissue.

PREVENTION OF LUNG CANCER BY LIMITATION OF SMOKING

Lars M. Ramström

National Smoking and Health Association, NTS
Stockholm, Sweden

I. INTRODUCTION

Considering well-known data on the relation between smoking and lung cancer it can be assumed that lung cancer death rates should decrease in a population where a large proportion of the smokers have stopped smoking. The general validity of this assumption has also been verified e.g. by the study of Doll and Hill regarding the mortality of British doctors.[1]

The purpose of the current study is to predict Swedish lung cancer death rates for the years 1980 and 1990 under different conditions regarding future smoking exposure, thereby making it possible to estimate to what extent lung cancer in Sweden can be prevented by smoking control action. This is a further development of an earlier study regarding men only.[2] Now women are included also and an improved method is used for expressing the level of exposure to tobacco smoke.

Earlier predictions of cancer mortality have generally been based purely on observations of mortality rates from bygone years, the prediction being just an extrapolation of recent trends. Such a prediction cannot reflect eventual future changes of the conditions that determine mortality rates in years to come. In the special case of lung cancer the role of certain exogenous aetiological factors are better known than for perhaps any other cancer. Therefore, the idea of this study is to use such factors as the basis for relating predicted, future mortality rates to those currently observed.

The most important factors in the aetiology of lung cancer are: 1) smoking 2) certain agents in some occupational environments. Smoking is the major factor, while the occupationally induced cases represent a much smaller percentage.[3] Since this study aims at estimating orders of magnitude rather than performing high precision calculations, those cases are neglected that are related to other exogenous factors than smoking, i.e. the calculations are carried out as if smoking were the only exogenous factor involved in the aetiology of lung cancer. The acceptability of using this approximation has been supported by the results of an earlier study that was based on the same assumption.[4] In that study the male population of the urban areas of Sweden was compared to the males living in rural areas. These populations differ both in smoking habits and in lung cancer death rates. Calculations were made to determine what ratio between urban and

781

rural lung cancer death rates that should be expected with regard to the differences in smoking habits. This smoking-related ratio coincided rather exactly with the ratio between the death rates that had actually been observed.

II. PROCEDURES AND MATERIALS USED

Similarly to the above-cited study the current one makes comparisons between different populations. But this time the populations that are compared do not differ with respect to living area but with respect to time. For men and women separately each one of the Swedish 1980 population and the 1990 population is compared to the 1970 population. Different presumptions are made regarding the development of smoking exposure after 1970, and in each case expected lung cancer death rates for the populations of 1980 and 1990 are calculated.

In Sweden cohorts under the age of 55 have very small age-specific lung cancer death rates, and so, regardless of their smoking habits, they contribute very little to the lung cancer death rate of the total population.[5] Therefore, the smoking habit characteristics of the 1970, the 1980 and the 1990 populations have in each case been defined as those of the cohorts 55 years and older in the year in question.

There have been studies on smoking habits in Sweden showing that there are wide differences between the smoking habits of men and women (except in cohorts born after 1950) and that among both men and women there are substantial differences between older and younger cohorts with respect to the following variables:[6,7]

   1) Percentage of smokers
   2) Average daily consumption per smoker
   3) Ordinary smoking methods (depth of inhalation etc)

In each one of these variables there is a continuous shift towards heavier exposure when we go from older to younger cohorts. This pattern applies to both sexes.

The first two variables obviously can constitute separate parameters in the calculations. Variable number 3 will be represented by another parameter so as it will be described later.

There are several epidemiological studies indicating a linear relationship between daily cigarette consumption and lung cancer death rate i.e.

$$R_N = k \cdot N \cdot R_0 \qquad (1)$$

where R_N = Lung cancer death rate of a population of smokers

   N = Daily consumption per smoker

   R_0 = Lung cancer death rate of a population of non-smokers

   k = Intensity factor

From a purely mathematical view-point the factor k is just a formula constant. In this specific connection, however, it should be interpreted as
an expression of both the general strength of the relationship, which is a
disease-related property, and such population-related properties that are
components of the above-mentioned smoking method variable. Since, in this
study, we are constantly considering the same disease, the factor k will
vary only as smoking methods vary between different populations. The factor k will be called "Intensity factor" and it will serve as a separate
.parameter in the calculations.

When determining numerical values of the intensity factor it has been
possible to use results of a 10-year (1963 - 1972) follow-up study of a
representative sample of the Swedish population.[8] These results include
lung cancer death rates registered separately for men and women, smokers
and non-smokers. Looking at males smoking cigarettes only the follow-up
study reports the relation $R_N = 7.0 \cdot R_0$. The average consumption level of
these men is 10 cigarettes per day. These data give us a value of k =
0.70, which is attributed to the male 1970 population. The k-values of the
female 1970 population and the other populations, have been estimated by
comparing data on inhalation habits of the different populations to the
corresponding data for the male 1970 population. According to data from
one large survey of Swedish smoking habits there is a 40 % prevalence of
deep inhalation among smokers in the male 1970 population.[6] The prevalence
figures for deep inhalation in the male 1980 and 1990 populations can be
estimated to 50 % resp. 60 %. Corresponding k-values have been determined
to be 0.85 resp. 1.0 presupposing that there should be approximately the
same ratios between the k-values as between the inhalation percentages.
For the female 1970, 1980 and 1990 populations the prevalence of deep inhalation among the smokers is 20 %, 30 % resp. 40 % and the corresponding
k-values have been determined to be 0.30, 0.50 resp. 0.70.

Another pertinent question is the role of pipe and cigar smoking. We know
that these conditions differ from country to country. The above-mentioned
follow-up study also permits an evaluation of the specifically Swedish
conditions in this respect. It indicates that pipe and cigar smoking in
Sweden has an equal effect on lung cancer death rates as smoking the same
amount of tobacco as cigarettes. Therefore, the daily consumption parameter, N, has been finally defined as the total number of grams of tobacco
smoked daily per smoker. Correspondingly the prevalence of smoking has
been defined as the percentage, P, of daily smokers of cigarettes or pipe
or cigars or any combination thereof.

Assuming the validity of formula (1) and applying the specific definitions
mentioned above, the lung cancer death rate of a population as a whole can
be expressed by the following formula:

$$R = R_0 (1 - 0.01 \cdot P + 0.01 \cdot k \cdot P \cdot N) \tag{2}$$

where R = Lung cancer death rate of the actual population as a whole

R_0 = Lung cancer death rate in a population of non-smokers

P = Percentage of smokers in the population

k = Intensity factor

N = Daily consumption per smoker

Formula (2) can easily be transformed in the following way:

$$\frac{R}{R_0} = C = 1 - 0.01 \cdot P + 0.01 \cdot k \cdot P \cdot N \qquad (3)$$

The ratio, C, will be called "Lung cancer mortality coefficient". It constitutes a specific measure of the smoking-related lung cancer mortality level of the population in question. Since this coefficient can be calculated for every one of the populations that are studied and the 1970 death rate is known, the death rate of any other population can be calculated. The size of the Swedish populations of 1980 and 1990 have been estimated.[9] By applying the expected death rates to estimated population sizes, expected number of lung cancer deaths can be calculated.

III. RESULTS

The calculations have been carried out in four alternatives representing different presumptions regarding future smoking-related characteristics. In all alternatives, however, the lung cancer death rate of non-smokers is presupposed to remain constant.

A. Alternative I

In this alternative it is presumed that no single individual will change his personal smoking habits and that there will be no change of average tar yield of the cigarettes. Both for males and females the 1980 and 1990 populations will differ from the 1970 population in cohort composition which means that there will be an increase in every one of the three basic parameters P, N, and k. Consequently, there will be a continuing increase in lung cancer deaths. Details will be found in table I.

B. Alternative II

In this alternative it is presumed that every second of those who were smokers in 1970 have stopped smoking in the first part of the 70´s, and, that in the first part of the 80´s, every second of those who are smokers in 1980, will stop. In the calculations these ex-smokers are taken together with non-smokers, since there are studies indicating that ex-smokers of less than 20 cigarettes per day, will approach the lung cancer mortality level of equal age non-smokers after 5 - 9 smoke-free years.[10] It is also presumed that those who continue to smoke have the same daily consumption and the same intensity factor as those who have stopped.

This alternative means a decrease in lung cancer mortality in men, while in women there is still an increase, but only a very slight one. Details will be found in table I.

C. Alternative III

In this alternative it is presumed, as in alternative I, that no single individual will change his personal smoking habits, but the average tar yield of cigarettes will decrease in the first decade after 1970 to 75 % and in the second decade to 50 % of its 1970 level. This presumption means that the daily consumption level, N, decreases in terms of the number of 1970-type cigarettes that should be consumed to give the actually presumed tar exposure. In women the final reduction of N is 25 % resp. 50 % because all the female consumption consists of cigarettes. In men the 25 % resp. 50 % reduction occurs only in that part of male consumption that consists of cigarettes (60 % in 1980 and 65 % in 1990).

This alternative means that, in both men and women lung cancer mortality will increase but the growth rate will be less than in alternative I. Details will be found in table I.

D. Alternative IV

In this alternative it is presumed that people stop smoking as in alternative II and that average tar yields of cigarettes goes down as in alternative III.

This alternative means that in men the mortality goes down faster than in any other alternative. In women there is still a slight increase up till 1980 but then we find, at last, a downward trend in women also. Details will be found in table I.

IV. DISCUSSION

Alternative I should be described as a prediction of an uninfluenced development from the 1970 situation which, in its turn, is characterized by lung cancer death rates that are intermediate for men and low for women. It seems that female lung cancer death rates have just recently begun to rise significantly above non-smokers level and the predicted increase between 1970 and 1980 is less than the predicted increase in males for the same period. During the following decade, however, the male lung cancer death rate will increase less than the female rate, which will increase more rapidly than during the decade before. This indicates, that if an uninfluenced development will go on up till 1990, we can expect male lung cancer rates by that time to begin approaching sort of a "saturation level" similarly to what has already been observed in some countries. Among women, on the other hand, we have to expect that an uninfluenced development will represent an increasingly steep rise in lung cancer mortality corresponding to the development among men several decades earlier. The whole of this pattern means, that in Sweden we have by now just reached an early stage of development in lung cancer mortality. But it also means, that we are in the process of approaching the situation of countries that do already carry a heavier burden of lung cancer deaths than Sweden does now.

Fortunately enough, there is some hope that the uninfluenced development will not become a reality. Alternative I therefore has its major significance as a frame of reference to which we can refer the other alternatives.

It is very difficult to assess what will be the most probable reduction of smoking habits or the most probable reduction of tar yield of cigarettes. Therefore it should be noted that alternatives II, III and IV have to be considered just as examples of calculation illustrating the order of magnitude of results that could be achieved if the presumptions in question became a reality.

When determining what reduction of smoking that should be presumed, the British doctors have served as a guideline. Since they, during a ten-year period, had managed to cut down the prevalence of smoking to about 50 % of its initial value, this seems to be a realistic reduction rate and that has been the reason for choosing the rather optimistic presumption that has been used in alternatives II and IV.

When determining what reduction of cigarette tar yield that should be presumed, the actual development up till now in some countries has served as a guideline. [11,12,13] These experiences indicate the possibility of achieving a 25 % reduction over a ten-year period and that's why this presumption has been used in alternatives III and IV. This should also be considered as an optimistic presumption, since there is a risk that part of the primary reduction will get lost because there is a possibility that a reduction of the tar and nicotine content of every single puff might influence smoking methods in a compensatory manner. [14]

From table I it can be derived how many lung cancer deaths that can be prevented in 1980 and 1990 if the presumptions of the alternatives II, III or IV would become a reality instead of the uninfluenced situation of alternative I. The approximate numbers of prevented deaths are given in the following summary.

	Men		Women	
	1980	1990	1980	1990
Alternative II	820	1740	90	310
Alternative III	260	800	60	250
Alternative IV	960	1940	130	370

If sufficiently powerful smoking control action is taken there might be both a reduced prevalence of smoking and a reduced tar yield of cigarettes as presumed in alternative IV. Then, in Sweden in 1980, we can prevent about 1,100 lung cancer deaths, i.e. about half the lung cancer mortality, that should be expected in an uninfluenced situation. Under the same conditions, it will be possible in Sweden in 1990 to prevent about 2,300 lung cancer deaths, i.e. about two thirds of the expected lung cancer mortality.

These calculations illustrate the obvious benefits in terms of lung cancer prevention that can be achieved by limitation of smoking supported by the development of less harmful cigarettes. They also illustrate, that smoking control efforts must be directed b o t h to adults and children. It is true that the long term solution of the public health problems related to smoking depends on the successfulness in preventing children from taking

up the smoking habit. But, as we see, that does not influence lung cancer
mortality until we reach the second or third decade of the next century.
If we want to reduce lung cancer mortality earlier than that, we have to
influence the smoking habits of today's adults also.

V. SUMMARY

The objective of this study is to predict Swedish lung cancer death rates
for the years 1980 and 1990 under different conditions regarding future
smoking habits and thereby to estimate to what extent lung cancer in
Sweden can be prevented by limitation of smoking. This is a further development of an earlier study regarding men only. Now women are included
also and an improved method is used for expressing the level of exposure
to tobacco smoke for different kinds of smokers.

Knowing the current smoking habits among both males and females in different cohorts of the Swedish population, models of the Swedish population
at 1980 and 1990 with regard to probable smoking habits have been constructed. Each one of these population models is then compared to the
actual 1970 population by applying a formula expressing the relative lung
cancer risk of a population with regard to its smoking habits. The comparison gives numerical relations to the known 1970 lung cancer death rates
and so rates for 1980 and 1990 can be calculated. This is done for several
alternative cases where different presumptions are made regarding the development of smoking habits and the development of average tar yield of
cigarettes.

The results indicate that, in the absence of changes in individual smoking
habits or average tar yield, the lung cancer death rates will rise substantially during the two decades that are studied, even more rapidly for
women than for men. Comparisons between different alternatives indicate,
that, in 1990, up to two thirds of the expected Swedish lung cancer mortality can be prevented by such limitation of smoking that seems to be quite
attainable if powerful smoking control action is carried through.

TABLE I. Definition of Variables (see text)

	Al-ter-nat.	Males			Females		
		1970	1980	1990	1970	1980	1990
Percentage	I	45.9	50.3	52.8	10.3	17.6	24.1
of smokers	II	45.9	25.2	13.2	10.3	8.8	6.0
in the	III	45.9	50.3	52.8	10.3	17.6	24.1
population	IV	45.9	25.2	13.2	10.3	8.8	6.0
Daily	I	11.2	12.8	14.0	8.5	8.8	9.0
consumption	II	11.2	12.8	14.0	8.5	8.8	9.0
per smoker	III	11.2	10.9	9.5	8.5	6.6	4.5
(g)	IV	11.2	10.9	9.5	8.5	6.6	4.5
Intensity factor	I-IV	0.70	0.85	1.00	0.30	0.50	0.70
Lung cancer	I	4.14	5.97	7.86	1.16	1.60	2.28
mortality	II	4.14	3.49	2.72	1.16	1.30	1.32
coefficient	III	4.14	5.16	5.49	1.16	1.40	1.52
	IV	4.14	3.08	2.12	1.16	1.20	1.13
Lung cancer	I	33.1	47.7	62.9	8.8	12.1	17.3
death rates	II	33.1	27.9	21.7	8.8	9.9	10.0
per 100 000	III	33.1	41.4	44.0	8.8	10.6	11.5
	IV	33.1	24.6	16.9	8.8	9.1	8.6
Size of pop. (millions)	I-IV	4.016	4.136	4.213	4.026	4.198	4.309
Number of	I	1,329	1,973	2,650	354	508	745
lung cancer	II	1,329	1,154	914	354	416	431
deaths	III	1,329	1,712	1,854	354	445	496
	IV	1,329	1,017	712	354	382	371

REFERENCES

1. Doll, R., and Hill, A.B. Mortality in Relation to Smoking: Ten Years' Observation of British Doctors. Brit. Med. J., 1:1399 and 1460, 1964.

2. Ramström, L.M. Prediction of Lung Cancer Incidence Rates in Sweden in Relation to Smoking Habits. XIth International Cancer Congress Abstracts, 4:763, 1974

3. Fraumeni, J.F. Chemicals in the Induction of Respiratory Tract Tumors. XIth International Cancer Congress Abstracts, 1:47, 1974

4. Ramström, L.M. The Urban/Rural Difference in Swedish Lung Cancer Rate in Relation to Differences in Smoking Habits. In: Abstracts of Papers: Second International Symposium on Cancer Detection and Prevention. Ed.: Cesare Maltoni et al. Excerpta Medica, Amsterdam, p. 111, 1973

5. Causes of Death 1969 and 1970 resp. 1971 (SOS). National Central Bureau of Statistics, Stockholm, 1972 resp. 1973

6. Smoking Habits in Sweden. Survey Research Center of the Central Bureau of Statistics, Stockholm, 1965

7. Jonsson, E., and Hibell, B. Undersökning av alkohol-, narkotika- och tobaksvanor i grundskolan och gymnasieskolan våren 1974. (Study of alcohol, drugs and tobacco habits in the comprehensive school and junior college in the spring of 1974.) Aktuellt från skolöverstyrelsen, 50:1-52, 1974/75

8. Cederlöf, R., Friberg, L., Hrubec, Z. and Lorich, U. The Relationship of Smoking and Some Social Covariables to Mortality and Cancer Morbidity. The Department of Environmental Hygiene, The Karolinska Institute, Stockholm, 1975

9. Statistical Abstracts of Sweden, 1974. National Central Bureau of Statistics, Stockholm

10. Hammond, E.C. Smoking in Relation to the Death Rates of 1 million Men and Women. In: Epidemiological Approaches to the Study of Cancer and Other Diseases. Ed.: W. Haenszel. U.S. Public Health Service, National Cancer Institute Monograph No. 19, Bethesda, pp. 127-204, 1966

11. Dontenwill, W. Search for a Less Hazardous Cigarette. In: Proceedings XI International Cancer Congress. Ed.: Pietro Bucalossi et al. Excerpta Medica, Amsterdam, 3:131-137, 1975

12. Gori, G.B. A Research Program to Decrease the Risk of Cancer and Other Diseases in the Tobacco Smoker. In: Proceedings XI International Cancer Congress. Ed.: Pietro Bucalossi et al. Excerpta Medica, Amsterdam, 3:151-156, 1975

13. Todd, G.F. Changes in Smoking Patterns in the U.K. In: Proceeding XI International Cancer Congress. Ed.: Pietro Bucalossi et al. Excerpta Medica, Amsterdam, 3:163-167, 1975

14. Turner, J.A.McM., Sillett, R.W., and Ball, K.P. Some Effects of Changing to Low-Tar and Low-Nicotine Cigarettes. Lancet, 2:737-738, 1974

LESS HAZARDOUS CIGARETTES

Gio B. Gori

Division of Cancer Cause and Prevention
National Cancer Institute
Bethesda, Maryland

I. INTRODUCTION

In the early 1960's, two reviews concluding that a relationship exists
between lung cancer and cigarette smoking were published independently
(1, 2). Since then several epidemiological studies have investigated
this relationship (3-14). The resulting evidence supports the earlier
reviews and indicates a dose-response relationship between inhalation
of cigarette smoke and the onset of lung carcinoma and cardio-pulmonary
diseases. Although educational programs have made this evidence available to the public, there has been no apparent decrease in cigarette
consumption. Publication of the Surgeon General's report and the banning
of cigarette advertising from television have had little impact on the
total number of cigarette smokers. In addition, although the tar and
nicotine levels of commercial cigarettes have been substantially reduced
during the past 20 years (1955 - 43 mg of tar, 2.8 mg of nicotine; 1975 -
18 mg of tar, 1.2 mg of nicotine), the average intake of cigarette smoke
per smoker has increased. The rate of increase for total number of
cigarettes sold appears to have stabilized over the last 13 years.
Number of cigarettes sold per smoker, however, is still rising.
Apparently the American public is resisting efforts to reduce cigarette
use.

Since the public persists in smoking cigarettes and other tobacco
products, the only course of action which remains is to develop a less
hazardous cigarette, which when smoked will not increase the risk of
smoking-related diseases. The Smoking and Health Program of the National
Cancer Institute has developed such a product. Today it is possible to

manufacture cigarettes significantly less hazardous than current commercial products. In their present state of development, these cigarettes
have one drawback - they are tasteless. To make them acceptable to a
cigarette user, flavor ingredients can be reintroduced to the tobacco
matrix. Substantial biological testing is necessary, however, to
establish the safety of these flavor additives before an acceptable
less hazardous cigarette can be released for general use.

Many areas of research were involved in the development of a less
hazardous smoking product. These include: 1) tobacco chemistry,
culture, and curing; 2) tobacco blending and processing; 3) epidemiology;
4) bioassay; 5) cigarette construction and physical characteristics of
burning cigarettes; and 6) organoleptic characteristics. Investigations
in these areas have been supported by the Smoking and Health Program of
the National Cancer Institute. This paper presents a summary of the
developments that have led to an acceptable less hazardous cigarette.

II. DEVELOPMENTS IN SMOKING AND HEALTH RESEARCH

A. Tobacco Chemistry, Culture, and Curing

Extensive chemical analysis has enabled identification of 1500 tobacco
constituents, only a few of which have been linked conclusively with
specific diseases. For example, several components of tar have been
shown to promote tumors (15-17) and adversely affect lung clearance
mechanisms (18-20). Development of cardiovascular diseases appears
to be enhanced by carbon monoxide and nicotine levels in inhaled
smoke (21-30). In addition, hydrogen cyanide, nitrogen oxides, phenols
and aldehydes, all constituents of tobacco, have been identified as
biologically toxic elements (21, 31-39).

New variants of tobacco, which yield leaf with reduced levels of tar,
nicotine and carcinogenic constituents and increased nitrate concentrations, have been developed by utilizing agronomic and genetic methods.
Smoke from burning these variants is less toxic than smoke from other
tobaccos (40-42). For example, Burley tobacco has a higher nitrate
content (precursor for compounds that inhibit pyrosynthesis of aromatic
hydrocarbons), lower amounts of nicotine, and a characteristically
higher burning rate, resulting in significantly lower biological

activity than Bright tobacco (33, 43-45). In addition, it has been
found that the position of the tobacco leaf on the stalk also determines
the concentration of toxic elements (45). Generally speaking, leaves
taken from higher positions on the plant stalk contain greater amounts
of harmful elements.

New techniques of tobacco curing and cultivation have also made possible
the production of tobacco with reduced concentrations of the precursors
for toxic pyrolytic products (46-48). Manipulation of the nitrogen
content in fertilizers is an example of such techniques (49). Cigarette
smoke condensate from tobacco grown with low-nitrogen fertilizer is less
biologically toxic than condensate from tobacco grown with high-nitrogen
fertilizers. Other examples of curing and cultivation techniques include
close cropping or high-density planting, whole-crop harvesting, and
freeze drying or extraction followed by fermentation. Utilization of
these techniques in combination with selective plant breeding has
produced tobacco low in known hazardous constituents.

B. Tobacco Blending and Processing

A significant and obvious method of reducing the biological hazards of
cigarettes is to remove a large portion of the tobacco. Although the
number of cigarettes smoked per person is still increasing, the number
of pounds of cigarette tobacco smoked per person is decreasing. Since
it has been shown that tobacco "tar" contains most of the hazardous
components in a cigarette, it is reasonable to expect that a reduction
in the amount of tobacco per cigarette will decrease toxicity.

Several processing techniques are available to reduce the tobacco content
of a cigarette. One method is to expand the leaf to half its normal
specific density (49-51). This does not reduce the concentrations of
the constituents of the whole tobacco, but it does decrease the smoke
concentration yield per cigarette. Extraction techniques using organic
solvents have been very successful in reducing tobacco toxicity. These
techniques decrease the wax layer of the leaf, which results in a reduction of the tumorigenic potential of the cigarette smoke (43, 44, 52, 53).
Use of reconstituted tobacco sheet is another promising technique. This
process utilizes "leftover" plant parts (i.e., stems, ribs, etc.) to
produce sheets of tobacco "paper" (54). These sheets are then shredded
and mixed with tobacco leaf. Since only the tobacco leaf has appreciable

levels of tar and nicotine, cigarettes produced in this manner have lower concentrations of these components (52, 55). In addition, the tobacco content of cigarettes can be reduced further by extension or dilution of the tobacco with inorganic fillers, artificial cellulose, humectants, and binders (50, 56). Tobacco reduction by these techniques can be so extensive that the resulting cigarette emits essentially hot air.

The Smoking and Health Program of the National Cancer Institute is producing several series of experimental cigarettes utilizing the above techniques for reducing tobacco content. As shown in Table I, the Institute has been very successful in producing a tobacco cigarette, Series IV, that is extremely low in tar (2.71 mg/cigarette). Series V represents a "chemical" cigarette containing no tobacco and, therefore, no tar. It is expected that the bioassay results of Series IV and V will indicate virtually no hazardous activity (i.e., no tumorigenesis, no cardio-pulmonary disease development, etc.). Data generated by testing these experimental cigarettes have been essential in producing a less hazardous smoking products.

C. Epidemiology

Continuing epidemiological and other studies involving human smokers have contributed information on inhalation patterns, smoking behavior changes, and type of cigarettes smoked and their relationship to carcinomas and other smoking-related diseases. Multifactorial analysis of available data indicates that the existence of a lower threshold for increased health risk is a function of the tar yield per cigarette, the frequency of puffs per cigarette, and the duration of the smoking habit (57, 58). Additional data indicate reduced risks to respiratory carcinomas when filter cigarettes are smoked in place of nonfilter cigarettes (14). This evidence suggests that a low level of smoking could be tolerated, given a sufficiently mild exposure to tobacco smoke constituents. Furthermore, prospective and retrospective studies provide data on the relative risks associated with use of modified cigarettes. Such data are necessary for developing safer cigarettes.

Studies on smoking patterns have provided information on the importance of nicotine in cigarette smoking. This substance appears to play a role in the depth and frequency of smoke inhalation as well as in the flavor and acceptability of cigarettes. When given cigarettes low in nicotine, humans smoke more cigarettes, take deeper and more frequent puffs, and rate the taste as less acceptable than when smoking cigarettes with high nicotine concentrations (59, 60). Such factors must be carefully considered when designing a less hazardous smoking product.

D. Bioassay Data

Bioassay techniques have been extremely useful in appraising candidate less hazardous cigarettes. The National Cancer Institute has sponsored several bioassay programs to evaluate their series of experimental cigarettes. The results of one of these programs are presented in Table II. Mouse dermal bioassay techniques were utilized to determine the probability of hazardous effects associated with the application of cigarette smoke condensate, and the index of tumorigenicity was based on the probability of skin tumor development. For the series of experimental cigarettes tested, on a gram per gram basis, a progressive reduction in biological activity of cigarette smoke condensate was found. Combining these results with those presented in Table I, it becomes increasingly clear that, as tar per cigarette is reduced, specific biological activity associated with the tar is also reduced.

In addition to testing whole smoke condensate, much useful information has been obtained from bioassays of individual smoke components and fractions (15-39). This information has led to the identification of smoke components as promoters and initiators. Knowledge of the interaction of these individual constituents has enabled the design of cigarettes with reduced biological activity.

E. Cigarette Construction

In designing less hazardous cigarettes, the physical characteristics of a cigarette are as important as the chemical constituents. Cigarette configuration and burning properties contribute to the pyrolytic formation of some hazardous components. Increasing air permeability dilutes the smoke and therefore reduces the inhaled concentration of several harmful smoke components (45). Smoke dilution is the only way to reduce CO levels, and this can be done by using perforated or high-porosity paper and/or aerated filter tips (45, 51, 61, 62). High-porosity paper increases the burning rate of the cigarette, thus reducing the level of volatile components such as tar, nicotine, phenols, etc. (46, 61).

795

The increasing popularity of filter cigarettes is also significant in reducing the hazards of smoking. These filters remove volatile components and particulate matter from the smoke. Studies supported by the Smoking and Health Program have tested the bioassay activity of several filter materials (63). Cellulose acetate, the most common filter, provides mechanical filtration of phenols and particulate matter. Charcoal particles can be added to the cellulose to aid in the selective removal of gases and vapors. Permanganate filters can be used to reduce NO in the inhaled smoke, and magnesium silicate can be used to remove aldehydes and other organic vapors. These cigarette modifications can change the composition of or dilute the smoke, thereby reducing the inhaled concentrations of smoke constituents. Utilizing the above knowledge, the National Cancer Institute has been able to produce cigarettes that when burned emit essentially hot air. Although such cigarettes are nonhazardous, they are also tasteless and unacceptable to the smoking public.

F. Organoleptic Characteristics

The Smoking and Health Program has supported research to analyze commercially acceptable cigarettes organoleptically (64). These analyses have resulted in the identification of a set of dimensions describing the range of acceptable cigarettes. Definition of these dimensions is extremely important in the development of an acceptable less hazardous cigarette. As stated above, a nonhazardous cigarette can now be produced, but it is virtually tasteless and is unacceptable to cigarette users. The National Cancer Institute is continuing to support research aimed at devising techniques for restoring flavor to these cigarettes. Such techniques include using pure chemicals as flavor additives, reintroducing extracted tobacco flavor compounds to the cigarette matrix, and using substitutes for tobacco constituents that contribute to cigarette flavor (e.g., nicotine substitutes). Studies are presently being conducted to determine the role of nicotine and other smoke constituents in cigarette acceptance. The preliminary results indicate that there are several means of reintroducing organoleptic characteristics to a cigarette matrix. With careful selection of reintroduced flavors, an acceptable less hazardous cigarette is a viable alternative for those people who persist in smoking.

III.   CONCLUSION

Research in diverse areas of smoking and health has made possible the
construction of a minimum cigarette. The properties of this cigarette,
as determined from research supported by the Smoking and Health Program,
are presented in Table III. Included in this table are alternative
methods for achieving these specifications. These methods are the result
of 1) advances in tobacco culture and curing techniques, which produce
tobaccos with reduced carcinogen precursors; 2) new tobacco blending and
processing regimens, which lead to the manufacture of cigarettes with
minimum tar; 3) epidemiological findings, which indicate that some minimum
amount of smoking may be acceptable and may result in a lower threshold
for increased health risk; 4) bioassay evidence, which shows that smoke
condensate tumorigenicity can be reduced by at least 80%, even on a gram
per gram basis; 5) alternative cigarette construction methods, which alter
burning temperature, burning rate, and smoke dilution in ways that at
least partially control the delivery of CO, NO_x, and other offending
constituents of cigarette smoke; and 6) flavor and acceptability research,
which identifies dimensions of acceptability and suggests new techniques
for reintroducing organoleptic characteristics without reintroducing
toxicity.

Now that the technology for producing an acceptable less hazardous cigarette is available, a substantial reduction in the incidence of and
mortality from smoking-related diseases can be expected. This expectation
is supported by the reduction in the risk of lung cancer associated with
the long-term use of filter cigarettes. Therefore, an acceptable less
hazardous cigarette presents a viable alternative to those people to
persist in smoking.

TABLE I. Minimum Condensate Tar Yields in National Cancer Institute Experimental Cigarettes

Experimental Series	Tar (mg/cigarette)[b]
SEB[a] (control)	24.5
I	10.36
II	9.91
III	6.06
IV	2.71
V	0

[a]SEB = standard experimental blend. This blend is reconstituted annually to represent the average commercially available blend.

[b]Based on average yield per cigarette for the four cigarette codes with the lowest yield in each series.

TABLE II. Results of Mouse Skin Painting Bioassays

National Cancer Institute Experimental Cigarettes	Index of Tumorigenicity[b]
SEB[a] (control)	0.47
Series I	0.23
Series II	0.31
Series III	0.12

[a]SEB = standard experimental blend.

[b]Based on probability of tumor development for lowest third of activity in low-dose group for each series.

TABLE III. Properties of Candidate Less Hazardous Cigarettes and
Alternative Methods to Achieve These Specifications

Specification	Method
Reduced tar and nicotine content	Use of a large proportion of tobacco sheet in the blend
	Use of inert fillers as tobacco extenders
	Use of tobacco varieties produced by selected culture and curing methods
Reduced CO and NO_x in cigarette smoke	Use of high-porosity paper as wrappers
	Use of filters and selected "best choice" smoke dilution devices
Reduction or elimination of specific biologically active constituents of cigarette smoke	Use of tobacco varieties produced by selected culture and curing methods
	Use of filters and selected "best choice" smoke dilution devices
	Use of tobacco extracted with water, hexane, or detergent

REFERENCES

1. Royal College of Physicians. Smoking and Health. Pitman Medical Publishing Co., London, 1962.

2. U.S. Public Health Service. Smoking and Health. Publication No. 1103. United States Government Printing Office, Washington, 1964.

3. Fletcher, C. M. and Horn, D. Smoking and Health. W.H.O. Chron., 24: 345-370, 1970.

4. World Health Organization. Prevention of Cancer: Report of a WHO Committee. W.H.O. Tech. Rep. Ser., 276: 3-53, 1964.

5. Hammond, E. C. Smoking in Relation to the Death Rates of One Million Men and Women. Natl. Cancer Inst. Monogr., 19: 127, 1966.

6. Hammond, E. C. Smoking Habits and Air Pollution in Relation to Lung Cancer. In: Environmental Factors in Respiratory Disease. Ed.: H. K. Lee. Academic Press, Inc., New York, 1972.

7. Doll, R. Cancers Related to Smoking. In: Proceedings of the 2nd World Conference on Smoking and Health. Ed.: R. G. Richardson. Pitman Press, London, p. 754, 1972.

8. Doll, R. and Hill, A. B. Mortality in Relation to Smoking. Br. Med. J., 1: 1399-1410 (Part 1) and 1: 1460-1467 (Part 2), 1964.

9. Kahn, H. A. Natl. Cancer Inst. Monogr., 19: 1-125, 1966.

10. Weir, J. M. and Dunn, J. E., Jr. Cancer, 25: 105-112, 1970.

11. Auerbach, O., Stout, A. P., Hammond, E. C., et al. Changes in Bronchial Epithelium in Relation to Cigarette Smoking and In Relation to Lung Cancer. N. Engl. J. Med., 265: 253, 1961.

12. Schneiderman, M. A. and Leirn, D. L. Trends in Lung Cancer. Mortality, Incidence, Diagnosis, Treatment, Smoking and Urbanization. Cancer, 30: 1320, 1972.

13. Wynder, E. L., Covey, L. S., and Mabuchi, K. Lung Cancer in Women: Present and Future Trends. J. Natl. Cancer Inst., 51: 391, 1973.

14. Wynder, E. L., Mabuchi, K., and Beattie, E. J., Jr. The Epidemiology of Lung Cancer. Recent Trends. J. Am. Med. Assoc., 213: 2221, 1970.

15. Hecht, S. S., Bondinell, W. E., and Hoffmann, D. Chrysene and Methylchrysenes: Presence in Tobacco Smoke and Carcinogenicity. J. Natl. Cancer Inst., 53: 1121-1133, 1974.

16. Kobayashi, N., Hoffmann, D., and Wynder, E. L. A Study of Tobacco Carcinogenesis. XV. Tumor Promoting Activity of Cigarette Smoke in the Larynx of Syrian Hamsters. Submitted to J. Natl. Cancer Inst.

17. Liu, Y. Y., Schmeltz, I., and Hoffmann, D. Quantitative Analysis of Hydrazine in Tobacco and Cigarette Smoke. Anal. Chem., 46: 885-889, 1974.

18. Battista, S. P. Cilia Toxic Components. In: Proceedings of the 3rd World Conference on Smoking and Health, in press.

19. Battista, S. P. and Kensler, C. J. Mucus Production and Ciliary Transport Activity. In Vivo Studies Using the Chicken. Arch. Environ. Health, 20: 326, 1970.

20. Dahlhamn, T. Some Factors Influencing the Respiratory Toxicity of Cigarette Smoke. J. Natl. Cancer Inst., 48: 1821, 1972.

21. U.S. Public Health Service. Harmful Constituents of Cigarette Smoke. Publication No. (HSM) 72-7516. United States Government Printing Office, Washington, p. 137, 1972.

22. Rylander, R. Environmental Tobacco Smoke Effects on the Nonsmoker. Report from a Workshop. Scand. J. Respir. Dis. Suppl., 91, 1974.

23. Schmeltz, I., Hoffmann, D., and Wynder, E. L. The Influence of Tobacco on Indoor Atmospheres. I. An Overview. Prev. Med., 4: 66, 1975.

24. Wald, N., Howard, S., Smith, P. G., and Kjeldsen, K. Association Between Atherosclerotic Diseases and Carboxyhemoglobin Levels in Tobacco Smokers. Br. Med. J., 1: 761, 1973.

25. Aronow, S. S., et al. Effect of Cigarette Smoking and Breathing Carbon Monoxide on Cardiovascular Hemodynamics in Anginal Patients. Circulation, 50: 340, 1974.

26. Anderson, E. W., Andelman, R. J., Strauch, J. M., Fortuin, N. J., and Knelson, J. H. Effect of Low-Level Carbon Monoxide Exposure on Onset and Duration of Angina Pectoris. A Study of Ten Patients with Ischemic Heart Disease. Ann. Intern. Med., 79: 46, 1973.

27. Anderson, E. W., Strauch, J. M., Andelman, R. J., Fortuin, N. J., and Knelson, J. H. Effects of Low-Level Carbon Monoxide Exposure on Human Cardiac Function. V. Subjects with Angina Pectoris. Preliminary Paper - Environmental Protection Agency with the C. V. Richardson Laboratory, 1972.

28. Aronow, W. S. Cigarette Smoking, Carbon Monoxide, Nicotine, and Coronary Disease. Prev. Med., 4: 952, 1975.

29. Aronow, W. S., Dendinger, J., and Rokaw, S. N. Heart Rate and Carbon Monoxide Level After Smoking High-, Low-, and Non-nicotine Cigarettes. A Study in Male Patients with Angina Pectoris. Ann. Intern. Med., 74: 697, 1971.

30. Greenspan, K., Edmands, R. E., Knoebel, S. B., and Fisch, C. Some Effects of Nicotine on Cardiac Automaticity, Conduction, and Inotropy. Arch. Intern. Med., 123: 707, 1969.

31. Kensler, C. J. and Battista, S. P. Chemical and Physical Factors Affecting Mammalian Ciliary Transport. Am. Rev. Respir. Dis., 93: 93, 1966.

32. Kensler, C. J. and Battista, S. P. Components of Cigarette Smoke with Ciliary Depressant Activity and Their Selective Removal by Filters Containing Activated Charcoal Granules. N. Engl. J. Med., 269: 1161, 1963.

33. Wynder, E. L. and Hoffmann, D. Tobacco and Tobacco Smoke: Studies in Experimental Carcinogenesis. Academic Press, Inc., New York, 1967.

34. Auerbach, O., Hammond, E. C., Kirman, D., and Garfinkel, L. Emphysema Produced in Dogs by Cigarette Smoking. U.S.A.E.C. Symp. Ser., 18: 375, 1970.

35. Freeman, G., Crane, S. C., Furiosi, N. J., Stephens, R. J., Evans, M. J., and Moore, W. G. Covert Reduction in Ventilatory Surface in Rats During Prolonged Exposure to Subacute Nitrogen Dioxide. Am. Rev. Respir. Dis., 106: 563, 1972.

36. Hecht, S. S. and Wynder, E. L. On the Identification of Carcinogens, Tumor Promoters, and Cocarcinogens in Tobacco Smoke. In: Proceedings of the 3rd World Conference on Smoking and Health, in press.

37. Stauffer, H. P. and Bourquin, J. Eine Spektralphotometrische Methode zur Bestimmunz von Formaldehyd im Vollrauch von Cigaretten. Beitr. Tabakforsch., 6: 21, 1971.

38. Brunnemann, K. D., Lee, H.-C., and Hoffmann, D. Determination of Catechols in Cigarette Smoke. In preparation.

39. Hecht, S. S., Thorne, R., Maronpot, R. R., and Hoffmann, D. A Study of Tobacco Carcinogenesis. XIII. Tumor Promoting Subfractions of the Weakly Acidic Fraction. J. Natl. Cancer Inst., 55: 1329, 1975.

40. Chaplin, J. F. Genetic Influence on Chemical Constituents of Tobacco Leaf and Smoke. In: Symposium on Chemical Requirements of the Tobacco Industry. Eds.: R. D. Deanin, I. Skeist, and P. G. Hereld. American Chemical Society, Chemical Marketing and Economics Division, Brooklyn, New York, pp. 239-257, 1975.

41. Matzinger, D. F. and Wernsman, E. A. Inheritance and Relationship Among Plant Characters and Smoke Constituents in Flue-cured Tobacco. In: Proceedings of the 5th International Tobacco Science Congress, Hamburg. pp. 68-75, 1970.

42. Tso, T. C., Sims, J. L., and Johnson, D. E. Some Agronomic Factors Affecting N-dimethylnitrosamine Content in Cigarette Smoke. Beitr. Tabakforsch., 8: 34-38, 1975.

43. Wynder, E. L. and Hoffmann, D. (eds.). Toward a Less Harmful Cigarette. Natl. Cancer Inst. Monogr., 28, 1968.

44. Wynder, E. L., Hoffmann, D., Ashwanden, P., and Wachsmuth, R. (eds.). Less Harmful Ways of Smoking. J. Natl. Cancer Inst., 48: 1739-1891, 1972.

45. Rathkamp, G., Tso, T. C., and Hoffmann, D. Smoke Analysis of Cigarettes Made from Bright Tobaccos Differing in Variety and Stalk Positions. Beitr. Tabakforsch., 7: 179-189, 1973.

46. Tso, T. C., Lowe, R., and De Jong, D. W. Homogenized Leaf Curing. I. Theoretical Basis and Some Preliminary Results. Beitr. Tabakforsch., 8: 44, 1975.

47. De Jong, D. W., Lam, J., Lowe, R., Yoder, E., and Tso, T. C. Homogenized Leaf Curing. II. Bright Tobacco. Beitr. Tabakforsch., 8: 93, 1975.

48. Roe, F. J. C., Clack, J. C., Bishop, D., and Peter, R. Comparative Carcinogenicity for Mouse Skin of Smoke Condensates Prepared from Cigarettes Made from the Same Tobacco Cured by Two Processes. Br. J. Cancer, 24: 107-121, 1970.

49. National Cancer Institute, Smoking and Health Program. Toward Less Hazardous Cigarettes, Report No. 2: the Second Set of Experimental Cigarettes. United States Government Printing Office, Washington, in press.

50. Gori, G. B. Approaches to the Reduction of Total Particulate Matter (TPM) in Cigarette Smoke. In: Proceedings of the 3rd World Conference on Smoking and Health, in press.

51. Johnson, W. H. New Processing Methods in the Premanufacturing of Tobacco. In: Proceedings of the 5th International Tobacco Science Congress, Hamburg. pp. 142-152, 1970.

52. Gori, G. B. (ed.). Toward Less Hazardous Cigarettes, Report No. 1: the First Set of Experimental Cigarettes. DHEW Publication No. (NIH) 76-905. United States Government Printing Office, Washington, 1976.

53. Tso, T. C. and Gori, G. B. Leaf Quality and Usability. Theoretical Model I. In: Symposium on Chemical Requirements of the Tobacco Industry. Eds.: R. D. Deanin, I. Skeist, and P. G. Hereld. American Chemical Society, Chemical Marketing and Economics Division, Brooklyn, New York, pp. 258-275, 1975.

54. Halter, H. M. and Ito, T. I. Reconstituted Tobacco. Smoking and Health Possibilities. J. Natl. Cancer Inst., 48: 1861-1883, 1972.

55. Hoffmann, D. and Wynder, E. L. Selective Reduction of Tumorigenicity of Tobacco Smoke. II. Experimental Approaches. J. Natl. Cancer Inst., 48: 1855-1868, 1972.

56. Gori, G. B. Artificial Tobacco Substitutes. J. Am. Med. Assoc., 234: 489-490, 1975.

57. Wynder, E. L. and Hoffmann, D. Tobacco and Tobacco Smoke. Semin. Oncol., <u>3</u>: 5, 1976.

58. Wynder, E. L. and Hoffmann, D. Less Harmful Ways of Smoking. J. Natl. Cancer Inst., <u>48</u>: 1749-1758, 1972.

59. Russell, M. A. H., Wilson, C., Patel, U. A., Feyerabend, C., and Cole, P. V. Plasma Nicotine Levels After Smoking Cigarettes with High, Medium and Low Nicotine Levels. Br. Med. J., <u>2</u>: 414, 1975.

60. Frith, C. D. The Effect of Varying the Nicotine Content of Cigarettes on Human Smoking Behavior. Psychopharmacologia, <u>19</u>: 188, 1971.

61. Norman, V. The Effect of Perforated Tipping Paper on the Yield of Various Smoke Components. Beitr. Tabakforsch., <u>7</u>: 282-287, 1974.

62. Richards, Y. C. and Owens, W. P. Effect of Porous Papers on the Yield of the Major Vapor Phase Components of Cigarette Smoke. <u>In</u>: Proceedings of the 20th Tobacco Chemists Research Conference, Winston-Salem, North Carolina. p. 13, 1966.

63. Gori, G. B., Battista, S. P., Thayer, P. S., Guerin, M. R., and Lynch, C. J. Chemistry and In Vitro Bioassay of Smoke from Experimental Filter Cigarettes. DHEW Publication No. (NIH) 76-1076. United States Government Printing Office, Washington, in press.

64. Smoking and Health Program, National Cancer Institute. Status Report. Bethesda, Maryland, January 1976.

Chapter 8

RADIATION

RADIATION INDUCED CANCER IN THE HEAD AND NECK REGION

Yujiro Matsumura

Yasushi Nomura, Sanetomi Eguchi, and Akio Horie

Division of Head and Neck Surgery
National Kyushu Cancer Center
Fukuoka, Japan

INTRODUCTION

The first report as to radiation-induced cancer had been described by Frieben (1) in 1902. It was only seven years after the discovery of X ray in 1895. Thereafter many papers concerning radiation cancer, for example, carcinomas of the skin (2), lung (3), larynx (4), pharynx (5,6), cervical esophagus (7) and thyroid (8) or leukemia (9,10) and sarkoma (11, 12) have been published up to now and they were professional radiation cancer (2, 13, 14) and cancer that developed in the patients irradiated for benign disease. However, lately the patients who must be treated with irradiation have been increasing, and as the five-year survival rate of the patients of cancer generally have become higher, the secondary other cancer in previously irradiated area (except leukemia) may occur more often. In fact, recently many reports in regard to radiation cancer which developed after treatment for malignant tumor have been increasing (15-19). In these years, twelve patients with radiation-induced cancer have been treated in our clinic. This paper was written to study on radiation-induced cancer and it was the purpose to prevent from occurring of radiation cancer from several facts. It might be difficult to define strictly the radiation cancer (20), however, the warning against imprudent irradiation for various diseases should be proposed (18, 19).

MATERIAL USED

Our twelve patients are divided into two groups A and B (Table I, II). The A group consists of eight patients (case 1 -8) treated with X ray for benign disease. The B group consists of four patients irradiated for malignant disease.

A group: The first case, a woman aged 64, had a big rough tumor (8x7x3cm) of the skin of the right cheek (Fig. 1). In 1926, at the age of 19, she had been irradiated for twenty minutes a day with moving radium plate (1.5x1.5cm) for port wine naevus on the right cheek of her face. Radiation had carried out six times a week at the intervals of three weeks for six months. Since seven years before admission to hospital she had felt itchy and after that the tumor which was of a poppy seed in size developed on her face. Then the tumor gradually became bigger. The tumor was completely excised on 19, September 1973 and showed a well in part moderately differentiated squamous cell carcinoma (Fig. 2). Intravenous injection of 30mg of Bleomycin was administered during operation to defend from permeating of cancer cells into the vessels. There was no evidence of recurrence for two and a half years after operation (Fig. 3).

The patients from the second to the eighth who had suffered from tuberculous lymphadenitis in the younger generation had been all treated with X ray and had almost similar clinical course. Induced tumors were located in the thyroid, hypopharynx, larynx and cervical esophagus respectively and surgical treatments for them were total thyroid lobectomy, pharyngo-laryngectomy or laryngo-esophagectomy with radical neck dissection and so on.

B group: The ninth case, a man aged 31, had complained of haemorrhage from a tumor of his right orbit. In 1962, at the age of 20, he had been irradiated with Cobalt-sixty 6000 rad after removal of the right maxillary tumor which showed reticulum cell sarcoma. The diagnosis of this time was confirmed by biopsy which showed a moderately differentiated squamous cell carcinoma.

The tenth case, a man aged 72, had complained of dysphagia for a month. X ray examination demonstrated a constriction of esophagus at C 6-7, with dilation above the narrowing (Fig. 4). In 1954, at the age of 53, he had been treated with X ray therapy after laryngectomy for a glottic cancer. In spite of surgical extirpation of the esophageal tumor, he died eight months later. The eleventh patient, a man aged 68, had been given X ray therapy after laryngectomy 16 years ago. He was found to have a big tumor of squamous cell carcinoma in the hypopharynx. One year after pharyngectomy with radical neck dissection no residual tumor could be detected.

The twelfth case, a man aged 56, was admitted to hospital with continual gingival bleeding, fever and tiredness for about a month. He was found on examination to be suffering from acute myeloid leukemia. In 1967, at the age of 49, he had been given radiation therapy of Cobalt-sixty 6000 rad for the left neck tumor (anaplastic carcinoma) and five years later again he had been given radiotherapy of Cobalt-sixty 8000 rad for cancer of the nasopharynx. Latent interval between the initial irradiation and the diagnosis of acute myeloid leukemia was seven years.

RESULTS

The age of the patient in A group was on an average 19 and it was 44 in B group. The latent interval between the initial irradiation and the diagnosis of radiation cancer in A group varied between 22 and 45 years with a mean of 33 years. The latent interval in B group varied between 7 and 19 years with a mean of 13 years. It was unable to obtain any correct quantitative estimation of total radiation dose in patients who were treated long years ago. According to statement of the patients, however, it was calculated that the total radiation dose was 2000 to 5000 R of X ray with conventional technique for tuberculous lymphadenitis, and it was 6000 to 8000 rad for malignant tumor in B group.

Most of the patients in A group have shown evidence of fairly remarkable damage to the skin. Changes to the skin of the neck were fibrosis, stigma, irregular pigmentation and leukoderma. On the other hand, the patients in B group have had slight dermatosis. Histological appearance of radiation cancer were in general anaplastic and each cancer cell could not be morphologically distinguished from individual cell of spontaneous cancer. As the tumor was relatively flat and had even thickness showing a extensive development, it was hardly able to recognize microscopically the primary site of cancer. Under layer of the growth was densely fibrous and there was little infiltration of the cancer cell.

DISCUSSION

The age when the patients of A group had been irradiated was generally younger than the age of the patients of B group. The mean of the age was 19 in the former and 44 in the latter. It shall be considered that the primary disease of the patients of B group was a spontaneous malignant tumor which occurred usually in an adult.

The latent interval has been estimated as the time between the initial irradiation and diagnosis of radiation cancer, as Goolden had described (21). The mean latent interval in A group was 33 years and it was 20 years longer than that (13 years) in B group. Cause of it might be supposed that the patient was older and the radiation dose was much in B group. Shortness of the latent interval in the patient who had been irradiated for malignant tumor was thought of important on the matter of radiation carcinogenesis.

Correct radiation dose in A group was obscure, however, there is high possibility of occurring of radiation cancer even after irradiation of a little dose. It will be suggested that the difference of damage of the skin in both A and B group depends on dose, sourse and field in radiation therapy. A few pathological views in regard to radiation cancer were observed. The tumor of radiation-induced cancer was spread diffusely and was thick uniformly. Microscopically the connective tissue under the tumor was firmly fibrous and

some cancer cell presented atypical shape. In the eighth
case, a 61-year-old male, cancers developed simultaneously in
the larynx and the oropharynx 39 years after the radiation
therapy for tuberculous lymphadenitis. Histological examination of the laryngeal tumor revealed a moderately differentiated squamous cell carcinoma and biopsy of the right soft
palate showed carcinoma in situ. That is, the multicentric
development of cancer was shown. These histological appear-
ances described above were thought to be a bit of the
characteristic nature of radiation cancer.

Biological difference of radiation cancer from spontaneous cancer is also interesting problem. Radiosensitivity and
malignancy of radiation cancer generally will be almost
similar to them of spontaneous cancer. Goolden (21) uttered
that prognosis of the patients of radiation cancer would be
well. Survivors in our series are four patients in A group
and one patient is alive in B group. From the histological
appearance it has been thought that radiosensitivity of
radiation cancer might be low. However, an exceptional case
existed in our series. The third patient, a man aged 42, was
treated with radiation therapy for local recurrence of the
residual tumor six months after operation. Four years later
to date he remained well with no evidence of recurrence or
distant metastasis. As Heilmann (7) also stated that the
radiation induced tumor was reacting well to a new radiotherapy, some of radiation cancer will react well to radiotherapy. Consequently if the operation would be possible,
early removal of the tumor should be done and radiotherapy
should be secondarily chosen.

As to histogenesis of radiation cancer, Berenblum's two
stage mechanism of carcinogenesis (22, 23) is partially able
to explain a development of radiation cancer, i. e. it will
be considered that radiation for the primary disease suddenly
acts as initiator making some latent or dormant tumor cells
and thereafter various factors affect the irreversibly
changed cells as promotor and then finally transformation to
cancer develops with a long duration.

For detection and prevention of radiation cancer, careful and repeated periodic examinations during the life of the patient who had been previously given a radiation therapy is necessary. Radiation therapy for cancer is today one of the most effective and valuable treatment, however, precaution against occurrence of radiation cancer also should be taken. As Lawson (19) indicated, especially radiation should not be used in the treatment for cancer of the larynx in persons under 50 years of age.

SUMMARY

1. Twelve patients with radiation-induced cancer were reported.
2. The average age when the patients in A group had been irradiated was younger than that of the patients in B group. On the contrary, the mean latent interval (33 years) of the patients irradiated for benign disease (A group) was longer than that (13 years) of the patients irradiated for malignant tumor (B group). No development of cancer had appeared less than seven years after radiation therapy in our series.
3. Radiation dose for primary disease was obscure in most of the patients, however, it might be presumable 2000-5000r of X ray for benign disease and it seemed to be 6000-8000 rad for malignant tumor.
4. As for the treatment of radiation cancer in the head and neck region, the operative procedure should be taken for the first choice.
5. In case of radiation therapy not only for the benign disease but also for the malignant tumor, possibility that the cancer might occur in the patient irradiated after a certain latent interval must be kept in mind all the time.

TABLE I. A Group: Patient Irradiated for Benign Disease

No.	Patient, age and sex	Primary disease	Radiation therapy and year treated	Age when irradiated	Latent interval	Induced cancer and site	Treatment for radiation cancer and result
1	K.S. 64 F	Port wine naevus	Radium, 6 months, dose? 1926	19	45 yrs	Scc* of cheek	Alive 2.5 yrs after operation
2	S.U. 31 F	T.B. lymph-adenitis	X ray, dose? 1948	9	22	Ad. ca. of thyroid	Alive 7 yrs after total lobectomy
3	H.T. 42 M	T.B. lymph-adenitis	X ray, twice a week, 1950	20	22	Scc of hypopharynx	Alive 4 yrs after operation and radiation
4	K.O. 52 M	T.B. lymph-adenitis	X ray, twice a week, 6 months, 1941	23	29	Scc of cervical esophagus	Died in 1971, operation
5	M.K. 51 M	T.B. lymph-adenitis	X ray, twice a week, 6 months 1932	17	34	Scc of hypopharynx	Died in 1971, operation and radiation
6	K.O. 57 F	T.B. lymph-adenitis	X ray, once a week, 3 years, 1937	20	37	Scc of hypopharynx	Alive 1 yr after operation
7	K.W. 60 F	T.B. lymph-adenitis	X ray, twice a week, 5 months, 1941	26	34	Scc of hypopharynx	unknown
8	E.O. 60 M	T.B. lymph-adenitis	X ray, once a week, 2 years, 1927	21	39	Scc of larynx and ca. in situ of oropharynx	Died in 1966 operation

* Scc... Squamous cell carcinoma

TABLE II. B Group: Patient Irradiated for Malignant Tumor

No.	Patient, age and sex	Primary disease	Radiation therapy and year treated	Age when irradiated	Latent interval	Induced cancer and site	Treatment for radiation cancer and result
9	M.S. 31 M	Reticulum c. sa. of maxilla	Co 6000 rads, 1962	20	11	Scc of orbit	Died in 1973, radiation
10	R.F. 72 M	Scc of larynx	X ray 6000 r, 1954	53	19	Scc of cervical esophagus	Died in 1973 operation
11	S.N. 68 M	Scc of larynx	X ray, dose? 1959	52	16	Scc of hypopharynx	Alive 1 yr after operation
12	M.M. 56 M	Ca. of naso-pharynx	Co 6000 (neck)1967 Co 8000 (epipharynx) 1972	49	7	Acute myeloid leukemia	Died in 1974, chemotherapy

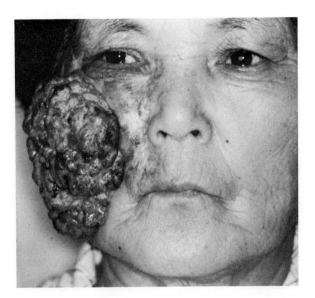

FIG. 1. Case 1. A big rough tumor with bleeding of the right cheek is shown. According to her statement, it seemed to be a poppy seed in size seven years ago. Leucoderma and radiation cicatrix are also seen.

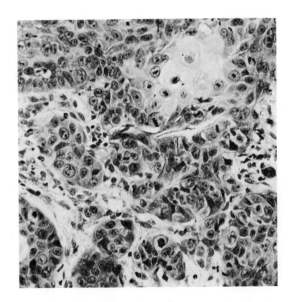

FIG. 2. Post-operative histological appearance of the tumor in Case 1. A well differentiated squamous cell carcinoma is shown and partially cancer cells present irregular arrangement, atypical shape and mitosis.

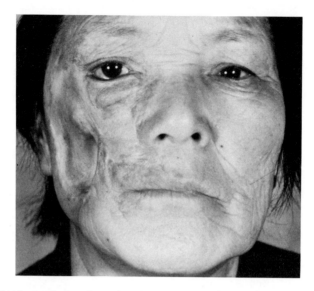

FIG. 3. Condition of the face in Case 1, two years after operation. Post-operative slight cicatrix and facial palsy are seen.

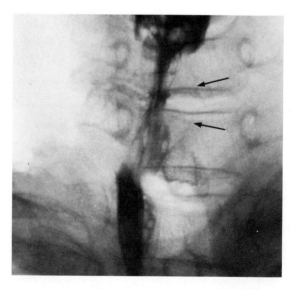

FIG. 4. Case 10. X ray examination revealed a tumor of the cervical esophagus C 6-7, 19 years after postoperative radiation for a glottic cancer.

REFERENCES

1. Frieben, A., Demonstration Eines Cancroid Des Rechten Handrueckens, Des Sich Nach Langdauernder Einwirkung Von Roentgenstrahlen Entwickelt Hatte. Fortschr. Roentgen str., 6: 106-112, 1902.

2. Porter, C.A., and White, C.J. Multiple Carcinomata Following Chronic X-ray Dermatitis. Ann. Surg., 46: 649-671, 1907.

3. Rostoski, O., Saupe, E., and Schmorl, G. Die Bergkrankheit Der Erzbergleute In Schneeberg In Sachsen (Schneeberger Lungenkrebs). Ztschr. f. Krebsforsch. 23: 360-684, 1926.

4. Jacques, P. Cancer Du Larynx Chez La Femme Apres Irradiation Thyroidienne Prolongee. Oto-rhino-laryngol. Int., 19: 277-278, 1935.

5. Kruchen, C. Spaetschaedigungen Durch Roentgenstrahlen. Strahlentherapie, 60: 466-475, 1937.

6. Goolden, A.W.G., and Morgan, R.L. Radiation Cancer Of The Pharynx. Acta Radiol., 3: 353-360, 1965.

7. Heilmann, H.P. Entstehung Eines Postkrikoidkarzinoms In Der Folge Mehrfacher Roentgenbestrahlungen Der Halsregion Wegen Lymphknoten-Tuberkulose. Strahlentherapie, 140: 388-391, 1970.

8. Simpson, C.L., and Hempelmann, L.H. The Association Of Tumors And Roentgenray Treatment Of The Thorax In Infancy. Cancer, 10: 42-56, 1957.

9. Court-Brown, W.M., and Doll, R. Leukemia And Aplastic Anaemia In Patients Irradiated For Ankylosing Spondylitis. Her Majesty's Stationary Office, London. Med. Res. Counc. Spec. Rep. 295, Ser. No. 259, 1957.

10. Watanabe, S. Nuclear Hematology Based On Experience With Atomic Explosions. Academic Press, New York, p. 485, 1965.

11. Cahan, W.G., Woodard, H.Q., Higinbotham, N.L., Stewart, F.W., Coley, B.L. Sarcoma Arising In Irradiated Bone; Report Of Eleven Cases. Cancer, 1: 3-29, 1948.

12. Feintuch, T.A. Chondrosarcoma Arising In A Cartilaginous Area Of Previously Irradiated Fibrous Dysplasia. Cancer, 31: 877-881, 1973.

13. Lewis, E.B. Leukemia, Multiple Myeloma And Aplastic Anaemia In American Radiologists. Science, 142: 1492, 1963.

14. Peller, S. and Pick, P. Leukemia In American Physicians.
    Acta Un. Int. Cancr., <u>11</u>: 292, 1955.

15. Sagerman, R.H., Cassady, J.R., Tretter, P., and Ellsworth,
    R.M. Radiation Induced Neoplasia Following External
    Beam Therapy For Children With Retinablastoma. Amer. J.
    Roentgenol., <u>105</u>: 529-535, 1969.

16. Nitze, H.R. Radiogene Tumoren Im HNO-Bereich. Arch. Klin.
    Exp. Ohr.-Nas.-u. Kehlk. Heilk., <u>199</u>: 634-638, 1971.

17. Som, M.L., and Peimer, R. Postcricoid Carcinoma As A
    Sequel To Radiotherapy For Laryngeal Carcinoma. Arch.
    Otolaryngol., <u>62</u>: 428-438, 1955.

18. Kikuchi, A., Watanabe C., Abe M., Kubota, H., Idogawa K.,
    and Ishikawa, T. Head And Neck Cancer Following
    Therapeutic Irradiation And A Brief Review On Those In
    Japan. Nippon Acta Radiologica, <u>34</u>: 491-503, 1974.

19. Lawson, W., and Som, Max. Second Primary Cancer After
    Irradiation Of Laryngeal Cancer. Ann. Otol, <u>84</u>: 771-775
    1975.

20. Holinger. P.H. and Rabbett, W.F. Late Development Of
    Laryngeal And Pharyngeal Carcinoma In Previously
    Irradiated Areas. Laryngoscope, <u>63</u>: 105-112, 1953.

21. Goolden, A.W.G. Radiation Cancer. A Review With Special
    Reference To Radiation Tumours In The Pharynx, Larynx,
    And Thyroid. Brit. J. Radiology, <u>360</u>: 626-640, 1957.

22. Berenblum, I., and Shubik, P. A New Quantitative
    Approach To The Study Of The Stages Of Chemical
    Carcinogenesis In The Mouse's Skin. Brit. J. Cancer, <u>1</u>:
    383-391, 1947.

23. Mayneord, W.V. Radiation Carcinogenesis. Brit. J.
    Radiol., <u>41</u>: 241-250, 1968.

CHRONIC MYELOGENOUS LEUKEMIA DEVELOPING
AFTER THYMIC IRRADIATION

Katsutaro Shimaoka and Joseph E. Sokal
Department of Medicine B
Roswell Park Memorial Institute
Buffalo, New York

Around the turn of the century, it was believed that an enlarged thymus gland could cause airway compression and respiratory distress. It was also thought that in some mysterious way, the thymus was involved in sudden death from trivial causes of previously well children, attributed to "status thymicolymphaticus." For these reasons, surgical removal of the gland was often undertaken, with high mortality. As x-ray equipment become generally available, the diagnosis of thymic enlargement was made frequently and radiation therapy replaced thymectomy. A variety of ports and dose schedules were used by different radiologists. Thymic irradiation was given preoperatively, or prophylactically, to asymptomatic infants and children with thymic enlargement.

Following an observation by Duffy and Fitzgerald of an association between malignant thyroid neoplasms and previous thymic irradiation (1), numerous studies of children who had received thymic irradiation were undertaken. Simpson et al

819

studied 1400 children who received thymic irradiation, and 1795 untreated siblings as controls. They reported an increased incidence of both thyroid cancer and leukemia in 1955 (2). This study has since been extended to cover 2872 treated children and 5055 untreated siblings, over 20 years of observation, and shows further occurrence of thyroid cancer, leukemia and other malignancies (3). In addition, there are several cohort analyses of children treated with thymic irradiation (4-7). All cases of leukemia reported in these studies have been acute leukemia. The development of chronic myelogenous leukemia (CML) in children and young adults following radiation exposure appears to be a rare event.

We have recently observed 2 young adults with CML who received thymic irradiation during infancy.

CASE REPORTS

Case 1

This white male was born in January 1949, after a normal pregnancy and delivery. At the age of 3 months, he underwent thymic irradiation for breathing difficulties and a widened superior mediastinum on chest x-ray. Radiation factors were 140 KV, 15mA at 50 cm distance through a port of 6x8 cm to the superior mediastinum. Three doses of 100r in air were given every other day, for a total of 300 r.

In December 1967, he noted areas of ecchymosis near the left knee, which prompted him to seek medical advice. A diagnosis of "acute leukemia" was made and he was referred to the Roswell Park Memorial Institute for further evaluation and treatment.

Physical examination revealed a palpable spleen tip, minor cervical adenopathy and areas of ecchymosis on both lower extremities. A diagnosis of CML was made on the basis of peripheral blood and bone marrow aspiration.

After an unsatisfactory response to an investigational agent, isopentenyl adenosine, treatment was changed to busulfan. This produced an excellent remission and he was maintained on intermittent busulfan therapy for the next 3 years. In June 1970, he entered an immunotherapy program, receiving repeated vaccinations with mixtures of BCG and cultured leukocytes of lines established from patients with myeloid leukemia (8).

In June 1972, 6-mercaptopurine was added to his therapeutic regimen because of basophilia of 14%. Subsequently, basophils ranged from 0 to 29%, but otherwise the patient remained in excellent clinical and hematologic status.

In November 1972, he was found to have a thyroid nodule in the right lobe which was "hypofunctioning" on radioiodine scan, and he was placed on suppressive therapy with 75 µg of Na liothyronine daily. Subsequently, the nodule was aspirated and cytological study showed follicular cells and abundant lymphocytes, many of which formed rosettes. There was no evidence of leukemic infiltration. These findings were interpreted as thyroiditis. In February 1973, the nodule was found to be 80% larger in cross-sectional area, and softer. In addition, another small, firm nodule was discovered.

Hematological deterioration was recorded in the fall of 1973 and in February 1974, he was considered to have entered the blastic stage of the disease. During the next 18 months, he was treated with various routines of combination chemotherapy, as well as radiation therapy, and underwent splenectomy. Partial remissions were obtained and he remained in good functional status for about a year, after which he was increasingly disabled by various complications of the disease, including leukemic infiltration of lymph nodes, nerve trunks and finally, the central nervous system. He expired on October 22, 1975.

Chromosomal analysis consistently yielded a pattern of 46XY with a single Ph' chromosome in all metaphases until September 1974, when some metaphases showed 47XY with two Ph' chromosomes. In subsequent examinations, the latter gradually became the dominant pattern and finally, the sole karyotype.

Case 2

This white male was born in January 1947. When he was 2 months old, he was given 3 weekly doses of radiation for an enlarged thymus. Radiation factors were: 100 KV, 5mA at a distance of 10 inches to a port of 10x10 cm, delivering 132 r in air, for a total dose of 396 r.

In March 1969, after rejection as a blood donor, he underwent a medical work-up. He was found to have an ecchymosis over the left upper quadrant of the abdomen and hepatosplenomegaly. A diagnosis of CML was made and was treated with busulfan and cyclophosphamide. He had a good partial remission, but developed thrombocytopenia. In June 1971, he was referred to the Roswell Park Memorial Institute.

Physical examination revealed the spleen tip to be palpable 2 cm below the left costal margin. Examination of peripheral blood and bone marrow aspirate confirmed the diagnosis. Chromosome analysis showed a pattern of 46XY with a Ph' chromosome in all metaphases. Antileukemic therapy was changed to a combination of hydroxyurea and 6-mercaptopurine. He continued to do well clinically, but mild splenomegaly persisted. In September 1971, he entered our immunotherapy program and received repeated vaccinations with BCG-cultured cell mixtures. He continued to do well until March 1973, when myeloblastic transformation was documented. Following partial control of the blastic state with cytosine arabinoside, splenectomy was performed. Subsequently, he was treated with combination chemotherapy. Improvement was incomplete and of short duration, and he died on August 14, 1973. Pulmonary hemorrhages were found at autopsy and considered to be the immediate cause of death.

Chromosome analysis during the blastic state showed a mode of 45 chromosomes, with deletion of one of the Group C chromosomes; a single Ph' chromosome was seen in all metaphases.

DISCUSSION

It is well known that exposure of human populations to
ionizing radiation is followed by an increased incidence of
various forms of leukemia, with the exception of chronic
lymphocytic leukemia. There are many reports of CML following
radiation exposure among adult populations (9-14). However,
CML has been recorded only rarely as a complication of
radiation exposure early in life, and most follow-up studies
of irradiated pediatric population report no cases (3-7,15,
16). Since CML following radiation exposure does not differ
from the "spontaneous" disease (17), there is no way at
present to identify an individual case of CML as radiation
induced.

The two patients reported here had typical CML. Their
survival was somewhat longer than average, but not different
from that of other patients in our immunotherapy program (8).
As is shown in Table I, CML is rare in younger age groups
and becomes much more common after the age of 30 (12,18-27).
Both our patients were rather young to have this disease. It
is of interest that one of these patients developed another
stigma of thymic irradiation--nodular goiter--a few years
after the diagnosis of leukemia. If thymic irradiation did,
in fact, induce these cases of leukemia, the incubation
periods to overt disease would be 18 and 22 years. These are
longer than those usually reported for radiation-induced CML,
but are not outside the range we have encountered in the past
(17) or which is reported in the data from Hiroshima (28).
Studies of that population exposed to the 1945 atom bomb
explosion indicate that excess cases of CML, and an abnormally
low AML/CML ratio in comparison to the Japanese average, were
still being recorded 25 years later (28,29).

Radiation exposure can cause both acute leukemia and CML.
However, for reasons not yet understood, chronic leukemia is
very rare in childhood and this age group appears to be particularly susceptible to acute leukemia. Table II shows a
survey of the pediatric literature for the frequency of CML;
this varies from 1 to 6% of all leukemias seen, with an

average of 3% (27,30-39). In the late teens and early 20's, the incidence of acute leukemia declines and that of CML increases slightly. Still, one would expect only one case of CML for every 10-20 cases of acute leukemia in populations followed to the early 20's. The total number of cases of acute leukemia reported in 5 follow-up studies of thymic irradiation (not all of which were continued until the subjects reached the adulthood) was 10 (3-7). Therefore, it is not surprising that no case of CML was found in these studies.

On the other hand, when cases of leukemia are studied for prior radiation exposure, the yield for the association becomes much higher, as in our experience. We have also found 2 other reports of CML following thymic irradiation; incubation periods for these cases were more typical, 9 and less than 5 years, respectively (35,37). In utero radiation exposure via pelvimetry has also been implicated as a possible cause of CML in one of the pediatric cases reported (34). Our series of CML patients also includes two who had had such exposure; CML was discovered at 11 and 20 years of age. It is of interest to note that all of these 3 cases had pelvimetry on two occasions.

In conclusion, the patients described in this report probably represent examples of radiation-induced CML. The paucity of reports of CML following thymic irradiation is probably due to (a) the much greater likelihood that acute leukemia will be induced, and (b) failure to obtain an accurate history of radiation exposure in many cases of leukemia. It is noteworthy that we would not have documented thymic irradiation in these cases, had it not been for the fact that one of them developed nodular goiter--which aroused suspicion of previous radiation exposure in the thyroid clinic. Following this incident, special inquiries regarding radiation exposure in utero and during childhood were made in all available cases in which CML had been diagnosed at an early age; this resulted in identification of the second patient as well as of several others with radiation exposure for diagnostic studies.

SUMMARY

Two cases of Ph'-positive chronic myelogenous leukemia
with a history of thymic irradiation are presented. Both
patients received radiation therapy from low voltage x-ray
equipment at 2-3 months of age. Leukemia developed 18 and 22
years later. Presentation, response to antileukemic therapy
and clinical course did not differ from that of other patients
with this disease treated in our department.

TABLE I. Age Distribution of CML Patients

INVESTIGATORS, Study Period / AGE	Ward (18) Up to 1917	Minot et al (19) 1898-1923	Hoffman & Craver (20) 1917-1930	McAlpin et al (21) 1919-1929	Leavel (22) 1917-1936	Wintrobe (23) 1926-1945	Bethell (24) 1927-1941	Krebs & Bichel (25) 1931-1946	Shimkins et al (26) 1910-1948	Gauld et al (27) 1938-1951	Gunz & Atkins (12) 1958-1961	Total 11 Studies	%
0- 9	7	3				1	1	1	1	1	2	17	1.3
10-19	12	6	2	1	2	2	6	3	8	5	3	50	3.8
20-29	25	30	18	2	9	8	12	5	43	13	5	170	13.0
30-39	84	51	26	8	25	18	27	11	33	21	6	310	23.7
40-49	60	37	15	7	23	8	32	13	59	48	13	315	24.1
50-59	30	23	13	5	20	13	32	15	40	37	9	237	18.1
60-69	22	15	6	1	6	8	18	5	24	28	17	150	11.5
70-79	5	1			2		2	2	4	16	19	51	3.9
80-89	2						1				4	7	0.5
Male	136	93	55	13	46	34	68	27	124	80	44	720	
Female	111	73	25	11	41	24	63	28	88	89	34	587	
Total	247	166	80	24	87	58	131	55	212	169	78	1307	

826

TABLE II. CML and Other Types of Leukemia in Pediatric
Population (Age Limit: 12-16)

Authors	Study Period	Institution	No. CML	No. Other Leukemia
Dale (30)	1932-1948	NY Hosp.	2	70
Rogers et al (31)	1932-1947	Toronto Child.	2	156
Cooke (32)	1931-1950	St. Louis Child.	15	279
Gauld et al (27)	1938-1951	Aberdeen Edingburgh	2	110
Lightwood et al (33)	1951-1957	London Child.	2	98
Barrett et al (34)	1952-1959	Walter Reed	4	116
Reisman & Trujillo (35)	1956-1962	LA Co & City of Hope	9	151
Gunz & Spears (36)	1953-1964	N. Zealand	8	288
Burgert et al (37)		Mayo Clinic	12	746
Rajani-Kantha et al (38)	1960-1971	Long Island Jewish	6	168
Hitzig (39)	1964-1973	U. Zurich	3	139

827

REFERENCES

1. Duffy, B.J., and Fitzgerald, P.J. Cancer of the thyroid in children: A report of 28 cases. J. Clin. Endoc. Metab., 10: 1296-1308, 1950.

2. Simpson, C.L., Hempelmann, L.H., and Fuller, L.M. Neoplasia in children treated with x-rays in infancy for thymic enlargement. Radiol. 64: 840-845, 1955.

3. Hempelmann, L.H., Hall, W.J., Phillips, M., Cooper, R.A., and Ames, W.R. Neoplasms in persons treated with x-rays in infancy: Fourth survey in 20 years. J. Nat. Cancer Inst. 55: 519-530, 1975.

4. Conti, E.A., Patton, G.D., Conti, J.E., and Hempelmann, L.H. Present health of children given x-ray treatment to the anterior mediastinum in infancy. Radiol. 74: 386-391, 1960.

5. Saenger, E.L., Silverman, F.N., Sterling, T.D., and Turner, M.E. Neoplasia following therapeutic irradiation for benign conditions in childhood. Radiol. 74: 889-904, 1960.

6. Pifer, J.W., Hempelmann, L.H., Dodge, H.J., and Hodges, F.J. Neoplasms in the Ann Arbor series of thymus-irradiated children. Am. J. Roent. 53: 13-18, 1968.

7. Janower, M.L., and Miettinen, O.S. Neoplasms after childhood irradiation of the thymus gland. J.A.M.A. 215: 753-756, 1971.

8. Sokal, J.E., Aungst, C.W., and Grace, J.T., Jr. Immunotherapy in well-controlled chronic myelocytic leukemia. New York State J. Med. 73: 1180-1185, 1973.

9. Court-Brown, W.M., and Abbatt, J.D. Incidence of leukaemia in ankylosing spondilitis treated with x-rays. Preliminary report. Lancet i: 1283-1285, 1955.

10. Doll, R., and Smith, P.G. The long term effects of irradiation in patients treated for metropathia hemorrhagica. Brit. J. Radiol. 41: 362-368, 1968.

11. Simon, N., Brucer, M., and Hayes, R. Radiation and leukemia in carcinoma of the cervix. Radiol. 74: 905-911, 1960.

12. Gunz, F.W., and Atkinson, H.R. Medical radiations and leukaemia: Retrospective survey. Brit. Med. J. i: 389-393, 1964.

13. DaSilva Horta, J., Abbatt, J.D., Cayolla da Motta, L., and Roriz, M.L. Malignancy and other late effects following administration of thorotrast. Lancet ii: 201-205, 1965.

14. Brill, A.B., Tomonaga, M., and Heyssel, R.M. Leukemia in man following exposure to ionizing radiation. Summary of findings in Hiroshima and Nagasaki, and comparison with other human experience. Ann. Int. Med. 56: 590-609, 1962.

15. Stewart, A., Webb, J., and Hewitt, D. Survey of childhood malignancies. Brit. Med. J. i: 1495-1508, 1958.

16. Stewart, A.M., and Kneale, G.W. Age distribution of cancers caused by obstetric x-rays and their relevance to cancer latent periods. Lancet ii: 4-8, 1970.

17. Shimaoka, K., Ezdinli, E., Han, T., and Fridman, M. Chronic myelocytic leukemia (CML) following irradiation. Proc. Am. A. Cancer Res. 12: 48, 1971.

18. Ward, G. The infective theory of acute leukaemia. Brit. J. Child. Dis. 14: 10-20, 1917.

19. Minot, G.R., Buckman, T.E., and Isaacs, R. Chronic myelogenous leukemia. J.A.M.A. 82: 1489-1494, 1924.

20. Hoffman, W.J., and Craver, L.F. Chronic myelogenous leukemia. J.A.M.A. 97: 836-840, 1931.

21. McAlpin, K.R., Golden, R., and Edsall, K.S. The roentgen treatment of chronic leucemia. Am. J. Roent. 26: 47-63, 1931.

22. Leavell, B.S. Chronic leukemia. Am. J. Med. Sci. 196: 329-340, 1938.

23. Wintrobe, M.M. Clinical Hematology, 2nd Edition. Lea & Febiger, Philadelphia, pp. 666-675, 1946.

24. Bethell, F.H. Leukemia. Ann. Int. Med. 18: 757-771, 1943.

25. Krebs, C., and Bichel, J. Results of roentgen treatment in chronic myelogenous leukemia. Acta Radiol. 28: 697-704, 1947.

26. Shimkin, M.B., Mettier, S.R., and Bierman, H.R. Myelocytic leukemia: An analysis of incidence, distribution and fatality, 1910-1948. Ann. Int. Med. 35: 194-212, 1951.

27. Gauld, W.R., Innes, J., and Robson, H.N. A survey of 647 cases of leukaemia, 1938-1951. Brit. Med. J. 1: 585-589, 1953.

28. Watanabe, S., Shimosato, Y., Ohkita, T., Ezaki, H., Shigemitsu, T., and Kamata, N. Leukemia and thyroid carcinoma found among A-bomb survivors in Hiroshima. In: Recent Results in Cancer Research. Eds.: E. Grundmann and H. Tulinius. Springer-Verlag, Berlin-Heidelberg-New York, 39: 57-83, 1972.

29. Ichimaru, M., and Ishimaru, T. Leukemia and related disorders. J. Rad. Res.(Suppl.) 16: 89-96, 1975.

30. Dale, J.H., Jr. Leukemia in childhood. J. Ped. 34: 421-432, 1949.

31. Rogers, C.L., Donohue, W.L., and Snelling, C.E. Leukaemia in children. Canad. Med. A. J. 65: 548-552, 1951.

32. Cooke, J.V. Chronic myelogenous leukemia in children. J. Ped. 42: 537-550, 1953.

33. Lightwood, R., Barrie, H., and Butler, N. Observations on 100 cases of leukaemia in childhood. Brit. Med. J. 1: 747-752, 1960.

34. Barrett, O., Jr., Conrad, M., and Crosby, W.H. Chronic granulocytic leukemia in childhood. Am. J. Med. Sci. 240: 587-592, 1960.

35. Reisman, L.E., and Trukillo, J.M. Chronic granulocytic leukemia of childhood. J. Ped. 62: 710-723, 1963.

36. Gunz, F.W., and Spears, G.F.S. Distribution of acute leukaemia in time and space. Brit. Med. J. 4: 604-606, 1968.

37. Burgert, E.O., Jr., Nieri, R.L., Mills, S.D., and Linman, J.W. Nonlymphocytic leukemia in childhood. Mayo Clin. Proc. 48: 255-259, 1973.

38. Rajani-Kantha, K.R., King, M., Levy, R.N., Sawitsky, A., and Rosner, F. Chronic myelogenous leukemia in childhood. N.Y. State J. Med. 75: 392-399, 1975.

39. Hitzig, W.H. Leukamien im Kindesalter. Schweiz M. Wschr. 105: 1088-1092, 1975.

TEMPORAL DISTRIBUTION OF RISK AFTER EXPOSURE

Charles E. Land

National Cancer Institute
Bethesda, Maryland   20014

Douglas H. McGregor

V.A. Center, Kansas City, and
University of Kansas Medical Center,
Kansas City, Kansas

INTRODUCTION

Latency, or time from exposure to diagnosis or death for a cancer
caused by that exposure, is a concept relevant both to hypotheses about
pathogenic mechanisms[1,2] and to assessments of the relationship between
level of exposure and consequent cancer incidence or mortality. For an
epidemiological study of cancer and occupational exposure histories, for
example, incidence or mortality rates may be based on a fixed interval of
observation for risk, while exposure may be given by a sequence of
measured or estimated levels of a carcinogen, identified by time relative
to the period of observation for risk. Latency considerations may play
a part in abstracting the sequence of carcinogen levels into a single
summary dose, which is then used to estimate a dose-response function, and
in interpreting the dose-response estimate in terms of lifetime risk for
a hypothetical occupational exposure history. For example, events
occurring shortly before the period of observation for risk may be
discounted because it is thought unlikely that a cancer caused by such
an event could be diagnosed or cause death during that period, or very
early events could be discounted because of a belief that any resultant
risk should largely be over before the beginning of the observation
period.

Because considerations other than latency play a part in estimating
the relationship between exposure and cancer incidence or mortality (e.g.,
the relative effects of continuous exposure at a low carcinogen level and

more infrequent exposures at higher levels), it may be difficult to make inferences about latency from data based on histories of repeated exposure to a carcinogen. In this respect the studies of A-bomb survivors carried out jointly by the Atomic Bomb Casualty Commission (ABCC) and the Japanese National Institute of Health (JNIH), and now being continued by their successor organization, the Radiation Effects Research Foundation (RERF), are particularly valuable. In these studies, based on an intensive surveillance for risk over time of a defined population following a single exposure to ionizing radiation, latency considerations are not required in the definition of dose, and latency and dose-response can be separated to an extent not possible with other material.

The studies of leukemia in A-bomb survivors, in particular, which showed an early dose-response gradient that has peaked and then diminished with time[3,4,5], have inspired others to hypothesize similar latency distributions for cancers resulting from occupational exposure. In their study of lung cancer mortality and exposure to radon daughter nuclides among U.S. uranium miners, Lundin et. al.[6] assumed that the time in years between initiation of a cancer and death was lognormally distributed with median equal to 10 years and standard deviation of logs equal to log 1.5. The distributional form and standard deviation were suggested by the distribution in time of leukemia cases among heavily exposed A-bomb survivors[3], while the median was estimated from the data on uranium miners. An "exposure" was defined to be a period of one month spent working in a uranium mine, with radon daughter dose estimated according to a series of measurements of that mine or similar mines. The weight given to an exposure was that part of the area under the assumed lognormal density curve beginning at the time of exposure that corresponded to the period of observation for risk (see Figure 1). The sum of weighted dose estimates was used as a summary measure of exposure (working-level months).

Other theoreticians, again inspired by the A-bomb survivors' leukemia history, but also by animal experiments in which quite high response rates were obtained, have proposed that the median time to response be assumed to be inversely proportional to the cube root of dose[7]. Such a model has recently been proposed by Enterline and Henderson[8] for studying lung cancer among asbestos workers.

Latency models based on the leukemia data have been constructed in the absence of sufficient data relating solid tumors to A-bomb exposure. In the future, as such data become available, we may expect latency

832

models to take them into account. The present study reviews latency data on lung cancer mortality and breast cancer incidence among A-bomb survivors, as well as leukemia mortality, for different age and exposure groups in an examination of the generality of the leukemia results.

PROCEDURES AND MATERIALS USED

The basis of the ABCC-JNIH-RERF studies is the extended Life-Span Study (LSS) sample, a probability sample selected on the basis of age and reported location at the time of the bomb (ATB) from the populations of Hiroshima and Nagasaki as of October 1, 1950*. Since the time of sample selection a continuing effort has produced estimates of radiation dose (kerma[9]) received by all but those with particularly complicated shielding histories. The distribution of the LSS sample by age ATB, exposure status, and estimated radiation dose is given in Table I[10].

Mortality follow-up by death certificate cause of death is complete, thanks to the unique Japanese family registry system[11]. The most recent reports on mortality, covering the periods October 1950-December 1970 and October 1950-December 1972, are the sources of the material presented here on leukemia and lung cancer mortality[10,12]. Incidence studies, in which clinical records, tumor registries, and other sources are searched for cases of specified diseases, are also tied to the extended LSS sample or to the somewhat more accessible clinical subsample, which receives periodic physical examinations. Information from a recent study of breast cancer incidence among female LSS sample members for the period October 1950-December 1969[13] is also presented.

The technique followed is to compare the distributions over time of the low-exposure (non-exposed + exposed with 0-9 rads) and high-exposure (100+ rads) deaths and incidence cases. This is done graphically by plotting cumulative proportions, adjusted for attenuation of the sample, for the two groups separately.

RESULTS

Leukemia mortality

A recent report by Ichimaru and Ishimaru, summarizing leukemia incidence in the LSS sample from October 1950 through December 1971[5],

---

*
Some of the non-exposed sample members were selected from the populations as of 1951 and 1953.

shows that heavily exposed A-bomb survivors have experienced much greater leukemia incidence, both chronic and acute, than those not in the city ATB or who were exposed to low levels of radiation. This is true for all age-ATB cohorts; however, age ATB has been an important factor determining both incidence level and latency. Chronic granulocytic leukemia peaked among the heavily exposed within the first 10 years after exposure and then declined; the sharpest peak and fastest decline occurred among those aged less than 15 ATB, while a much less pronounced peak and slower decline took place among those over 30 ATB. Acute leukemia peaked around 1950-51 for heavily exposed subjects under 15 ATB, and around 1955, 1960, and 1965 for those aged 15-29, 30-44, and 45 or more ATB, respectively. Moreover, the sharpness of the peak and steepness of decline following the peak both decrease as age ATB increases. The latency distributions for acute leukemia, in particular, are reminiscent of a family of log-normal densities with constant standard deviation of logs and increasing median (Figure 2).

Since leukemia is generally a rapidly progressing disease of high fatality, the pattern over time of leukemia mortality can be expected to follow that of leukemia incidence. In Figure 3 cumulative plots over the period October 1950-December 1972, adjusted for sample attenuation, are given for deaths from all types of leukemia among heavily exposed (100+ rads) and non-exposed and lightly exposed (0-9 rads) survivors, by age ATB cohort. Since the heavily exposed groups have high relative risks (39.6, 10.2, 16.2, 6.4, and 12.8 in the 0-9, 10-19, 20-34, 35-49, and 50+ age ATB cohorts, respectively) with significance levels less than .00001 in all cases, Figure 3 can be considered to contrast leukemia induced by A-bomb radiation with naturally occurring leukemia. For the 0-9, 10-19, 20-34, and 35-49 age ATB cohorts, the tendency for leukemia attributable to A-bomb radiation to occur earlier than "natural" leukemia is apparent. For those aged 50 and over ATB, however, the two distributions are indistinguishable.

Lung cancer mortality

Evidence for a dose-specific A-bomb effect on respiratory cancer is strong only for cancers of the trachea, bronchus, and lung, which make up about 80 percent of the LSS respiratory cancer deaths recorded through December 1972[12]. Both low-dose and high-dose deaths occurred in substan-

tial numbers only among those aged over 34 ATB, with relative risks of 1.6
(p < .04) in the 35-49 ATB cohort and 2.4 (p < .003) in the 50+ ATB cohort.
Cumulative proportions for high and low exposure deaths in these two
cohorts are shown in Figure 4.

Comparison with the cumulative plots for leukemia mortality is
complicated by the much lower proportions of radiation-induced cancer
mortality in the high-dose curves in Figure 4. However, there is no
evidence that mortality from cancer of the bronchus, trachea and lung
induced by A-bomb radiation has occurred earlier than that induced by
more usual causes.

Breast cancer incidence

Female breast cancer is a major A-bomb radiation effect whose case
fatality rate is considerably below those of leukemia and lung cancer.
Although LSS sample mortality analyses have shown breast cancer to
increase with increasing dose[10,12], incidence information is greatly
preferable for studies of time trends. The 1968 report by Wanebo et. al.[14],
covering 31 cases in the ABCC-JNIH clinical subsample, prompted an
intensive search for cases among the entire LSS sample. In all, 231
cases were found with diagnosis during the period October 1950-December
1969[13]. No cases were found among those exposed to A-bomb radiation
before age 10, but excessively high rates were found among those exposed
to 100 rads or more in the older cohorts. Relative risks of 6.1
(p < .00001), 3.5 (p < .00001), 2.1 (p=.07) and 3.2 (p < .05) were obtained
for the 10-19, 20-34, 35-49, and 50+ ATB cohorts, respectively; however,
only 7 and 4 high-dose cases, respectively, were observed for the 35-49
and 50+ ATB cohorts. The cumulative plots for breast cancer incidence in
Figure 5 show no tendency for breast cancer to appear earlier in the high
dose groups; the contrast between Figures 3 and 5 is especially impressive
for the 10-19 ATB cohort, since the relative risk obtained for breast
cancer in this cohort approaches that obtained for leukemia. The 50+ ATB
comparison, on the other hand, has little significance since it is based
on only 4 high-dose breast cancer cases.

DISCUSSION

The evidence of Figures 3-5 is that there is no universally applicable
latency rule for cancers resulting from A-bomb radiation. The assumption

that latency tends to decrease with increasing dose does not appear to hold for lung cancer and breast cancer, nor even for leukemia in the oldest age ATB cohort, although it seems valid for leukemia in those aged less than 50 ATB. Even here, however, age at exposure is an important factor, with the earliest latencies occurring among those who were youngest ATB. The evidence for lung and breast cancer suggests that the effect of exposure to A-bomb radiation is to increase the rates of these cancers, but not to change their age distributions.

Doll's remark that cancers resulting from a single exposure appear in a "wave" of limited duration[2] is not necessarily contradicted by the data presented here. The tendency for lung cancer and breast cancer to occur at higher rates among the heavily exposed, but at the same ages as among those with little or no exposure to A-bomb radiation, is consistent with the hypothesis that several exposures are required for these cancers, the final ones being associated with increasing age. The same conjecture could also be made about leukemia, in the sense that leukemia occurring naturally among the aged may well be caused by age-related exposures. For example, the tendency for median leukemia latency among the heavily exposed A-bomb survivors to increase with increasing age ATB, corresponding roughly to the lognormal densities in Figure 2, could result from a mixture of a wave effect for leukemias due solely to the radiation and age-dependent leukemias whose rate is increased by radiation exposure without changing the age distribution.

The implications of these data for epidemiological studies of cancer resulting from occupational exposure are, first, that latency models of the wave type, based on analogy with leukemia among heavily exposed A-bomb survivors, may have little relevance in many cases. In particular, for cancers normally associated with aging, it is reasonable to hope that it may be possible largely to ignore latency when grouping by similar ages at risk and roughly similar ages at exposure, and thus focus attention on other considerations, such as frequency of exposure, for abstracting exposure history into a summary dose value.

SUMMARY

Observed latencies for leukemia, lung cancer, and breast cancer among heavily exposed A-bomb survivors and controls are compared, by age at the time of the bomb (ATB). The previously observed tendency for leukemia to occur earlier in the heavily exposed than in controls of the same age ATB is confirmed, for those under 50 ATB but not for those aged 50 and over ATB. The latencies for high-dose lung cancer deaths and high-dose breast cancer incidence are similar to those among controls, even though these cancers occurred at higher rates among the heavily exposed. It is suggested that this contrast may be due to differences in the causation of these cancers: that many leukemias may have been caused solely by A-bomb radiation whereas lung and breast cancer, and other leukemias, may have been caused by radiation followed by other, age-related exposures. It is further suggested that in epidemiological studies relating cancer to occupational exposure history, latency models based on analogy to the occurrence of leukemia in heavily exposed A-bomb survivors may be inappropriate.

TABLE I. Numbers of persons, extended LSS sample, by age ATB, exposure status, and estimated dose in rads

Age ATB	Exposure Status						Total
	Not exposed	Exposed					
		0-9 rads	10-99 rads	100+ rads	Unk		
0-9	5015	10759	3687	820	302		20583
10-19	5978	11815	3398	1621	1117		23929
20-34	5671	10836	3599	1232	775		22113
35-49	6161	12664	4544	1313	583		25265
50+	3698	9060	3075	690	354		16877
Total	26523	55134	18303	5676	3131		108767

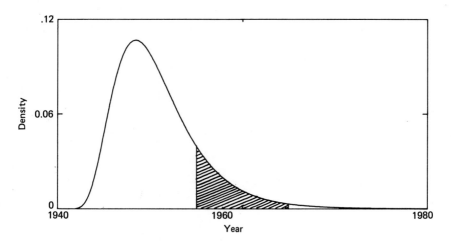

FIG. 1. Density function for lognormal latency distribution with 10-year median and log 1.5 standard deviation of logs, for an exposure in 1940. The shaded area under the curve is the weight to be given to the exposure for a 1955-1964 period of observation for risk, according to the method of Lundin, et al[6].

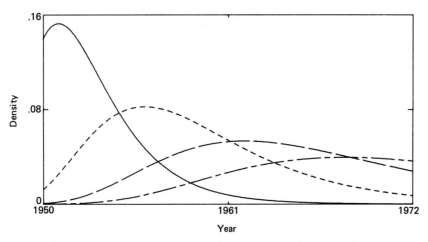

FIG. 2. Lognormal density curves, with common origin at 1945, standard deviation of logs = log 1.5, and separate medians = 7, 13, 20, and 27 years.

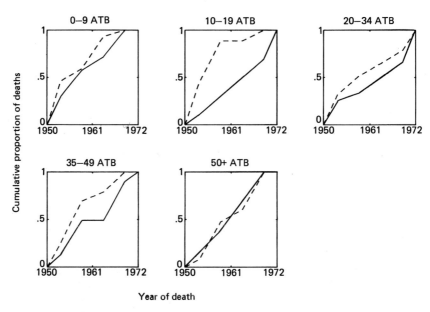

FIG. 3. Cumulative proportions over time of leukemia mortality, 1950-1972, by age ATB and dose: non-exposed + 0-9 rads (solid lines) vs. 100+ rads (dashed lines).

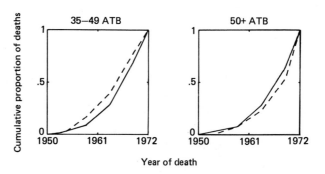

FIG. 4. Cumulative proportions over time of mortality from cancer of the bronchus, trachea, and lung, 1950-1972, by age ATB and dose: non-exposed + 0-9 rads (solid lines) vs. 100+ rads (dashed lines).

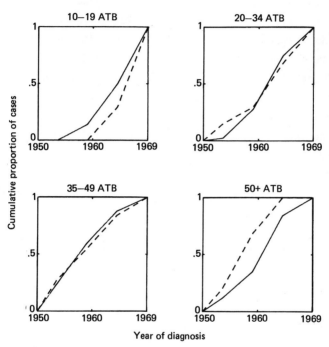

FIG. 5. Cumulative proportions over time of female breast cancer incidence, 1950-1969, by age ATB and dose: non-exposed + 0-9 rads (solid
line) vs. 100+ rads (dashed line).

REFERENCES

1. Armitage, P. and Doll, R.: Stochastic models for carcinogenesis. Proc. Fourth Berkeley Symposium on Mathematical Statistics and Probability, 4, 19-38. Berkeley and Los Angeles, University of California Press, 1961.

2. Doll, R.: Cancer and aging: the epidemiological evidence. Oncology 1970, Proceedings of the 10th International Cancer Congress, 5, 1-30. Chicago, Year Book Medical Publishers, 1971.

3. Bizzozero, O.H., Jr., Johnson, K.G. and Ciocco, A.: Distribution, incidence, and appearance time of radiation-related leukemia, Hiroshima-Nagasaki 1946-64. N Engl J Med 274: 1059-1102, 1966.

4. Ishimaru, T., Hoshino, T., Ichimaru, M., Okada, H., Tomiyasu, T., Tsuchimoto, T. and Yamamoto, T.: Leukemia in atomic bomb survivors, Hiroshima-Nagasaki, 1 October 1950 - 30 September 1966. Radiat Res 45: 216-233, 1971.

5. Ichimaru, M. and Ishimaru, T.: Leukemias and related disorders. J Radiat Res 16, Supplement: 89-96, 1975.

6. Lundin, F.E., Jr., Wagoner, J.K. and Archer, V.E.: Radon daughter exposure and respiratory cancer: quantitative and temporal aspects. Report from the Epidemiological Study of United States Uranium Miners. Nat. Inst. for Occup. Safety and Health, Nat. Inst. of Environ. Health Sciences Joint Monograph No. 1, 1971.

7. Albert, R.E. and Altshuler, B.: Considerations relating to the formulation of limits for unavoidable population exposures to environmental carcinogens. Radionuclide Carcinogenesis, Ballou, J.E. et. al. (Eds.), AEC Symposium Series, CONF-72050, NTIS, Springfield, Va., 233-253, 1973.

8. Enterline, P. and Henderson, V.: A model for extrapolating to low levels of asbestos exposure (Abstract). Presented at Conference on Problems of Extrapolating the Results of Laboratory Animal Data to Men and Extrapolating the Results from High Dose Level Experiments to Low Dose Level Exposure, Pinehurst, N.C., March 11, 1976.

9. Kerr, G.D.: Report of liaison studies with the Atomic Bomb Casualty Commission - Hiroshima, Japan, August 20, 1974 to September 17, 1974. ORNL-TM-4830, Oak Ridge National Laboratory, Oak Ridge, Tennessee, 1975.

10. Jablon, S. and Kato, H.: Studies of the mortality of A-bomb survivors. 5. Radiation dose and mortality, 1950-1970. Radiat Res 50: 649-698, 1972.

11. Beebe, G.W., Kato, H. and Land, C.E.: Studies of the mortality of
    A-bomb survivors, 4. Mortality and radiation dose, 1950-66. Radiat
    Res 613-649, 1971.
12. Moriyama, I. and Kato, H.: JNIH-ABCC life span study report 7,
    Mortality experience of A-bomb survivors. 1970-72, 1950-72. ABCC
    Technical Report 15-73, 1973.
13. McGregor, D.H., Choi, K., Tokuoka, S., Liu, P.I., Wakabayashi, T.,
    Land, C.E. and Beebe, G.W.: Breast cancer incidence among atomic
    bomb survivors, Hiroshima and Nagasaki, 1950-1969. In preparation.
14. Wanebo, C.K., Johnson, K.G., Sato, K. and Thorslund, T.W.: Breast
    cancer after exposure to the atomic bombings of Hiroshima and
    Nagasaki. N Engl J Med 279: 667-671, 1968.

Chapter 9

OCCUPATIONAL HAZARDS

FURTHER OBSERVATIONS ON CANCER MORTALITY AMONG CHEMISTS

Robert G. Olin M.D.

Department of Safety and Health
Royal Institute of Technology
Stockholm, Sweden

INTRODUCTION

The chemical industry has developed rapidly in recent decades, and
the use of chemicals has increased markedly in other branches of
industry as well. In Sweden, this development started out from a
relatively low level of chemical industrialization, but has now
kept pace with the development in other industrialized countries.
The acute hazards in the handling of chemicals, and these include,
for example, the dangers of fires and explosions, have been
recognized for a long time and have received due consideration in
the planning of work routines. The long-term hazardous effects of
chemicals on the other hand, have, in general, been ignored or
underestimated. This is probably due to a lack of knowledge of
toxicology and it´s practical applications amongst chemists, and
as a result chemists have generally disregarded possible long-term
hazards both when working in chemical laboratories themselves and
when participating, often in management positions, in the planning,
development and supervision of chemical processes. This often
fundamental lack of knowledge of the long-term effects of chemicals,
separately and in various combinations, constitutes primarily a
hazard for chemists themselves. Subsequently, however, a much larger

group of people are also exposed to varying degrees of risk in the
handling of these same chemicals, not only industrial workers, but
possibly even the consumers of the finished products.

PROCEDURES AND MATERIALS USED

The cohort consisted of those chemists who graduated from the
School of Chemical Engineering at the Royal Institute of Technology
(KTH) Stockholm, Sweden, between 1930 and 1950. 530 male students
graduated during this 21 year period. Their average age at the time
of graduation was 24.6 years.

The members of the group were traced through various registers until
December 1974. In these registers it was possible to trace 517 persons
belonging to the group whereas reliable information was not available for the remaining 13 persons (2,5 % of the sample). 58 had died
during the observation period and death certificates for these 58
chemists were received and examined. (Each of these certificates
was made out in Sweden). The study also contains an attempt to
investigate the occupational level of exposure to chemicals among
the chemists. A senior professor in analytical chemistry at the
Royal Institute of Technology, who has taught at this school since
the mid 1930´s felt that he could supply information on the occupations of the chemists in this study, subsequent to their graduation.
It should be mentioned that Sweden is a relatively small country
and that during the years investigated in this study, most of the
high-school chemists who subsequently pursued higher education in
chemistry in Sweden, did so at KTH. It was agreed that he would
operationally distinguish between persons who had been active with
any sort of laboratory work after graduation and those who had not
been. The latter group of so-called "non-chemists" contained for
instance chemists who had taken up management positions of some
kind. The distinctions were made without access to information on
wether the chemists in question were still alive or had died. The
"non-chemists" group consisted of 109 individuals and the other
group, the so called "chemist" group, consisted of 408 individuals.

"Life Tables from the Decade 1961-1970"[8] was used in order to determine the age-adjusted number of deaths in the population. To determine the specific mortality rates "Causes of Death"[4] from 1973 was used. (Here the relative frequency of cancers was higher in a comparison with earlier editions.) Chi-square values were computed to estimate the relative numbers of deaths due to different causes. For small numbers the Poisson distribution was applied. z-values and t-values were computed to estimate differences between various subgroups in the material.

RESULTS

In the study group there were 58 deaths, when 67 deaths were expected by comparison with the general population. (Table I). This difference is not significant. But there was a significantly high frequency of cancer deaths in the cohort, 22 cases whereas 13 were expected ($P < 0.02$). This difference was due to an excess of deaths from malignant lymphoma, 6 deaths compared with the 1.7 deaths expected ($P < 0.001$). Half of these tumours, or 3 deaths were attributed to Hodgkins disease. Cancers of the urinary organs (I.C.D. 188-189) were also more numerous ($P < 0.08$). No other cancer cause of death differed in frequency from the general population.

The high relative frequency of cancer deaths in the cohort was necessarily associated with a lower percentage of deaths in other categories, particularly the group accidents and suicides ($P < 0.05$).

The cohort was divided into a "chemist" and a "non-chemist" group. In the former there were 49 deaths compared with 9 deaths in the latter ($z=0.45$, not significant). But there were 21 deaths from cancer in the "chemist" group compared with just one death from cancer in the "non-chemist" group ($z=2.95$, $P < 0.002$).

During the observation period the average life span reduction was 1.75 years in the " chemist" group. For the "non-chemist" group the reduction was much smaller, 0.44 years ($t=2.16$, dF 500, $P < 0.05$).

849

DISCUSSION

With many good reasons there has lately been much speculation about
the effects of occupation on the health of the working class.[5,9,10]
However, until the study of King[6] there was little information about
the relationship between occupation and health among the learned
professions, such as medicine, law, teaching and the ministry. On
the basis of official statistics and study findings in 6 countries
over the past century King demonstrated consistent differences in
mortality from low among teachers and clergymen to relatively
high among lawyers and physicians. This was particularly true for
such causes as coronary heart disease, suicide and vascular lesions
of the central nervous system.

The Swedish chemists appear to exhibit a tendency to a lower mortality rate in comparison with the general population but this
difference is not significant. Here it must be pointed out that the
observation period so far is limited to 24-44 years after the year
of graduation which means that the oldest chemists in the study
were just above 70 years of age. As for the causes of death there
was a lower rate of death due to accidents. This result is not
surprising - a group of college-educated chemists very possibly
lead lives which in this context are more protected and privileged
than the general Swedish male population.

In a comparison of aneathesiologists with the general population
Bruce et al[3] found high mortality rates for suicides and malignancies of the lymphoid and reticuloendothelial tissues. In a national
study[2] in the USA the data suggest an increased ocurrence of cancer,
particularly of leukemia and lymphoma among the female members in
an operating room-exposed group. But this increased occurrence of
cancer was not verifiable in exposed male respondents. In 1969 Li
et al[7] studied the causes of death of 3.637 members of the American
Chemist Society who died between 1948 and 1967. (The study covered
78 % of the known decedents.) A significantly higher proportion of
deaths from cancer was found compared with the frequency among
other professional men. Nearly half the excess cancer deaths were
attributed to malignant lymphomas and cancer of the pancreas.

The increase in mortality as a result of neoplasms in general, and
the even more distinct increase in the frequency of malignant
lymphomas or leukaemias and especially of Hodgkin's disease, is
interesting. Chemical hazards as a contributing or decisive factor
in carcinogenesis, has in later years become a serious if disputed
hypothesis[5]. In the past year leuchaemias have been reported to
occur in an increasing number amongst certain chemical industry
workers, as well as in the populations living in the vicinity of
certain industries[11]. Theories other than the chemical carcinogenesis theory predominate in the case of Hodgkin's disease, but
there do exist studies[1] that have pointed to a role played by
chemical carcinogenesis even here. The hypothesis that contact with
chemical agents was the main reason for the excess cancer mortality
was strengthened when the history of chemical exposure was studied
retrospectively for the nine individuals (Table II) who had died
either of lymphoma or of cancer of the urinary organs (the kidney
or the bladder). Of the 9 chemists, 8 had been working within the
domain of organic chemistry for at least some years after graduation. (The 9th, who died of reticulosarcoma had taken up a management position in the chemical industry immediately after graduation
and had subsequently never had any known exposure to chemicals).

It must be pointed out that this study has some imperfections. The
total number of deaths was small. The number of deaths for certain
sub-groups of cancers was still smaller. It was impossible to
evaluate retrospectively the history of chemical exposure more than
arbitrarily for the college-educated chemists under observation.
For obvious reasons it has been impossible to evaluate retrospectively the smoking habits in the cohort. Table I shows, however, that
the frequency of lungcancer is low rather than high.

However, on the positive side, it was possible to trace almost
everyone in the study. Further, the results obtained here are in
good accordance with those of Li et al[7] and complement their results.
Specifically, those college-educated chemists who continue working
with organic compounds after graduation run an increased risk of

lymphoma/leukemia and possibly cancer of the urinary organs. - The study is currently expanded to include the approximately 350 chemists that were educated during the same period of time at Chalmers School of Chemical Engineering in Gothenburg, Sweden.

SUMMARY

The causes of death among the 58 chemists, who belonged to a cohort of 517 men who graduated from the School of Chemical Engineering at KTH, Stockholm during the years 1930 to 1950 were studied. The group was followed until the end of 1974. There was a significant increase of cancers, particularly of lymphomas (P < 0.001). Half of the latter cases were Hodgkin's disease. The study suggested that those chemists who continued with laboratory work for at least some years after their graduation and who then specifically worked with organic compounds exhibited an increased frequency of death from cancer, as well as a significant shortening of life.

TABLE I. Observed and Expected Deaths, Grouped According to the Cause of Death, Among Swedish College-educated Chemists Educated During 1930-1950 (group followed until Dec. 31, 1974)

Cause of death (I.C.D. no[*])		Obs	Exp	Chi-square values
Malignant neoplasms	(140-207)	22	13.0	6.39 (P < 0.02)
Digestive	(150-159)	6	4.5	-
Respiratory system	(160-164)	1	2.4	-
Urinary organs	(188-189)	3	1.0	(P < 0.08)[**]
Lymphatic/ haematopoetic	(200-207)	6	1.7	10.91 (P < 0.001)[***]
[Hodgkin's disease]	(201)	(3)	(0.3)	(P < 0.01)[**]
Circulatory	(390-458)	14	20.7	-
Ischaemic	(410-414)	7	15.2	4.56 (P < 0.05)
Respiratory	(460-519)	3	1.8	-
Digestive	(520-577)	2	4.0	-
Accidents, Suicides	(E800-959)	9	18.0	4.66 (P < 0.05)
All other causes		8	9.5	-
All		58	67	-

[*]   I.C.D. eigth revision

[**]   Poisson distribution

[***] using Poisson distribution, P 0.01

TABLE II. Causes of Death and Age Characteristics for Important
Neoplastic Deaths

CASE	DIAGNOSIS	I.C.D.	YEAR OF BIRTH	YEAR OF EXAM	YEAR OF DEATH
1.	Tumor renis	180.0	1907	1931	1960
2.	Tumor renis	180.0	1917	1941	1967
3.	Tumor vesic. urin.	181.0	1918	1942	1972
4.	Retikulosarcoma	200.0	1920	1943	1964)
5.	Lymphosarcoma	200.1	1913	1937	1939
6.	Lymphogran.mal.	201	1910	1933	1962
7.	Lymphogran.mal.	201	1914	1937	1947
8.	Lymphogran.mal.	201	1926	1949	1955
9.	Leukaemia myeloides	205.9	1917	1941	1949

REFERENCES

1. Aksoy M., Erdem S., Dincol K., Hepyüksel T. and Dincol G.:
   Chronic Exposure to Benzene as a possible Contributary
   Etiologic Factor in Hodgkin's Disease. Blut 28: 293-298, 1974.

2. ASA Ad Hoc Committee: Occupational Disease among Operating
   Room Personnel Anesthesiology, 41: 321-340, 1974.

3. Bruce D.L., Eide K.A., Linde H.W. and Eckenhoff J.E.: Causes
   of Death among Anesthesiologists: A 20-year survey. Anesthesiology, 29: 565-569, 1968.

4. Causes of Death 1973. Official Statistics of Sweden. Stockholm,
   1974.

5. Epstein S.S.: Environmental Determinants of Human Cancer.
   Cancer Research, 34: 2425-2435, Oct 1974.

6. King H.: Health in the Medical and Other Learned Professions.
   J. Chron. Dis., 23: 257-281, 1970.

7. Li F.P., Fraumeni J.F., Mantel N. and Miller R.W.: Cancer
   Mortality among Chemists. J. Natl. Cancer Inst., 43: 1159-1164,
   1969.

8. Life Tables from the Decade 1961-1970. Official Statistics of
   Sweden. Stockholm, 1974.

9. Selikoff I.J.: Recent Perspectives in Occupational Cancer.
   Ambio, 4: 14-17, 1975.

10. Stellman J.M., Daum S.M.: Work is Dangerous to Your Health.
    Vintage Books, New York, 1973.

11. Vigliani E.C.: Benzene and Leukemia. In: The New Multinational
    Health Hazards. ICF. Geneve, pp.196-201, 1975.

POTENTIAL CANCER RISK IN THE GRAPHIC ARTS AND TEXTILES INDUSTRIES[1,2]

Kingsley Kay, M. A., Ph.D.
Environmental Sciences Laboratory - Department of Community Medicine
Mount Sinai School of Medicine of the City University of New York
Fifth Avenue and 100th Street, New York, New York 10029

There have been epidemiological reports concerning elevated cancer incidence in the graphic arts industry. However, carcinogenicity evaluation of the chemicals characteristic of the industry has not been made on a comprehensive basis reflecting the many technical innovations in recent years. Studies on cancer incidence in textile dyeing, printing and finishing personnel appear not to have been made, yet many of the chemicals used in the graphic arts are also employed in preparing textiles for market. Accordingly, occupational environments in fifty printing, printing ink formulation, textile dyeing, printing and finishing concerns were surveyed in order to describe the current range of chemicals in use. The potential cancer risk was then assessed.

THE GRAPHIC ARTS INDUSTRY

Epidemiological studies on cancer in graphic arts personnel are summarized in Table 1. Some evidence of above-normal lung and laryngeal cancer incidence among printers in England was uncovered in 1947 by Kennaway and Kennaway(1). In 1955, Ask-Upmark (2) found the bronchogenic cancer incidence of a group of typographers to be eighteen times higher than normal (without adjustment for smoking habits.) Dunn and Weir (4) followed the cancer experience of several United States occupations progressively

1. Supported by - National Institute of Environmental Health Sciences
    Grant - ES 00928 and American Cancer Society Grant - R-53.

2. Portions of this paper dealing with the graphic arts will appear in
   Clinical Toxicology 9 (3), 1976.

and concluded in 1965 that printers did not show higher than normal incidence. Badger (3) has noted that printers employed in security work have been reported to have developed bladder tumors from exposure to benzidine used in security paper impregnation and printing materials in order to produce a visible stain when treated with fluids used in forgery. Beginning in 1970, the mortality of newspaper printers was examined by two investigating groups in New York (5,6). No significant differences between exposed and unexposed groups were found. Cole et al. (7) in a study of occupation and cancer of the lower urinary tract, did not find an excess of such cancers among printers. This confirmed the findings of Greenberg (8) from a 1952-1966 study of a group of 670 London newspaper workers which, however, showed a statistically significant excess of lung cancers without smoking adjustment. This finding was confirmed by Moss et al (9) in a group of 2000 newspaper worker deaths which included the 670 of Greenberg (8); excess of lung cancer was also found among 652 deaths of newspaper workers in Manchester (9). White collar worker deaths in the newspapers of these two areas showed no excess above normal. Concurrently, Lloyd et al. (10) compared observed and expected cancer deaths of 2,604 newspaper and commercial printing pressmen in the United States. Newspaper pressmen experienced a significant excess of buccal and pharyngeal cancers and an excess of emphysema deaths. Commerical printing pressmen (ages 20-54) had a significant excess of cancer of the pancreas, and an excess for rectal cancer with the estimated rate more than double expectation after age 64.

As Benzene (13-20), chloroform (21-2) and carbon tetrachloride (23-27) have been found carcinogenic, the foremost in man. A tentative finding of rodent carcinogenicity for trichlorethylene has been announced (28). Benzene was in use in rotogravure printing twenty-five years ago, at which time leucopenia cases occurred (29). Although the use of benzene in rotogravure was discontinued, Viadana and Bross (11) found evidence of an excess of leukemia incidence for printers over the years 1959-1962. No evidence linking chlorinated hydrocarbon solvents to cancer in graphic arts personnel has been uncovered.

Last year, Hoover and Fraumeni (12) found positive gradients for bladder and liver cancers associated with printing ink manufacturing areas.

Chemicals in the graphic arts industry.

The survey of printing and printing ink establishments[1] clearly showed that the number of pigments and dyes used in the graphic arts was almost overwhelming, in particular because each customer's specifications for the color and texture of the printed substrates had to be met. However, only a limited number of color compounds were used in substantial quantities. In the situation, the president of a major New York printing ink concern cooperated by analyzing the extent of use of color components in the manufacture of his printing inks. A list of thirty-seven used in largest quantity was provided. These are shown in Tables 2a-2c along with the data available for carcinogenic evaluation. The list was reviewed by the National Association of Printing Ink Manufacturers and was considered to be representative.

As shown in summarizing Table 3, there were four components cancer-positive in man or animals, 15 probable by virtue of chemical class and five were negative. The evidence was conflicting for four and on nine, no information could be found. The most important single positive was lead chromate, which alone, and in association with the molybdate salt, was used to the extent of 60% of the amount of titanium dioxide, the major ingredient of printing ink.

There were eleven azo colorants, with a degree of probability as carcinogens, since many azo compounds have been identified as neoplasia - producing. (41). The implications of this aspect will be examined in the discussion section.

Recent findings on laboratory animals introduce the possibility of nonmalignant kidney damage in persons exposed to not only lead pigments (78-81), but also benzidine-based colorants (82-85) and 2-aminoanthraquinone (86).

Several years ago 22 printing inks of unidentified composition were tested in England by subcutaneous injection in mice (87). Seventeen were negative. Five caused injection site neoplasms of which two showed metastases to the lung. Indeed as long ago as 1929, Steinbruck (88,89) painted mouse skin with a printing ink and produced skin epitheliomas with lung metastases, and lymphomas.

1. Anthony F. Sessa, N. Y. Typographic Union, No. 6 and Pat Dejanero, Local 447, Printing Pressmens' Union arranged plant visits.

Carbon black

Carbon black is used in large quantities in printing inks. It was noted in the printing ink establishments surveyed, that the manipulation of carbon black was highly contaminating to the handlers and generally was carried out in a separate room. Furthermore in newspaper printing, ink was seen to be heavily dispersed into the atmosphere - to such an extent that clean paper placed on printing equipment was very soon blackened by atmospheric fallout. Clearly printing ink was entering the lungs of exposed personnel. In 1950, Ingalls (90) examined the cancer experience of 677 carbon black workers and 353 associated service employees and failed to find a difference. No positive evidence for the carcinogenicity of carbon black in man has since been reported with the exception of unpublished results referred to by Gold (91) in which excess stomach cancer was found among rubber tire workers with a high carbon black exposure. Subsequent to the report of Ingalls (90) much investigation of the carcinogenicity of carbon black was carried out (49-56). It would appear that apart from source differences, biological activity is dependent on particle size and adsorptivity (52). Carbon blacks of average particle diameter 17mμ tenaciously held added benzo[a]pyrene and were biologically inactive. However, the presence of the eluent tricaprylin evoked carcinogenicity at site of subcutaneous injection. It would have to be determined whether the high boiling oils used with carbon black in inks would also act as eluents for cancer-producing chemicals adsorbed on the carbon. Nau et al. (55) found no malignancies in monkeys lengthily exposed to carbon black by inhalation notwithstanding that extracts of carbon black produced cancer when applied to the skin of mice (54). More recently injection site fibrosarcomas have been produced in mice (8). An extensive range of polycyclic aromatic hydrocarbons has been found in benzene eluents but only after many hours of refluxing (91-93). However, not all are carcinogens (94).

Solvents

In the printing establishments visited, the chlorinated hydrocarbon solvents, methyl chloroform and methylene chloride were employed for hand cleaning of typeface. It was an operation with substantial, albeit intermittent, exposure for the typeface cleaner and adjacent workers.

High volatility solvents are used in formulation of inks for flexography
and gravure where fast drying is required. Benzene was featured in these
applications until its high toxicity toward the blood and blood forming
organs was recognized (13-20). None was found during the plant survey,
having apparently been replaced by toluene which, however, is usually
contaminated with samll quantities of benzene. An extensive range of
petroleum hydrocarbon solvents was seen in use, but none had been reported
carcinogenic. Nevertheless the occurrence of a number of cases of rare
Reye's syndrome following spraying with petroleum solvent-based material,
has been reported from Nova Scotia. Subsequent experiments with mice
showed that their susceptibility to virus infection was greatly increased
(95).

Polymers and solventless ink

Many well-known polymers are used in printing inks to bind pigment to the
printed surface. Conventional plasticizers and oxidation accelerators
are also ink ingredients. The newest development in the graphic arts
industry at the time of this survey was vinyl-based solventless ink cured
by addition polymerization with ultraviolet radiation. This ink was for
use in photolithography and plate coatings. Solventless ink formulas are
proprietary so the patent literature was relied upon by Vanderhoff (96)
who reported on the subject this year. Among an extensive array of solventless ink chemicals were, formaldehyde resins, halogenated photoin-
itiators, benzophenone, anthraquinone and styrene, all with chemical
relatives that, have been found cancer associated. Another component,
minor by weight proportion (a few per cent) was Michler's ketone shown to
be mutagenic to Drosophila larvae as long ago as 1946 (97).

Ball point and felt-pen inks

Ink making and filling of ball point and felt pens ia an aspect of the
writing instruments industry. Ink flow clog resistance and drying present
unique application problems. A review of recent patents indicates that
alkylene glycols are widely used as vehicles. Pigments and dyes are comparable to those used in printing inks. Binders include allyl alcohol -
styrene polymers, formaldehyde - ketone and urea - formaldehyde resins.

TEXTILE DYEING, PRINTING AND FINISHING

Studies on cancer incidence in textile dyeing, printing and finishing
personnel appear not to have been made, yet many of the chemicals used in
the graphic arts are also employed in preparing textiles for market. For
this reason, technological developments that might bear on safety and
health of persons in these occupational categories have been examined by
plant surveys of fifteen establishments in the New York - New Jersey area.
Additionally, consultations have been held with managements, engineering
specialist, chemists, the American Association of Textile Chemists and
Colorists, the American Dye Manufacturers Association, National Cancer
Institute and the International Agency for Research on Cancer. Tie dyeing
chemicals and techniques were explored with New York crafts specialists.
The plant survey was arranged through the auspices of Mr. Eric Frumin of
the Textile Workers Union.

From the plant visits it was apparent that textile printing and finishing
are frequently carried out in the same space as dyeing. Furthermore, it
seemed likely that certain combinations of conditions in all three processes will be hazardous to health even though gross ill-effects are not
being reported in the medical literature currently. Craft specialists
work at home customarily. Contamination of living space with colorants
seems to be prevalent.

Technical observations

The processes of dyeing, printing and finishing have been designed according to the physics and chemistry of fiber types, dyes and finishing
materials. Thus, a wide variety of chemicals was found being applied under a wide variety of conditions, as indicated in Table 4. It was observed that elevated temperatures were frequently used in open vats and ovens,
this being conducive to the dissemination of chemicals into the work
environment. Preparation of fabric for dyeing or printing was found to
require chemical and enzyme (amylolytic) detergents, alkalis, sodium per-
oxide and hypochlorite bleaches, and organic solvents to remove waxes
from natural fibers, sizes (polysaccharides, and polyvinyl alcohol, poly-
acrylics and methacrylics), and spinning oils from both natural and synthetic fibers. Hot solutions are used at most stages of cleaning as well
as dyeing. It was noted in the plants visited, that air was hot, humid
and of poor quality because most of the processes are open.

Dyeing

Dyeing (and printing) is accomplished by selecting colorant which is chemically and physically compatible with fibers. Other chemicals are used to promote the coloring process with the different classes of dyes. Among the many assisting chemicals, mention may be made of sulfuric acid, used to promote acid dye retention in wool; sodium ethylenediaminetetra-acetate and sodium thiocyanate for protecting dyes against metal ions originating from metal equipment; sulfonated wetting agents to assist in penetration of dyes; sodium dichromate pretreatment for fixing dye in fibers; optical brighteners such as diaminostilbenes and vinylene bis-benzimidazoles to combat discoloration (see section on optical brighteners). Formaldehyde and dichromates are used as after-treatment chemicals for dye fixing.

Textile printing

Textile printing has for some years consisted of surface application of dyes in paste form (localized dyeing) by photogravure or extrusion through appropriately designed screens. The liquid component of the pastes has been water and some water-miscible hygroscopic solvents (alcohols) to increase the solubility of the dye and to absorb moisture during subsequent steaming. Another component is thickener, generally alginate or gum to produce a sharp outline and smooth coverage of the printed design. As in dyeing there are assistant or auxiliary chemicals. Dried prints are generally not fast to washing. Ageing with steam to fix dyes in prints, and chemical after-treatment to develop colors, are common. There are three notable differences between textile printing and dyeing. The water of the dyebath is replaced by steam. The time required to fix the dye inside the fiber is comparatively short in printing. The dye in printing is highly concentrated hence many dyes have too low a solubility for application as a paste.

Dyes, like many other organic substances, vaporize below their melting points and condense on nearby cold surfaces (sublimation). Transfer printing a recently developed and much-favored printing process, is based upon sublimation of dye from printed paper to adjacent textile by use of heat or vacuum. Consultation with the heat transfer specialists of a prominent ink company indicates that the hazard from inhalation of vaporized dye by operators of this process has not been evaluated.

Finishing

Finishing (sometimes meant to include dyeing, printing and coating) refers mainly to crease resistance and water repellancy treatments with chemicals. Mechanical finishing involves tentering to restore desired width after processing and surface mechanical treatment to increase hairiness or luster.

Water repellants of many types are applied in finishing as, for instance. waxes, silicones, alkanolamines and fluoroacrylate polymers. The most commonly used crease-proofing agents are urea-based as for instance, DMEU (dimethylolethylene urea). Methylol carbamates are also employed as well as melamines. Production of resin with formaldehyde must take place within the fibers. Zinc boron fluoride is one catalyst in the process and there are other assistant chemicals. Application of resins from chlorinated hydrocarbon solvents has shown technical advantage.

During the course of the investigation, the National Institute of Occupational Safety and Health reported the finding of the potent cancer-producing chemical bis-chloromethylether in the atmospheres of several dyeing and finishing plants. It has been known for some time that formaldehyde, commonly used in dyeing and finishing, can under certain circumstances combine with chlorine to form this potent carcinogen (98). It was found that magnesium chloride has been widely used as a catalyst in finishing and could represent a source of chlorine.

Carcinogenicity of textile dyes

While pigments predominate in ink formulation, dyes are generally used as textile colorants. However, pigments can be used for textile printing if bonded to the fabric with resins. For instance, glass fibers will not take up dyes but can be colored with resin-bonded pigments. As was the case in printing ink manufacture, textile dyes are formulated to each customer's specification. Hence the formulating laboratories of the establishments surveyed had literally thousands of dyes in stock but, owing to proprietory considerations, it was not possible to secure a list of dyes used most frequently and in largest amounts. As an alternative, the statistics on production and sale of dyes issued by the International Tariff Commission were relied on (99). The 46 used in largest quantity had been selected in 1971 for an on-going American Dye Manufacturer's

Institute study of water pollution control by the industry (100). An attempt was made to evaluate these dyes for carcinogenicity by literature search as well as by consultation with the National Cancer Institute and the International Agency for Research on Cancer. Carcinogenic data was found on only three out of the 46 (see Table 5) but 22 had cancer-associated chemical relatives. Available experimental data has been summarized in Table 6. No human data was found on any of the forty six. The structures of the six dyes on which experimental data was uncovered, are shown in Fig. 1. Rinde and Troll (40) had fed three of these dyes - Direct black 38, Direct brown 95 and Direct Blue 6 to Rhesus monkeys and identified carcinogenic benzidine as a urinary metabolic product, corresponding to around 1% of the ingested dye. The significance will be explored in the discussion to this paper. Direct blue 6 had many years before been found to produce injection site tumors (groin) without metastases in two out of ten rats treated weekly over a period of 200 days (103), indicating a weak carcinogenic response in the probable presence of carcinogenically active benzidine (40) as a direct blue 6 metabolite.

Another 320 compound in the list of 46 - Disperse yellow 3, formed by azotization of aminoacetanilide and p-cresol - produced bladder cancers in mice on implantation (102). Reports of tests of two other dyes in the list were found in the literature. One of these, Vat green 1, an anthraquinone derivative (see Tables 5, 6 and fig. 1) was found negative in rats after subcutaneous injection in an experiment of 300 days duration (101). Another compound, Basic green 4, proved positive on the basis of subcutaneous implantation of mammary and lung cancers from treated female rats into their progeny (104).

Flame retardants (FR)

Government standards of fire resistance for textiles (e.g. The 1967 amendment to the Flammable Fabrics Act of 1953) have stimulated active development of treatment chemicals particularly of the durable and semi-durable types. Furthermore, the widening variety of man-made textile fibers has increased the technical complexity of the problem because FR chemicals have different suitabilities and effectiveness depending upon the composition of the textiles. The result has been that hundreds of FR treatment chemicals have been introduced over a relatively short period of time (105), some to be padded, on others incorporated into the polymer mix when fibers are spun. However, only a limited number of entities have proved commercially viable. For example, although LeBlanc (105) lists 13 durable finishes for cellulosic apparel, nine are based on tetrakis (hydroxymethyl) phosphonium chloride (THPC) or derivatives; for polyesters and polyester/cotton blends, tris (2,3-dibromopropyl) phosphate (TRIS) has the bulk of the current market including children's sleepwear. Chlorinated paraffin wax (40 to 70% chlorine) with antimony oxide as an afterglow inhibitor, have been widely used in outdoor military and industrial applications (106).

Direct carcinogenicity assessment of FR chemicals appears not to have been part and parcel of their preparation for the textile market - or for that matter an aspect of their acceptability under law, inspite of the fact of their intimate contact with wearers' skin and their escape into the air as part of respirable fibers and particles resulting from wear abrasion.

Notwithstanding, the foregoing evidence on carcinogenicity of some structural relatives of FR chemicals has recently alerted governments to the importance of carcinogenicity testing in the FR field. Mutagenicity studies on several flame retardants were recently initiated by EPA (107) and have already shown the compound TRIS to be mutagenic for histidine - deficient strains of Salmonella typhimurium, TA-100 and TA-1535 (base pair substitution mutations). Three known contaminants of TRIS were also found mutagenic (TA-1535) viz; 1,2-dibromo-3-chloropropane; 1,2,3-tribromo-propane; and 2,3-dibromopropanol (108).

Tables 7 and 8 (from ref. 106) show the variety of halogenated and organophosphorus flame retardants currently available. In this context it is important to recall that there are a substantial number of carcinogenic chemical relatives of such compounds. Neoplasia - inducing halogenated hydrocarbons (rodents) have been described in recent years among the chlorinated hydrocarbon solvents (chloroform (21-2), trichlorethylene (28) and carbon tetrachloride (23-27), and the pesticides (DDT)(109-115), aldrin(116-117), dieldrin (109,116-119), the benzene hexachlorides (109, 120-122), polychlorinated biphenyls and triphenyls (123-125), pentachloronitrobenzene, Mirex, Strobane and ethyl 4,4-dichlorobenzilate (112), Kepone (126), the fumigants, ethylene dibromide and 1,2-dibromo-3-chloropropane (127-130). The propellant vinyl chloride has proved to be carcinogenic in both man (131) and laboratory models (132). Vinyl chloride as well as the FR copolymer, vinyl bromide, have been found to have alkylating metabolic products (132a).

The pesticidal organic phosphates, Dipterex (phosphonic acid (2,2,2-trichloro-1-hydroxyethyl) - dimethylester and dimethoate (0,0-dimethyldithiophosphorylacetic acid) have been found carcinogenic (133-135). Dichlorvos (phosphoric acid, 2,2-dichlorovinyl dimethylester) has been repeatedly shown to be alkylating in vitro (136-139), in E. coli (140) in mice (140) and in rats (141). It has been shown to induce abnormalities in rat sperm (142). Nevertheless, dichlorvos has not yet been found carcinogenic, possibly because of its high rate of in vivo metabolism (143). In this respect a parallel with alkylating and mutagenic formaldehyde exists (144).

It has been noted experimentally (p. 4-18, ref 106) that some of the THPC finishes give off formaldehyde, hydrogen chloride and anticholinesterase organic phosphorus compounds for up to two months after textile finishing. The possibility that the carcinogen, bis-chloromethyl ether, may be formed (98) during or after finishing has to be entertained pending necessary confirmatory experimental work.

As stated before, tetrakis (hydroxymethyl) phosphonium compounds dominate cotton FR finishing along with Ciba-Geigy's Pyrovatex FR (based on N-methylol dimethyl phosphonopropionamide). This latter treatment is applied by padding on the fabric, drying and curing briefly at 175°C. It is used with a triazine resin (106). As will be seen in Table 9, there are a number of THPC treatments which also involve the use of the triazine derivatives, trimethylolamine and TEPA (2,4,6-tris [1-aziridinyl] phosphine oxide). It is well known that TEPA has mutagenic (145), tumor inhibitory (146) and antifertility properties (147-148). On this account it must be regarded as a potentially hazardous substance for use in treatment of clothing textiles. Similarly, trimethylolmelamine has been reported to have mutagenicity for Drosophila (149,150), antitumor (151,152) and cytostatic activity (153-154). Tests for carcinogenicity gave equivocal results (153). Nevertheless, carcinogenic activity has been demonstrated for nitrogen mustards (155,156) to which trimethylolmelamine compares by virtue of its tumor inhibitory and cytotoxic activity. Trimethylolmelamine produced chromosome fragmentation in Walker 256 tumors and "bridge" formation qualifying the compound as radiomimetic. Its cytotoxic effects were also pronounced in proliferating tissues such as bone marrow, lymphoid and germinal epithelium.

Attention is directed to Table 10 (from ref. 106) listing a number of inorganic chemicals used in non-durable flame and glow-proofing. Only sodium arsenate used to the extent of 33 parts by weight per 100 parts fabric
might engender concern in light of recent findings on arsenical cancer
associates (157).

Fluorescent whitening agents (FWA)

These agents, used to correct discoloration and to enhance whiteness and
brightness, have been applied widely, especially with polymeric substances.
Fluroescence of the violet-blue bands produced by these agents, is best
for correcting yellow discoloration. The materials may be applied to textiles in detergents, at the dyeing and finishing stages by padding and
curing - or can be incorporated into synthetic fibers during polymerization in the melt, in solvent solution, or after spinning while the
fiber is in a swollen condition. Concentrations around one-tenth percent
are used. Reactive brighteners may be copolymerized with monomers or
prepolymers (158). Clearly there is exposure of the skin and respiratory
tract to fluorescent whitening agents in textiles. Hence their toxicolog-
ical and carcinogenic evaluation is important.

Table 12 lists fluorescent whitening agents used by major detergent manufacturers. Figure 2 gives the structures of 14 types differing widely in
chemical composition. Table 12 lists the chemical names of the 14
structures (from ref. 158).

Neukomm and DeTrey (159), Snyder et al (160), Bingham and Falk (161,162)
and Forbes and Urbach (163-165) have tested various fluorescing agents
for carcinogenicity with negative results. However Bingham and Falk (161)
found that the three agents 3-benzyl-4-methyl-7-hydroxycoumarin; disodium
4,4'-bis-(2,4-dimethoxybenzamido)-2,2'-stilbenedisulphonate; and disodium
4,4'-bis-(4,6-dianilino-s-triazin-2-yl)amino-2,2'-stilbenedisulphonate,
enhanced the carcinogenic potency of germicidal ultraviolet radiation
using mice, results which Forbes and Urbach (163-165) were unable to confirm last year using four different stilbene derivatives, sodium 2-(4-
styryl-3-sulphophenyl)-2H-naphtho[1,2-d[triazole;disodium 4,4-bis-[(4-
anilino-6-morpholino-1,3,5-triazin-2-yl)amino]stilbene-2,2'-disulphonate;
disodium 4,4'-bis-([4-anilino-6-(N-methyl-2-hydroxyethylamino)-1,3,5-

triazin-2-yl]amino)stilbene-2,2'-disulphonate;disodium4,4'-bis-(2-sul-
phostyryl)biphenyl.

Apart from the possibility that further demonstrations of synergism between ultraviolet radiation and fluorescent brightening agents may be
made, it is noteworthy that the most widely used agents contain both triazinyl and stilbene moieties which have been central in certain reported
carcinogens (p.8 and p.280, ref. 41) The existing literature on carcinogenicity testing of FR agents consitutes a meager examination of the
potential carcinogenicity of the wide variety of chemicals used in such
intimate contact with the body, especially since governmental regulations
dictate the use of FR chemicals in the clothing of the very young.

DISCUSSION

Table 13 shows that many chromophores are cancer-associated in pigments
and dyes. However,reference to Tables 3 and 5 will show how few pigments
and dyes have been tested for carcinogenicity on animals models or evaluated as etiological agents of cancer in man. Furthermore, 37 out of the
83 pigments and dyes covered in the Tables belong to chemical classes in
which carcinogens have been found. Notably, 30 of the 37 are colorants
containing the azo chromophore (-N=N-) first found cancer-associated in
a disazo dye, Scarlet Red, in 1924 (167). Many years before, Scarlet Red
had been used to promote the healing of epithelial wounds and had been
shown to be tissue-proliferating in a manner reminiscent of malignant
growth (168). Stoeber (169) and Hayward (170) established that the pro-
liferation-inducing segment of Scarlet Red was o-aminoazotoluene identified many years later as a carcinogen (171). This Scarlet Red fragment
could only have been produced by breaking the double bond in one azo group.
Shortly thereafter Butter Yellow, a dye of simpler structure -4- dimethyl-
aminoazobenzene(DAB) was found potently carcinogenic in rodents (172).

Stevenson et al (173) then showed that DAB was metabolized to urinary N-
acetyl-p-aminophenol and N,N'-diacetyl-p-phenylenediamine, indicating reductive cleavage of the azo linkage, ring hydroxylation and N-demethyla-
tion. These processes have since been identified, along with N-oxygen-
ation, in the metabolism of other azo dyes. For example carcinogenic 3,3-
dimethylbenzidine was shown to occur in metabolism of tryptan blue indicating cleavage of the two azo linkages (174).

869

It was shown by Kensler (175,176) in 1947 that the azo linkage in DAB was reduced by rat liver slices and that riboflavin content directly correlated with the reductive cleavage. Further work, by Mueller and Miller (177-179) indicated the existence of a hepatic microsomal reductase enzyme. However there is conflicting evidence as to whether the level of this enzyme correlates quantitatively with carcinogenicity (p.243, ref 41).

As noted previously, Rinde and Troll (40) showed last year that some disazobenzidine dyes fed to monkeys were metabolized to benzidine in small proportion (1 percent of ingested) as evidenced by the finding of urinary benzidine. Three of their disazobenzidine dyes direct black 38, direct brown 95 and direct blue 6 are included in Table 6. There were two diasotized 3,3'dichlorobenzidine colorants among the 37 major ink constituents (Tables 2a and 2c). 3,3-dichlorobenzidine has been shown to be carcinogenic - thus far only in rats (39).

Gut microorganisms also play a role in the metabolism of azo dyes. This was demonstrated in vivo by Radomski and Mellinger (180) using water-soluble azo food dyes and by Yoshida and Miyakawa (181) with azotized benzidine dyes.

The carcinogenic significance of the metabolism of the azo dyes by whatever route, rests in part on whether the diazotized constituents were themselves carcinogens. Benzidine is a well-known human and animal bladder carcinogen. While it has not been demonstrated in laboratory models that the occurrence of urinary benzidine correlates with production of bladder cancer when diazotized benzidine is ingested, it is perhaps significant that Yoshida and Miyakawa (181) observed a high incidence of bladder concer in Japanese kimono painters using azobenzidine dyes under personal conditions conducive to ingestion of the dyes (licking paint brushes to a point).
Obviously further investigation will be required to improve the data base for estimating the carcinogenic implications in the conversion of azobenzidine dyes to benzidine by bacteria of the duodenum (181) and or microsomes of the liver (182). In regard to the stilbene dyes, it should be noted that the ethylenic linkage (Table 13) does not undergo metabolic cleavage (p.247, ref 41).

The two azoic dyes shown in Table 13, Para Red and Dinitroaniline Orange

are p-nitroaniline and 2.4-dinitroaniline monazo pigments, azotized with
2-naphthol.(There is no evidence of their carcinogenicity in the literature). Presumably they can be cleaved at the azo linkage by bacterial and
hepatic microsomal enzyme action. This would yield 1-amino-2-naphthol in
both instances, and the original aniline associates would be regenerated.
Neither of the aniline compounds has been reported to be carcinogenic but
1-amino-2-naphthol has been found carcinogenic by bladder implantation
(166). As with the azotized benzidine dyes, the neoplastic significance
will presumably rest, at least in part, on the amount ingested and the
extent of conversion by azo cleavage.

TABLE 1. Studies of Cancer Among Graphic Arts Workers, 1955-1975

Investigators	Occupation	Target organ	Ref.
Kennaway and Kennaway, 1947	Printers	Lung and larynx	1
Ask-Upmark, 1955	Typographers	Bronchogenic	2
Badger, 1962	Printers-security work	Bladder	3
Dunn and Weir, 1965	Printers	Negative	4
Goldstein et al., 1970	Newspaper printers	Negative	5
Pasternack and Ehrlich, 1972	Newspaper printers	Negative	6
Cole et al., 1972	Printers	No urinary tract	7
Greenberg, 1972	Newspaper printers	Lung	8
Moss et al., 1972	Newspaper printers	Lung	9
Lloyd et al., 1972	Newspaper, commercial printers	Buccal, pharyngeal, pancreas, rectum	10
Viadana and Bross, 1972	Printers	Leukemia	11
Hoover and Fraumeni, 1975	Printing ink makers	bladder, liver	12

TABLE 2. A Summary of Findings on the Carcinogenicity of Thirty-Seven Major Printing Ink Constituents

Name of Component	Generic name	CI number[1]	Chemical class	Usage as % TiO_2	Species	Route of entry to the body	Exposure or dose level	Duration	Target organs	Lit.refs.
Titanium dioxide	CL pigment white 6	77891	Inorganic	100	-	-	-	-	-	No refs.
Lead chromate	No name	77600	$PbCrO_4$	40	Man rats	Inhalation subcatan.	Occupatnl. 10% aqu.	Years 37 weeks	Lung Inj. site	30-33
Molybdate orange	CI pigment red 104	77605	$PbCrO_4$-$PbMoO_4$	20	See above	See above	See above	See above	See above	30-33
Phthalo-cyanine blue	CI pigment blue 15	74160	Copper complex	20	Mice	Sub-cutaneous	0.5mg/wk.	8 months	Nil	34
Calcium carbonate	No name	No number	$CaCO_3$	20	-	-	-	-	-	No refs.
Diarylide	CI pigment yellow 12	21090	Disazo benzidine[2]	15	Some disazobenzidines reduce (hepatic azoreductase) to carcinogenic 3,3'-dichlorobenzidine.					35-40 41(p.241)
Alkali blue	CI acid blue 110	42750	Triphenyl methane deriv	15	A variety of members of this chemical class have been found to be carcinogenic					41(p. 22) 42-47
Clay	No name	No number	Silicates	15	-	-	-	-	-	No refs.
Barium sulfate	CI pigmen red 49	77120	$BaSO_4$	15	-	-	-	-	-	No refs.
Lithol red	CI pigmer red 49	15630	Monoazo Na sal	10	Rats	Ingestion	0-1% of diet	2 years	Nil	48
Iron blue	CI pigment blue 27	77510	Ferric Ferroxyanide	10	-	-	-	-	-	No. ref.
Carbon	No name	No number	Elemental	10	Mice	Skin surf. subcatan.	Various	To 20 mos.	Skin Injec. site	49-56

1. Assigned by British Society of Dyers and Colourists, and the American Association of Textile Dyers and Colorists. Published as the Color Index.

2. 3,3'-dishlorobenzidine → acetoacetanilide.

TABLE 2 (Continued)

Name of Components	Generic name[1]	CI number[1]	Chemical class	Usage as % TiO_2	Species	Route of entry to the body	Exposure or dose level	Duration	Target organs	Lit Refs.
Magnesium carbonate	CI pigment white 18	77713	Inorganic	10	-	-	-	-	-	No refs.
Red lake C	CI pigment red 53	15585	Monoazo Ba salt	7	Rats	Ingestion	0-1% diet Ba salt	2 years	Nil	57
Lithol rubine	CI pigment red 57	15850	Monoazo Ba salt	7	Related members of this chemical class found carcinogenic.					41(p.200)
BON red	CI pigment red 52	15860	Monoazo Ba salt	7	Related members of this chemical class found carcinogenic.					41(p.200)
Red 2B	CI pigment red 48	15865	Monoazo Ba salt	5	Related members of this chemical class found carcinogenic.					41(p.200)
Rhodamine[2]	CI basic red 1	45160	Xanthene derivative	5	Conflicting experimental evidence					41(p.23)58
Methyl Violet	CI basic Violet 1	42535	Triaryl methane	5	Conflicting experimental evidence					41(p.22) 42-47,59
Victoria blue	CI basic blue 7	42595	Triaryl methane	5	A variety of members of this chemical class have been found to be carcinogenic.					41(p.22) 42-47
Phythalocyanine green	CI pigment green 7	74260	Chlorinated Cu complex	5	-	-	-	-	-	No refs.
Aluminum hydrate	CI pigment white 24	77002	Al_2O_3 and $Al_2(SO_4)_3(OH)_2$	5	Various experimental protocols				Nil	60-65
Phloxine red	CI acid red 87	45380	Xanthene derivitive	3	Conflicting experimental evidence					41(p.23)
Naphthol red	CI pigment red 22	12315	Monoazo	2	Related members of this chemical class found carcinogenic.					41(p.200)

1. Assigned by British Society of Dyers and Colourists, and the American Association of Textile Dyers and Colorists. Published as the Color Index.

2. Constitution number covers rhodamine 6G in the Color Index.

Name of component	Generic name[1]	CI number[1]	Chemical class	Usage as % TiO$_2$	Species	Route of entry to the body	Exposure or dose level	Duration	Target organs	Lit. refs.
Magenta[2]	CI basic violet 10	45170	Xanthene deritivite	2	Conflicting experimental evidence					41(p.23),46, 47,58,66-70
Hansa Yellow	CI pigment yellow 1	11680	Monoaze	2	Related members of this chemical found carcinogenic					41(p.200)
Bronze powder	CI pigment metal 2	77400	Copper-zinc - iron alloy	2	-	-	-	-	-	No refs.
Aluminum powder	No name	No number	Elemental	2	Various experimental protocols				Nil	62, 64, 71-73
Silica aerogel	No name	No number	SiO$_2$ amorphous	2	-	-	-	-	-	No refs.
Cadmium red	CI pigment red 108	77196	Cadmium selenide	<1	Other cadmium salts have been found carcinogenic to animals					32, 74, 75
Fire red	CI pigment red 4	12085	Monoazo	<1	Related members of this chemical class found carcinogenic					41(p.200)
Para red	CI pigment red 1	12070	Monoazo	<1	Related members of this chemical class found carcinogenic					41(p.200)
Toluidine red	CI pigment red 3 13	12120	Monoazo	<1	Related members of this chemical class found carcinogenic					41(p.200)
Diarylide orange	CI pigment orange 13	21110	Disazo benzidine[3]	<1	Some disazobenzidines reduce (hepatic azoreductase) to carcinogenic 3,3'-dichlorobenzidine					35-40 and 41(p.241)
Dinitroaniline orange	CI pigment orange 5	12075	Monoazo	<1	Related members of this chemical class found carcinogenic					41(p.200)
Cadmium yellow	CI pigment yellow 37	77199	Cadmium sulfide	<1	Rats	Subcutan. intramusc.	25mg single 50mg single	Up to 15 months	Injection site	74-75
Talc	-	-	Silicate	<1	Man	Inhalation	Various	Years	Lungs	76-77

1. Assigned by British Society of Dyers and Colourists, and the American Association of Textile Dyers and Colorists. Published in the Color Index. 2. The constitution number covers rhodamine B in the Color Index, where magenta is either CI basic violet 14 (42510) or the phosphotungstomolybdic acid salt of rhodamine B (45170:2) listed as magenta lake B. CI basic violet 14 is a triphenylmethane triamino derivitive.
3. 3,3-dichlorobenzidine → 3-methyl-1-phenyl-5-pyrazolone.

TABLE 3. Condensed Assessment of the Carcinogenicity[1] of 37 Printing Ink Color-related Components Including Usage as Percentage of TiO$_2$ Used

Positive	% TiO$_2$	Probable	% TiO$_2$	Conflicting evidence	% TiO$_2$	Negative[3]	% TiO$_2$	No Information[4]	% TiO$_2$
Lead chromate	40	2 disazo benzidines	15 <1	3 xanthenes	10	Phthalo-cyanine blue	20	Titanium dioxide	–
Lead chromate-lead moly-bdate	20	2 triaryl methanes	20	1 triaryl methane	3	2 Monoazos	17	Calcium carbonate	20
Carbon black	10	9 Monoazos	25			Aluminum hydrate	5	Clay	15
Cadmium sulfide	<1	Cadmium selenide	<1			Aluminum powder	2	Barrium sulfate	15
		Talc	<1					Ferric Ferrocyanide	10
								Magnesium carbonate	10
								Chlorinated copper complex	5
								Bronze powder	2
								Silica aerogel	2
Total 4	70+	Total 15	60+	Total 4	15	Total 5	44	Total 9	79

1. In man and/or laboratory animals. 2. A variety of members of these chemical classes have been found carcinogenic. 3. Negative to the extent tested (see Tables 2a to 2c for details). 4. No information on these or related members of their chemical classes.

TABLE 4. A Digest of the Processes Observed in Textile Dyeing, Printing and Finishing New York - New Jersey 1975

Processes	Potentially toxic chemicals
Fabric preparation	
bleaching boiling singeing mercerizing(cotton)	spinning oils wax solvents hypochlorites sizes(acrylics and polyvinyl alcohol)
Dyeing and Printing	
formulating coloring rinsing fixing curing drying	Azo and other dyes, formic, acetic and sulfuric acids, hydro- sulfites, sodium sulfide, chromium fluoride and dichromate fixatives, stilbene and triazine fluorescent brighteners, antidulling thiocyanate, chloride assistants, etc.
Finishing	
tentering hairiness and lustre development water repellency crease resistance fire retardant treatment	dimethylolethyleneurea, formaldehyde, carbamates, zinc boron fluoride catalyst, chlorinated hydrocarbon resin solvents, alkanolamines, fluoroacrylate polymers, vinylbromide co- polymers, organic phosphates

TABLE 5. Condensed Information Currently Available on the Carcinogenicity[a] of 46 Major Dyes Including Annual Production as Millions of Pounds[b]

Positive	Pds. x 10^6	Probable[c]	Pds. x 10^6	No Information[e]	Pds. x 10^6
Disperse yellow 3 (monoazo)	2.6	Direct black 38 (azobenzidine)	6.1	Three structure unknown	3.5
Direct blue 6 (azobenzidine)	0.6	Direct brown 95 (azobenzidine)	0.8	Disperse yellow 42 (nitro)	1.4
Basic green 4 (triarylmethane)	0.5	Fluorescent brightener 28 (aminostilbene)	1.7	10 anthraquinones[d]	16.1
		Basic violet 1 (triarylmethane)	1.3	Direct blue 218 (azodianisidine)	1.2
		Acid black 52 (azochromium)	0.9	Basic yellow 11 (methine)	1.1
		16 azo dyes see ref. 100	8.8	Direct blue 86 (phthalocyanine)	1.0
		Direct yellow 11 (stilbene)	--	Disperse yellow 54 (quinoline)	0.7
				Basic blue 3 (oxazine)	--
				Two phenols and sulfides	--
Total 3	3.7	Total 22	19.6	Total 21	10.0

a. In man and/or laboratory animals.
b. Selected by the American Dye Manufacturers Institute (see ref. 100).
c. A variety of members of these chemical classes have been found carcinogenic.
d. Vat green 1 was negative to the extent tested (see Table 6 for details).
e. No information on these or related members of their chemical classes.

TABLE 6. A Summary of Findings on the Carcinogenicity of the Six Dyes, Out of the Forty-six Used in Largest Quantities, That Have Been Reported on in the Literature

Name of Component	CI number[2]	Chemical class	Pounds used 1969	Species	Route of entry to the body	Exposure or dose level	Duration of Experiment	Target Organs	Lit. refs.
Direct black 38	30235	Trisazo benzidine	6112000	Rhesus monkeys	Stomach tube	Single dose[3]	72 hours	see footnote 4	40
Vat green 1	59825	Anthraquinone	3667000	Rats	Subcut. 10 doses	Total 460-550 mg.	300 days	Negative	101
Vat green 1	59825	Anthraquinone	3667000	Rats	Oral	0.1% in food	400 days	Negative	101
Disperse yellow 3	11855	Monoazo	2608000	Mice	Bladder implant	No info.	25 weeks	Bladder	102
Direct brown 95	30145	Trisazo benzidine	785000	Rhesus monkeys	Stomach tube	Single dose[3]	72 hours	See footnote 4	40
Direct blue 6	22610	Disazo benzidine	612000	Rhesus monkeys	Stomach tube	Single dose[3]	72 hours	See footnote 4	40
Basic green 4	42000	Triaryl methane	483000	Rats Mice	Intraven.	30mg/kg monthly	6 mos. see footnote 5	Lung mamm. mice	104

1. Ref. 99, 100.
2. Assigned by British Society of Dyers and Colourists, and the American Association of Textile Dyers and Colorists. Published in the Color Index.
3. Direct black 38 fed at two levels 13 and 63 mg benzidine moiety in the compound; Direct brown 95-7 and 35mg; Direct blue 6-8 and 40mg.
4. Pooled urine for 72 hours after feeding was analyzed for benzidine which was present to the average extent of 1.25 percent of the dye ingested.
5. This paper (ref. 104) also describes the breeding of dye-sensitive rats and tumor transplantation from one generation to another.

TABLE 7. Some Organophosphorus Flame Retardants[1]

Tris (2,3 Dibromopropyl) Phosphate

Bis (2,3-Dibromopropyl) Allyl Phosphate

Bis (2-Chloroethyl) Vinyl Phosphonate

Diethyl Vinyl Phosphate

Dialkylchloromethyl Phosphonates

Diallyl-2-3-Dibromopropyl Phosphate

Diallylphenyl Phosphonate

Triaryl Phosphates

Polychlorophosphonates

Triallylphosphene Oxide

N-Methylol Dimethyl Phosphonopropionamide

From ref. 106.

TABLE 8. Halogenated Monomers for Flame Retarding[1] Textile Polyesters, Polyamides, and Modacrylics

Diol Moiety Modification	–	Pentaerythritol Dichloride
	–	Chloropropanediols
	–	Mono-, Di - and Trichlorobutanediol
	–	Epoxylated Tetrachlorohydroquinone
	–	Halogenated Bisphenol A
	–	Glycidyl Ether of Pentahalophenol
Phthalic Anhydride Moiety Modification	–	Tetrachlorophthalic Anhydride
	–	Tetrabromophthalic Anhydride
	–	Chlorendic Anhydride
Vinyl Monomers	–	Vinyl Chloride
	–	Vinylidene Chloride
	–	Vinyl Bromide

From ref. 106

TABLE 9. Fire Retardant Treatments Based on Tetrakis(Hydroxymethyl)phosphonium Chloride(THPC) and Tetrakis(Hydroxymethyl)phosphonium Hydroxide (THPOH)[1,2]

THPC, methylol melamine, urea, heat

THPC, methylol melamine, urea, partial heat cure,
    partial NH_3 cure

THPC & tris(1-aziridinyl)phosphine oxide with heat

THPC + NaOH, methylol melamine, urea, heat

THPC + NaOH, amide, partial heat cure, partial NH_3 cure

THPC + NaOH, methylol melamine, urea, copper

THPC + NaOH, NH_3 cure

1. THPC can be reacted 1:1 with NaOH to produce THPOH.

2. From ref. 106.

TABLE 10. Amount of Retardant Required to Prevent[1] Flaming and Glowing (Nondurable Finishes)

Retardant	Minimum add-on %[2]
Ammonium bromide, NH_4Br	7
Ammonium molybdate, $(NH_4)_2MoO_4$	7
Sodium tungstate, $Na_2Wo_4 \cdot 2H_2O$	9
Diammonium phosphate, $(NH_4)_2 HPO_4$	12
Phosphoric acid, H_3PO_4	12
Zinc chloride, $ZnCl_2$	12
Ammonium iodide, NH_4I	14
Calcium chloride, $CaCl_2 \cdot 6H_2O$	14
Magnesium chloride, $MgCl_2$	16
Ammonium sulfate, $(NH_4)_2So_4$	18
Sodium stannate, Na_2SnO_3	18
Sodium aluminate, $NaAlO_2$	19
Sodium silicate, $Na_2SiO_3 \cdot 9H_2O$	20
Ammonium chloride, NH_4Cl	22
Ammonium borate, NH_4BO_3	24
Sodium bisulfate, $NaHSO_4 \cdot H_2O$	30
Sodium arsenate, $Na_3AsO_4 \cdot 12H_2O$	33
Borax, $Na_2B_4O_7 \cdot 10H_2O$	60

1. Table 3-1 from ref. 106.

2. Parts by weight added per 100 parts fabric.

TABLE 11.   Fluorescent Whitening Agents Used by Major Detergent
Manufacturers

---

bis (anilino-morpholino-triazinylamino) stilbene
disulfonate

bis (anilino-hydroxyethylmethylamino-triazinylamino)
stilbene disulfonate

bis (anilino-dihydroxyethylamino-triazinylamino)
stilbene disulfonate

naphthotriazolyl-stilbene sulfonate

bis (anilino-methylamino-triazinylamino) stilbene
disulfonate

bis (styrylsulfonate) biphenyl

bis (phenyl-triazolyl) stilbene disulfonate

All of these compounds are sold as the trans
isomer. However, when these FWA's are irradiated
in solution they are converted to a mixture of the
nonfluorescent cis form and the trans isomer.

TABLE 12. Chemical Names of 14 Optical
Brighteners Illustrated in Fig. 2

---

1. Derivatives of bistriazinyl-4,4'-diaminostilbene
   -2,2'-disulfonic acid, in which R may be C_6H_5NH-,
   m or p $HO_3SC_6H_4NH-$, $(HOCH_2CH_2)_2N-$, $O(CH_2CH_2)N-$,
   $HOCH_2CH_2O-$ or $Cl-$

2. Closely related to 1 are the acyl and ureido derivatives of 4,4'-diaminostilbene-2,2'-disulfonic acid,
   where R is C_6H_5CO-, C_6H_5NHCO- or $O-CH_3OC_6H_4CO-$. These
   compounds are symmetrical.

3. A class of unsymmetrical brighteners of considerable
   importance is derived from stilbenenaphthotriazole
   (4-naphthotriazolylstilbene) where X may be $-SO_3H$,
   $-SO_2OC_6H_5$, $-SO_2NR_2$, $-CN$ or $SO_2NHCH_2CH_2N-(CH_3)_2$.

4. Another important group is the bisazoles such as
   vinylenebisbenzimidazoles where R is a hydroxyalkyl
   group or where the vinylene

5. may be replaced by stilbene and the vinylenebis-
   benzoxazoles where R is alkyl or where the vinylene
   is replaced by a thiophene ring.

6. 4-methyl-7-hydroxycoumarin (-methylumbelliferone)
   still used, led to the development of the closely
   related but far more useful 4-alkyl-7-dialkyl-
   aminocoumarins......

7. and the 3-phenyl-7-aminocoumarins where R is acyl,
   triazinyl etc.

8. Benzidinesulfone disulfonic acids - where R is
   $CH_3OC_6H_4CO-$

9. Diphenylpyrazolines where X is $-SO_3H, -SO_2NR_2$,
   $-COOH, -CONR_2$ and R is H, alkyl or aryl.

10. Cationic oxacyanines

11. Imidazolones

12. Pyrazines

13. Aminonaphthalimides

14. Oxadiazoles where R is $-CH=CHC_6H_4SO_3H$

TABLE 13. Main Carcinogenicity-related Chromophores

Chromophore	Structural moiety	Typical colorants	References
Azo[1]	$-N=N-$ one to three units	Disperse yellow 3 and Direct black 38	102 40
Azoic		Para red and Dinitroaniline orange	Footnote 3
Triarylmethane Amines		Parafuchsin and Crystal Violet	p.22, ref. 41 42-47, 59
Stilbene[2] Amines		Footnote 4	161
Xanthene		Rhodamine B	p.23, ref.41 46,47,58, 66-70
Chromate	Hexavalent Chromium	Lead chromate $PbCrO_4$	30-33

---

1. Azo and anthraquinone dyes account for roughly two-thirds of synthetic dye production. The anthraquinone chromophore has not yet been found cancer-related.

2. Occurs with the carcingenicity-related moiety, triazinyl, to produce fluorescent brightening agents (see test).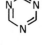

3. No literature evidence for the carcinogenicity of these compounds has been found but the azo linkage may break in vivo to form carcinogenic 1-amino-2 naphthol (166).

4. (Disodium 4,4'-bis-[4,6-dianilino-S-triazin-2-yl]amino 2,2'-stilbene disulfonate)$_2$.

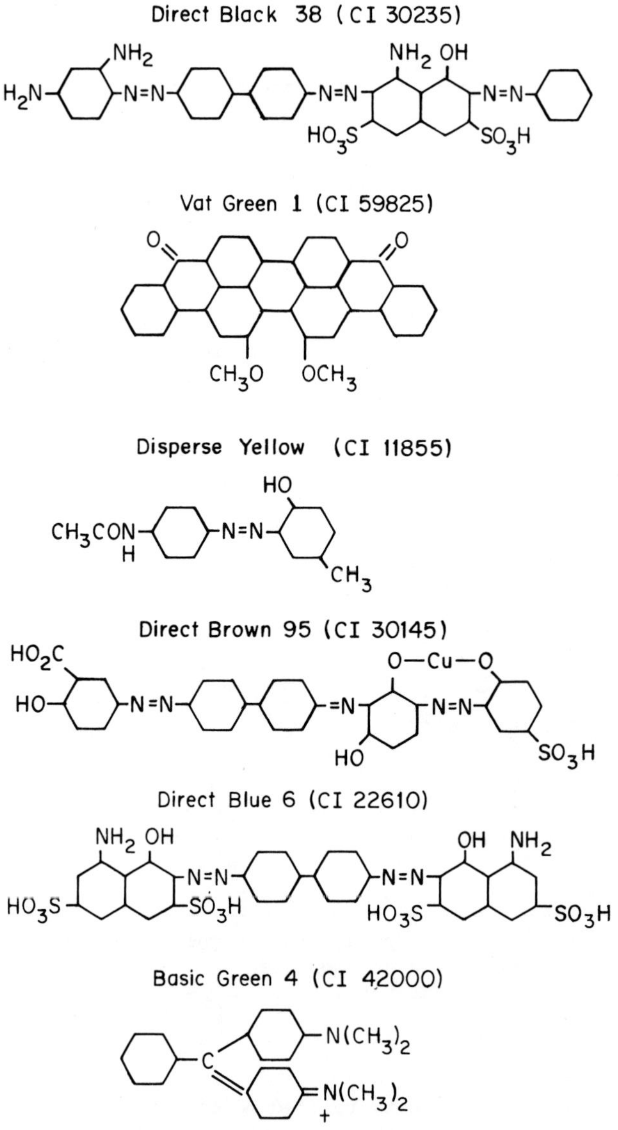

Direct Black 38 (CI 30235)

Vat Green 1 (CI 59825)

Disperse Yellow (CI 11855)

Direct Brown 95 (CI 30145)

Direct Blue 6 (CI 22610)

Basic Green 4 (CI 42000)

FIG. 1. Six dyes among the 46 most widely used[1] on which carcinogenicity data has been reported.

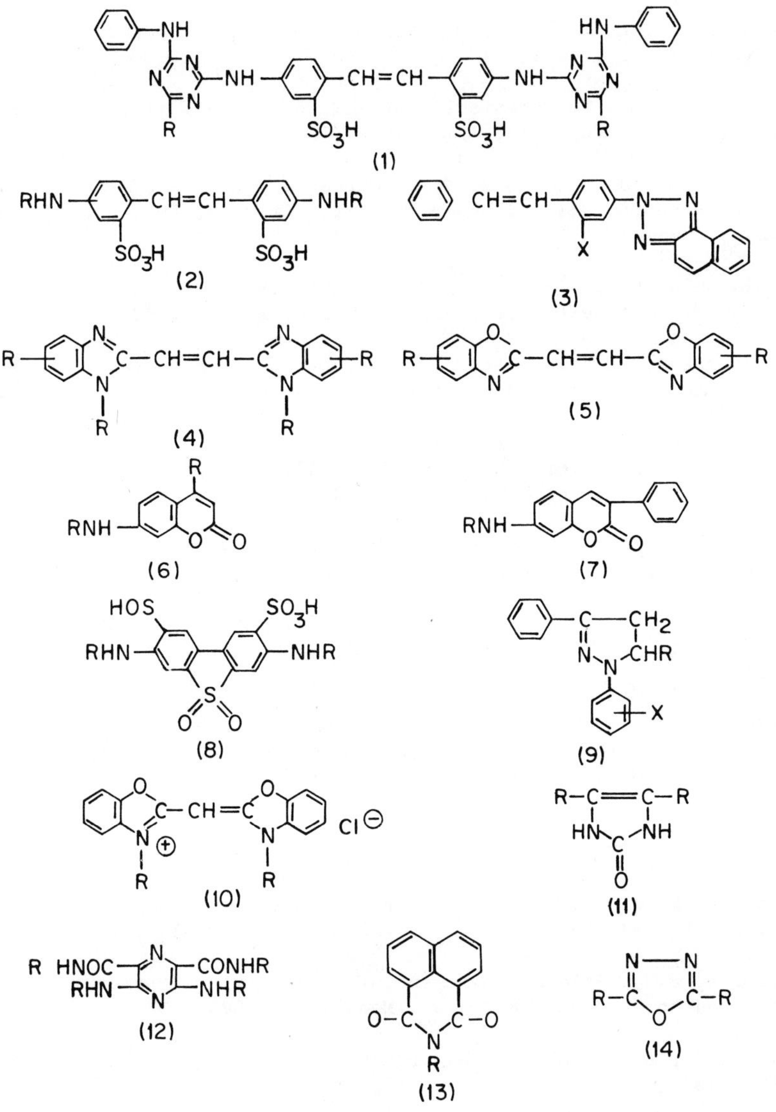

FIG. 2. Types of optical brighteners.[1] From ref. 158.

References

1. Kennaway, E. L. and Kennaway, N. M. A further study of the incidence of cancer of the lung and larynx. Brit. J. Cancer 1, 260-298, 1947.

2. Ask-Upmark, E. Bronchiolarcarcinoma in printing workers. Dis. Chest. XXVII: 427-435, 1955.

3. Badger, G. M. The chemical basis of carcinogenicity. C.E. Thomas Publisher, Springfield, Ill. 1962.

4. Dunn, J.E., Jr. and J. M. Weir, Cancer experience of several occupational groups followed progressively. Amer. J. Pub. Hlth. 55:1367-1375, 1965.

5. Goldstein, D. H., J.N. Benoit and H. A. Tyroler. An epidemiologic study of an oil mist exposure. Arch. Environ. Hlth. 21:600-603, 1970.

6. Pasternack, B. and L. Ehrlich. Occupational exposure to an oil mist atmosphere. A 12-year mortality study. Arch. Environ. Hlth. 25:286-294, 1972.

7. Cole, P., R. Hoover, and G. H. Friedell. Occupation and cancer of the lower urinary tract. Cancer 29:1250-1260, 1972.

8. Greenberg, M. A proportional mortality study of a group of newspaper workers. Brit. J. Ind. Mcd. 29:15-20, 1972.

9. Moss, E., T.S. Scott and G.R.C. Atherley. Mortality of newspaper workers from lung cancer and bronchitis 1952-1966. Brit. J. Ind. Med. 29:1-14, 1972.

10. Lloyd, J.W., P. Decoufle and L.G. Salvin. Unusual mortality experience of printing pressmen. Paper presented at Annual Meeting, American Industrial Hygiene Association, San Francisco, California 18 May 1972.

11. Viadana, E. and I.D.J. Bross. Leukemia and occupations. Prev. Med. 1:513-521, 1972.

12. Hoover, R. and J.F. Fraumeni, Jr., Cancer mortality in U.S. counties with chemical industries. Environ. Res. 9, 196-207, 1975.

13. Thorpe, J.J. Epidemiologic survey of leukemia in persons potentially exposed to benzene. J. Occup. Med. 16:375-383, 1974.

14. Vigliani, E.C. and Saita G. Benzene and leukemia. N.E.J. Med. 271:872-876, 1964.

15. Aksoy, M., Erdem, S. and Dincol, G. Leukemia in shoe workers exposed chronically to benzene. Blood 44:837-841, 1974.

16. Forni, A. Pacifico, E. and Limonta, A. Chromosome studies in workers exposed to benzene or toluene or both. Arch. Env. Hlth. 22:373-378, 1971.

17. Forni, A.M., Cappellini, A., Pacifico, E. and Vigliani, E.C. Chromosome changes and their evolution in subjects with past exposure to benzene. Arch. Env. Hlth. 23:385-391, 1971.

18. McMichael, A.J., Spirtas, R., Kupper, L.L. and Gawble, J.F. Solvent exposure and leukemia among rubber workers: An epidemiological study. J. Occup. Med. 17:234-239, 1975.

19. Forni, A. and Moreo, L. Chromosome studies in a case of benzene-induced erythroleukemia. Europ. J. Cancer. 5:459-463, 1969.

20. Ward, J.M., J.H. Weisburger, R.S. Yamamoto, T. Benjamin, C.A. Brown and E.K. Weisburger. Long-term effect of benzene in C57BL/6N mice. Arch. Env. Hlth. 30:22-25, 1975.

21. Eschenbrenner, A.B. and Miller, E. Induction of hepatomas in mice by repeated oral administration of chloroform, with observations on sex differences. J. Nat. Cancer Inst. 5:251-255, 1944/45.

22. Carcinogensis program, Division of Cancer Cause and Prevention, National Cancer Institute, National Institutes of Health, Bethesda, Md. Report on carcinogenesis assay of chloroform. Mar. 1, 1976.

23. Della Porta, G., Terracini, B. and Shubik, P.J. Induction with carbon tetrachloride of liver cell carcinomas in hamsters. J. Nat. Cancer Inst. 26:855-863, 1961.

24. Eschenbrenner, A.B. and Miller, E. Studies on hepatomas. I. Size and spacing of multiple doses in the induction of carbon tetrachloride hepatomas. J. Nat. Cancer Inst. 4:385-388, 1943.

25. Edwards, J.E., Heston, W.E. and Dalton, A.J. Induction of the carbon tetrachloride hepatoma in strain L mice. J. Nat. Cancer Inst. 3:297-301, 1942.

26. Edwards, J.E. and Dalton, A.J. Induction of cirrhosis of the liver and of hepatomas in mice with carbon tetrachloride. J. Nat. Cancer Inst. 3: 19-41, 1942.

27. Edwards, J.E. Hepatomas in mice induced with carbon tetrachloride. J. Nat. Cancer Inst. 2:197-199, 1941.

28. Carcinogenesis program, Division of Cancer Cause and Prevention, National Cancer Institute, National Institutes of Health, Bethesda, Md. Memorandum of alert-trichlorethylene. Mar. 20, 1975.

29. Greenburg, L., M.R. Mayers, L. Goldwater and A.R. Smith. Benzene (benzol) poisoning in the rotogravure printing industry in New York City. J. Ind. Hyg. Toxicol. 21:395-420, 1939.

30. Maltoni, C., Sinibaldi, C. and Annoscia, C. Insorgenza di sarcomi sottocutanei nel ratto in sequito a iniezione locale di giallo e arancio chromo. Tumori 57:213, 1971.

31. Langard, S. and Norseth, T. A cohort study of bronchial carcinomas in workers producing chromate pigments. Brit. J. Ind. Med. 32:62-65, 1975.

32. International Agency for Research on Cancer. IARC monographs on the evaluation of carcinogenic risk of chemicals to man. Some inorganic and organometallic compounds. Vol. 2, Lyon, 1973.

33. Worker exposure to chromate pigments can lead to "unusually" high cancer risks. C&EN p. 8, Oct. 13, 1975.

34. Haddow, A. and Horning, E.S. On the carcinogenicity of an iron-dextran complex. J. Nat. Cancer Inst. 24:109-127, 1960.

35. Spitz, S., Maguigan, W.H. and Dobriner, K. The carcinogenic action of benzidine. Cancer 3:789-804, 1950.

36. Scott, T.S. The incidence of bladder tumours in a dyestuffs factory. Brit. J. Ind. Med. 9:127-132, 1952.

37. Zavon, M.R., Hoegg, V. and Bingham, E. Benzidine exposure as a cause of bladder cancer. Arch. Env. Hlth. 27:1-7, 1973.

38. Pliss, G.B. On some regular relationships between carcinogenicity of aminodiphenyl derivatives and the structure of substance. Acta Un. Int. Contra Cancrum 19:499-501, 1963.

39. Pliss, G.B. The blastomogenic action of dichlorobenzidine. Vopr. Onkol. 5:524-533, 1959.

40. Rinde, E. and Troll, W. Metabolic reduction of benzidine azo dyes to benzidine in the Rhesus monkey. J. Nat. Canc. Inst. 55:181-182, 1975.

41. Arcos, J.C. and Argus, M.F. Chemical induction of cancer. Structural bases and biological mechanisms. Vol. IIB. Academic Press, New York 1974.

42. Druckrey, H. and Schmähl, D. Cancerogene wirkung von 4-dimethylamino triphenylmethan bei subkutaner gabe an ratten. Naturwissenschaften 42: 215, 1955.

43. Druckrey, H., Nieper, H.A. and Lo, H.W. Carcinogene wirkung von para-fuchsin im injektionsversuch an ratten. Naturwissenschaften 43:543-544, 1956.

44. Kaump, D.H., Schardein, J.L., Woosley, E.T. and Fisken, R.A. Tris (p-aminophenyl)-carbonium pamoate and tumor induction in albino rats. Cancer Res. 25:1919-1924, 1965.

45. Kinosita, R. Studies on the cancerogenic and related compounds. Yale J. Biol. Med. 12:287-300, 1939-1940.

46. Wilhelm, R. and Ivy, A.C. A preliminary study concerning the possibility of dietary carcinogenesis. Gastroenterol. 23:1-19, 1953.

47. Bonser, G.M., Clayson, D.B. and Jull, J.W. The induction of tumours of the subcutaneous tissues, liver and intestine in the mouse by certain dyestuffs and their intermediates. Brit. J. Cancer 10:653-667, 1956.

48. Davis, K.J. and Fitzhugh, O.G. Pathologic changes in rats fed D&C Red. no. 10 [monosodium salt of 2-(2-hydroxy- 1 -naphthylazo) -1-naphthalene-sulfonic acid for two years. Toxicol. Appl. Pharmacol. 5:728-734, 1963.

49. Falk, H.L., Steiner, P.E., Breslow, A. and Hykes, R. Carcinogenic hydro-carbons and related compounds in processed rubber. Cancer Res. 11:318-326, 1951.

50. Falk, H.L., Steiner, P.E. and Goldfein, S. Carcinogenic hydrocarbons in processed rubber and in carbon black. Cancer Res. 11:247, 1951.

51. Von Haam, E. and Malette, F.S. Studies on the toxicity and skin effects of compounds used in the rubber and plastics industries. III Carcinogenicity of carbon black extracts. A.M.A. Arch. Indust. Hyg. 6:237-242, 1952.

52. Steiner, P.E. The conditional biological activity of carcinogens in car-bon blacks and its elimination. Cancer Res. 14:103-110, 1954.

53. Nau, C.A., J. Neal and V.A. Stembridge. A study of physiological effects of carbon black. I. Ingestion. A.M.A. Arch. Ind. Hlth. 17:21-28, 1958.

54. Nau, C.A., J. Neal and V.A. Stembridge. A study of the physiological effects of carbon black. II. Skin contact. A.M.A. Arch. Ind. Hlth. 18:511-520, 1958.

55. Nau, C.A., J. Neal, V.A. Stembridge and R.N. Cooley. Physiological effects of carbon black. IV. Inhalation. Arch. Environ. Hlth. 4:415-31, 1962.

56. Neal, J. and N.M. Trieff. Isolation of unknown carcinogenic polycyclic hydrocarbon from carbon black. Health Lab. Sci. 9:32-38, 1972.

57. Davis, K.J. and Fitzhugh, O.G. Pathologic changes noted in rats fed D and C red No. 9 for two years. Toxicol. Appl. Pharmacol. 4:200-205, 1962.

58. Umeda, M. Experimental study of xanthene dyes as carcinogenic agents. Gann 47:51-78, 1956.

59. Schaeppi, H.U. Versuche über Krebs - und leukämieerzeugende eigenschaften des methyl violetts. Z Umfallmed Berufskr. 1:48-68, 1955.

60. Engelbrecht, F.M., Byers, P.D., Stacy, B.D., Harrison, C.V. and King, E.J. Tissue reactions to injected aluminium and alumina in the lungs of mice, rats, guinea-pigs and rabbits. J. Path. Bact. 77:407-416, 1959.

61. Stacy, B.D., King, E.J., Harrison, C.V., Nagelschmidt, G. and Nelson, S. Tissue changes in rats' lungs caused by hydroxides, oxides and phosphates of aluminium and iron. J. Path. Bact. 77:417-426, 1959.

62. Klosterkötter, W. Effects of ultramicroscopic gamma-aluminum oxide on rats and mice. Arch. Ind. Hlth. 21:458-472, 1960.

63. Shafer, W.G. Experimental salivary gland tumorigenesis. J. Dent. Res. 41:117-124, 1962.

64. Kobayashi, N., Ide, G., Katsuki, H. and Yamane, Y. Effect of aluminium compound on the development of experimental lung tumor in mice. Gann 59:433-436, 1968.

65. Kobayashi, N., Katsuki, H. and Yamane, Y. Inhibitory effect of aluminum on the development of experimental lung tumor in mice induced by 4-nitroquinoline 1-oxide. Gann 61:239-244, 1970.

66. Bonser, G.M., Bradshaw, L., Clayson, D.B. and Jull, J.W. A further study of the carcinogenic properties of orthohydroxyamines and related compounds by bladder implantation in the mouse. Brit. J. Cancer 10:539-546, 1956.

67. Bonser, G.M., Clayson, D.B., Jull, J.W. and Pyrah, L.N. The carcinogenic activity of 2-naphthylamine. Brit. J. Cancer 10:533-538, 1956.

68. Umeda, M. Experimental production of sarcoma in rats by injection of rhodamine B. Gann 43:120-122, 1952.

69. Umeda, M. Experimental production of sarcoma in rats by injections of rhodamine B. (IInd report) Gann 46:369-371, 1955.

70. Umeda, M. Production of rat sarcoma by injections of propylene glycol solution of M-toluylenediamine. Gann 46:597-602, 1955.

71. Dworski, M. Prophylaxis and treatment of experimental silicosis by means of aluminum. Arch. Ind. Hlth. 12:229-246, 1955.

72. Furuya, Y. and Eiseiin, K. Tissue reactions produced by aluminum dusts and the effect of aluminum on the development of silicosis. Bull. Inst. Public Health (Tokyo) 7:19-28, 1958.

73. King, E.J., Harrison, C.V., Mohanty, G.P. and Yoganathan, M. The effect of aluminium and of aluminium containing 5% quartz in the lungs of rats. J. Path. Bact. 75:429-434, 1958.

74. Kazantzis, G. Induction of sarcoma in the rat by cadmium sulphide pigment. Nature 198:1213-1214, 1963.

75. Kazantzis, G. and Hanbury, W. J. The induction of sarcoma in the rat by cadmium sulphite and by cadmium oxide. Brit. J. Cancer 20:190-199, 1966.

76. Kay, K. Inorganic particles of agricultural origin. Env. Hlth. Persp. 9:193-195, 1974.

77. Rohl, A.N. Asbestos in talc. Environ. Hlth. Persp. 9:129-132, 1974.

78. Goyer, R.A. The renal tubule in lead poisoning. 1. Mitochondrial swelling and aminoaciduria. Lab. Investig. 19:71-77, 1968.

79. Lilis, R., N. Gavrilescu, B. Nestorescu, C. Dumitriu and A. Roventa. Nephropathy in chronic lead poisoning. Brit. J. Ind. Med. 25:196-202, 1968.

80. Hirsch, G.H. Effect of chronic lead treatment on renal function. Toxicol. Appl. Pharmacol. 25:84-93, 1973.

81. Cramer, K., R.A. Goyer, R. Jagenburg and M.H. Wilson. Renal ultrastructure, renal function, and parameters of lead toxicity in workers with different periods of lead exposure. Brit. J. Ind. Med. 31:113-127, 1974.

82. Dunn, T.B., H.P. Morris and B.P., Wagner. Lipemia and glomerular lesions in rats fed diets containing N-N' -diacetyl and 4,4-4',4'-tetramethylbenzidine. Proc. Soc. Exptl. Biol. Med. 91:105-107, 1956.

83. Bremner, D.A. and J.D. Tange. Renal and neoplastic lesions after injection of N-N' -diacetylbenzidine. Arch. Pathol. 81:146-151, 1966.

84. Harman, J.W., E.C. Miller and J.A. Miller. Chronic glomerulonephritis and nephrotic syndrome induced in rats by N,N'-diacetyl-benzidine. Amer. J. Pathol. 28:529-530, 1952.

85. Harman, J.W. Chronic glomerulonephritis and the nephrotic syndrome induced in rats with N,N'-diacetylbenzidine. J. Pathol. 104:119-158, 1971.

86. Bater, J.R., E.R. Smith, Y.H. Yoon, G.G. Wade, H. Rosenkrantz, B. Schmall, J. H. Weisburger and E. K. Weisburger. Nephrotoxic effect of 2-aminoanthraquinone in Fischer rats. J. Toxicol. Env. Hlth. 1:1-11, 1975.

87. Carter, R.L., B.C.V. Mitchley and F.J.C. Roe. Preliminary survey of 22 printing inks for carcinogenic activity by the subcutaneous route in mice. Fd. Cosmet. Toxicol. 7:53-58, 1969.

88. Steinbrück, Kunstliche krebserzeugung durch drückerschwarze. Berl. Tierärztl. Wschr. 45:525-527, 1929.

89. Steinbrück and Carl. Ibid. 46:161-165, 1930.

90. Ingalls, T.H. Incidence of cancer in the carbon black industry. Arch. Ind. Hyg. Occup. Med. 1-2, 662-676, 1950.

91. Gold, A. Carbon black adsorbates: separation and identification of a carcinogen and some oxygenated.polyaromatics. Anal. Chem. 47:1469-1972, 1975.

92. Wallcave, L., D.L. Nagel, J.W. Smith and R.D. Waniska. Two pyrene derivatives of widespread environmental distribution: cyclopenta(c,d) pyrene and acepyrene. Env. Sci. Technol. 9:143-145, 1975.

93. Qazi, A.H. and C.A. Nau. Identification of polycyclic aromatic hydrocarbons in semi-reinforcing carbon black. A.I.H.A.J. 36:187-192, 1975.

94. Kay, K. Liquid chromatography analysis in air pollution. In: Chromatographic analysis of the environment. ed. Robert L. Grob. Marcel Dekker Inc., New York 1975.

95. Rare children's disease tied to solvents used in pesticides. N.Y. Times, Apr. 10, 1976.

96. Vanderhoff, J.W. Ultraviolet light-cured printing inks -- a review. Paper presented to Division of Organic Coatings and Plastics, American Chemical Society, 169th Meeting April 7-11, 1975. Philadelphia, Pa.

97. Rapoport, I.A. Carbonyl compounds and the chemical mechanism of mutations. Compt. rend acad. sci. URSS. 54, 65-67, 1946.

98. Kallos, G.J. and Solomon, R.A. Investigations of the formation of bis-chloromethylether in simulated hydrogen chloride-formaldehyde atmospheric environments Amer. Ind. Hyg. Assoc. J. 34, 467-473, 1973.

99. International Trade Commission. Synthetic Organic Chemicals, United States Production and Sales, 1969. TC Publication 412, 1971. Washington, D. C.

100. American Dye Manufacturers Institute. Dyes and the environment. Reports on selected dyes and their effects. Vol. 1, Sept. 1973. New York.

101. Umeda, M. Studies in carcinogenesis of indanthrene dyes. Gann 47:597-599, 1956.

102. Boyland, E., E.R. Busby, C.E. Dukes, P. L. Grover and D. Manson. Further experiments on implantation of materials into the urinary bladder of mice. Brit. J. Cancer 18:575-581, 1964.

103. Fujita, K., T. Mine, S. Iwase, T. Mizuno, T. Takayanagi, Y. Sugiyama and T. Arai. The carcinogenicity of certain compounds related to tryptan blue. Brit. J. Exptl. Pathol. 38:291-296, 1957.

104. Werth, G. Transplantationsergebnisse mit durch malachitgrun erzeugten tumoren. Zeit. Krebsforchung 64:234-244, 1961.

105. LeBlanc, R.B. What's available for flame retardant textiles. Textile Industries 140, 29-31, 35,37,39,41,43,88, 1976.

106. McGeehan, T.J. and Maddock, J.T. A study of flame retardants for textiles. Final report AUER-2200-TR-4, Auerbach Assoc. Inc. 121 North Broad St. Philadelphia, Pa. 19107. Dec. 31, 1975.

107. Prival, M.J. Information available to date relevant to the mutagenicity of tris(2,3-dibromopropyl) phosphate. Dec. 2, 1975. Office of Toxic Substances, Environmental Protection Agency. Washington, D. C. 20460

108. Prival, M. Flame retardant chemicals and the Toxic Substances Control Act. Paper presented to the National Academy of Sciences, Jan. 27, 1976. Office of Toxic Substances, Environmental Protection Agency. Washington, D.C. 20460.

109. Thorpe, E. and Walker, A.I.T. The Toxicology of Dieldrin(HEOD). II. Comparative Long-term Oral Toxicity Studies in Mice with Dieldrin, DDT, Phenobarbitone, beta-BHC and gamma-BHC. Food Cosmet. Toxicol. 11:433-442, 1973.

110. Fitzhugh, O.G. and Nelson, A.A. Chronic Oral Toxicity of DDT(2,2-bis(p-chlorophenyl)-1,1,1-trichloroethane). J. Pharmacol. Exp. Therap. 89: 18-30, 1947.

111. Halver, J.E. Crystalline aflatoxin, and other vectors for trout hepatoma. Trout Hepatoma Conference Research papers: U.S. Fish and Wildlife Service Res. Rep. 70:78-102, 1967.

112. Innes, J.R.M., Ulland, B.M., Valerio,M.G., Petrucelli, L., Fishbein, L., Hart, E.R., Pallotta, A.J., Bates, R.R., Falk, H.L., Gart, J.J., Klein, M., Mitchell, I. and Peters, S. Bioassay of Pesticides and Industrial Chemicals for Tumorigenicity in Mice: A Preliminary Note. J. Natl. Cancer Inst. 42:1101-1114, 1969.

113. Kemeny, T. and Tarjan, R. Investigation on the Effects of Chronically Administered Small Amounts of DDT in Mice. Experientia 22:748-749, 1966.

114. Shabad, L.M., Kolesnichenko, T.S. and Nikonova, T.V. The Effects of Transplacental Administration of DDT on Organ Cultures of Foetal Mouse Lung Tissue. Intern. J. Cancer 9:365-373, 1972.

115. Tomatis, L., Turusov, V., Day, N. and Charles, R.T. The Effect of Long-term Exposure to DDT on CF-1 Mice. Intern. J. Cancer 10:489-506, 1972.

116. Fitzhugh, O.G., Nelson, A.A. and Quaife, M.L. Chronic oral toxicity of Aldrin and Dieldrin in rats and dogs. Food Cosmet. Toxicol. 2:551-562, 1964.

117. Davis, K.J. and Fitzhugh, O.G. Tumorigenic Potential of Aldrin and Dieldrin for Mice. Toxicol. Appl. Pharmacol. 4:187-189, 1962.

118. Walker, A.I.T., Thorpe, E. and Stevenson, D.E. The Toxicology of Dieldrin (HEOD). Long-term Oral Toxicity Studies in Mice. Food Cosmet. Toxicol. 11:415-432, 1973.

119. Hunt, P.F., Stevenson, D.E., Thorpe, E. and Walker, A.I.T. Mouse Data. Letter to Editor. Food Cosmet. Toxicol. 13:597-598, 1975.

120. Nagasaki, H., Tomii, S., Mega, T., Marugami, M. and Ito, N. Development of Hepatomas in Mice Treated With Benzene Hexachloride. Gann 62:431-433, 1971.

121. Nagasaki, H., Tomii, S., Mega, T., Marugami, M. and Ito, N. Hepato-carcinogenic Effect of Alpha, Beta, Gamma and Delta Isomers of Benzene Hexachloride in Mice. Gann 63:393, 1972.

122. Nagasaki, H., Kawabata, H., Miyata, Y., Inoue, K., Hirao, K., Aoe, H. and Ito, N. Effect of Various Factors on Induction of Liver Tumors in Animals by the Alpha Isomer of Benzene Hexachloride. Gann 66:185-193, 1975.

123. Allen, J.R. and Norback, D.H. Polychlorinated Biphenyl- and Triphenyl-Induced Gastric Hyperplasia in Primates. Science 179:498-499, 1973.

124. Nagasaki, H., Tomii, S., Mega, T., Marugami, M. and Ito, N. Hepato-carcinogenicity of Polychlorinated Biphenyls in Mice. Gann 63:805, 1972.

125. Kimbrough, R.D., Squire, R.A., Linder, R.E., Strandberg, J.D., Montali, R.J. and Burse, V.W. Induction of Liver Tumors in Sherman Strain Female Rats by Polychlorinated Biphenyl Arochlor 1260. J. Natl. Cancer Inst. 55:1453-1459, 1975.

126. Franklin, B.A. Pesticide Peril: Inaction and Ills. p. 14, New York Times, Janusry 28, 1976.

127. Brem, H., Coward, J.E., and Rosenkranz, H.S. i,2-dibromoethane-Effect on the Metabolism and Ultrastructure of Escherichia Coli. Biochem. Pharmacol., 23:2345-2347, 1974.

128. Olson, W.A., Habermann, R.T., Weisburger, E.K., Ward, J.M. and Weisburger, J. H. Induction of Stomach Cancer in Rats and Mice by Halogenated Aliphatic Fumigants. J. Natl. Cancer Inst., 51:1993-1995, 1973.

129. Rosenkranz, H.S. Genetic Activity of 1,2-dibromo-3-chloropropane, A Widely-Used Fumigant. Bull. Environ. Contam. Toxicol., 14:8-12, 1975.

130. Amir, D. The Sites of the Spermicidal Action of Ethylene Dibromide in Bulls. J. Reprod. Fertility, 35:519-525, 1973.

131. Creech, J.L. and Johnson, M.N. Angiosarcoma of liver in the manufacture of polyvinyl chloride. J. Occup. Med. 16, 150-151, 1974.

132. Maltoni, C. and Lefemine, G. Carcinogenicity bioassays of vinyl chloride: i Plan of the project and early results. Environ. Res., 7, 387-405, 1974.

132a. Barbin, A., Bresil, H., Croisy, A., Jacquinon, P., Malaveille, C., Montesano, R. and Bartsch, H. Liver-microsome-mediated formation of alkylating agents from vinyl bromide and vinyl chloride. Biochem. Biophys. Res. Commun. 67, 596-603, 1975.

133. Preussmann, R. Direct Alkylating Agents as Carcinogens. Fd. Cosmet. Toxicol., 6:576-577, 1968.

134. Gibel, W. Tierexperimentelle Untersuchungen Uber die Hepatotoxische und Kanzerogene Wirkung Phosphoroganischer Verbindungen. I. Mitteilung: Trichlorphon. Arch. Geschwulstforsch., 37:303-312, 1971.

135. Gibel, W., Lohs, Kh., Wildner, G.P., Ziebarth, D. and Stieglitz, R. Uber die Kanzerogene, Hamatotoxische und Hepatotoxische Wirkung Pestizider Organische Phosphorverbindungen. Arch. Geschwulstforsch., 41: 311-328, 1973.

136. Schrader, G. Konstitution und Wirkung Organischer Phosphorverbindungen. Z. Naturforsch., 186:965-975, 1963.

137. Hilgetag, G. and Teichmann, H. The Alkylating Properties of Alkyl Thiophosphates. Angew. Chem. Internatl., 4:914-922, 1965.

138. Preussmann, R., Schneider, H. and Epple, F., Untersuchungen zum Nachweis Alkylierender Agentien. II. Der Nachweis Verschiedener Klassen Alkylierender Agentien mit Einer Modifikation der Farbreaktion mit 4-(4-Nitro-Benzyl)-Pyridin(NBP). Arzneimittel-Forsch., 19:1059-1073, 1969.

139. Loefroth, G., Kim, Ch. and Hussain, S. Alkylating Property of 2,2-Dichlorovinyl Dimethyl Phosphate - A Disregarded Hazard. Environ. Mutagen. Soc. News Letter, 2:21-27, 1969.

140. Wennerberg, R. and Loefroth, G. Formation of 7-Methylguanine by Dichlorvos in Bacteria and Mice. Chem.-Biol. Interactions, 8:339-348, 1974.

141. Loefroth, G. and Wennerberg, R. Methylation of Purines and Nicotinamide in the Rat by Dichlorvos. Zeit. Naturforsch., 61:651, 1974.

142. Wyrobek, A.J. and Bruce, W.R. Chemical Induction of Sperm Abnormalities in Mice. Proc. Natl. Acad. Sci. 72:4425-4429, 1975.

143. Blair, D., Hoadley, E.C. and Hutson, D.H. The distribution of Dichlorovs in the Tissues of Mammals After its Inhalation or Intravenous Administration. Toxicol. Appl. Pharmacol. 31:243-253, 1975.

144. Poverenny, A.M., Siomin, Yu., A., Saenko, A.S. and Sinzinis, B.I. Possible Mechanisms of Lethal and Mutagenic Action of Formaldehyde. Mutation Res. 27:123-126, 1975.

145. Epstein, S.S. and Shafner, H. Chemical mutagens in the human environment. Nature 219, 385-387, 1968.

146. Buckley, S.M., Stock, C.C., Parker, R.P., Crossley, M.L., Kuh, E. and Seeger, D. R. Inhibition studies of some phosphoramides against Sarcoma 180. Proc. Soc. Exptl. Biol. Med. 78, 299-305, 1951.

147. Borkovec, A.B. Sexual sterilization of insects by chemicals. Science 137, 1034-1037, 1962.

148. Borkovec, A.B. Insect chemosterilants: their chemistry and application. Residue Rev. 6, 87-103, 1964.

149. Röhrborn, G. Chemische konstitution und mutagene wirkung. II Triazinderivative. Z. Verbungslehre 93, 1- , 1962.

150. Ibid Drosophila Inform. Serv. 33, 156, 1959.

151. Walpole, A.N. The Walker carcinoma 256 in the screening of tumour inhibitors. Brit. J. Pharmacol. 6, 135-154, 1951.

152. Rose, F.L., Hendry, J.A. and Walpole, A.L. Newcytotoxic agents with tumour - inhibitory activity. Nature 165, 993-996, 1950.

153. Hendry, J.A., Rose, F.L. and Walpole, A.L. Cytotoxic agents: I. Methylolamides with tumour inhibitory activity and related inactive compounds. Brit. J. Pharmacol. 6, 201-234, 1951.

154. Hendry, J.A., Homer, R.F., Rose, F.L. and Walpole, A.L. Cytotoxic agents: II, Bis-epoxides and related compounds. Brit. J. Pharmacol. 6,235-255, 1951.

155. Boyland, E. and Horning, E.S. The induction of tumours with nitrogen mustards. Brit. J. Cancer 3, 118-123, 1949.

156. Haddow, A. Mode of action of the nitrogen mustards - a new working hypothesis and its possible relation to carcinogenesis. Proc. Nat. Cancer Conf. 88-94, 1949.

157. Kay, K. Conference on toxicology-epidemiology-health effects of pesticides. A review of the problem. Clin. Toxicol. 8, 289-300,1975.

158. Brighteners, optical. pp. 606-613, Vol. 2 Encyclopedia of Polymer Science and Technology. Interscience Publishers, New York, 1965.

159. Neukomm, S. and De Trey, M. Study of some optical azo dyes from the point of view of their carcinogenic and co-carcinogenic activity. Medicina Experimentalis 4, 296-306, 1961.

160. Snyder, F.H., Opdyke, D.L. and Rubenkoenig, H.L. Toxicologic studies on brighteners. Toxicol. Appl. Pharmacol. 5, 176-183, 1963.

161. Bingham, E. and Falk, H.L. Combined action of optical brighteners and ultraviolet light in the production of tumours. Fd. Cosmet. Toxicol. 8, 173-176, 1970.

162. Falk, H.L. and Bingham, E. Interaction of fluorescent whitening agents and ultraviolet radiation. Ambio 2, 22-25, 1973.

163. Forbes, P.D. and Urbach, F. Experimental modification of photo-carcinogenesis. I. Fluorescent whitening agents and short-wave UVR. Fd. Cosmet. Toxicol. 13, 335-337, 1975.

164. Forbes, P.D. and Urbach, F. Experimental modification of photo-carcinogenesis. I. Fluorescent whitening agents and simulated solar UVR. Fd. Cosmet. Toxicol. 13, 339-342, 1975.

165. Forbes, P.D. and Urbach, F. Experimental modification of photo-carcinogenesis. III. Simulation of exposure to sunlight and fluorescent whitening agents. Fd. Cosmet. Toxicol. 13, 343-345, 1975.

166. Bonser, G.M., Clayson, D.B. and Jull, J.W. The potency of 20-methylcholanthrene relative to other carcinogens on bladder implantation. Brit. J. Cancer 17, 235-241, 1963.

167. Schmidt, M.B. Uber vitale fettfarbung in geweben und sekreten durch Sudan und geschwulstartige wucherungen der ausscheidenden drusen. Virchow's Arch. Pathol. Anat. 253, 432-451, 1924.

168. Fischer, B. Die experimentelle erzungung atypischer epithelwucherungen und die entstehung bosartiger geschwulste. Münch. Med. Wochschr 53, 2041-2047, 1906.

169. Stoeber, H. Experimentelle untersuchungeuber die erzeugung atypischer epithelwucherungen. Munch. Med. Wochschr 56, 129-131, 1909.

170. Hayward, E. Weitere Klinische erfahrungen uber die anwendung der scharlachfarbstoffe und deren komponenten zur beschleunigten epithelialisierung granulierencer flachen. Munch. Med. Wochschr 56, 1836-1838, 1909.

171. Yoshida, T. Histopathological studies with aminoazotoluene (o-tolueneazo-o-toluidine). II. Further observations on the epithelial metaplasia of guinea - pig thyroid gland and the experiment of oral administration in rats. Trans. Japan. Pathol. Soc. 22, 934-937, 1932.

172. Kinosita, R. Researches on cancerogenesis of various chemical substances. Gann 30, 423-426, 1936.

173. Stevenson, E.S., Dobriner, K. and Rhoads, C.P. The metabolism of dimethylaminoazobenzene (butter yellow) in rats. Cancer Res. 2, 160-167, 1942.

174. Mecke, R., Jr. and Schmähl, D. Die spaltbarkeit der azo-brücke durch hefe. Arzneimittelforsch. 7, 335-340, 1957.

175. Kensler, C.J. Effect of diet on the production of liver tumors in the rat by N,N'-dimethyl-aminoazobenzene. Ann. NY Acad. Sci.49, Art 1, 29-40, 1947.

176. Kensler, C.J. The influence of diet on the ability of rat-liver slices to destroy the carcinogen N,N'-dimethyl-p-aminoazobenzene. Cancer 1, 483-488, 1948.

177. Mueller, G.C. and Miller, J.A. The metabolism of 4-dimethylaminoazobenzene by rat liver homogenates. J. Biol. Chem. 176, 535-544, 1948.

178. Mueller, G.C. and Miller, J.A. The reductive cleavage of 4-dimethylaminoazobenzene by rat liver: the intracellular distribution of the enzyme system and its requirement for triphosphopyridine nucleotide. J. Biol. Chem. 180, 1125-1136, 1949.

179. Mueller, G.C. and Miller, J.A. The reductive cleavage of 4-dimethylaminoazobenzene by rat liver reactivation of carbon dioxide treated homogenates by riboflavin-adenine dinucleotide. J. Biol. Chem. 185, 145-154, 1950.

180. Radomski, J.S. and Mellinger, T.J. The absorption, fate and excretion of the water-soluble azo dyes, FD&C red no. 2, FD&C red no. 4 and FD&C yellow no. 6. J. Pharmacol. Exptl. Therapeut. 136, 259-266, 1962.

181. Yoshida, O. and Miyakawa, M. Etiology of bladder cancer: metabolic aspects. In Analytical and Experimental Epidemiology of Cancer Eds. Nakahara, W., Hirayoma, T., Nishioka, K., et al. Baltimore Univ. Park Press, pp. 31-39, 1973.

182. Walker, R. The metabolism of azo compounds: a review of the literature. Fd. Cosmet. Toxicol. 8, 659-676, 1970.

CANCER MORTALITY AMONG CARPENTERS IN HAWAII

Ann M. Budy and M. Nabil Rashad

Pacific Biomedical Research Center, Department of
Genetics and Cancer Center of Hawaii
University of Hawaii

INTRODUCTION

This study was designed to compare cancer mortality experience of
carpenters before and after the introduction of water soluble arsenical
wood preservatives in Hawaii. The only wood preservative used in Hawaii
from 1935 to 1969 was FCAP, a Tanalith preservative containing disodium
arsenate (Table I). In 1970, CCA-B and CCA-C were introduced; these
preservatives are copper-chrome-arsenates, either arsenic acid or pentavalent arsenic compounds.

Usage of arsenic wood preservatives increased gradually over the
years from an initial figure of 1 million board feet of treated construction lumber to a high, in 1973, of 74 million board feet. Because carpenters work mainly in the construction industry, the majority would be
exposed to most of the available arsenate-treated wood.

We were particularly interested in the mortality rate of cancer of
the lung and the leukemia group. Because of the latent period for the
development of lung cancer and the history of arsenic-treated wood usage,
we have made two assumptions. First, the unexposed group of carpenters
who died during 1949-51 had little, if any, exposure to arsenate-treated
wood. Second, the exposed group of carpenters who died during 1970-73
would have had chronic exposure to arsenate, based on the increased usage
of treated lumber.

PROCEDURES AND MATERIALS

Microfilms of death certificates were reviewed for two designated
periods of four years each. The years between January 1948 through
December 1951 (Group A) was a period of very low usage of arsenate wood

901

preservative; the years between January 1970 through December 1973 (Group B) was a period of heavy usage.

Data collected consisted of: date of death, sex, race, marital status, birth and causes of death. To provide for adjustment for race and age, index cases were matched with non-carpenter controls of the same sex, age (± 5 yrs) and the year of death with the next record in sequence.

All cancers entered on death certificates were recoded using the International Classification of Diseases (ICD), 8th revision. No distinction was made as to the primary or secondary cause of death by cancer. All deaths for carpenters and controls within the two periods were tabulated by age-interval and race.

Age-specific death rates were computed using U.S. census data; the 1950 figure for the early period and the 1970 figure for the later period. Chi square tests were done to test for significance among and between the two groups of carpenters and controls. Results are stated on the basis of excess cancer mortality, i.e., the expected value in the general population.

RESULTS

Microfilms of 11,860 death certificates were reviewed for the first period and 17,385 for the second period. The review of the mortality file over the eight years yielded a total of 520 recorded carpenters; 227 in Group A and 293 in Group B.

The number of deaths and the number of cancers among carpenters by race and age-interval are presented in Table II for Group A and in Table III for Group B. The mean age for carpenters in Group A was 61.46 yrs; in Group B, 66.36 yrs. The mean age for controls in Group A was 61.52 yrs; in Group B, 66.00 yrs.

Major racial composition consisted of Caucasian, Japanese, Chinese, Hawaiian including part-Hawaiian, Filipino and Korean. Residual ethnic groups are included in the column headed by Other; these are: Samoan, Micronesian, Puerto Rican and Negro as well as biracial and triracial combinations of all races.

Neoplasms among carpenters and controls are presented in Table IV for all races and ages. In comparing mortality of carpenters with that of the matched controls (Table V), cancer among carpenters was higher than the controls only in the early groups; the excess of cancer was statistically significant (P<.05). Results of chi square tests between

902

and among carpenters and controls were not significant for either cancer of trachea, bronchus and lung (ICD 162) or cancer of lymphatic and hematopietic tissue (ICD 200-209).

Denominator data, obtained from the 1950 and 1970 census data of Hawaii are presented in Table VI. Age-specific death rates, based on the census data, were computed to estimate the age distribution and characteristics of the population at risk (Table VII). Cancer among carpenters is compared with the general population for excess of cancer.

Comparison of the death rate among carpenters with total death rate in the general population showed a significant increase in deaths among the carpenters (Table VIII). The excess of cancer death rate was consistent in the two periods studied. For the early period the relative risk for total death for carpenters was 2.15; for the later period the relative risk was 2.29. The relative risk for cancer death among carpenters was 3.58 for Group A and 2.72 for Group B.

DISCUSSION

It is common knowledge that environmental or occupational cancer may involve many organs and tissues and that the site of the cancer depends not only on the type of the carcinogenic agent, but also on the kind of exposure.

Although arsenical cancer has been known since 1820, the first cases of industrial or occupational cancer were reported by Nutt et al[6] in 1913, where two men had developed epitheliomatous growths after working for 20 years in a factory making arsenical sheep dip. Studies over the years have indicated that chronic exposure to soluble inorganic arsenicals predisposes to carcinomas of the skin. Epidemiologic evidence has been provided by Yeh et al[7] in a study of skin cancer among Taiwanese exposed to arsenic in their drinking water.

The situation with arsenical-induced cancers of other organs has met with some degress of uncertainty. The association of arsenicals with lung cancer dates back to 1878 when Härtig and Hesse[3] reported the occurrence of pulmonary carcinoma among miners working with cobalt arsenide ore. It was long believed that the causative agent was arsenic in the ore, with perhaps some contributions by cobalt. This belief was challenged after the discovery of radium. The carcinogenic agent was not arsenic, but the high level of radioactivity in mines that caused the high incidence of pulmonary carcinoma among miners.

903

With the increased use of arsenicals in wood preservatives, interest has been renewed in the possible association of arsenicals and lung cancer. Arsenicals have been suspect because carpenters have the highest cancer mortality experience of all occupational groups studied, as reported by Dublin and Vane[2]. As yet, there is no evidence either for or against such a hypothesis. However, there does appear to be some evidence that natural wood contains substances that may be carcinogenic.

Milham and Hesser[5], in case-control studies have provided evidence that carpenters and other wood workers have a high cancer mortality. Our methodology is very similar to that of Milham and Hesser; however, their work does not implicate any wood treatment chemicals. They presented evidence that Hodgkin's disease is related to an occupational exposure to wood, suggesting that deaths from Hodgkin's disease may be due to exposure to an environmental agent associated with wood. The report by Acheson et al[1] that carcinoma of the nasal cavity and accessory sinuses is more common in woodworkers than in workers in other occupations lends increased credibility to the findings of Milham and Hesser.

In a later study, Milham[4] examined current mortality patterns in a large wood-exposed population, with particular attention directed to possible wood-cancer relationships. His study identified a number of areas of excessive mortality among union members and supports the hypothesis that wood contains cancer causing agents. The associations reported were: excess lung cancer in acoustical tile applicators and insulators; excess gastrointestinal cancer in pile drivers; excess leukemia-lymphoma group cancers in millwrights, millmen, lumber and sawmill workers, and cabinet makers; excess lung and stomach cancer in construction workers with greater excesses seen in major urban areas.

Our study is in agreement with Milham's and others with respect to excess cancer deaths among carpenters. However, the relative risk for cancer among carpenters exposed to arsenate-treated wood does not show a significant excess for the periods studied.

SUMMARY

Comparison of the death rate among carpenters with total death rate in the general population showed a significant increase in deaths among the carpenters. The excess of cancer death rate was consistent before the introduction of arsenate-treated wood and during a period of substantial exposure to treated wood. For the early period the relative risk for total death for carpenters was 2.15; for the later period the relative risk was 2.29. The relative risk for cancer death among carpenters during the unexposed period was 3.58; that for the exposed period was 2.72. These ratios do not show a significant excess for the two periods studied.

ACKNOWLEDGMENT

This investigation was supported in part by a grant-in-aid from the American Wood Preservers Institute and in part through a contract with the Epidemiologic Studies Program, Health Effects Branch, Office of Pesticide Programs, Technical Service Division, U.S. Environmental Protection Agency, Washington, D.C., 20460.

We gratefully acknowledge the cooperation of Dr. Thomas Burch, Chief, Research & Statistics Division, State of Hawaii Department of Health for permission to review the microfilms of death certificates.

TABLE I. Volume of Waterborne Salt-treated Wood,
in Million Board ft/yr, Used in Hawaii

Year	FCAP	CCA-B	CCA-C	Total
1935–1939	1			1
1939–1944*	6			6
1945–1955	2			2
1956	2			2
1957	4			4
1958	7			7
1959	5			5
1960	8			8
1961	6			6
1962	8			8
1963	12			12
1964	13			13
1965	18			18
1966	14			14
1967	16			16
1968	26			26
1969	37			37
1970	26	2		28
1971	49	6		55
1972	18	8	36	62
1973	6	10	58	74

*Amount used throughout the Pacific for war effort.
FCAP, Tanalith preservative containing disodium
arsenate. CCA-B, CCA-C are copper-chrome-arsenates,
either arsenic acid or pentavalent arsenic compounds.

Supplied by courtesy of R. D. Arsenault, Technical
Director, Koppers Company, Inc. (unpublished).

TABLE II. Summary of Deaths Among Carpenters in Group A. Upper Half: Number of Deaths by Race and Age; Lower Half: Number of Cancers Recorded on Death Certificates

Race	Age Interval									
	15-24	25-34	35-44	45-54	55-64	65-74	75-84	85-94	95-104	Total
Caucasian	1	2	1	6	9	9	5	1	-	34
Japanese	4	12	4	11	34	48	23	5	1	142
Chinese	-	1	1	3	-	4	1	2	-	12
Hawaiian/part-Hawaiian	1	-	2	3	6	8	1	1	-	22
Filipino	2	-	2	2	3	1	1	-	-	11
Korean	-	-	1	-	-	3	1	-	-	5
Other	-	-	-	-	-	1	-	-	-	1
Total	8	15	11	25	52	74	32	9	1	227
Caucasian	-	-	1	-	2	2	2			7
Japanese	-	2	-	5	14	20	4			45
Chinese	-	-	-	2	-	1	-			3
Hawaiian/part-Hawaiian	-	-	-	1	1	-	-			2
Filipino	-	-	-	-	1	-	1			2
Korean	-	-	-	-	-	1	-			1
Other										0
Total	-	2	1	8	18	24	7			60

TABLE III. Summary of Deaths Among Carpenters in Group B. Upper Half: Number of Deaths by Race and Age; Lower Half: Number of Cancers Recorded on Death Certificates

Race					Age Interval					
	15-24	25-34	35-44	45-54	55-64	65-74	75-84	85-94	95-104	Total
Caucasian	2	3	1	8	8	11	9	3	–	45
Japanese	2	2	6	27	32	34	33	34	5	175
Chinese	–	–	–	–	–	3	7	1	1	12
Hawaiian/part-Hawaiian	4	2	4	2	5	2	2	1	–	22
Filipino	2	1	1	2	1	9	6	1	–	23
Korean	–	–	–	–	1	–	–	4	–	5
Other	2	–	1	1	1	3	2	1	–	11
Total	12	8	13	40	48	62	59	45	6	293
Caucasian	–	–	–	1	1	4	3	1	–	10
Japanese	–	–	1	7	12	12	5	4	1	42
Chinese	–	–	–	–	–	–	2	–	–	2
Hawaiian/part-Hawaiian	1	–	2	1	2	–	1	–	–	7
Filipino	–	–	–	–	–	–	–	1	–	1
Korean	–	–	–	–	1	–	–	1	–	2
Other	–	–	–	–	1	2	–	–	–	3
Total	1	0	3	9	17	18	11	7	1	67

TABLE IV. Neoplasms Among Carpenters (CAR) and Controls (CON)

Neoplasms Recorded	ICD	Group A		Group B	
		CAR	CON	CAR	CON
Buccal Cavity & Pharynx	140-149				
Tongue	141	1		1	
Salivary gland	142			1	
Oropharynx	146				1
Nasopharynx	147	1		1	
Pharynx unspecified	149	1		1	
Digestive Organs & Peritoneum	150-159				
Esophagus	150	5	2	3	2
Stomach	151	16	15	9	13
Small intestine & duodenum	152			1	
Large intestine	153	3	1	3	8
Rectum & rectosigmoid junction ...	154			3	3
Liver & intrahepatic bile ducts ..	155	4	3	3	2
Gallbladder & bile ducts	156		2	1	3
Pancreas	157	4	2	4	2
Respiratory System	160-163				
Mastoid	160.1				1
Larynx	161	2	2	1	
Trachea, bronchus & lung	162	11	5	13	9
Bone, Connective Tissue, etc.	170-174				
Osteosarcoma	170.7		1		
Connective & other soft tissue ...	171	1			
Melanoma	172.9	1			
Genitourinary Organs	180-189				
Prostate	185	1		3	6
Testis	186	1			1
Bladder	188		1	3	
Kidney	189			2	
Other & Unspecified Sites	190-199				
Brain	191	3	1		2
Thyroid	193				1
Second. - respir. & digest. systems	197	1			
Without specification of site	199	2	1	5	4
Lymphatic & Hematopoietic Tissue ..	200-209				
Lymphosarcoma/retic.-cell sarcoma	200			2	
Hodgkin's disease	201			1	2
Multiple myeloma	203	1		1	1
Lymphocytic leukemia	204		1		
Myeloid leukemia	205	1	1	2	2
Other & unspecified leukemia	207			3	
Total Malignant Neoplasms	140-209	60	38	67	63

909

TABLE V. Comparison Between and Among Carpenters and Controls

Description	X^2	P
Total cancer		
Among groups, carpenters vs. controls:		
Group A	5.74	<.05
Group B	.09	NS
Between groups, Group A vs. Group B:		
Carpenters	.70	NS
Controls	1.56	NS
Cancer of trachea, bronchus & lung (ICD 162)		
Among groups, carpenters vs. controls:		
Group A	1.62	NS
Group B	.43	NS
Between groups, Group A vs. Group B:		
Carpenters	.00	NS
Controls	.11	NS
Cancer of lymphatic & hematopoietic tissue (ICD 200-209)		
Among groups, carpenters vs. controls:		
Group A	.00	NS
Group B	.66	NS
Between groups, Group A vs. Group B:		
Carpenters	2.00	NS
Controls	.20	NS

TABLE VI. Carpenter Population in Hawaii: Data from U.S. Census in Hawaii

Age interval	1950	1970
16-19	43	131
20-24	389	516
25-34	1927	1128
35-44	1266	1201
45-54	687	1792
55-59	147	647
60-64	186	324
65+	71	80
Total:	4716	5819

TABLE VII. Age-specific Death Rate per 100,000 for Neoplasms
Among Carpenters, by Age-interval, All Races

Age Interval	Cancer Deaths	Average Annual Rates	Total Deaths	Average Annual Death Rates
GROUP A:				
16-24	0	0	8	462.9
25-34	2	25.9	15	194.55
35-44	1	19.75	11	217.25
45-54	8	291.12	25	909.77
55-64	18	1351.3	52	3703.9
65+	31	10915.1	116	40843.5
Total:	60	318.05	227	1203.3
. . . .				
GROUP B:				
16-24	1	38.63	12	463.7
25-34	0	0	8	177.3
35-44	3	62.4	13	270.6
45-54	9	502.2	40	558.0
55-64	17	437.7	48	1235.8
65+	37	11562.5	172	53750.0
Total:	67	287.90	293	1258.8

TABLE VIII. Death Rate per 100,000 in the General Population During Periods of the Study

Period	Cancer Deaths*	Rate	Total Deaths	Rate
Group A				
1948	441	61.6	3104	574.3
1949	413	86.0	2965	616.0
1950	450	90.0	2919	583.0
1951	457	97.0	2872	461.0
	----	------	------	------
1948-1951	1761	88.65	11,860	558.6*
Group B				
1970	747	97.7	4206	538.5
1971	778	105.1	4365	583.5
1972	897	110.9	4494	555.8
1973	909	109.2	4320	519.1
	----	------	------	------
1970-1973	3331	105.7*	17,385	549.2

*Average annual rates. The "cancer death rate" given here is not the conventional cancer-specific mortality rate, which is based on the underlying cause of death given in Part I of the death certificate. Rather, it is an enumeration of death certificate with any mention of cancer.

REFERENCES

1. Acheson, E. D., Cowdell, R. H., Hadfield, E. & Macbeth, R. G.: Nasal cancer in woodworkers in the furniture industry. *Brit. Med. J.*, *2*: 587-596, 1968.

2. Dublin and Vane, cited in Milham, Ref. 4.

3. Härtig and Hesse. Der Lungenkrebs, die Bergkrankheit der Schneeberger Gruben. See Leuenberger, S.J.L Die unter dem Einfluss der synthetischen Farbenindustrie beobachtete Geschwulstentwickelung. *Beitr. z. klin. Chir.* *80*: 269, 1951.

4. Milham, S., Jr. *Mortality Experience of the AFL-CIO United Brotherhood of Carpenters and Joiners of America, 1969-1970.* HEW Publication No. (NIOSH) 74-129, July 1974.

5. Milham, S., Jr. and Hesser, J. E.: Hodgkin's disease in woodworkers. *Lancet* *2*: 136-137, 1967.

6. Nutt, Beattie and Pye-Smith: Arsenic cancer. *Lancet* *2*: 210, 1913.

7. Yeh, S., How, S. W. and Lin, C. S.: Arsenical cancer of skin: histologic study with special reference to Bowen's disease. *Cancer, N.Y.* 21: 312-339, 1968.

URINARY AND TISSUE GLYCOSAMINOGLYCAN
PATTERNS IN HEPATIC ANGIOSARCOMA

Charles E. Kupchella and Carlo H. Tamburro

Cancer Center and Department of Medicine
University of Louisville School of Medicine
Louisville, Kentucky 40201

I. INTRODUCTION

The recent discovery of a relationship between vinyl chloride and angiosarcoma of the liver has received much attention (1-3). Although there are now systematic detection programs for vinyl chloride workers (3,4), there is as yet no specific chemical abnormality that serves as a good indicator of early, vinyl-chloride-induced liver injury and angiosarcoma. Alpha feto-protein has been a relatively valuable serological marker for hepatocellular carcinoma (5), but is has not as yet proven useful in the detection of angiosarcoma (6). New leads are needed if more specific tests are to be developed for angiosarcoma.

The literature suggests that the glycosaminoglycans in the urine and/or blood should be evaluated as a possible aid in early detection. The production of sulfated glycosaminoglycans is characteristic of malignant vascular tumors of the skin and some pathologists use this feature as a diagnostic aid (7). Barr and Bonin (8) observed a strong positive alcian-blue, glycosaminoglycan staining reaction in human angiosarcoma tissue and suggested than an attempt be made to qualitate and quantitate the production of glycosaminoglycans in the neoplasms, serum, and urine of those at risk. They pointed out that the urinary glycosaminoglycans may have diagnostic significance in angiosarcoma and, if so, a glycosaminoglycan spot test might easily be employed as a gross screening test of vinyl chloride production workers.

A number of other observations place the glycosaminoglycans in a relevant position with regard to angiosarcoma. Angiosarcoma is accompanied by connective tissue abnormalities (2,9) and changes in tissue, urinary, and blood glycosaminoglycans have been found to occur in many connective-tissue disorders -- including connective tissue disorders of the liver (10-14) -- as well as in hepatic cancer (15-17).

Supported in part by grants from the B. F. Goodrich Company and the American Cancer Society (IN-111) and a contract with the National Cancer Institute (NO1-CN-55212).

The purpose of this study was to make a preliminary determination of the glycosaminoglycan patterns in tissue and urine associated with angiosarcoma of the liver and with vinyl-chloride-induced liver injury other than angiosarcoma and to compare these patterns with those in normal controls and those associated with other liver disease. Our goal was to evaluate the use of glycosaminoglycan patterns in the early detection of vinyl-chloride-induced liver injury and angiosarcoma and to explore the role of the glycosaminoglycans in the etiology of vinyl chloride injury.

II. PROCEDURES AND MATERIALS USED

Urine specimens were collected as occasional samples from: 9 normal controls; 9 individuals with histories of occupational exposure to vinyl chloride and having abnormal, liver, biochemical studies; 6 with "other" cancers prior to surgery; 3 with angiosarcoma; 8 with active viral hepatitis; 6 with cirrhosis; 2 with lung-liver metastases; and 4 with metabolic disorders of the liver (congenital and indirect hyperbilirubinemia).

In one case of angiosarcoma, 24-hr urines were collected on alternate days beginning 2 weeks prior to death.

Urine samples were collected without preservative and frozen at -76° until analysis. Specimens were divided into two 25 ml samples and one 5 ml sample. Urinary creatinine was measured on the 5 ml sample using a Technicon Autoanalyzer. The degree of urinary glycosaminoglycan polymerization was estimated by dialyzing one 25 ml sample for 24 hours in tap water; the sample was then treated identically to an undialyzed sample by the method of DiFerrante (18) using cetylpyridinium chloride as a precipitant. After resolubilization of the glycosaminoglycans in water, duplicate samples were assayed for total uronic acid by the modified carbozole reaction of Bitter and Muir (19). The remaining glycosaminoglycans were reprecipitated with cetylpyridinium chloride and separated into the wash, hyaluronic acid, chondroitin sulfate, and heparin fractions as described by Schiller et. al.(20). Each of the fractions was assayed for uronic acid (μg per mg of creatinine).

Autopsy tissue was obtained in 2 cases of hepatic angiosarcoma (tumor tissue and non-tumor tissue adjacent to tumor), 2 cases of cirrhosis, and in 3 control cases (gun-shot wound victims without liver pathology) and analyzed for glycosaminoglycans by a previously reported modification (21) of the method of Schiller et. al. (20). Uronic acid was determined in each of the hyaluronic acid, chondroitin sulfate, and heparin fractions.

Pieces of tissue were subjected to alcian-blue-periodic-acid-Schiff staining with and without hyaluronidase and diastase pretreatment. These procedures were carried out according to the methods described by Mowry (22).

Ascitic fluid was also obtained at autopsy in one case of angiosarcoma and analyzed for glycosaminoglycans. The fluid was centrifuged

and the sediment analyzed as tissue above. The supernatant was treated
by the method for urine described above.

III. RESULTS

A summary of the urinary glycosaminoglycan measurement is given in
Table I. Normal controls had the least urinary glycosaminoglycans
(measured as uronic acid) of all groups. All other groups showed some
elevation. The levels in angiosarcoma, hepatitis, cirrhosis, and liver
metastases were significantly elevated ($P < .05$) over normal controls.
The cirrhotic group exhibited the greatest variance in urinary glycosaminoglycans. No significant differences were found in urinary creatinine
levels between groups.

There were no significant differences between groups in either the
percentage of the total glycosaminoglycans that was dialyzable (Table I)
or in the percentage of the unfractionated total that appeared in the
hyaluronic acid, chondroitin sulfate, and heparin fractions.

Seven of 9 vinyl-chloride-exposed individuals other than those
with angiosarcoma had positive chondroitin sulfate fractions with negative hyaluronic acid and heparin fractions. This was true in only 3 of
32 other urines evaluated in this same manner.

The pattern of daily glycosaminoglycan excretion prior to death
due to angiosarcoma in one individual is given in Figure 1.

Total tissue glycosaminoglycan levels for angiosarcoma tumors,
fibrotic tissue adjacent to tumors, cirrhotic liver tissue and normal
liver tissue are shown in Figure 2. Fractional hyaluronic acid, chondroitin sulfate, and heparin levels are given in Figure 3.

Histochemically, angiosarcomatous tissue exhibited a strong alcian-
blue positive staining reaction. Alcian-blue staining was only slightly
less in "non-tumor" tissue adjacent to tumor masses. The staining
reaction in tissue from normal liver was very weak and only slightly
stronger in cirrhotic liver tissue. The strong alcian-blue reaction in
angiosarcomatous tissue did not occur if sections were pretreated with
hyaluronidase.

Ascitic fluid sediment was uronic-acid-positive in only the
hyaluronic acid fraction -- 112 μg uronic acid per gram of dry, defatted
sediment; ascitic fluid supernatant contained 1.7, 1.2, and 0.2 μg
uronic acid per ml in the hyaluronic acid, chondroitin sulfate, and
heparin fractions, respectively.

IV. DISCUSSION

The literature indicates that normal male creatinine excretion is
1.5 g per 24 hrs (23). Thus, our normal mean (Table I) of $3.2 \pm .4$ μg
cetylpyridinium chloride-precipitable uronic acid per mg creatinine falls
in the middle of the normal ranges reported by Varma et. al. (24),

917

2.6 - 4.7 µg/mg; DiFerrante and Rich (25), 2.9 - 4.8 µg/mg; and Kao and Leslie (26), 1.8 - 4.9 µg/mg.

Although our study was not controlled for age, Goldberg and Cotlier (27) have shown that urinary glycosaminoglycan excretion is constant from ages 20-70. Manley et. al. (28) have shown that the proportion of urinary glycosaminoglycans in the chondroitin sulfate fraction is constant from ages 20-70. Manley et. al. also reported that the chondroitin sulfate fraction is highest at birth and that it gradually drops until age 20, suggesting that urinary chondroitin sulfate reflects tissue growth.

The fact that we found no differences between groups in the creatinine concentration is significant in that it indicates that occasional samples do reflect 24-hour excretion when normalized to creatinine. Precedent for expressing glycosaminoglycan measurements as a function of creatinine content in occasional urine samples has been established by DiFerrante and Rich (25) and Pennock (29). Manley et. al. (28) have shown that the creatinine/uronic acid ratio is steady from ages 20-70.

Our results indicate that the liver diseases evaluated are accompanied by elevated urinary glycosaminoglycan excretion. Our tissue data suggests that this reflects liver-tissue glycosaminoglycan elevation and conforms to the reports by others that both hepatic connective tissue disorders (10-14) and hepatic cancer (15) result in increased hepatic glycosaminoglycan levels. It may be significant that the angiosarcoma patients had half the urinary glycosaminoglycan excretion of patients with liver metastases and that our analysis of angiosarcomatous tumor tissue exhibited half the glycosaminoglycan content reported by Kojima et. al. (15) for hepatocellular carcinoma.

While our data suggest that liver disease results in a decrease in the proportion of highly polymerized glycosaminoglycans, variance was large within each group and none of the differences between groups were statistically significant.

Although we have not completed the characterization of isolated glycosaminoglycan fractions, our data indicate: 1) that the chondroitin sulfates are the primary urinary glycosaminoglycans in both normal controls and in disease states; 2) that the chondroitin sulfates and heparin are the dominant glycosaminoglycans in normal and cirrhotic livers (Figure 3). Chondroitin sulfate is elevated in the fibrotic, non-tumor, portions of angiosarcomatous livers while heparin is the predominant glycosaminoglycan in tumor tissue. Hyaluronic acid is also apparently elevated relative to chondroitin sulfate in angiosarcomatous tumors (Figure 3); and 3) that hyaluronic acid is the sole glycosaminoglycan in ascites fluid sediment.

These qualitative data are in general agreement with those reported by others. Goldberg and Cotlier (27), Douglas et. al. (30), and Varma et. al. (24) have reported that the chondroitin sulfates are the predominant urinary glycosaminoglycans. Varma et. al. reported that 2/3 of urinary glycosaminoglycans are chondroitin-4-and chondroitin-6-sulfate and this agrees with our data on normal controls and on those with liver disease.

Kojima et. al. (15) reported that in hepatocellular carcinoma

918

tissue, chondroitin sulfates and hyaluronic acid were increased 33 and 10 times, respectively, over amounts found in healthy livers; the heparin and heparan sulfate proportions dropped. This contrasts with our data on angiosarcoma tissue, i.e. heparin and hyaluronic acid increased 5 and 10 times, respectively, over normal tissue; chondroitin sulfate levels rose but fell in proportion to other glycosaminoglycans. Galambos and Shapira (10) reported that the chondroitin sulfates are dominant in normal livers and in hepatic fibrosis, but Kojima et. al. (15) report that chondroitinase-resistant and hyaluronidase-resistant glycosaminoglycans are dominant. Kuroda et. al. (31) also reported that heparan sulfate is the dominant glycosaminoglycan in the normal liver. Our histochemical observation that nearly all of the increased alcian-blue positive material in angiosarcomatous livers was susceptible to hyaluronidase digestion suggests that the observed chondroitin sulfate elevation is due to chondroitin-4- and/or chondroitin-6-sulfate.

The increases in liver and urinary glycosaminoglycans may well reflect an important role of these substances in the process of fibrogenesis and in tumor growth. Galambos and Shapira (10) reported that hyaluronic acid was elevated during hepatic fibrogenesis. If a similar fibrotic process is operative in angiosarcoma, it may be that the observed tumor-tissue heparin increase is reflective of tumor growth. We did observe a four- to six-fold greater heparin level in tumor tissue than in adjacent, non-tumor tissue.

The observation that the chondroitin sulfates tend to be the exclusive uronic-acid-positive constituents in the urine of individuals is paradoxical in that those glycosaminoglycan fractions that are most elevated in angiosarcomatous tissue are those that are absent from the urine of individuals who may well have early, vinyl-chloride-induced liver injury. This pattern may be due to the selective action of lysosomal, glycolytic enzymes in the liver and/or may reflect the role of the chondroitin sulfates in early fibrotic changes in the liver. Certainly the potential usefulness of this pattern in early detection warrants the more complete evaluation now ongoing in our laboratory.

V. SUMMARY

Glycosaminoglycans were measured in urine and tissue of patients with hepatic fibrosis and hepatic cancer including vinyl-chloride-exposure-associated liver injury and angiosarcoma. Angiosarcoma, hepatitis, cirrhosis, and liver metastatic patients exhibited significantly elevated glycosaminoglycan excretion. Angiosarcoma tissue exhibited elevated glycosaminoglycan levels with the greatest increases in the heparin fraction. Histochemically, angiosarcomatous tissue gave a strong alcian-blue staining reaction which could be prevented by pretreatment with hyaluronidase. Although vinyl-chloride-exposure-associated liver injury other than angiosarcoma was not accompanied by a significantly elevated glycosaminoglycan excretion, this condition tended to be associated with a urinary glycosaminoglycan excretion pattern in which the chondroitin sulfate fraction was the only uronic-acid-positive fraction.

TABLE I.   Urinary Glycosaminoglycan Levels in µg Uronic Acid per mg
Creatinine by Liver Diseases Category

Patient group	Cases	ug uronic acid per mg creatinine (± 1 S.E.)	% uronic acid not dialyzable (± 1 S.E.)
normal control	9	3.2 ± .4	65 ± 5
vinyl chloride exposed	9	4.1 ± .4	39 ± 6
other cancer	6	4.5 ± 1.5	39 ± 6
other liver disease	4	5.1 ± 0.8	37 ± 13
angiosarcoma	3	7.6 ± 1.6	41 ± 22
hepatitis	8	8.5 ± 1.8	52 ± 14
cirrhosis	6	12.7 ± 3	53 ± 9
liver metastasis	2	13.8 ± .9	42

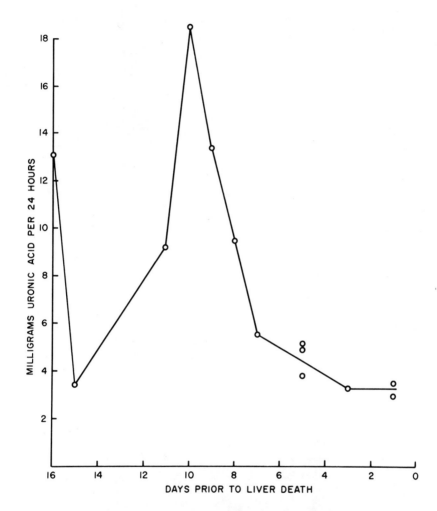

FIG. 1. Urinary glycosaminglycan output in one angiosarcoma patient during the 16-day period prior to death.

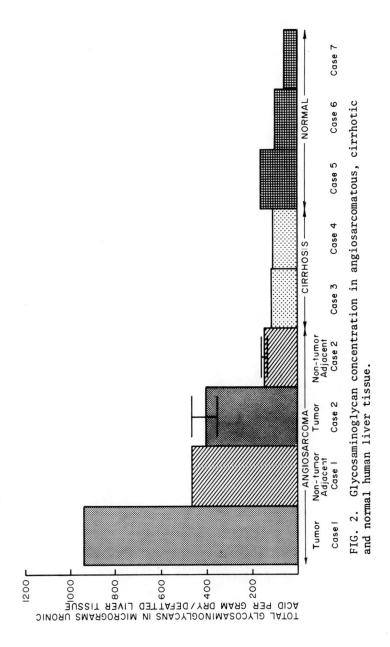

FIG. 2. Glycosaminoglycan concentration in angiosarcomatous, cirrhotic and normal human liver tissue.

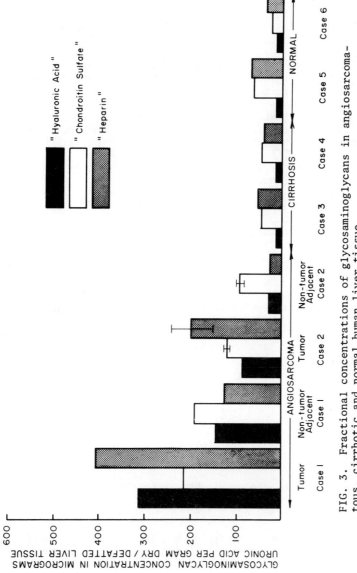

FIG. 3. Fractional concentrations of glycosaminoglycans in angiosarcomatous, cirrhotic and normal human liver tissue.

VI. REFERENCES

1. Creech, J. L. and Johnson, M. N. Angiosarcoma of the Liver in the Manufacture of Polyvinyl Chloride. J. Occup. Med. 16: 150-151, 1974.

2. Falk, H., Creech, J. L., Heath, D. W., Johnson, M. N., and Key, M. M. Hepatic Disease Among Workers at a Vinyl Chloride Polymerization Plant. JAMA 230: 59-63, 1974.

3. Makk, L., Creech, J. L., Whelan, J. G., and Johnson, M. N. Liver Damage and Angiosarcoma in Vinyl Chloride Workers: A Systematic Detection Program. JAMA 230: 64-68, 1974.

4. Creech, J. L., Makk, L., Whelan, J. and Tamburro, C. H. Hepatotoxicity Among Polyvinyl Chloride Production Workers During First Year of Surveillance Program. Gastroenterology 67: 786, 1974.

5. Kohn, J. and Weaver, P. C. Serum Alpha Fetoprotein in Hepatocellular Carcinoma. Lancet 2: 334-336, 1974.

6. Tamburro, C. H., Makk, L. and Creech, J. L. Unpublished observation.

7. Girard, D., Johnston, W. C., and Grahm, J. H. Cutaneous Angiosarcoma. Cancer 25: 868-883, 1970.

8. Barr, R. and Bonin, M. "Letters." JAMA 231(9): 914, 1975.

9. Popper, H., and Thomas, L. B. Alterations of Liver and Spleen Among Workers Exposed to Vinyl Chloride. Ann. NY Acad. Sci. 246: 172-194, 1975.

10. Galambos, J. T., and Shapira, R. Natural History of Hepatitis: IV Glycosaminoglycuronans and Collagen in the Hepatic Connective Tissue. J. Clin. Invest. 52(11): 2952-2962, 1973.

11. Koizumi, T., Nakamura, N., and Abe, H. Changes in Acid Mucopolysaccharide in the Liver in Hepatic Fibrosis. Biochim. Biophys. Acta. 148: 749-756, 1967.

12. Kojima, J. Studies on the Metabolism of Hepatic Connective Tissue in Fibrosis of the Liver. Med. J. Osaka Univ. 16: 419-429, 1964.

13. Rubin, E. Autoradiographic Characterization of Sulfated Acid Mucopolysaccharides in Experimental Cirrhosis. J. Histochem. Cytochem. 14: 688-689, 1966.

14. Patrick. R. S. and Kennedy, J. S. The Synthesis of Sulfated Mucopolysaccharide at Sites of Hepatic Fibrosis Induced by Carbon Tetrachloride, Amyloidosis, and the Implantation of Catgut. J. Pathol. Bacteriol. 88: 549-555, 1964.

15. Kojima, J., Nakamura, N., Kanatani, M. and Ohmori, K. The Glycosaminoglycans in Human Hepatic Cancer. Cancer Res. 35(3): 542-547, 1975.

16. Anghileri, L. J. Metabolism of Acid Mucopolysaccharides in Hepatoma and in Normal Liver. Oncology 30: 304-317, 1974.

17. Yamamoto, K., and Teryama, H. Comparison of Cell Coat Acid Mucopolysaccharides of Normal Liver and Various Ascites Hepatoma Cells. Cancer Res. 33: 2257-2264, 1973.

18. DiFerrante, N. M. The Measurement of Urinary Mucopolysaccharides. Anal. Biochem. 21: 98-106, 1967.

19. Bitter, T., and Muir, H. A Modified Uronic Acid Carbazole Reaction. Anal. Biochem. 4: 330-334, 1962.

20. Schiller, S., Slover, G. A., and Dorfman, A. A Method for the Separation of Acid Mucopolysaccharides: Its Application to the Isolation of Heparin from the Skin of Rats. J. Biol. Chem. 236(4): 983-987, 1961.

21. Kupchella, C., and Steggerda, F. The Distribution of Acid Mucopolysaccharides in the Canine Gastrointestinal Mucosa. Trans. NY Acad. Sci. 34: 351-360, 1971.

22. Mowry, R. W. Alcian Blue Techniques for the Histochemical Study of Acidic Carbohydrates. J. Histochem. and Cytochem. 4: 407, 1956.

23. Sunderman, F. W. and Boerner, F. Normal Values in Clinical Medicine. W. B. Saunders. Philadelphia, p. 353, 1949.

24. Varma, R. S., Varma, R., Allen, W. S., and Wardi, A. H. Urinary Excretion of Acid Mucopolysaccharides in Schizophrenia. Biochem. Med. 11(4): 358-369, 1974.

25. DiFerrante, N. and Rich, C. The Determination of Acid Aminopolysaccharide in Urine. J. Lab. Clin. Med. 48: 491-494, 1956.

26. Kao, K. and Leslie J. Micro Fractionation and Determination of Urinary Glycosaminoglycans. Biochem. Med. 9(4): 317-326, 1974.

27. Goldberg, J. and Cotlier, E. Specific Isolation and Analysis of Mucopolysaccharides (Glycosaminoglycans) from Human Urine. Clin. Chim. Acta. 41: 19-27, 1972.

28. Manley, G., Severn, M. and Hawksworth, J. Excretion Patterns of Glycosaminoglycans and Glycoproteins in Normal Human Urine. J. Clin. Pathol. 21: 339-345, 1968.

29. Pennock, C. A. A Modified Screening Test for Glycosaminoglycan Excretion. J. Clin. Path. 22: 310, 1969.

30. Douglas, C., Nowak, J. and Danes, B. Mucopolysaccharides in Urine During Normal Human Development. Pediatr. Res. $\underline{7}$: 724-727, 1973.

31. Kuroda, J., Saito, S., Seno, N., Nagase, S., and Anno, K. Isolation and Chemical Characterization of Mucopolysaccharides from Rat Tumors. Cancer Res. $\underline{34(2)}$: 308-312, 1974.

IMMUNOPATHOLOGIC OBSERVATIONS IN LIVER ANGIOSARCOMA

Enrique Espinosa, M.D.

Department of Pathology
University of Louisville School of Medicine
Louisville, Kentucky

I. INTRODUCTION

In hepatic fibrosis and angiosarcoma associated with vinyl chloride exposure of industrial workers, manifestations of the disease could not be detected in most cases until the process was far advanced (1). Normal values of liver function tests were reported in a case with significant vinyl chloride hepatic fibrosis (2), and only a small percentage of workers of a plant unit where seven cases of liver angiosarcoma were diagnosed had abnormal blood screening tests (3). Thus, conventional liver function tests do not appear to be sensitive indicators of vinyl chloride liver disease. Development of more sensitive methods for detecting the disease in early stages would be of great importance. An approach to this may be provided by immunologic studies. In such a study the question arises whether the fibrotic and angiosarcomatous livers contain antigens that are different from those present in normal tissue and whether such changes could stimulate an immunologic response. The purpose of this study was to search for antigenic changes in the angiosarcomatous tissue and to test for possible presence of an antibody response in the host.

II. PROCEDURES AND MATERIALS USED

A. Patients' Sera and Tissue Specimens

Serum samples from B.F. Goodrich Co. workers with histories of vinyl chloride exposure of several years included samples from two individuals with liver angiosarcoma, ten with liver dysfunction with fibrosis and ten with normal liver function tests. The patients with angiosarcoma died and the diagnosis was confirmed at autopsy and portions of tumor and neighboring liver tissues were obtained at autopsy. Patients with liver dysfunction with fibrosis included individuals with

927

abnormalities in liver function tests and fibrosis detected at biopsy. Tissues were also obtained from coroner's autopsies of healthy individuals a few hours after death by gunshot wounds.

B. Tissue Extracts and Antisera

Liver angiosarcoma and adjacent liver tissue and post-mortem tissues considered to be normal were frozen and stored at -70°C until used. Portions were cut, thawed and homogenized in 2-3 volumes of distilled water in a Potter-Elvehjem grinder in an ice bath until a smooth suspension was obtained. After centrifugation at 20,000 x G for 30 min, the supernatant fluid containing the aqueous extract was lyophilized. Albino rabbits were immunized with the tumor or normal liver extracts in Freund's complete adjuvant and sera collected and stored following procedures detailed elsewhere (4). Reaction of these immune sera with human serum or plasma was eliminated by absorption with 100 mg of lyophilized, pooled normal human serum /ml antiserum. Antisera were routinely absorbed in this manner prior to use. Additional absorption with tissue extracts was carried out with 100 mg lyophilized extract/ml antiserum. Absorptions followed a procedure described previously (5).

C. Treatment of Tissue Extracts

Enzymatic treatment of tissue extracts was carried out with Pronase and trypsin as previously described (6). Periodate oxidation was done according to Rajam et al. (7). Ammonium sulfate and cold ethanol fractionations were carried out as detailed (8).

D. Immunodiffusion and Immunofluorescence

Double immunodiffusion was carried out in 0.8% agarose in phosphate-buffered saline pH 7.2 (PBS) containing 0.1% sodium azide. Circular wells, 2 mm in diameter, 3 mm apart were used. Immunoelectrophoresis was performed according to Scheidegger (9) using 0.8% agarose in 0.025 M Veronal buffer at pH 8.2.

In immunofluorescent studies cryostat sections of rat kidney, stomach or intestine and liver (4 microns) were used as substrate for antimitochondrial, antismooth muscle and antinuclear antibodies. Liver sections from rats exposed 4, 8 and 14 days to 1-2% vinyl chloride for 4 hr/day were also used. The sections were covered with dilutions of patients' sera for 45 min at room temperature, washed twice in PBS for 10 min and then covered with fluorescein conjugated IgG fraction of rabbit anti-human immunoglobulins serum (Cappel Laboratories, Inc.) for 45 min and washed as before prior to examination. Cryostat sections of liver angiosarcoma and liver tissue considered to be normal (4 microns) were washed twice in PBS for 10 min to wash off nonfixed immunoglobulins. After drying, sections were stained with fluorescein conjugated IgG fractions of rabbit anti-human IgG serum and goat anti-human IgM serum (Cappel Laboratories, Inc.). Sections were washed as above and examined under the fluorescent microscope. Representative frozen sections were stained with hematoxylin and eosin to allow correlation between immunofluorescence and the histological findings. The antigenic preservation of the tissues was indicated by the demonstration of their staining by antinuclear factor according to the indirect immunofluorescent procedure.

E. Elution of Tumor-bound IgG

The tumor and liver tissues were extracted five times with PBS to wash off nonfixed immunoglobulins and then extracted at pH 2.5 to release bound IgG according to a procedure applied in the elution of renal-bound antibody (10).

F. Circulating Tissue Antigens

Liver-specific antigen LSA (8), tissue antigens of wide organ distribution (4) and bile antigens (11) were tested in the patients' sera by immunodiffusion as described previously.

III. RESULTS

A. Angiosarcoma-related Antigen

To test for presence of new antigens appearing in liver angiosarcoma, antiangiosarcoma serum was absorbed with human serum and liver extract and tested by immunodiffusion with extracts of both normal liver and angiosarcoma tumor at varying concentrations. This absorption eliminated all reactivity with liver extracts prepared from five normal individuals but not with the angiosarcoma extracts where one line of precipitation remained (Fig. 1). This line of precipitation could still be seen after additional absorption of the antiserum with kidney extract. In contrast, absorption with the tumor extracts eliminated completely the angiosarcoma-related line of precipitation. Absorption with spleen and lung extracts also eliminated this line of precipitation. Thus, the antigen appeared to be of restricted tissue distribution and not angiosarcoma specific. The antigen was inactivated by trypsin and Pronase and thus appeared to be a protein or closely associated to protein. Incubation of the tumor extracts for 1 hr at 4°C in citrate buffer, pH 2.5, resulted in inactivation of the antigen whereas incubation in phosphate buffer, pH 5.0, neutral or alkaline pH up to pH 10.0, did not affect it. The antigen was shown to be relatively thermolabile. Incubation of the tumor extracts for 30 min in PBS at 25° and 56°C did not affect the antigen whereas incubation at 70°C and higher completely inactivated it. The antigen precipitated mainly at 20-30% saturated ammonium sulfate and at ethanol concentrations of 30-70% (Table I).

B. Absence of a Normal Tissue Antigen in Angiosarcoma

Antiliver serum absorbed with human serum gave several arcs of precipitation in immunoelectrophoresis with extracts of normal liver and angiosarcoma tissue (Fig. 2a). These lines could not be seen following additional absorption of the antiserum with normal liver. In contrast, absorption with liver angiosarcoma extract failed to eliminate one of the arcs of precipitation (Fig. 2b). Thus, the tissue antigen related to this arc of precipitation appeared to be absent in the angiosarcomatous tissue whereas the antigens corresponding to the other arcs were present. The absent antigen in angiosarcoma was shown to be present in kidney and lung extracts in addition to liver by absorption and direct immunodiffusion tests. Physicochemical characterization studies indicated this antigen to be unaffected by Pronase and trypsin and inactivated by periodate treatment. The antigen was relatively thermostable withstanding incubation at 70°C for 30 min in PBS. The antigen was destroyed following incubation of the liver extract in citrate buffer at pH 2.5 or lower for 1 hr at 4°C; incubation at pH 5.0 or higher (up to pH 10.0) did not affect it. This antigen precipitated over a wide range of ammonium sulfate and ethanol concentrations (Table I).

C. Angiosarcoma-bound IgG

IgG fluorescent staining appeared in a linear pattern in the peripheral portion of the tumor cells suggesting in vivo binding by the tumor of the immunoglobulin. This staining is illustrated in Fig. 3. Fig. 4 shows the angiosarcomatous cells surrounding irregular vascular spaces. Relatively coarse, linear fluorescence was also present along some hepatic cords and strands of connective tissue. There was no evidence of IgM. Control post-mortem liver tissue did not show any significant fluorescence of bound IgG. Staining for IgG of the tumor sections did not change after several washings at pH 7.2 indicating that the IgG was firmly bound to the tumor. In contrast, sections showed marked diminution of staining after washing at pH 2.5. Elution of bound IgG from saline-extracted tumor homogenates was thus attempted at acid pH. With the five successive saline extractions the amount of saline soluble IgG gradually diminished to nondetectable levels; and at acid pH bound IgG was released from the homogenate. Similar treatment of liver homogenates did not demonstrate presence of bound IgG (Table II).

D. Circulating Autoantibodies and Tissue Antigens

Serum autoantibodies to nuclei, mitochondria and smooth muscle were negative in all patients examined. In addition, serum from these patients did not show reactivity with liver from rats exposed to vinyl chloride. Liver-specific antigen LSA (8), bile antigens (11) and other tissue antigens (4) associated with liver damage were not detected in these patients.

IV. DISCUSSION

The immunologic characteristics of cancer have been under intense investigation during recent years, and antigenic differences between normal and malignant tissue are considered to be fundamental factors in the immunologic approach to cancer therapy and diagnosis. Liver angiosarcomatous tissue was thus analyzed in this work for presence of neoantigens, normal tissue antigens and tumor-bound immunoglobulins. Several normal tissue antigens were found by immunodiffusion to be present in the tumor, but one antigen of rather wide organ distribution was not detected. These findings are in agreement with observations in other tumors indicating that tumor cells contain many of the antigens of their original hosts and lack some normal tissue antigens. For example, immunohistochemical studies have shown the loss of kidney antigens in stilbestrol- and x-ray-induced kidney tumors (12), of skin antigen in 3-methylcholanthrene-induced mouse squamous cell carcinoma (13) and of certain muscle antigens in 20-methylcholanthrene-induced rat rabdomyosarcoma (14). By far the most extensively studied class of tumors are the chemically induced hepatomata where deletion of liver antigens have been shown in tumors induced with 4-dimethylaminoazobenzene (15, 16), diethylnitrosamine (15) and 2-acetomidofluorene in the rat (15, 17) and o-aminoazotoluene in the mouse (18). In human carcinoma, loss of antigens have been reported in squamous cell carcinoma (12, 19), loss of the ABH blood group isoantigens in some solid tumors (20, 21) and of HL-A isoantigen in lymphoma (22). In addition, it has been well documented that as cells transform from a normal state to malignancy they may gain new antigenic specificities. Tumor-specific transplantation antigens have been demonstrated in a number of experimentally induced tumors (23-26) as well as in spontaneous tumors in man (27-29). In the present report immunodiffusion analyses of liver angiosarcoma and other human tissues with rabbit antiangiosarcoma serum did not indicate the presence of a tumor-specific antigen but rather of an antigen found in lung and spleen but not in liver and kidney. This antigen is being further characterized in our laboratory.

Of particular interest is the demonstration of tumor-bound IgG by immunofluorescence and elution experiments. This finding must however be interpreted with caution and should be confirmed in biopsy specimens. The tumor-bound IgG may represent specific antitumor antibody, antibody fixed by the tumor tissue "nonspecifically" or part of both. Further speculation is premature until it has been shown that the staining pattern

is due to the deposition of a specific antibody, that the eluted antibody is specific or until the relevant antigen has
been identified. Work is in progress to determine the precise
significance of the finding of IgG in the tumor.

V. SUMMARY

Immunodiffusion analyses of human liver angiosarcoma associated with vinyl chloride exposure indicated presence in the
tumor of an antigen not detected in normal liver and kidney
but found to be present in lung and spleen. This antigen was
shown to be a protein, inactivated by Pronase and trypsin,
relatively susceptible to heating and to acid pH and precipitated mainly at 20-30% saturated ammonium sulfate and at 30-
70% ethanol concentrations. The tumor was shown to contain
several antigenic constituents of normal tissue but one normal
tissue antigen was not detected. This antigen was characterized as a substance unaffected by Pronase and trypsin and inactivated by periodate. It was relatively thermostable, affected by acid pH and precipitated over a wide range of ammonium sulfate and ethanol concentrations. Tumor specimens obtained at autopsy contained bound IgG as shown by immunofluorescence and elution experiments suggesting possible in vivo
binding of IgG to the tumor.

Acknowledgements: The author wishes to thank Drs. W. M.
Christopherson, G. R. Schrodt and P. H. Carstens for fruitful
discussion and advice about the histologic sections and Drs.
C. Tamburro and L. Maak for providing serum samples and autopsy material. I also wish to thank Miss M. VanBraun and
Mrs. V. Petrey for skilled technical assistance. This work
was supported in part by a grant from B. F. Goodrich, Co.

TABLE I. Angiosarcoma-related Antigen and Antigen Absent
from the Tumor in Ammonium Sulfate and Ethanol Fractions

	Presence of[a]	
Fraction tested	Angiosarcoma-related antigen[b]	Antigen absent from Angiosarcoma[c]
Ammonium sulfate:		
0-20% saturation	+	-
20-30% saturation	++	+
30-50% saturation	-	+++
50-70% saturation	-	++
Ethanol:		
0-20%	-	++
20-30%	-	+++
30-50%	++	+++
50-70%	++	++
SN[d]	-	+

[a]
 +++, ++, + indicate strength of double diffusion reaction
in dilution assay.
[b]
 Detected in angiosarcoma fractions.
[c]
 Detected in liver fractions.
[d]
 SN = supernate of the 70% ethanol precipitation, dialyzed
and lyophilized.

TABLE II. IgG in Saline and Acid Extracts of Angiosarcoma and Liver Tissues

Preparation tested	Weight solid extracted from 1 gm (wet weight) tissue (mg)	Presence of IgG[a]
Angiosarcoma:		
Saline extract 1	29.8	+++
Saline extract 2	8.6	++
Saline extract 3	6.2	+
Saline extract 4	5.6	−
Saline extract 5	6.1	−
Acid extract	6.1	++
Liver:		
Saline extract 1	47.4	+++
Saline extract 2	14.5	+++
Saline extract 3	8.6	+
Saline extract 4	7.4	−
Saline extract 5	6.4	−
Acid extract	9.0	−

[a] Tested by immunodiffusion at concentrations of the eluates ranging up to 2%. Present at concentrations 0.05-0.1% (+++); 0.2-0.5% (++); 1-2% (+); negative at 2% (−).

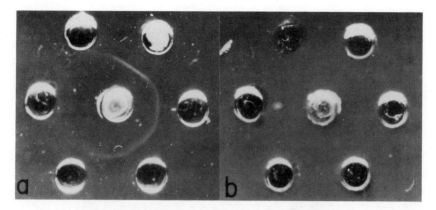

FIG. 1. Demonstration of angiosarcoma-related antigen. Peripheral wells
have 2-fold serial dilutions of liver angiosarcoma extract (a) and normal
liver extract (b). Dilutions are clockwise and start at 100 mg/ml in the
upper right well. Central wells in each plate contain rabbit antiangiosarcoma serum absorbed with normal human serum and liver extract.

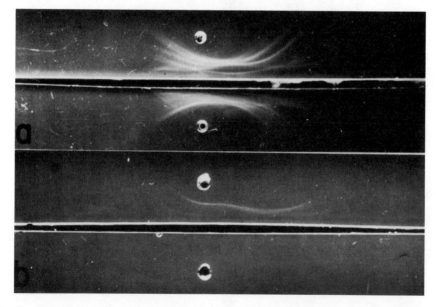

FIG. 2. Demonstration of tissue antigen absent in angiosarcoma. (a)
Trough contains rabbit antihuman liver serum absorbed with normal human
serum. (b) Trough contains the antiliver serum additionally absorbed with
angiosarcoma extract. In both plates top wells have 10% solution of liver
extract and lower wells angiosarcoma extract. Anode is to the right.

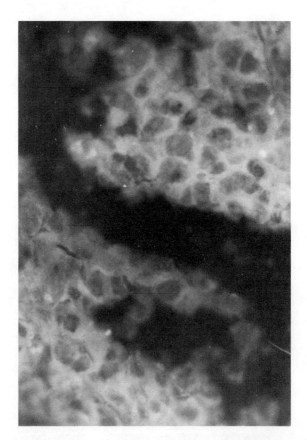

FIG. 3. Immunofluorescent staining of liver angiosarcoma by fluorescein conjugated IgG fraction of rabbit antihuman IgG serum (x 400).

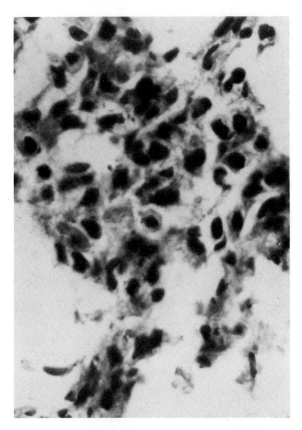

FIG. 4. Cryostat section of angiosarcoma tumor stained with hematoxylin-eosin (x 400).

REFERENCES

1. Heath, C.W., Jr., Falk, H., and Creech. J.L. Character-
   istics Of Cases Of Angiosarcoma Of The Liver Among Vinyl
   Chloride Workers In The United States. Ann. N.Y. Acad.
   Sci., 246:231-236, 1975.
2. Berk, P.D., Martin, J.F., and Waggoner, J.G. Persistence
   Of Vinyl Chloride-Induced Liver Injury After Cessation Of
   Exposure. Ann. N.Y. Acad. Sci., 246:70-77, 1975.
3. Wyatt, R.H., Kotchen, J.M., Hochstrasser, D.L., Buchanan,
   J.W., Jr., Campbell, D.R., Slaughter, J.C., and Doll,
   A.H. An Epidemiologic Study Of Blood Screening Tests And
   Illness Histories Among Chemical Workers Involved In The
   Manufacture Of Polyvinyl Chloride. Ann. N.Y. Acad. Sci.,
   246:80-87, 1975.
4. Espinosa, E. Circulating Tissue Antigens. I. Tissue
   Antigens In Serum Of Patients With Diseases Involving Injury Of The Liver And Of Other Organs. Clin. Exp. Immunol., 16:153-162, 1974.
5. Espinosa, E., and Kaplan, M.H. Antigenic Analysis Of
   Human Heart Tissue. Identification Of Antigens With
   Specificity Restricted To Heart And Skeletal Muscle In
   Acid Extracts Of Myocardium. J. Immunol., 100:1020-1031,
   1968.
6. Espinosa, E., and Kaplan, M.H. Antigenic Analysis Of
   Human Heart Tissue. Antigens With Restricted Organ Distribution In Acid Extracts Of Human Myocardium. J. Immunol., 105:416-425, 1970.
7. Rajam, P.C., Gaudreau, C.J., Grady, A., and Rundlett,
   S.T. Preparation, Derivation And Partial Characterization Of Organ-Specific Antigens From Human Brain. Immunology, 17:367-385, 1969.
8. Espinosa, E. Circulating Tissue Antigens. II. Studies
   On An Organ-Specific Antigen Of Human Liver. Lab.
   Invest., 29:556-561, 1973.
9. Scheidegger, J.J. Une Micro-Méthode De L'Immuno-Électro-
   phorèse. Internat. Arch. Allergy, Basel, 7:103-110,
   1955.
10. Krishnan, C., and Kaplan, M.H. Immunopathologic Studies
    Of Systemic Lupus Erythematosus. II. Antinuclear Re-
    action of γ-Globulin Eluted from Homogenates and Isolated
    Glomeruli Of Kidney From Patients With Lupus Nephritis.
    J. Clin. Invest., 46:569-579, 1967.
11. Espinosa, E. Circulating Tissue Antigens. III. Identi-
    fication And Characterization Of Antigens Of Limited And
    Of Wide Body Distribution In Human Gallbladder Bile.
    Presence In Serum Of Patients With Acute Hepatitis.
    Submitted for publication.
12. Nairn, R.C., Richmond, H.G., McEntegart, M.G., and Foth-
    ergill, J.E. Immunological Differences Between Normal
    And Malignant Cells. Br. Med. J., 2:1335-1340, 1960.
13. Carruthers, C., and Baumler, A. Immunochemical Staining
    With Fluorescein-Labeled Antibodies As An Aid In The
    Study Of Skin Cancer Formation. J. Natl. Cancer Inst.,
    34:191-200, 1965.

938

14. Fel, V.J., and Tsikarishvili, T.N.   Reduction Of Normal Muscle Antigens In Rat Tumors Of Muscle Origin Induced By Intramuscular Injections Of 20-Methylcholanthrene. Cancer Res., 24:1675-1677, 1964.

15. Baldwin, R.W., and Barker, C.R.   Antigenic Deletions In Carcinogen-Induced Rat Hepatoma.   Nature, 214:292-293, 1967.

16. Kalnins, V.I., and Stick, H.F.   Loss Of Liver Cell Antigens In Azo-Dye Induced Hepatomas Of Rats.   Nature, 200: 189-190, 1963.

17. Hiramoto, R., Bernecky, J., Jurandowski, J., and Pressman, D.   Immunohistochemical Staining Properties Of The N-2-FAA Rat Hepatoma.   Cancer Res., 21:1372-1376, 1961.

18. Abelev, G.I., Khramkova, N.I., and Postnikova, Z.A.   The Antigenic Structure Of Mouse Hepatomas.   I.   Organ-Specific Antigens Of The Liver And Immunoelectrophoretic Study Of Their Occurrence In Hepatomas.   Neoplasma, 9: 123-130, 1962.

19. Hillemans, H.G.   Serological And Immunological Studies On The Pathogenesis Of Cervical Cancer.   Z. Naturforsch., 17B:240-261, 1962.

20. Kay, H.E.M.   A And B Antigens In Normal And Malignant Cells.   Br. J. Cancer, 11:409-414, 1957.

21. Davidsohn, I., and Ni, L.Y.   Loss Of Isoantigens A, B And H In Carcinoma Of The Lung.   Am. J. Pathol., 57:307-314, 1969.

22. Seigler, H.F., Kremer, W.B., Metzgar, R.S., Ward, F.E., Haung, A.T., and Amos, D.B.   HL-A Antigenic Loss In Malignant Transformation.   J. Natl. Cancer Inst., 46:577-583, 1971.

23. Cryan, W.S., Hide, R.M., and Garb, S.   Demonstration By Gel Diffusion Of Antigen In Spontaneous Mouse Tumors. Cancer Res., 26:1458-1465, 1966.

24. Heppner, G.H., and Pierce, G.   In Vitro Demonstration Of Tumor-Specific Antigens In Spontaneous Mammary Tumors In Mice.   Internat. J. Cancer, 4:212-218, 1969.

25. Isojima, S., Yagi, Y., and Pressman, D.   Antigens Common To Rat Hepatoma Induced With 2-Acetylaminofluorene. Cancer Res., 29:140-144, 1969.

26. Kahan, B.D., Holmes, E.C., Reisfeld, R.A., and Morton, D.L.   Water Soluble Guinea Pig Transplantation Antigen From Carcinogen-Induced Sarcomas.   J. Immunol., 102:28-36, 1969.

27. Hughes, L.E., and Litton, B.   Antigenic Properties Of Human Tumors: Delayed Cutaneous Hypersensitivity Reactions.   Br. Med. J. 1:209-212, 1964.

28. Itakura, K.   Studies On Human Cancer Antigens By Gel Diffusion Methods.   Gann, 54:93-104, 1963.

29. McKenna, J.M., Sanderson, R.P., and Blakemore, W.S.   Extraction Of Distinct Antigens From Neoplastic Tissue. Science, 135:370-371, 1962.

Chapter 10

ENVIRONMENTAL CARCINOGENESIS

SHORT-TERM ASBESTOS EXPOSURE AND DELAYED CANCER RISK

Herbert Seidman, M.B.A.*, Ruth Lilis, M.D.**
and Irving J. Selikoff, M.D.**

From the *American Cancer Society
777 Third Avenue, New York, New York 10017
Environmental Sciences Laboratory**
Mount Sinai School of Medicine
of the City University of New York
Fifth Avenue and 100th Street, New York, New York 10029

I. INTRODUCTION

The relationship of lung cancer and mesothelioma of the pleura and peritoneum with asbestos exposure has been well documented by numerous epidemiologic studies in various countries. The awareness of this risk has
led to concern regarding relatively low-level and/or short-term asbestos
exposure, especially since experiences with "neighborhood" and "household"
exposures have been reported to result in mesothelioma (Newhouse(1),
Wagner(2), Anderson(3).

Cancer of the lung, while less specific for the asbestos carcinogenic
effect is, nevertheless, several times more frequent a cause of death in
asbestos-exposed workers. Definition of the minimum asbestos exposure
that would lead to a significant increase in lung cancer is an unanswered
question of high theoretical and practical importance.

II. MATERIALS AND METHODS

The requirements of the U.S. Navy for asbestos insulation for pipes,
boilers and turbines of its ships led to the establishment of an amosite
asbestos factory in Paterson, New Jersey just before the entry of the
United States into World War II. From 1941 through 1945, 933 men were

Supported in part by Grants from the National Institute of Environmental
Health Sciences, ES 00928 and the American Cancer Society, R-53C.

943

recruited to work in this plant which continued in operation through 1954. Though non-whites were employed in the latter years of the plant's operation, the initial group was almost entirely white. Wartime conditions had a marked influence on the composition of this work force. Younger and fitter men having been siphoned off by the Armed Services, these men tended to be older than is usual for men entering a new line of work. There were very few "career" men and only 19 had worked with asbestos previously; they have been omitted from the present analysis. In contrast to other groups of asbestos workers that have been studied, composed largely of those who continued to work in the industry once they started, a large proportion of the remaining 914 men drifted off to other employment after a while, and others left to enter the Armed Services, as the need for men increased.

This resulted in a unique body of data; experiences of men with a very limited duration of asbestos work exposure. Thus, there were 65 who worked in the plant less than a month; 101, worked one month; 103, two months; 165, 3-5 months; and 151, 6-11 months. We know that this plant had poor ventilation as detailed by review of conditions with workers and management, and examination of ventilation engineering plans. Examination of tissues obtained at autopsy (A.M. Langer) has shown that even short periods of exposure sufficed to leave the men with a lifetime burden of a large number of asbestos fibers in their lungs.

Our approach in this study has been to examine the mortality experience of these men in each year through 30 years after onset of work, in comparison with a hypothetical group of men of identical age at outset, subject to age specific death rates prevailing for white males in the general population of New Jersey in each relevant calendar year 1941-1974.

Table I shows the status of the 914 men at various intervals subsequent to entry. We took 1943 as the average starting point, 1948 as the 5 year point, etc. The setting in time has great significance for many reasons including the kinds of cigarettes available at the particular time.

Age 40 may be taken as roughly the age at which the frequency of cancer begins to be of appreciable magnitude. Despite the dwindling total number of men, we can see that for much of the period of observation there was actually an increase in the number of "effective" men (i.e., those 40 or over) at risk, as the younger men became older.

The "withdrawals alive" include 52 men lost to followup, mostly in the early years of the study, 17 men terminated from observation in this study at a time at which they accepted asbestos work elsewhere, and 36 men who had begun work in 1945 but who had not yet finished their 30th year of observation by December 31, 1974.

The "expected" number of men at risk are the number of survivors from the original group of 914 men depleted on the basis of mortality for white males in New Jersey,* allowing for "withdrawals alive." Subtracting the actual number of men at risk from the "expected" number yields what we have termed "net susceptibles", or more precisely "net susceptibles at the level of asbestos exposure experienced." Besides being a measure of the excess mortality among the asbestos workers, the fact that these "susceptibles" were not available for observation in subsequent time periods means that some understatement was likely in such periods in the cumulative probabilities of death data we will show for the asbestos workers.

We have used followup study life table methods to estimate the probabilities of death in various parts of the first year after onset of work, and year by year thereafter. To obtain these probabilities we adopted the approach by Chiang(11) and Littel (12) in which P_t, the probability of surviving a small time interval t was computed from λ, the death rate per man-year for the interval, through the relationship $P_t = e^{-t\lambda}$. Chain multiplication of these probabilities gave the cumulative probability of surviving from some initial point of time to some later point of time. Subtracting the cumulative probability of surviving from 1 results in the cumulative probability of dying from all causes.

The cumulative probabilities of death for cancer and lung cancer were derived by summing over the various intervals the products obtained by multiplying the part of the probability of death during that interval attributable to cancer or lung cancer by the cumulative probability of surviving to that interval.

---

*The depletions were calculated by interpolation and extrapolation of single year of age l_x from published life tables for New Jersey white males for 1940(4), 1950(5) and 1960(6). The 1970 life table is not yet available so we developed one(7,8) from mortality data for the years 1969-1971(9) and population data from the 1970 census(10).

In order to start the cumulative probabilities of death for all subgroups from the date of onset of work, each subgroup was given the mortality experience for all men during the period less than one month after onset. Subgroups which worked one month or more were given the mortality experience of all such men for month 1. Subgroups which worked two months or more were given the mortality experience of all such men for month 2.

Through 1971, mortality data for New Jersey were available from the annual vital statistics publications of the National Center for Health Statistics (9). Annual populations were estimated by interpolating and extrapolating decennial population data(10,13-15). The kind cooperation of the National Center for Health Statistics provided us with unpublished mortality data for 1972-1973(16). The 1974 data not yet being available, we extrapolated for 1974 from 1967-1973.

The coding for cause of death in this study is that of the VI through VIII revisions of the International List in use in the United States from 1949 on. The observed deaths were coded in two ways. First, according to death certificate information but then also according to verified diagnosis, established from additional information available for the decedent from autopsy, surgical specimens, x-ray films and clinical information. For this analysis we have utilized the verified diagnosis. To obtain total cancer death rates on a consistent basis for New Jersey prior to 1949, we extrapolated from rates for 1949-1955.

For New Jersey white males, age specific death rates were available for total cancer of the respiratory system but not for lung cancer specifically, although this neoplasm constitutes the major part of the category. However, the all ages total for lung cancer were at hand. We estimated the age-specific lung cancer rates as follows: For each age group, to the United States lung cancer death rates for 1949 on, we applied the ratio of New Jersey to United States total respiratory cancer rates in order to obtain first estimates of lung cancer rates for New Jersey. These first estimates were multiplied against population figures for New Jersey and the resulting implied numbers of deaths were summed to obtain the totals. These were then compared with the actual total numbers. There was excellent agreement and only small adjustments were required between the first and final estimates.

III. RESULTS

The results for small subgroups are subject to substantial sampling variation. Even so, for the 65 men who worked less than a month, the indications were for favorable mortality for all causes of death during the 30
year period of observation(Fig. 1). No cancer death was observed until
the 22nd year and no lung cancer death until the 25th year but in the
probabilities thereafter there is the hint that even in these men the
time bomb of "residence asbestos exposure" (residual retained asbestos in
tissues) was ticking away.

When we proceed to the findings for the men who worked a month or more,
the mortality after a number of years was consistently unfavorable
(Figs. 2-7).

Table II provides a summary for all causes of death at various points of
time after onset of work, of the absolute and the relative differences
between the observed and expected cumulative probabilities of death for
the several subgroups. Underneath the lines and in the unshaded area, the
observed mortality is consistently unfavorable. For those who worked 1,
2 and 3-5 months, this became evident at 20 years while for those who
worked longer, it is evident earlier.

Table III provides a similar summary for total cancer. The absolute differences were smaller and the relative differences larger than those for
all causes of death. The smaller absolute differences for cancer compared
with all causes means that cancer did not account for all of the excess
mortality in these asbestos workers. For those who worked 1-11 months it
took longer for cancer **than** for all causes for the excess mortality to
become evident.

In the summary for lung cancer in Table IV the relative differences are
clearly much larger than those in Tables II and III. As compared with the
respective absolute differences for total cancer, lung cancer sometimes
accounted for all of the excess cancer mortality and sometimes for only
a part of the excess.

Figure 8 shows the relative differences 30 years after onset of work in
the observed compared with expected cumulative probabilities of death
from all causes for the various subgroups. Relative differences of observed to "expected" of 1.3, 1.4 and 1.5 may not seem impressive, but it

947

must be remembered that as "expected" cumulative probability of death approached 50%, the largest possible relative difference was 2. Figure 9 shows these data for all cancer and Figure 10 for lung cancer.

IV. DISCUSSION

The fact that direct asbestos exposure of short duration (less than one year), results in significant excess risk of lung cancer, together with the development of mesothelioma after minor (neighborhood or household) asbestos exposure, is of considerable interest for the evaluation of the "minimum carcinogenic dose" for asbestos.

It is also evident that the asbestos exposure in "residence" is immensely important. Calculations of asbestos dose which consider only the initial direct exposure dose deal with the visible tip of the iceberg and ignore the bulk of the mass which is out of sight(17).

Since tissues continue to be exposed after cessation of the individual's direct exposure, the disease outcome is influenced by the duration of post-employment tissue exposure ("residence time"); epidemiologically, this becomes evident only with long post-employment observation.

The lengthy interval between the direct dosage and the emergence of cancer poses the challenge to use this time in some way to intervene and abort the cancer process in those we know to be high risk persons. To date, the opportunity may be there, but not the know-how of how to take advantage of it.

In coding cause of death using all of the information compiled for the 494 decedents among this group of 914 men, we classified 142 deaths in the category "total cancer" including 76 as lung cancer. Based on death certificate information alone, 135 deaths would have been classified as cancer and 65 as lung cancer. Some investigators assert that for greater comparability only death certificate information for coding causes of death should be used. Of course, it would be optimal if causes of death in the general population were also to be coded with all of the relevant records at hand. This not being feasible, we believe our approach is well justified because of the unique problems in asbestos workers. For instance, with careful effort it is not unusual to detect mesothelioma in an asbestos worker, mesothelioma which was probably unrecorded on death certificates. In the general population with equal effort it would be rare to detect mesothelioma because it simply is only rarely there to be detected and recorded.

V. SUMMARY

Workers exposed to amosite asbestos for merely a month showed a clear excess risk of cancer. With longer direct exposure (i.e., 2 months, 3 months, 6 months, etc.) the cancer risk became greater. Moreover, with very brief direct exposure, increased cancer risk was found only after 25 years. Longer employment resulted in cancer after shorter post-exposure observation.

Thus, brief asbestos employment (less than one year) resulted in important excess cancer mortality.

In evaluating cancer hazards of asbestos exposure, it is necessary to include post-employment observation of adequate duration, since the retained asbestos results in tissue exposure long after employment ceases.

Acknowledgements: We wish to thank Stephen L. Smith, Ashley Bodden and Edwin Silverberg of the American Cancer Society, for their assistance in processing the data of this study.

TABLE I. Status of All 914 Men With Respect To Elapsed Time After Onset of Work, 1941-1945

Item	Number of Elapsed Years Since Onset of Work						
	0	5	10	15	20	25	30
Middle calendar year	1943	1948	1953	1958	1963	1968	1973
Number of men at risk	914	814	760	686	584	472	337
Mean years of age per man	37.3	42.0	46.1	49.9	53.0	56.0	59.1
Number of men age 40 or more at risk	382	440	487	521	522	472	337
Number of deaths in ensuing 5 years	38	51	74	101	110	108	...
Number of withdrawals alive	62	3	0	1	2	37	...
"Expected" number of men at risk	914.0	814.9	767.0	712.5	647.9	573.7	458.3
Cumulative "net susceptibles" already dead	...	0.9	7.0	26.5	63.9	101.7	121.3

TABLE II. Observed Compared With Expected Cumulative Probability Of Death Through 30 Elapsed Years Since Onset Of Work In An Amosite Asbestos Factory, 1941 - 1945, by Length of Time Worked. ALL CAUSES OF DEATH

Elapsed Number Of Years Since Onset Of Work

Length Of Time Worked	5		10		15		20		25		30	
	O-E (%)	O/E	O-E (%)	O/E	O-E (%)	O/E	O-E (%)	O/E	O-E (%)	O/E	O-E (%)	O/E
<1 Month	-1.72	0.48	-5.39	0.23	-8.58	0.27	-14.70	0.18	-14.23	0.44	-7.71	0.77
1 Month	0.19	1.04	-0.88	0.91	-0.94	0.94	5.32	1.22	8.45	1.26	9.44	1.23
2 Months	1.63	1.26	2.01	1.16	2.34	1.11	4.10	1.14	9.00	1.23	15.31	1.32
3-5 Months	2.53	0.53	-3.10	0.73	-0.09	1.00	4.54	1.17	15.76	1.44	15.19	1.34
6-11 Months	1.57	1.36	4.56	1.49	4.50	1.30	15.12	1.68	16.21	1.54	17.42	1.47
1 Year	2.22	1.62	-1.95	0.97	4.79	1.38	5.40	1.29	7.36	1.29	17.92	1.54
2+ Years	-2.45	0.53	1.06	1.09	5.71	1.29	10.76	1.37	15.27	1.39	21.04	1.43

TABLE III. Observed Compared With Expected Cumulative Probability Of Death Through 30 Elapsed Years Since Onset Of Work In An Amosite Asbestos Factory, 1941 - 1945, by Length of Time Worked.
ALL CANCER

Length Of Time Worked	Elapsed Number Of Years Since Onset of Work											
	5		10		15		20		25		30	
	O-E (%)	O/E	O-E (%)	O/E	O-E (%)	O/E	O-E (%)	O/E	O-E (%)	O/E	O-E (%)	O/E
<1 Month	-0.50	0.00	-1.19	0.00	-2.15	0.00	-3.40	0.00	-1.74	0.65	-0.28	0.96
1 Month	0.23	1.29	0.26	1.15	0.03	1.01	3.79	1.84	2.07	1.33	2.34	1.29
2 Months	-1.01	0.00	0.05	1.02	-1.54	0.60	0.19	1.03	3.07	1.41	7.16	1.76
3-5 Months	-0.22	0.76	-1.37	0.33	-1.46	0.58	0.95	1.18	5.24	1.75	5.46	1.62
6-11 Months	0.02	1.03	-0.19	0.89	0.12	1.06	3.14	1.76	5.24	1.92	7.29	1.99
1 Year	-0.55	0.00	-1.29	0.00	1.04	1.46	1.48	1.43	4.15	1.84	10.79	2.63
2+ Years	-0.84	0.00	0.41	1.20	5.35	2.42	9.09	2.62	11.10	2.45	16.65	2.72

TABLE IV. Observed Compared With Expected Cumulative Probability Of Death Through 30 Elapsed Years Since Onset Of Work In An Amosite Asbestos Factory, 1941 - 1945, by Length of Time Worked. LUNG CANCER

Length Of Time Worked	Elapsed Number Of Years Since Onset Of Work											
	5		10		15		20		25		30	
	O-E (%)	O/E	O-E (%)	O/E	O-E (%)	O/E	O-E (%)	O/E	O-E (%)	O/E	O-E (%)	O/E
<1 Month	-0.09	0.00	-0.24	0.00	-0.48	0.00	-0.83	0.00	0.26	1.13	2.93	2.52
1 Month	-0.14	0.00	-0.35	0.00	0.39	1.59	3.13	3.96	2.62	2.66	3.09	2.44
2 Months	-0.18	0.00	-0.45	0.00	-0.83	0.00	-0.14	0.89	1.75	1.95	5.95	3.49
3-5 Months	-0.16	0.00	-0.40	0.00	-0.74	0.00	0.17	1.14	1.68	1.99	1.79	1.78
6-11 Months	-0.12	0.00	-0.31	0.00	0.16	0.28	1.99	3.15	4.42	4.13	4.62	3.37
1 Year	-0.09	0.00	-0.24	0.00	2.00	5.20	3.33	5.15	4.54	4.62	7.34	5.10
2+ Years	-0.43	0.00	-0.20	1.25	3.77	3.92	8.33	7.45	10.80	6.84	15.27	7.22

953

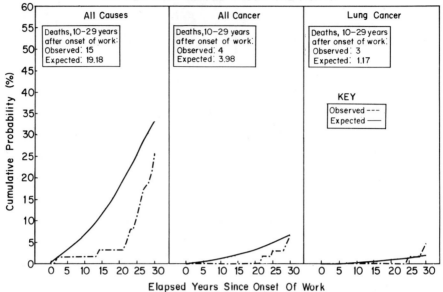

FIG. 1. Cumulative observed and expected probability of dying from all causes, all cancer, and lung cancer for 65 men who worked less than 1 month, through 30 elapsed years since onset of work in an amosite asbestos factory, 1941-1945.

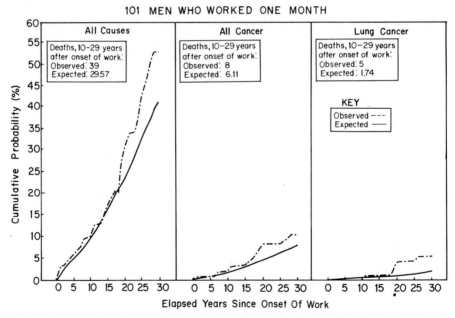

FIG. 2. Cumulative observed and expected probability of dying from all causes, all cancer, and lung cancer for 101 men who worked one month, through 30 elapsed years since onset of work in an amosite asbestos factory, 1941-1945.

954

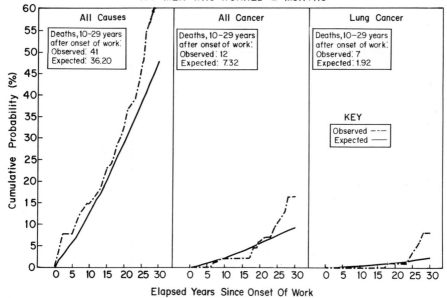

FIG. 3. Cumulative observed and expected probability of dying from all causes, all cancer, and lung cancer for 103 men who worked 2 months, through 30 elapsed years since onset of work in an amostie asbestos factory, 1941-1945.

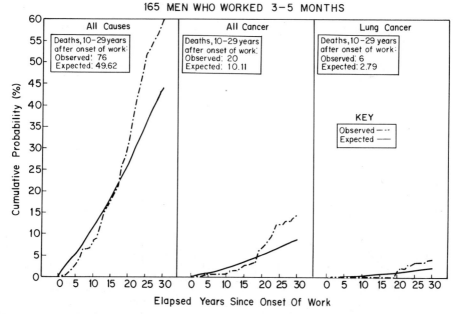

FIG. 4. Cumulative observed and expected probability of dying from all causes, all cancer, and lung cancer for 165 men who worked 3-5 months, through 30 elapsed years since onset of work in an amosite asbestos factory, 1941-1945.

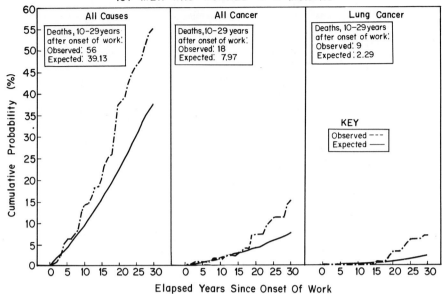

FIG. 5. Cumulative observed and expected probability of dying from all causes, all cancer, and lung cancer for 151 men who worked 6-11 months, through 30 elapsed years since onset of work in an amosite asbestos factory, 1941-1945.

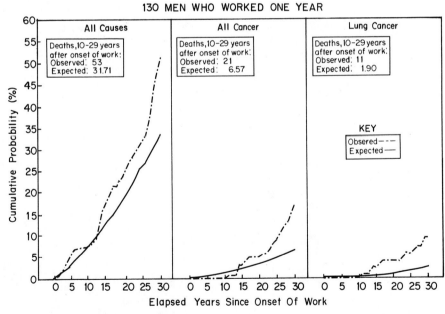

FIG. 6. Cumulative observed and expected probability of dying from all causes, all cancer, and lung cancer for 130 men who worked 1 year, through 30 elapsed years since onset of work in an amosite asbestos factory, 1941-1945.

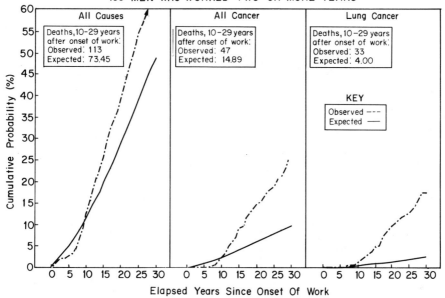

FIG. 7. Cumulative observed and expected probability of dying from all causes, all cancer, and lung cancer for 199 men who worked 2+ years, through 30 elapsed years since onset of work in an amosite asbestos factory, 1941-1945.

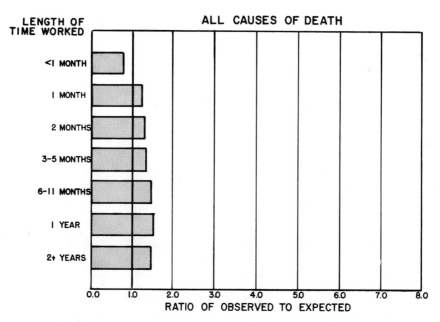

FIG. 8. Ratio of observed to expected cumulative probability of deaths at 30 elapsed years since onset of work.

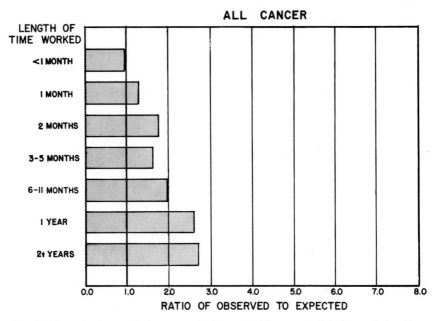

FIG. 9. Ratio of observed to expected cumulative probability of deaths at 30 elapsed years since onset of work.

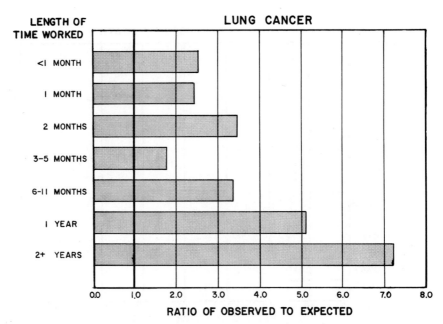

FIG. 10. Ratio of observed to expected cumulative probability of deaths at 30 elapsed years since onset of work.

References

1. Newhouse, M.L. and Thompson, H. Mesothelioma of the pleura and peritoneum following exposure to asbestos in the London area. Br. J. Industr. Med. 22: 261-269, 1965.

2. Wagner, J.C. Sleggs, C.A. and Marchand, P. Diffuse pleural meso-thelioma and asbestos exposure in the N.W. Cape Province. Br. J. Industr. Med. 17: 260-271, 1960.

3. Anderson, H.A. Lilis, R. Daum, S.M. Fischbein, A.S. and Selikoff, I.J. Household - contact asbestos neoplastic risk. Ann. N.Y. Acad. Sci., 271: 311-323, 1976. In Press.

4. U. S. Federal Security Agency - Public Health Service, National Office of Vital Statistics, State and Regional Life Tables 1939-41 (New Jersey) U. S. Government Printing Office, Washington, D.C., 1948, pp. 182-185.

5. U. S. Department of Health, Education, and Welfare - Public Health Service: National Office of Vital Statistics, State Life Tables (New Jersey), 1949-51. Vital Statistics - Special Reports, 41: 265-280 (Suppl. 34), 1956.

6. U. S. Department of Health, Education, and Welfare - Public Health Service: National Vital Statistics Division. 1966. Life Tables: 1959-61, Volume 2 - No. 32, New Jersey, State Life Tables: 1959-61, Public Health Service Publication No. 1252. U. S. Government Printing Office, Washington, D.C., 1966, pp. 495-508.

7. Reed, L.J. and Merrell, M. A short method for constructing an abridged life table. Vital Statistics - Special Reports, 9: 683-712, 1949.

8. Wolfenden, H.H. Population Statistics and Their Compilation, University of Chicago Press, Chicago, 1954.

9. U. S. Public Health Service, National Vital Statistics Division: Vital Statistics of the United States, Annual 1941-1971. Govern-ment Printing Office, Washington, 1943-1975.

10. U. S. Bureau of the Census: Census of the Population: 1970, General Population Characteristics. Final Report PC(1)-B32, New Jersey. U. S. Government Printing Office, Washington, 1971.

11. Chiang, C.L. A stochastic study of the life table and its appli-cations: III. The follow-up study with the consideration of competing risks. Biometrics, 17: 57-78, 1961.

12. Littel, A.S. Estimation of the T-year survival rate from follow-up studies over a limited period of time. Human Biology, 24: 87-116, 1952.

13. U. S. Bureau of the Census: Sixteenth Census of the United States:
     1940. Population, Volume II. Characteristics of the Population.
     Part 4: Minnesota-New Mexico. U. S. Government Printing Office,
     Washington, 1943.

14. U. S. Bureau of the Census: U. S. Census of Population: 1950.
     Vol. II, Characteristics of the Population. Part 30, New Jersey.
     U. S. Government Printing Office, Washington, 1952.

15. U. S. Bureau of the Census. U. S. Census of Population: 1960.
     General Population Characteristics, New Jersey. Final Report
     PC(1)-32B. U. S. Government Printing Office, Washington, 1961.

16. U. S. Public Health Service, National Vital Statistics Division:
     Unpublished tabulations.

17. Selikoff, I.J. and Hammond, E.C. Lapsed Time (Editorial) Environ.
     Res. 4: i-ii, April 1971.

"ADULT TYPE" CANCER IN CHILDREN AND ADOLESCENTS

Charles B. Pratt, M.D.
Warren W. Johnson, M.D.
H. Omar Hustu, M.D.

St. Jude Children's Research Hospital
332 North Lauderdale
Memphis, Tennessee 38101 USA

Pediatric oncologists concerned with the diagnosis and treatment of childhood cancer patients have directed their efforts toward patients with the most common malignant diseases of children and adolescents — leukemia, Hodgkin's disease, non-Hodgkin's lymphoma, neuroblastoma, Wilms' tumor, brain tumors and bony and soft-tissue sarcomas.[9-11,14,15,17]

With referral of increasing numbers of patients to childhood cancer centers, there has become evident an increased need for pediatric oncologists to be prepared to treat tumors rarely encountered in pediatric patients. Recent referral patterns suggest an increase in the frequency of adult-type cancer in children. The purpose of this report is to detail the incidence of adult cancers seen in a pediatric oncology center.

PROCEDURES AND METHODS

Between March 1962 and January 1976, 1009 children with malignant solid neoplasms have been admitted to St. Jude Children's Research Hospital. Fifty-eight of these patients, ages 3 months to 19 years, have had tumors usually encountered only in adults. Median age of the 58 patients was 12 years 9 months. Distribution of pathologic diagnoses of these patients is detailed in Table I. Thirty-seven of these 58 patients had carcinomas, and 21 patients had sarcomas of the types more commonly seen in adults than in children. During the same period of time 960 children were seen with acute lymphocytic leukemia and 269 children with the diagnosis of nonlymphocytic leukemia were encountered. Among the solid tumor patients, 150 had Hodgkin's disease, 142 had neuroblastomas, 127 had non-Hodgkin's lymphoma, 99 patients had Wilms' tumor, and 99 patients had rhabdomyosarcoma, 74 patients had osteosarcoma, 57 had Ewing's sarcoma, and 51 had retinoblastoma.

Of 58 patients with adult cancers, 22 were encountered in Caucasian boys, 18 in Caucasian girls, 11 in black males, and 7 in black females.

Age distribution, diagnosis and survival are presented in Table II. Distribution of diagnoses for patients by age group is presented in Table II. It will be noted that 30 of the 58 patients with adult cancers are surviving from 3 months to more than 11 years following diagnosis.

Annual accrual of patients with adult cancers is presented in Figure 1 and compared with the annual admission of patients with malignant solid tumors. It can be noted that after 1968 there was an increase in the number of solid tumor admissions with the exception of the year 1970.

RESULTS

CARCINOMAS

Colorectal carcinoma: The most commonly encountered adult cancer seen in these 58 children and adolescents was carcinoma of the colon. Single patients with this diagnosis were admitted in 1964, 1966 and 1973. A 15-year-old black girl was admitted with the diagnosis of carcinoma of the rectum in 1969. Nine patients with carcinoma of the colon were admitted between October 1974 and November 1975. None of these patients were persons considered to be at high risk for the development of colorectal cancer, i.e., persons with familial polyposis, ulcerative colitis, prior bowel cancer, with bowel cancer in a close relative, or prior breast or genital cancer.[5,7]

Comparison of the times of admission of patients with adult cancers and patients with colorectal cancer are presented in Figure 2. Five of these patients were black boys, 5 were black girls and 3 were white girls. Except for the patient with adenocarcinoma of the rectum, the histology of the colon lesions was that of a mucin-producing carcinoma.[7] Three patients had carcinoma of the cecum. The primary tumors of the other patients were the splenic flexure 3, the transverse colon 1, the descending colon 2, the sigmoid colon 1, and the rectum 1. The median age of these patients was 15 5/12 years. These patients were born between June 1953 and September 1966; they ranged in age at the time of diagnosis from 8 years 11 months to 19 years, with a median age of 15 5/12 years. Median time of their birth was April 1969. The place of residence from which these patients were referred to this hospital is demonstrated in Figure 3. Only 3 of these 13 patients were from towns or cities with populations exceeding 10,000.

Of the four patients referred between 1964 and 1974, only the patient with carcinoma of the rectum survives; she remains free of tumor 6½ years following diagnosis following successful treatment with preoperative radiation therapy, abdomino-perineal resection and intravenous 5-fluorouracil which was administered for 1 year.

Of the nine patients who were treated in 1974 and 1975, 5 patients are surviving of whom 2 are living with evidence of disease, and 3 have had no apparent disease for 4+ months, 6+ months, and 18+ months, following definitive surgery and chemotherapy with vincristine, methyl CCNU and oral 5-fluorouracil administered in monthly courses.[13]

Hepatocellular carcinoma: The 6 patients with hepatocellular carcinoma included in this series were 3 boys and 3 girls. One girl developed hepatocellular carcinoma and cholangiocarcinoma in association with acute lymphocytic leukemia; this patient had received treatment with androgens for the diagnosis of aplastic anemia. The sites of hepatocellular carcinoma in this patient were multifocal.

Four of the other 5 patients with hepatocellular carcinoma had involvement of both lobes of the liver. The only patient for whom complete resection of the right lobe of the liver could be performed is surviving 8 years following resection. Therapeutic measures, including radiation therapy and multiple-drug chemotherapy, were of little benefit to patients with unresectable primary hepatocellular carcinoma.

The ages of the patients with hepatocellular carcinoma range from 9 months to 16 years 3 months (median 4 years 5 months). In comparison to 13 patients with hepatoblastoma, whose ages ranged from 3 months to 7 years 1 month (median age at diagnosis for patients with hepatoblastoma was 2 years 1 month), 5 of the 13 patients with hepatoblastoma continue to survive from 1 year to 9+ years.

Adrenocortical carcinoma: Three patients with this diagnosis have been admitted to this hospital in the past 13 years. The ages of these patients at the time of diagnosis was 3 months, 10 years 6 months, and 14 years 6 months. Two of the 3 patients are surviving for 2+ months and for more than 2 years.

Melanoma: Three of the patients in this series have the diagnosis of melanoma. Two of the patients were white boys, ages 14 years each. One patient had a primary tumor site involving the right ear; another patient had metastatic disease involving the lymph nodes of the neck and an undetermined primary site. These patients had radical neck dissections and have remained tumor free for 1 and 7 years respectively.

The third patient with this diagnosis was a black girl who presented with a large right flank mass. This mass represented a melanoma of the adrenal cortex. The patient's therapy consisted of multiple chemotherapeutic agents, which were given without success. She died with pulmonary insufficiency caused by enlarging pulmonary metastases.

Carcinoma of the pancreas: This condition was encountered in 2 white girls, each aged 1 year 8 months at the time of diagnosis. The first patient had adenocarcinoma of the body of the pancreas and responded briefly to vincristine and cyclophosphamide before death 1 year 7 months following diagnosis.

The second patient had nonfunctioning islet cell carcinoma of the tail of the pancreas, which was completely resected except for a single metastasis involving the right lobe of the liver. This metastasis has responded satisfactorily to treatment with Bis-chlorethyl nitrosurea (BCNU) and 5-fluorouracil.

Dysgerminoma: Two girls, ages 8 and 16 years, have been treated for this diagnosis; following resection of the ovarian tumor, both patients received total abdominal radiation and are now 3- and 4-year survivors respectively.

Teratocarcinoma: This diagnosis was encountered in two boys, ages 8 months and 15 years. The primary site of the 8-month-old boy was the chest wall. He failed to survive because of extension of the tumor into the chest. The second patient, whose mixed germ cell tumor of the testis had extended to the mediastinum and periaortic lymph nodes, continues to receive treatment for his metastases following orchiectomy.

Carcinoma of the parotid: One patient had mucin-producing carcinoma of the left parotid gland with metastases of the cervical lymph nodes and lungs; he failed to respond to treatment with radiation therapy to the neck. There was no response following multiple-drug chemotherapy, and he died from pulmonary insufficiency 6 months following diagnosis.

Carcinoma of the thyroid: Papillary carcinoma of the thyroid was encountered in an 11-year-old white girl who has now survived free of disease for more than 5 years following thyroidectomy and radical neck dissections followed by radiation therapy to the neck and mediastinum.

Carcinoma of the kidney (hypernephroma): An 11-year-old girl with unresectable carcinoma involving the right kidney was admitted to this hospital in 1971. She had progressive enlargement of the primary abdominal tumor as well as pulmonary metastases before her death 4 months following diagnosis.

Seminoma: A 14-year-old white boy was admitted to this hospital in June 1974 with markedly enlarged cervical lymph nodes. He had a large anterior mediastinal mass and there was a diffuse lymphangitic pattern of metastatic disease throughout the lung fields. There was also radiographic evidence of abdominal lymph node enlargement. Biopsies of the cervical lymph nodes and mediastinal mass were consistent with the diagnosis of seminoma. Orchiectomy was performed because of a questionable nodule in the right testis; no tumor was found within the testis. The patient responded satisfactorily with clearing of all evidence of disease following vincristine-cyclophosphamide-dactinomycin and radiation therapy delivered to the mediastinal and periaortic node areas. He developed recurrence of disease in the mediastinum and retroperitoneal node areas 18 months following diagnosis and has now been treated with vinblastine and Bleomycin with a second complete response.

Choriocarcinoma: This diagnosis was encountered following abdominal exploration of a 14-year-old white boy for a large left retroperitoneal mass. The patient additionally had multiple pulmonary metastases. For a 4-month period there has been disappearance of the abdominal mass and almost complete resolution of the pulmonary metastases following vincristine-cyclophosphamide-dactinomycin chemotherapy.

Adamantinoma: One patient, a 15-year-old white boy, was admitted in January 1974 with this diagnosis following biopsy of the right tibia. The patient has remained free of any evidence of metastases following above-the-knee amputation.

SARCOMAS

Liposarcoma: Liposarcoma is the most frequently encountered soft-tissue sarcoma of adults.[14] Nine of our patients have had this diagnosis. Three of the 9 patients were boys. Each of the girls with this diagnosis was Caucasian. Primary tumor sites were in the retroperitoneal area of 4 patients, in the thigh of 2 patients, in the thigh and pelvis of 1 patient, in the foot of 1 patient, and in the intercostal area of 1 patient. At the time of diagnosis, 1 patient had localized disease, 7 had unresected regional disease, 1 had generalized disease which included pulmonary metastases. One patient, who has been the subject of a previous report from this hospital, is now surviving 11 years following irradiation and vincristine-cyclophosphamide chemotherapy.[8]

Three additional patients are surviving free of tumor following partial resection and chemotherapy-radiation therapy. Durations of the followup of these patients have been 1½ years, 4 years, and 4 years respectively.

Synovial sarcoma: Five patients, 1 black boy and 4 white boys, have been admitted with this diagnosis. Each of the lesions involved an extremity. Two patients had localized, completely resectable disease at the time of diagnosis; one patient had regional disease which was completely resected, and 2 patients presented with generalized disease, including pulmonary metastases. Therapy for 4 patients has consisted of resection (amputation for 3 patients, complete surgical removal for the 4th patient). Three patients are surviving 1, 5 and 5 years respectively, following these procedures. One patient died following complete response with vincristine-cyclophosphamide-dactinomycin and radiation therapy; this patient's survival time was 2 years. One patient is currently surviving with evidence of generalized pulmonary metastases 4 months following diagnosis.

Schwannoma: Two patients, 1 girl and 1 boy, ages 14 and 16 years, both with the typical characteristics of neurofibromatosis, have been treated for Schwannoma. Both of these patients had extensive primary tumors which were unresectable and both had evidence of distant spread of the tumor. These patients failed to respond to radiation therapy or multiple-drug combination chemotherapy.

Alveolar soft part sarcoma: This tumor has been encountered in two white children. The first, an 11-year-old Amish boy, had a primary tumor of the right ethmoid sinus with metastasis to the right cervical lymph nodes. The tumor failed to respond to treatment with combination chemotherapy. Following complete excision of the tumor and right radical neck dissection, the patient has remained free of evidence of disease for more than 1 year.

The second patient with this diagnosis, an 18-month-old white girl, has been followed 6 months after resection and radiation therapy for primary tumor of the left forearm. She has had no evidence of local recurrence or distant spread.

Histiocytoma: This recently described tumor of the bone was encountered in one patient, a white boy with primary tumor of the left acromion. Following confirmation of the diagnosis a left forequarter amputation was performed and the patient has received adjuvant chemotherapy with vincristine, cyclophosphamide, dactinomycin and adriamycin for a 6-month period, during which time he has remained free of evidence of pulmonary and other metastases.

Angiosarcoma: One patient, a 13-year-old boy, had primary tumor of the left pelvis; he developed generalized metastatic deposits following response to the primary tumor to radiation therapy and chemotherapy. He survived 2 years following diagnosis.

Mesenchymoma: A 4-year-old black boy was admitted with this diagnosis in 1973. Primary tumor site was the liver. His presenting characteristics were massive

964

hepatomegaly and ascites. Therapy consisting of radiation therapy to the entire abdomen and multiple-drug chemotherapy produced a transient response; however, the patient died of progressive disease 6 months following diagnosis.

DISCUSSION

The 58 patients encountered over a 13-year period in this hospital with cancers usually found in adult patients constitute 5% of the total number of solid tumor admissions to this hospital. Although almost all tumors which are more commonly seen in adults may occur in children, the occurrence of these rare tumors is of potentially greater importance in regard to the implications of the changing diagnostic categories of patients referred to pediatric oncology centers. There has not been a change in the referral patterns to this institution from various geographic areas.

Mucin-producing carcinoma is seen in only 5% of all adult patients with colon cancer[6]; this histologic subtype appears to be the predominant type encountered in children,[12,16] and was the histologic subtype encountered in each of our patients with colon carcinoma.

Along with increased numbers of patient referrals to this institution from 1963 to 1975 with the exception of 1973, there has been an increased number of pediatric patients with adult-type cancers admitted in 1974 and 1975. Twenty-five of the 58 patients were admitted in 1974 and 1975 and account for 8% of the total admissions of pediatric tumor patients during those 2 years. By Chi-square analysis, there is as yet no indication that more pediatric patients are being referred for adult-type cancers. However, the admission of nine patients with carcinoma of the bowel within a 15-month period is highly suggestive that there is an increasing frequenty of large bowel cancer in pediatric patients and that environmental circumstances may have had a major role in the development of this tumor in these young patients.[2-4]

SUMMARY

Between March 1962 and January 1976, 1009 children with malignant solid tumors have been admitted to St. Jude Children's Research Hospital. Fifty-eight of these patients (5.7%) had malignant tumors rarely encountered in pediatric patients. Thirty-seven patients had carcinomas and 21 had sarcomas. Of the patients with carcinomas, 12 had carcinoma of the colon and 1 had carcinoma of the rectum; nine of these 13 patients were admitted between October 1974 and November 1975. Adult-type cancers accounted for 8% of the total solid tumor admissions in the years 1974 and 1975. There is no indication that more pediatric patients are being referred with "adult-type" cancers. However, the admission of nine patients with carcinoma of the bowel within a 15-month period suggests an increasing frequency of this tumor in pediatric patients.

Supported by USPHS Childhood Cancer Research Center Grant CA08480 and by A LSAC.

Address for reprints: Charles B. Pratt, M.D., St. Jude Children's Research Hospital, P.O. Box 318, Memphis, Tennessee 38101.

TABLE I

Adult Cancers in Children and Adolescents

St. Jude Children's Research Hospital

1962–1975

Carcinomas		Sarcomas	
Colon	12	Liposarcoma	9
Hepatocellular	5	Synovial	5
Adrenal	3	Schwannoma	2
Melanoma	3	Alveolar Soft Part	2
Pancreas	2	Histiocytoma	1
Dysgerminoma	2	Angiosarcoma	1
Teratocarcinoma	2	Mesenchymoma	1
Parotid	1		
Thyroid	1		
Cholangiohepatocellular	1		
Kidney	1		
Rectum	1		
Seminoma	1		
Choriocarcinoma	1		
Adamantinoma	1		
	37		21

TABLE II

Adult Cancers in Children and Adolescents

Age	Diagnosis	No. Surviving/Total	Age	Diagnosis	No. Surviving/Total
0–2	Hepatocellular	1/2	11–15	Colon	3/6
	Carcinoma of Pancreas	1/2		Melanoma	2/2
	Adrenal	1/1		Synovial Sarcoma	2/2
	Liposarcoma	1/1		Liposarcoma	1/2
	Teratocarcinoma	0/1		Hepatocellular	0/2
		4/7		Rectum	1/1
				Thyroid	1/1
2–5	Liposarcoma	1/3		Seminoma	1/1
	Synovial Sarcoma	1/1		Adamantinoma	1/1
	Alveolar Soft Part	1/1		Histiocytoma	1/1
	Hepatocellular	0/1		Choriocarcinoma	1/1
	Mesenchymoma	0/1		Kidney 0/1	
		3/7		Adrenal	0/1
				Schwannoma	0/1
6–10	Colon	1/2		Angiosarcoma	0/1
	Liposarcoma	1/2			14/24
	Dysgerminoma	1/1			
	Alveolar Soft Part	1/1	16–20	Colon	1/4
	Adrenal	0/1		Synovial	2/2
	Parotid	0/1		Dysgerminoma	1/1
	Cholangio-Hepatocellular	0/1		Teratocarcinoma	1/1
	Melanoma	0/1		Liposarcoma	0/1
		4/10		Schwannoma	0/1
					5/10

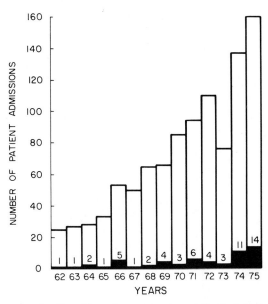

FIG. 1. Annual accrual of pediatric patients with "adult" cancers is compared with the annual accrual of all patients with solid tumors from 1962 through 1975.

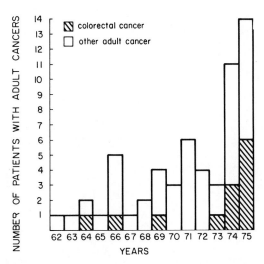

FIG. 2. Comparison of year of admission of children and adolescents with colorectal cancers with annual accrual of patients with other "adult" cancer types.

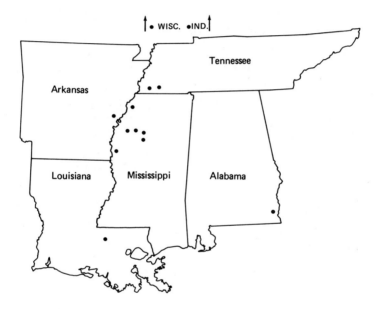

FIG. 3. Geographic distribution of patients with colorectal carcinoma referred to St. Jude Children's Research Hospital from 1964 through 1975. Most patients were referred from the rural areas of Mississippi and Tennessee.

REFERENCES

1. Andersen, D.H. Tumors of Infancy and Childhood. I. A Survey of Those Seen in the Pathology Laboratory of the Babie's Hospital During the Years 1935–1950. Cancer, 4:890–906, 1951.

2. Berg, J.W., Haenszel, W., and Devesa, S.S. Proceedings: Epidemiology of Gastrointestinal Cancer. Proc. Natl. Cancer Conf., 7:459–464, 1973.

3. Burkitt, D.P. Epidemiology of Cancer of the Colon and Rectum. Cancer, 28: 3–13, 1971.

4. Burkitt, D.P. An Epidemiologic Approach to Cancer of the Large Intestine: The Significance of Disease Relationships. Dis. Colon Rectum, 17:456–461, 1974.

5. Chabalko, J.J., and Fraumeni, J.F. Colorectal Danger in Children: Epidemiologic Aspects. Dis. Colon Rectum, 18:1–3, 1975.

6. Falterman, K.W., Hill, C.B., Markey, J.D., Fox, J.S., and Cohn, I. Jr. Cancer of the Colon, Rectum and Anus: A Review of 2313 Cases. Cancer, 34:951–959, 1974.

7. Fraumeni, J.F. Jr., and Mulvihill, J.J. Who is at Risk of Colorectal Cancer? In: Cancer Epidemiology and Prevention. Ed.: D. Shottenfeld. Charles C. Thomas, Springfield, pp. 404–415, 1975.

8. James, D.H. Jr., Johnson, W.W., and Wrenn, E.L. Jr. Effective Chemotherapy of an Abdominal Liposarcoma. J. Pediatr., 68:311–313, 1966.

9. Kiesewetter, W.B., and Mason, E.J. Malignant Tumors in Childhood. JAMA, 172: 1117–1121, 1960.

10. Miller, R.W. Fifty-two Forms of Childhood Cancer: United States Mortality Experience, 1960–1966. J. Pediatr., 75:685–689, 1969.

11. Miller, R.W., and Dalager, N.A. U.S. Childhood Cancer Deaths by Cell Type, 1960–68. J. Pediatr., 85:664–668, 1974.

12. Middlekamp, J.N., and Hoffner, H. Carcinoma of the Colon in Children. Pediatrics, 32:558:571, 1963.

13. Moertel, C.G., Schutt, A.J., Hahn, R.G., and Reitemeier, R.J. Therapy of Advanced Colorectal Cancer with a Combination of 5-fluorouracil, Methyl-1,3-cis(2-chlorethyl)- 1-nitrosurea, and Vincristine. J. Natl. Cancer Inst., 54:69–71, 1975.

14. Morton, D.H. Soft Tissue Carcinomas. In Cancer Medicine. Ed.: J.F. Holland and E. Frei, III. Lea and Febiger, 1973, Philadelphia, pp. 1845–1861, 1973.

15. Pearson, D., and Steward, J.K. Malignant Disease in Juveniles. Proc. Roy. Soc. Med., 62:685–688, 1969.

16. Sessions, R.T., Riddell, D.H., Kaplan, H.J., and Foster, J.H. Carcinoma of the Colon in the First Two Decades of Life. Ann. Surg., 162:279–284, 1965.

17. Young, J.L. Jr., and Miller, R.W. Incidence of Malignant Tumors in U.S. Children. J. Pediatr., 86:254–258, 1975.

RETICULUM CELL SARCOMAS AS SEQUELAE OF CO_2-TREATMENT OF NORMAL TISSUE

A. E. Goldsmith and G. F. Ryan

National Cancer Cytology Center
Melville, New York

INTRODUCTION

Concern evidenced in the literature for the rising atmospheric con-centrations of carbon dioxide (1) adds pertinence to the study of the long term clinical effects of its abnormal accumulation in the body. Appreciable changes in the external environment may alter structure and function of cellular constituents by an alteration in their micro-environment. Certain disease states also tend to change the local environment of tissue cells. For example, congestive heart failure, chronic obstructive pulmonary disease and renal diseases associated with metabolic alkalosis tend to increase the carbon dioxide (CO_2) tissue tension. An earlier experimental finding of an abnormal carbonate-rich calcium alkali phosphate in the bone mineral of a premalignant lesion, Paget's Osteitis Deformans (2), focused attention upon the possible importance of the CO_2 tissue tension and its fluctuations in controlling formation and function of body constituents. Once evidence was accumu-lating that "...the reactions of CO_2 release are reversible, and that CO_2 may be liberated or absorbed, depending upon conditions, in a wide variety of organisms" (3), it was realized too that even in human physiology there is a "complex relation between CO_2 of tissues and the external environment" (3). Unhydrated CO_2 (4) diffuses across the cell membrane giving rise to hydrogen ions <u>inside</u> the cell (5); its rate of penetration is determined by the pressure of the gas dissolved within a tissue, pCO_2 (6). This direct, local action of the CO_2 molecule within tissue cells (5,7-9) has been repeatedly held responsible for the numerous, diverse symptoms of acute and chronic hypercapnia (10,11) and other diseases (12). It caused some authors to comment: "...the only way of rapidly changing intracellular pH is through CO_2 diffusion, and this change in intracellular pH may be one of the fundamental mechanisms of body regulations" (5). Others view the CO_2 tissue tension as a "physiological regulator of cell multiplication" (13) and differentiation, and of embryonic growth (14). In 1920 (15) the distinction between the effect of the local pCO_2 (8) and that of the extracellular fluid pH was established by the production of hydrogen ions inside the cell by CO_2-containing neutral and alkaline solutions (7). Lower concentrations of CO_2 stimulate and higher ones retard cell respiration (13,16-19). At higher tensions malignant cells, unlike fibroblasts, compensate for their respiratory energy loss (16,19) by the simultaneous stimulation of glycolysis (13). High CO_2 concentrations in vitro produce numerous

971

mitotic abnormalities and dedifferentiation of cells (9,14,23). These and their nuclei are greatly enlarged (20-22) appearing similar to those found in vivo under conditions of hypercapnia (12). CO_2 is, therefore, a most important variable which, according to concentration (9), may act as a stimulant or a brake of the numerous cellular processes it influences (24). Recognition of the dual role of CO_2, not only as a physiological regulator and substrate for cellular synthesis, but also as a pathogenic agent, prompted this attempt to learn more about CO_2 as a pathogen. This is a report of this attempt.

PROCEDURES AND MATERIALS USED

A. Mice

Young adult virgin female mice, age 4-6 weeks, were used as donors; 20-23 day old ones as recipients. Two inbred strains, BALB/c and CBA and one noninbred group, Swiss albino mice, S/W were employed in all transplantations. Inbred strains were derived from colonies which had been maintained by continuous, single-line, brother-to-sister mating. Samples of each strain had been regularly checked for homozygosity by skin grafting. The Swiss mice, obtained from the Purina Chow Company, were random bred in a closed colony in the laboratory. All mice were kept on a standard pellet diet and water ad libitum.

B. Pre-transplantation Treatments and Grafting Procedure

For the exposure of tissues before transplantation to approximately 45-48% CO_2 in air at room temperature, a vacuum desiccator was used, connected to a CO_2-gas cylinder on the one hand, and a manometer and vacuum pump on the other. Since the desiccator had to be partially evacuated before running in CO_2 gas, the same procedure was followed with the grafts that were to be exposed only to the culture environment, before finally closing the desiccator. Thus, identical treatment of the two sets of tissues was insured, apart from the presence of CO_2 in the atmosphere of the one, in case reduced pressure affected the cells. Grafts were kept in Waymouth's culture medium in plastic Petri dishes. The exposure period to the two different culture environments was 24 hours. Fourth mammary gland and inguinal lymph node tissue was cut into pieces about 1 mm^3 or less. They were then exposed to culture environment either in the CO_2/air mixture or in room air only and transplanted into syngeneic hosts (pure strains) or allogeneic hosts (noninbred Swiss mice only). Some mammary gland and lymph node tissue in each strain was also grafted directly from donor to host without exposure to culture environment or any contact, however brief, with culture medium. The clinical effects of transplantation alone should be evident in these syngeneic hosts. The transplantation site for these grafts was the fourth mammary fat pad cleared of mammary epithelium immediately before transplantation. The method used for the tail skin autografts has been previously described (25).

C. Experimental Design

Table I lists the 28 experimental groups of mice in the complete study. This report, however, is confined to a discussion of the available results in the following groups. Skin autografts: BALB/c, Swiss, CO_2-grafts and air-grafts; mammary gland isografts: BALB/c, CO_2-grafts, air-grafts and untreated grafts; lymph node isografts: BALB/c, CO_2-grafts, air-grafts and untreated grafts; mammary gland allografts: noninbred Swiss, CO_2-grafts, air-grafts and untreated grafts; lymph node allografts: noninbred Swiss, CO_2-grafts, air-grafts and untreated grafts. Percentage incidences of observed lesions in Table III are cumulative incidences. A group of completely untreated animals of each strain served as controls. Mice were observed until death, or killed when moribund. All experimental and untreated control mice were autopsied and the following tissues removed for histological examination: spleen, peripheral and mesenteric lymph nodes, thymus, liver, pancreas, kidneys, ovaries, uterus, lungs and any other tissue with visible lymphomatous involvement. Tissues were fixed in buffered formalin and stained with hematoxylin and eosin.

D. Two Pilot Studies

(a) Ten embryos of strain CBA were exposed to gaseous CO_2 intermittently throughout their intra-uterine life after the first 7 days. The gas was introduced directly into the maternal peritoneal cavity for 1-2 minutes per day. (b) In 12 one-month old BALB/c mice gaseous CO_2 was introduced directly into the peritoneum continuously for 7-12 days, at the level of the spleen in the subphrenic area, by means of narrow tubing. The tubes were then disconnected and the mice observed without further experimentation.

Abbreviations: CO_2-grafts: grafts cultured in the CO_2/air mixture
                       air-grafts: grafts cultured in air only
                none-grafts: grafts transplanted directly from
                              donor to host

RESULTS

Table III lists the incidences of lesions most frequently observed in the recipients of the various grafts and in their untreated controls. In the experimental animals of all strains of mice examined, the morphological changes in lymphoreticular and renal tissues predominated. Complete histological examination for every experimental group cited in Table I is not yet available. As a result, Table III is as yet incomplete but it serves to demonstrate the major trends that emerge from a comparison of the incidences of the main lesions in the different groups of graft recipients in inbred strain BALB/c and the noninbred Swiss mice. The results obtained with tail skin autografts in pure strains BALB/c and CBA and noninbred Swiss mice have been reported elsewhere (25), but were included in Table III for comparison. The results obtained with the two pure strains BALB/c and CBA were very similar, and only those obtained with the former are given in this table.

A. Malignant Lymphomas

The dominant experimental findings of this complete study are evident from Table III. (a) The lymphoma incidence in all CO_2-treated

973

graft recipients was significantly higher than the spontaneous incidence in that strain. This was the case in all strains and hybrid groups examined. (b) Irrespective of the pre-transplantation treatment of the graft or the type of tissue grafted, all recipients of the isografts (inbred strains) had a high lymphoma incidence, ranging from 20-61%. (c) The noninbred Swiss mice have a spontaneous incidence of 8% in the age range 5-13 months; the incidence increases above this age. (d) In contrast to the inbred strains, and possibly due to their higher spontaneous incidence, the lymphoma occurrence in the Swiss rises to high levels (63-88%) in all graft recipients, irrespective of the following three factors: pre-transplantation treatment, type of graft (autograft or allograft - as noninbred mice) or type of tissue grafted (tail skin, mammary gland, lymph node - the latter to be reported later). (e) In the two pure strains, the skin autograft recipients respond very differently from their isograft recipients on the one hand, or the noninbred autograft recipients on the other. The pre-transplantation treatment of the graft appears to be critical for the clinical outcome of the transplantation, since only the CO_2-graft recipients have a high lymphoma incidence in the BALB/c mice (33%), while the grafts exposed to culturing-in-air only elicit no lymphomas in their hosts. The great majority of these lymphomas were reticulum cell sarcomas, type C according to Dunn's nomenclature (26); they correspond to malignant lymphomas, lymphocytic or lymphoblastic in man. There were also a few reticulum cell sarcomas, type A and type B (the murine Hodgkin's-like lesion) (26) and two giant follicular lymphoma-like tumors.

B. Other Lesions

Other lesions of interest were (Fig. 1): (a) Amyloidosis: Its incidence ranges from 15% in some of the Swiss mice to 63% in CO_2-graft recipients of the BALB/c mice. (b) Myocarditis, which did not occur in any untreated controls, appeared relatively frequently in all recipients, particularly in the BALB/c mammary gland and lymph node isograft recipients (e.g. 41%, 22%). (c) Glomerular lesions are similar in all graft recipients of both types of mice. (d) Pyelonephritis: these incidences range from 10% in some of the Swiss groups to 88-97% in the BALB/c lymph node graft recipients. (e) The pulmonary adenocarcinoma incidence does not appear to be significantly affected by the transplantations in either strain.

C. Lymphoid Hyperplasia and Atrophy

The previous study with skin autografts in the same strains drew attention to the high incidence, more than 50%, of lymphoid hyperplasia with concomitant atrophy, even within the same organ, occurring in the CO_2-graft recipients (25). It was also histologically apparent that the periarteriolar and interfollicular areas of spleen and lymph nodes showed frequently marked proliferation of the lymphoid cells, while the follicular mantle was often atrophic (25). In order to ascertain the significance of these findings, the BALB/c recipients of the lymph node isografts were selected for a more detailed study of the morphological distribution of lymphoid hyperplasia and atrophy. In each case of lymphoid hyperplasia and/or atrophy the distinction was made on a morphological basis alone, whether it was chiefly a T-cell or B-cell abnormality. In cases of considerable destruction of architecture by widespread lymphoma or of abundant deposits of amyloid, mainly in the spleen, the distinction between

T-cell rich and B-cell rich areas in lymph nodes and spleen was not possible. It should be emphasized that this is the merest attempt at a morphological, not immunological, distinction between predominantly T-cell hyperplasia and predominantly B-cell hyperplasia. This attempt seems justified despite its limitations. The T-cell and B-cell rich areas in lymph nodes and spleen were assigned according to the literature (27). While comparing the incidences of T-cell and B-cell hyperplasia in experimental animals with those in the untreated controls, it should be noted that the degree of hyperplasia in the experimental mice was marked and much greater than that in the controls. This was reflected in the thickness of the periarteriolar sheath and the follicular mantle, respectively. Also of interest is the fact that a significant number of animals in the controls shows both splenic and nodal T-cell hyperplasia in contrast to the experimental group. A comparison of the incidences of T-cell and B-cell hyperplasia and atrophy in spleens and lymph nodes of lymphoma-bearing mice with those in non-lymphoma-bearing controls gives the following information (Table IV and Figure 2): (a) The incidence of T-cell atrophy in spleen and nodes and in experimental and control mice is zero. The incidences of B-cell atrophy as well as of T-cell and B-cell hyperplasia vary greatly in spleens and nodes of the experimental and control animals. (b) The highest incidence of T-cell hyperplasia occurs in the experimental spleens. The incidence of B-cell atrophy is almost the same as that of B-cell hyperplasia. (c) The incidence of T-cell hyperplasia in the control spleens is only a third of that in the experimental spleens. This relatively low T-cell hyperplasia is accompanied by a zero incidence of B-cell hyperplasia. This is the opposite of the situation in the experimental spleens. These splenic trends are reversed in the lymph nodes. (d) In the nodes of the experimental mice the incidence of T-cell hyperplasia is almost zero, contrasting with the very high splenic incidence. This appears to indicate an abnormal rise in splenic T-cell activity, coupled with an abnormal decrease in the nodes of the experimental animals. The incidences of nodal T-cell and B-cell hyperplasia in the controls are several times as high as those in the experimental mice (almost eight and four times, respectively). (e) While nodal and splenic T-cell hyperplasia are almost the same in the controls, the incidence of B-cell hyperplasia is highest in the nodes; it is zero in their spleens. The controls have almost the same incidences of nodal and splenic B-cell atrophy.

D. Two Pilot Studies

The malignancies observed when CO_2 gas was introduced intra-peritoneally into BALB/c mice are given in Table II. It is of interest to note that 3 out of 12 mice developed lymphomas, but spontaneous pulmonary adenocarcinoma incidence was more than doubled (33%) in these mice. This contrasts with the finding in the graft recipients, in which the pulmonary tumor incidence seemed unaffected by the different transplantations. Six out of 10 CBA embryos, exposed to gaseous CO_2 during intra-uterine life, developed lymphomas at the age of six months. This is young compared to the age at which graft recipients developed lymphomas (8-12 months) and probably represents a somewhat shorter latent period. Some senile hyperkeratosis also occurred. Their gross appearance too was very abnormal, looking as these mice normally do at the age of 15 months with prematurely greying hair, severe alopecia and ruffled fur.

975

DISCUSSION

Although this study is not yet complete certain general trends are already apparent. At least seven factors, interacting, affected not only the occurrence of malignant lymphomas but also that of other lesions noted. They are: (a) type of pre-transplantation treatment of graft, (b) type of tissue grafted, (c) type of graft, (d) genome of host, (e) site and route of transplantation, (f) form of transplant, (g) duration of pre-transplantation treatment of graft. The nature of the treatment of the graft and the genetic constitution of the host appeared to have the strongest influence. The results in the two pure strains are similar, particularly the lymphoma incidences, while those in the non-inbred Swiss mice differ widely from both. They were the only mice studied which spontaneously developed lymphomas with age. Whatever the etiology of this pronounced susceptibility, it is thought to be responsible for the fact that in the Swiss mice alone the incidence of lymphoreticular neoplasias is similar and near its maximum in <u>all</u> graft recipients. Thus, lymphoma development in these animals appears to be independent of four of the seven factors: nature of graft treatment, type of tissue grafted, type of graft and duration of treatment. The lymphoma incidence is always markedly higher in the Swiss than in the corresponding recipient group of another strain. This seems to indicate that even a weak stimulus, such as might be exerted by an autograft exposed to culturing only, may cause the appearance of maximum numbers of a lesion in susceptible groups of animals. The influence on the clinical outcome of the transplantations of some of the factors mentioned is briefly considered.

A. Host Genome

Some clinical response, frequently a long-term effect, is elicited to most transplantations, but it differs in the various strains. This variation, possibly genetic, in the response of the lymphoreticular tissue to the chronic stimulation seemingly exerted by most types of grafts, is expressed in the different strains as differences in the incidences of the lymphoreticular abnormalities: atrophy, hyperplasia and neoplasia. The predisposition of various strains for different syndromes is indicated by their increased occurrence under stress in the experimental animals. For instance, carcinomas of the eye not found in any other strain examined, appeared only in the CO_2-graft recipients of the CBA mice.

B. Treatment Period

Exposures to the CO_2/air mixture of isografts for only 1-2 hours, greatly increased the appearance of lymphomas in their recipients. In the two pure strains, the incidence increases stepwise until the maximum is reached by approximately 4-5 hours' exposure. The Swiss mice, seemingly due to their spontaneous predisposition, reach their maximum incidence after only one hour's exposure of their grafts.

C. Type of Graft and the Nature of its Treatment

With autografts, the pre-transplantation treatment of the grafted tissue determines the lymphoma incidence in the hosts, in the absence of a spontaneous susceptibility. This is shown by the fact that in the BALB/c mice the CO_2-treated skin autografts elicited a 33% lymphoma incidence in their recipients in comparison with the zero incidence caused by the grafts that were cultured only. In the susceptible Swiss mice, both graft treatments induced in their hosts maximum lymphoma incidences (79-88%). The influence of the treatment is not as clear with the BALB/c isografts and Swiss mice allografts. In the susceptible Swiss recipients there is no significant difference between the high lymphoma incidences in the three different treatment groups: CO_2-treated, cultured only and untreated grafts; thus, autografts and allografts elicited similar, high incidences in these mice. The CO_2-isograft recipients of the pure strains, however, tended to have higher lymphoma incidences than the hosts of non-CO_2-treated grafts. Therefore, the consequences of isografting in the pure strains differ markedly from those of autografting, in contrast to the Swiss mice.

The appearance in significant numbers in the graft recipients of lesions known to be associated with altered immunological status, such as glomerular lesions, amyloidosis and myocarditis (Table III, Fig. 1), suggests that immunological mechanisms are involved in the formation of the lymphomas, even if they may not be the primary cause. The study, therefore, of the morphological distribution of the T-cell and B-cell hyperplasia and atrophy in lymphoma-bearing recipients and non-lymphoma-bearing controls seemed justified and revealed complex relationships illustrated in Table IV and Fig. 2. Their significance is still obscure but the briefest summary underlines dominant trends.

1. T-CELL HYPERPLASIA

In lymphoma-bearing mice the splenic incidence is highest and twenty times that of the nodal incidence. In non-lymphoma-bearing mice splenic and nodal incidences of T-cell hyperplasia are almost the same and only one third of that in the experimental spleens.

2. B-CELL HYPERPLASIA

In lymphoma-bearing mice the splenic incidence is also high and at least twice that in the nodes. In non-lymphoma-bearing controls this incidence is zero, in contrast to the nodal incidence of B-cell hyperplasia, which is the highest encountered.

3. T-CELL HYPERPLASIA AND B-CELL ATROPHY

It is possible to detect a hint of an interrelationship between T-cell hyperplasia and B-cell atrophy (Table IV). The highest incidence of T-cell hyperplasia in the experimental spleens is accompanied by the highest incidence of B-cell atrophy (Fig. 2). The lowest incidence of T-cell hyperplasia in the experimental nodes is associated with an equally low incidence of B-cell atrophy. Moderate incidences of splenic and nodal T-cell hyperplasia in the controls are matched by moderate incidences of B-cell atrophy in spleen and nodes.

The observations in the non-lymphoma-bearing controls are the reverse of those in the lymphoma-bearing mice. The overall impression gained is one of increased lymphoid activity in both T- and B-cell lines in the spleens of the lymphoma-bearing animals. This increase in splenic activity contrasts sharply with the decrease in nodal activity. It is of interest in this context to note that, analogous to the human situation, the lymphomas appeared predominantly in the lymph nodes; splenic involvement seems to be a later development and occurs in widespread cases only. Additional corroborative evidence for the involvement of T-cells in the formation of these lymphomas may be the finding that skin autografts cultured in phytohemagglutinin containing medium doubled the occurrence of malignant lymphomas in their hosts. Since phytohemagglutinin-responding cells are chiefly the cortisone-resistant subpopulation of T-cells (28) the possibility of their participation exists.

While a predominantly T-cell hyperplasia in the spleens of lymphoma-bearing mice may not be surprising, this splenic T-cell response was also observed, to a lesser extent, in the spleens of non-lymphoma-bearing isograft recipients of BALB/c mice. Since these were grafts between syngeneic animals, stimulation could not have been caused by a difference in the major histocompatibility antigens. The question thus arises: what is the reason for the apparent immunogenicity to their hosts of all, even completely untreated isografts, and of the CO_2-treated autografts? All these grafts induced lymphomas in their inbred hosts. Autografts that were only cultured, however, induced no lymphomas.

In the case of isografts, the possibility may exist that even with syngeneic mice there are some minor antigenic differences that are capable of eliciting a host response. This cannot explain, however, the immunogenicity of the CO_2-treated autografts. Culture treatment of tissues before transplantation may modify lymphocyte proteins and excite thymus-derived cell-mediated cytotoxicity in their hosts against the modified proteins. That such an "In vitro induction of thymus-derived cell-mediated cytotoxicity to trinitrophenol-modified syngeneic lymphocyte surface proteins" exists has been described by Shearer (29). He also demonstrates that cortisone-resistant thymocytes are involved in this process. Shearer (29) suggested that the proteins modified by trinitrophenol were controlled by genes within distinct regions of the major histocompatibility complex. Although trinitrophenol and CO_2 are not likely to affect cell surface proteins in exactly the same manner, antigenic sites that would not normally be active, may have been uncovered by the CO_2. Thus, similar mechanisms may have been initiated with similar consequences in the case of the CO_2 altered cells in this study.

The predominantly T-cell response, which occurred chiefly in the spleens of graft recipients and lymphoma-bearing mice, as well as the previously mentioned phytohemagglutinin effect on the lymphoma incidence tempt some speculation. Chronic antigenic stimulation of the cortisone-resistant thymocytes proceeding from the grafts and the accompanying activity of the cortisone-sensitive T-cells, which have a "predilection for splenic localization" (30,31) may cause the observed hyperplasia in the spleens of these recipients and result in an abnormal non-functional T-cell system. Support for this view may be the very high incidence of pyelonephritis ($\sim$97%) in the lymph node graft recipients, which may indicate an injured immunological system. The modulating role of the cortisone-sensitive thymocytes, which take part in the DNA synthetic response to antigen, has been shown to be dose-dependent (30). Thus, varying the antigenic dose "...could cause the influence of the cortisone-sensitive cells to change from helper to suppressor" (30). Chronic stimulation by a graft might represent such a variation in antigenic dose.

The possibility thus exists that the CO_2-treatment played a similar role to that described for trinitrophenol by Shearer (29). The cell surface proteins modified by in vitro treatment subsequently act as immunogens with the resulting generation of cytotoxic effector cells in vitro, demonstrated by Shearer, and thymus-derived cell-mediated cytotoxicity in vivo, as proposed in this investigation. This immune process, once started in the host, appeared to have lymphoma production as its sequel. It may have the character of an autoimmune-type mechanism when using autografts. Not even a hypothesis may be advanced for the intermediate steps.

However, a hint of the possible involvement of autoimmune-type mechanisms in some tumor production may be derived from the neoplastic sequelae of the two pilot studies: (a) lymphomas followed CO_2-exposure in utero and (b) pulmonary adenocarcinomas (33%) and lymphomas followed the direct introduction of gaseous CO_2 into the subphrenic area. When considering the causal relationship between cigarette smoke and pulmonary tumors, this increase in lung tumor incidence following exposure to CO_2 of certain tissues should not be ignored. May this smoke not contain other active constituents in addition to the tars? Is it not possible that a part is also played by the chronic exposure of tissues to the abnormal CO_2 concentrations, necessarily present as a result of burning organic material?

The role of a primary carcinogen which causes malignant transformations in the cells of its target tissue is not postulated here for CO_2. Had this been the case, skin and mammary gland malignancies should have developed within the grafted tissues, since the grafts were the primary target tissue of the abnormal CO_2 concentrations in this study. It appears more plausible that CO_2, in common with many endogenous substances, may influence the microenvironment of cells in those tissues in which pathological conditions may cause its prolonged presence in abnormal concentrations. Carcinogens or other factors may then arise from this abnormal environment within a primary target tissue and cause tumor formation in the secondary target tissue. In these circumstances, the primary target tissue might merely be considered as that tissue within which a physiological substance is chronically present in unphysiological concentrations. The role proposed for CO_2 in the lymphoma production described in this study is merely one for setting the stage for the formation of other carcinogens or pre-carcinogens.

SUMMARY

This investigation into the long term clinical effects of abnormal CO_2 concentrations in the tissues was prompted by the increased CO_2 tissue

979

tensions found in certain disease states, the rising atmospheric concentrations of CO_2 and the dual role of CO_2, not only as a substrate for cellular synthesis but also as a pathogenic agent. Different tissues were exposed in vitro to a concentration of 45% CO_2 in air and transplanted as isografts and autografts. The findings of the complete study were: (a) The incidence of malignant lymphomas in all CO_2-treated graft recipients, even autograft, was significantly higher than the spontaneous incidence in that strain. (b) Recipients of non-CO_2-treated isografts also incurred lymphoma incidences higher than the spontaneous ones, but lower than the CO_2-treated graft recipients. Comparison of the incidences of malignant lymphomas and other lesions in inbred, noninbred and hybrid mice showed that these were affected by at least 7 factors, of which the nature of the pre-transplantation treatment of the graft, the genome of the host and the type of graft were the most important. Predisposition for different syndromes in various strains is indicated by their increased occurrence, under stress, in the experimental animals. Even a weak stimulus, such as an autograft, cultured for only 24 hours, may cause maximum numbers of a lesion in susceptible mice. The high lymphoma incidences in all graft recipients in the noninbred Swiss mice, are an example. Appearance in the recipients of significant numbers of lesions associated with altered immunological status, particularly glomerular lesions and myocarditis, pointed to an involvement of immunological mechanisms in the formation of these lymphomas. Increased lymphoid activity in T- and B-cell lines was observed in the spleens of lymphoma-bearing mice, contrasting sharply with the decrease in nodal activity. Findings in the non-lymphoma-bearing controls were the reverse: incidence of lymphoid hyperplasia, particularly B-cell, was higher in the nodes than in the spleen. An interrelationship appeared between T-cell hyperplasia and B-cell atrophy. The highest incidences of both occurred in the experimental spleens and the lowest in the experimental nodes. On the other hand, moderate incidences of both occurred in control spleens and nodes. Autoimmune-type mechanisms in some tumor productions were suggested by the development of lymphomas following CO_2-exposure in utero and of pulmonary adenocarcinomas (33%) and lymphomas following direct introduction of gaseous CO_2 into the subphrenic area. The role of a primary carcinogen was not proposed for CO_2 but rather that its chronic abnormal accumulation in the tissues may so alter the microenvironment of cells as to cause the formation of abnormal immunogenic cells or other factors with carcinogenic properties.

TABLE I.   Pretransplantation Treatment

AUTOGRAFT			ISOGRAFT						ALLOGRAFT (NONINBRED SWISS)	
SKIN			MAMMARY GLAND		LYMPH NODE		LYMPH NODE CELL SUSPENSION		MAMMARY GLAND	LYMPH NODE
SWISS	BALB/c	CBA	BALB/c	CBA	BALB/c	CBA	BALB/c	CBA	SWISS	SWISS
CO_2	CO_2	CO_2	CO_2	CO_2	CO_2	CO_2	CO_2	CO_2	CO_2	CO_2
AIR	AIR	AIR	AIR	AIR	AIR	AIR	AIR	AIR	AIR	AIR
			NONE	NONE	NONE	NONE			NONE	NONE

TABLE II. Malignancies in CO_2-Treated BALB/c and CBA Mice

	Number of mice in group	Mean age Months	Percentage Incidences	
			Reticulum Cell Sarcoma, Type C	Pulmonary Adenocarcinoma
BALB/c				
CO_2-treated (i.p.)	12	10	25(3)	33(4)
Untreated controls	16	20	0	13(2)
CBA				
CO_2-treated (in utero)	10	6	60(6)	0
Untreated controls	15	15	0	0

Number of mice in parentheses.

TABLE III. Major Lesions in Graft Recipients and Controls (the Figures Represent Percentage Cumulative Incidences)

	BALB/c MICE												NONINBRED SWISS MICE					
	Con-trols	Skin Autografts		Mammary Gland Isografts			Lymph Node Isografts			Con-trols	Skin Autografts		Mammary Gland Allografts		
		CO_2	Air	CO_2	Air	None	CO_2	Air	None		CO_2	Air	CO_2	Air	None
Mean age months	20	10	11	13	13	11	10	11	10	13	13	11	14	13	13
Number of mice in group	35	25	28	22	20	21	30	25	20	40	22	20	22	20	24
Malignant lymphomas	0	33	0	40	20	29	45	48	61	8	88	79	68	64	63
Amyloidosis	2	30	0	31	46	29	63	16	38	3	10	0	18	23	15
Myocarditis	0	12	0	9	23	41	7	4	22	0	2	0	20	23	0
Glomerular lesions	0	18	0	9	7	17	7	12	16	14	12	0	4	17	2
Pyelonephritis	28	43	32	36	46	52	97	88	94	9	80	8	40	11	9
Pulmonary adenocarcinomas	14	8	6	9	7	0	7	8	0	0	0	0	22	23	0

Abbreviations: CO_2 = CO_2-graft recipients
Air = air-graft recipients
None = untreated graft recipients

983

TABLE IV. T- and B-Cell Abnormalities in Lymphomatous and Non-Lymphomatous Groups

| | Lymphomatous | | | | Non-lymphomatous | | | |
| | Spleen | | Node | | Spleen | | Node | |
	T	B	T	B	T	B	T	B
Hyperplasia	59	28	3	12	19	0	23	42
Atrophy	0	25	0	3	0	15	0	15

984

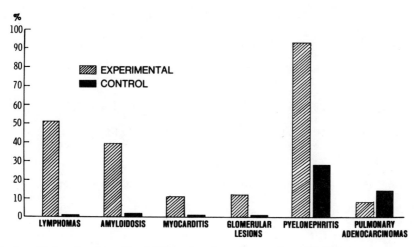

FIG. 1. Major lesions in BALB/c lymph node graft recipients + controls.

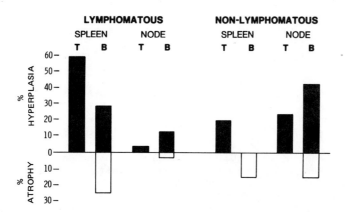

FIG. 2. T + B Cell abnormalities in lymphomatous + non-lymphomatous groups.

REFERENCES

1. Broecker, W.S. Climatic Change: Are We On The Brink Of A Pronounced Global Warming? Science, 189: 460-463, 1975.
2. Goldsmith, A.E. Paget's Osteitis Deformans: A Carbonate-Rich Calcium Alkali Phosphate In The Pre-Malignant Bone Mineral And Implications For Lymphoma Production By CO_2. Bioinorganic Chemistry, in press.
3. Goddard, D.R. The Biological Role Of Carbon Dioxide. Anesthesiology, 21: 587-596, 1960.
4. Nichols, G.,Jr. Solubility Of Carbon Dioxide In Body Fat. Science, N.Y., 126: 1244-1245, 1957.
5. Ligou, J.C. and Nahas, G.G. Comparative Effects Of Acidosis Induced By Acid Infusion And CO_2 Accumulation. Am. J. Physiol., 198: 1201-1206, 1960.
6. Loomis, W.F. pCO_2 Inhibition Of Normal And Malignant Growth. J. Natn. Cancer Inst., 22: 207-217, 1959.
7. Jacobs, M.H. The Production Of Intracellular Acidity By Neutral And Alkaline Solutions Containing Carbon Dioxide. Am. J. Physiol., 53: 457-463, 1920.
8. Jacobs, M.H. Effects Of Carbon Dioxide On The Consistency Of Protoplasm. Biol. Bull., Mar. Biol. Lab., Woods Hole, 42: 14-19, 1922.
9. Mottram, J.C. The Role Of Carbon Dioxide In The Growth Of Normal And Tumour Cells. Lancet ii: 1232-1234, 1927.
10. Nichols, G.,Jr. Serial Changes In Tissue Carbon Dioxide Content During Acute Respiratory Acidosis. J. Clin. Invest., 37: 1111-1122, 1958.
11. Schaefer, K.E. Atmung Und Säure-Basengleichgewicht Bei Langdauerndem Aufenthalt In 3% CO_2. Pflügers Arch. Ges. Physio., 251: 689-715, 1949.
12. Kloos, K. Kohlensäure Als Pathogenetischer Faktor. Ärztl. Wschr., 14: 825-831, 1959.
13. Kieler, J., Nissen, N.I., and Bicz, W. Investigation Of The Cytostatic Function Of O_2 And CO_2 Tension. Acta Un. Int. Cancr., 18: 228-233, 1962.
14. Loomis, W.F. Feedback Control Of Growth And Differentiation By Carbon Dioxide Tension And Related Metabolic Variables. In: Rudnick Cell, Organism And Milieu. Ronald Press, New York, 1959.
15. Jacobs, M.H. To What Extent Are The Physiological Effects Of Carbon Dioxide Due To Hydrogen Ions? Am. J. Physiol., 51: 321-331, 1920.
16. Bicz, W. The Influence Of Carbon Dioxide Tension On The Respiration Of Normal And Leukemic Human Leukocytes. Influence On Endogenous Respiration. Cancer Res., 20: 184-190, 1960.
17. Kieler, J. Influence Of CO_2 Tension On The Respiration Of Yoshida Ascites Tumor Cells. J. Natn. Cancer Inst., 25: 161-176, 1960.
18. Kieler, J., Bicz, W., and Mosbech, J. Influence Of CO_2 Tension On Leukemia Cell Metabolism. Proc. Congr. European Soc. Haematol., 8: No. 120, 4p, 1961.
19. Nissen, N.I. Influence Of CO_2 On Respiratory Metabolism Of Ehrlich Ascites Tumor. Proc. Soc. Exp. Biol. Med., 104: 446-448, 1960.
20. Bauer, J.T. The Effect Of Carbon Dioxide On Cells In Tissue Cultures. Bull. Johns Hopkins Hosp., 37: 420-427, 1925.

21. Frank, B. Atypische Wuchsform Von Retinaepithel Vom Embryonalen Hühnerauge Nach Vorbehandlung Mit Kohlensäure. Z. Krebsforsch., 50: 496-500, 1940.
22. Mottram, J.C. On The Division Of Cells Under Varying Tensions Of Carbon Dioxide. Br. J. Exp. Path., 9: 240-244, 1928.
23. Mottram, J.C. Carbon Dioxide Tension In Tissues In Relation To Cancerous Cells. Nature, Lond., 121: 420-421, 1928.
24. Larner, J. Intermediary Metabolism And Its Regulation. Prentice Hall, Englewood Cliffs, 1971.
25. Goldsmith, A.E., and Narvaez, R. Lymphomas As Sequelae Of The Transplantation Of CO_2-Treated Skin Autografts In Mice. Oncology, 32: 247-265, 1975.
26. Dunn, T.B. Normal And Pathologic Anatomy Of The Reticular Tissue In Laboratory Mice, With A Classification And Discussion Of Neoplasms, J. Natn. Cancer Inst., 14: 1281-1433, 1954.
27. Eisen, H.N. Immunology. Harper And Row, Inc., Hagerstown, p. 459, 1974.
28. Weber, W.T. Difference Between Medullary And Cortical Thymic Lymphocytes Of Pig In Their Response To Phytohemagglutinin. J. Cell Physiol., 68: 117-126, 1966.
29. Shearer, G.M. In Vitro Induction Of Thymus-Derived Cell-Mediated Cytotoxicity To Trinitrophenol-Modified Syngeneic Lymphocyte Surface Proteins. Ann. N.Y. Acad. Sci., 249: 47-53, 1975.
30. Cohen, P., and Gershon, R.K. The Role Of Cortisone-Sensitive Thymocytes In DNA Synthetic Responses To Antigen. Ann. N.Y. Acad. Sci., 249: 451-461, 1975.
31. Lance, E.M., and Cooper, S. Hormones And The Immune Response. Ciba Foundation Study Group, 36: 73-95, 1970.

Chapter 11

TRANSPLACENTAL AND PERINATAL EXPOSURE TO CARCINOGENS

CHARACTERISTICS OF MOTHERS AT HIGH RISK
OF LEUKEMIA DEVELOPING IN THEIR CHILDREN

Mary G. McCrea Curnen, MD, DPH
Livia Turgeon, MS

Divisions of Epidemiology and Biostatistics
Columbia University School of Public Health
New York, New York   .

John T. Flannery, BS

Connecticut Tumor Registry
Hartford, Connecticut

Andre A. O. Varma, MD, MS

Department of Community Medicine
State University of New York
Stony Brook, New York

INTRODUCTION

Children who develop cancer early in life are especially well suited
for the study of prenatal factors likely to be associated with the
development of the disease. Miller reported on 78 infants in the USA
who died of cancer on the first day of life and 138 additional children
who died between the first and 28th day of life.[1] These neoplasms
presumably originated during intrauterine life.

In a study based on data from the Connecticut Tumor Registry, we
tested the hypothesis of a transplacental viral mechanism in the etiology
of childhood leukemia.[2] We did not find a significant variation
among the leukemia rates in children by year of birth nor by place of
birth. Furthermore, there was no clustering of these births in time and
space. We were also unable to demonstrate an increased risk of leukemia
in the offspring of mothers who were more likely than other mothers to
have been exposed to infectious diseases during pregnancy.

Because susceptibility to infectious diseases is related to age
(younger mothers being more likely than older ones to be susceptible),
the relation of maternal age and birth order to childhood leukemia was
investigated. Among those who studied these factors previously,
MacMahon and Newill in 1962 reported on a series of approximately 2,000
children born in New England and the Middle Atlantic states between 1947
and 1954 who had died of leukemia under age 12.[3] The risk of leukemia
appeared to be 40 percent higher in children of women over 40 years of
age than in those of women under 20. In 1966, Stark and Mantel published

a report on 706 children who were born in Michigan between 1950 and 1964 and who died of leukemia prior to age 15.[4] They found a significant positive association between childhood leukemia and age of the mother for children born in the 1950-54 period but not in the two later periods studied, 1955-59 and 1960-64.

SOURCE OF DATA

A. <u>Cross-sectional study</u>. We identified from the Connecticut Tumor Registry 389 children with leukemia who were born in Connecticut between 1946 and 1964. We grouped the leukemic children by year of birth into two consecutive time periods: those born from 1946-54 and from 1955-64. Our first period coincided with the one used in studies by MacMahon et al. and Stark et al., thus facilitating comparisons. For each child with leukemia, mother's age at delivery was classified into three groups: under 20, 20-34, and 35 years and older. Birth order was divided into five categories: 1, 2, 3, 4, 5 and greater. These data were analyzed in an attempt to detect a "cross-sectional" effect in time which would be manifested by affecting <u>all</u> mother irrespective of their age.

B. <u>Maternal birth cohort study</u>. In contrast to a cross-sectional effect, a maternal birth cohort effect would be apparent at all reproductive ages but at different chronological times in individual mothers. A series of 500 children from the Connecticut Tumor Registry was obtained by identifying those children born in Connecticut between 1935 and 1964 who developed leukemia during their first ten years of life. This series included 222 girls and 278 boys, all but 14 were white. Their distribution by histological type of leukemia was as follows: 57% lymphocytic, 15% myelocytic, and 28% "other" (monocytic, stem cell, unspecified types).

RESULTS

A. <u>Cross-sectional study</u>. The leukemia rates by <u>maternal age</u> for time period I and II are shown in Figure 1. They were higher for the very young mothers (under 20) in both time periods. In the first period, the rate of 74 per 100,000 live births in mothers under 20 was significantly higher than that found in mothers 20 years of age and older (X_1^2 = 5.65 with P <.02).

Figure 2 illustrates the leukemia rates by <u>birth order</u>. No definite pattern is evident in either time period. The rates were high for birth order 1 and 5 in time period I; rates in birth order 5, however, were unstable since they were based on a proportionally small number of births in this category.

In nature, maternal age and birth order are strongly correlated; a mother under 20 is unlikely to have a fifth child. Thus we did not aim at eliminating a birth order effect from a maternal age effect by adjusting rates to a standard population especially as leukemia rates by birth order, as illustrated in Figure 2, did not reveal statistically significant variations between birth order groups.

Because of the possible effect of birth weight on the subsequent development of leukemia, we computed the average birth weights by sex,

mother's age and birth order for a random sample of the Connecticut white
live birth population for the years 1959-62 (N=13,921). The average
birth weights by sex, mother's age and birth order of the 205 white
leukemic children for whom birth weight was available were compared to
those of the population sample. There were no remarkable differences in
average birth weight between these two groups.

B. Maternal birth cohort study. It is evident that young mothers in
time period I will move to an older age group in time period II. In the
cohort analysis, missing data on the early offspring of older mothers in
time period I are irretrievable because the Connecticut Tumor Registry
was not in existence prior to 1935. At present, data are also missing
for the young mothers in time period II who have not lived long enough
to complete their reproductive years. These data, however, will be
obtainable in the future.

Figure 3 illustrates by year of birth of mothers the set of live
births for infants born in Connecticut from 1935-64. Mother's year of
birth is indicated along the abscissa. The figure should be read upwards
in order to add up the infants delivered at different ages by women
belonging to the same birth cohort. The three age groups at which mothers
delivered their children are represented by different shadings. Clearly
not all maternal birth cohorts have their full reproductive history
represented here for reasons just mentioned. The shape of the figure,
however, contains the Connecticut live born infants who, in our study,
were used as the denominators to compute the leukemia rates.

In Figure 4, we have represented in a similar way in the bottom
half of the graph the 500 leukemic children by year of birth of mother
and her age at delivery.

Leukemia rates by year of birth of mother and age group at delivery
are shown in the upper half of Figure 4. Although these maternal birth
cohorts have still an incomplete follow-up, it is noteworthy that for
mothers born in the same year leukemia rates were consistently higher in
children born of mothers under 20 as compared to those born to mothers
from the same cohort when they were older. This striking finding for
young mothers under 20 is particularly noticeable for women born in
certain years (1932, 1934 and 1940).

DISCUSSION

In both analyses, leukemia rates were higher in children born of
young mothers under 20 than of mothers 20 years of age and older. This
was particularly striking in the cross-sectional analysis of children
born in the first time period, from 1946 to 1954. Although our leukemia
cases are included in MacMahon et al.'s larger series, they represent
less than 8% of those cases. Our observation differs from those of
MacMahon et al. and Stark et al. who, for a similar time period, found a
positive association between childhood leukemia and advancing maternal
age. Rates by birth order did not vary significantly during the study
period.

We did not find that the cases of lymphocytic leukemia were responsible for the higher rates of leukemia in the offspring of mothers under

20. Although in the cohort analysis, leukemia rates by year of birth of the mother and by age group at delivery were also higher for mothers under 20, this finding did not carry over when women of the same cohort delivered at older ages. The follow-up is still incomplete, however, so a cohort phenomenon cannot as yet be definitely excluded.

The finding that mothers under 20 are more at risk than older mothers to bear a child who will develop leukemia in the first 10 years of life is compatible with the hypothesis that these very young mothers are also those most likely to be susceptible to infectious agents. No pattern emerged when stillbirth rates for Connecticut women were compared with leukemic rates by year of birth for children born in Connecticut who developed the disease before age 10. Although young pregnant women may have been subjected more frequently than older women to X-ray for pelvimetry, we do not have this information for the mothers in our series. We also cannot estimate the possible effects of the anesthesia and drugs which these mothers may have received.

SUMMARY

A higher incidence of leukemia in the offspring of mothers under 20 years of age as demonstrated in data from Connecticut remains unexplained. The simultaneous search for a cross-sectional and a cohort effect in mothers of children who develop leukemia may offer a promising approach to the elucidation of maternal factors in childhood cancer.

ACKNOWLEDGEMENTS

We dedicate this work to the memory of Dr. Barbara Christine, past Director of the Connecticut Tumor Registry, who died earlier this year. She provided us with constant aid and encouragement.

This work was supported by Public Health Service Grant CA 13696 to the Cancer Research Center, Columbia University College of Physicians and Surgeons, from the National Cancer Institute.

We wish to thank Suri Harris, MPH, for her help in the early stage of this study. We are grateful to Dr. M. Honeyman and Mr. H. Burdo and staff for making available essential vital statistics from the Connecticut State Department of Health. We appreciate the constructive criticism provided to us by Dr. M. Susser and his staff in the Division of Epidemiology at Columbia University School of Public Health. We are grateful for the invaluable suggestions by Dr. E. Curnen, Jr. and to Ms. M. Keigher and A. Thomsen for their skillful assistance in preparing this paper.

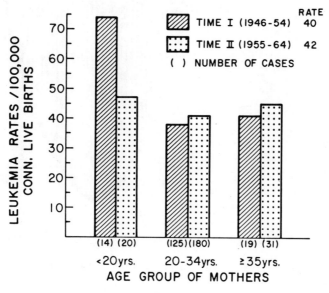

FIG. 1

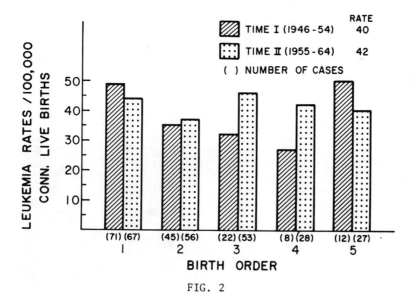

FIG. 2

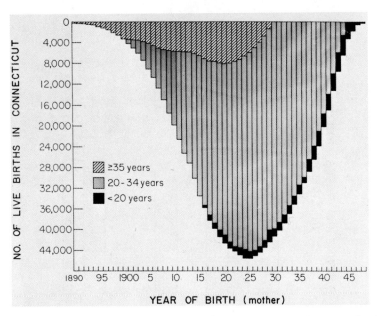

FIG. 3. Number of live births in Connecticut (1935-1964) by mother's year of birth and age at delivery.

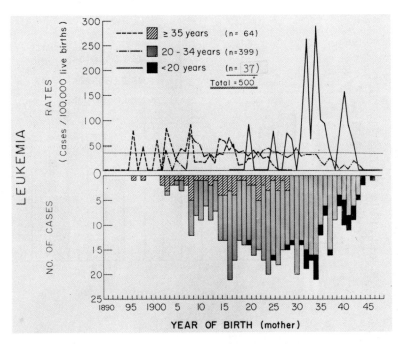

FIG. 4. Leukemia rates, with number of leukemic children born in Conn. (1935-1964), by mother's year of birth and age at delivery.

REFERENCES

1. Miller, R. W. Prenatal Origins Of Cancer In Man: Epidemiological Evidence. In: Transplacental Carcinogenesis. Ed.: L. Tomatis and V. Mohr. International Agency For Research On Cancer, Scientific Publications No. 4, Lyon, pp 175-180, 1973.

2. Curnen, M. G. McCrea, Varma, A. O., Christine, B. W., and Turgeon, L. R. Childhood Leukemia And Maternal Infectious Diseases During Pregnancy. J. Natl. Cancer Inst. 53: 943-947, 1974

3. MacMahon, B., and Newill, V. A. Birth Characteristics Of Children Dying Of Malignant Neoplasms. J. Natl. Cancer Inst. 28: 231-244, 1962.

4. Stark, C. R., and Mantel, N. Effects Of Maternal Age And Birth Order On The Risk Of Mongolism And Leukemia. J. Natl. Cancer Inst. 37: 687-698, 1966.

INFLUENCE OF TRANSPLACENTAL 3-METHYLCHOLANTHRENE ON ARYL HYDROCARBON HYDROXYLASE ACTIVITY OF MOUSE LUNG

William G. Hunt, Stephen E. Knight and Lester F. Soyka

Department of Pharmacology
University of Vermont
Burlington, Vermont

I. INTRODUCTION

The mixed function oxygenase aryl hydrocarbon hydroxylase, which is involved in the activation and detoxification of aromatic polycyclic hydrocarbon carcinogens, is present in many tissues, including the lung (Conney, 1967; Burki et al., 1973). Lung aryl hydrocarbon hydroxylase activity can be induced in strains of mice in which hepatic aryl hydrocarbon hydroxylase is relatively resistant to induction by polycyclic hydrocarbons (Nebert and Gelboin, 1969; Gelboin et al., 1972; Wiebel et al., 1973).

The mouse lung is highly susceptible to pulmonary adenoma formation following exposure to chemical carcinogens (Shimkin, 1955) and to squamous cell carcinomas of the respiratory tract as a result of intra-tracheal exposure (Nettesheim et al., 1971).

It is important to know whether aryl hydrocarbon hydroxylase activity in target tissues such as lung and experimentally induced or genetically controlled differences in its activity correlate with tumor type or incidence. Therefore, studies were undertaken to define lung aryl hydrocarbon hydroxylase activity and its response to induction by pheno-barbital and 3-methylcholanthrene in mice exposed in utero to doses of 3-methylcholanthrene known to produce lung adenomas during late adulthood (Tomatis et al., 1971). Such factors as strain, sex, inducibility and age were investigated. A companion paper deals with these effects on hepatic microsomal aryl hydrocarbon hydroxylase and other prototype mixed-function oxidase reactions (Soyka et al., in press).

II. PROCEDURES AND MATERIALS USED

A. Animals

Pregnant outbred Swiss-Webster mice were obtained from Canadian Breeders, St. Constant, Quebec. Mice used in breeding our hybrid strains were obtained from the Jackson Laboratory, Bar Harbor, Maine.

All mice were maintained in plastic cages with softwood bedding and fed from the same lot of Purina Lab chow. Studies in mice bedded in various materials revealed that the bedding material used did not act as an inducer.

B. Chemicals

The cofactors, 3-methylcholanthrene and benzo(a)pyrene were purchased from Sigma Chemical Company, St. Louis, Missouri.

C. Experimental Protocol

Pregnant mice were treated with two doses, 24 hours apart, of 3-methylcholanthrene (4 mg in 0.2 ml olive oil) administered subcutaneously two to four days prior to delivery. Control animals received olive oil at the same times.

Offspring were killed by cervical dislocation in three different age groups; neonates (10 and 20 days postpartum), young (9 - 12 weeks) or old (16 - 18 months) adults. Lungs were removed, rinsed in cold normal saline and connective tissue and major bronchi excised by blunt dissection. The tissue was homogenized in 4.5 ml sucrose-EDTA-Tris buffer, pH 7.6, using a 10 ml Potter-Elvehjem tissue grinder with teflon pestle resulting in a 5 - 10% by weight lung homogenate.

For induction studies, mice were treated with 3-methylcholanthrene (100 mg/kg, i.p.) 24 hours prior to assay or with sodium phenobarbital (80 mg/kg, i.p.) for five days.

A second type of experiment was designed to compare the exposure to 3-methylcholanthrene (and/or its metabolites) transplacentally to that via the milk during suckling. Thirty timed pregnant Swiss-Webster mice were divided into four groups: seven pregnant mice received two subcutaneous doses of olive oil and nursed their own offspring (Group A); eight mice received olive oil but their offspring (Group B) were nursed by mothers treated with 3-methylcholanthrene; eight pregnant mice received two subcutaneous injections of 3-methylcholanthrene in olive oil 48 hours apart and their progeny (Group C) were nursed by control mothers; seven mice were injected with 3-methylcholanthrene and nursed by their own own progeny (Group D). The mothers were switched within two hours of delivery which virtually eliminated cross-exposure in the various groups. Lung aryl hydrocarbon hydroxylase activity was assayed at 10 and 20 days of age.

D. Enzyme Assay

Aryl hydrocarbon hydroxylase activity was measured using a modification of the method of Nebert and Gelboin (1968). The room was protected from sunlight and dim yellow fluorescent light was used. The incubation mixture (total volume 1.05 ml) contained 0.70 ml Tris-MgCl$_2$ buffer, pH 7.5, 0.2 ml cofactor solution (2 μmoles NADPH and 2 μmoles NADH in 0.1 M Na$_2$HPO$_4$·2H$_2$0 buffer, pH 7.4), and 0.1 ml lung homogenate. The reaction was begun by the addition of 50 μl freshly prepared benzo(a)pyrene (80 μM) in acetone. For the kinetic studies benzo(a)pyrene concentrations from 2.5 to 100 μM were prepared by dilution. Samples in 10 ml

Erlenmeyer flasks were shaken in air at 37° for 30 minutes in an
Eberbach shaker. The reaction was stopped by addition of 1 ml cold
acetone and the mixture extracted with 3.25 ml hexane with shaking at 37°
for ten minutes. A 1 ml aliquot of the organic phase was removed and
shaken for ten seconds with 3 ml of 1 N NaOH and the alkaline phase was
read immediately.

The fluorescence due to phenolic products was measured using an
Aminco-Bowman spectrophotofluorometer with excitation wavelength 396 nm
and emission wavelength 522 nm. A 1 µg/ml solution of quinine sulfate in
0.1 N H_2SO_4 was used as a standard for daily calibration of the instrument.
Aryl hydrocarbon hydroxylase activity was expressed as fluorescent units/
mg protein/30-minute incubation period.

Protein was determined according to the method of Lowry et al. (1951)
with bovine serum albumin as the standard.

E. Statistical Procedures

Student's paired t-test was used with the level of significance
chosen to be $P < 0.05$. Data from the cross-foster study were subjected
to factorial analysis of variance (ANOVA and Newman-Keuls).

III. RESULTS

A. Lung Aryl Hydrocarbon Hydroxylase Levels as a Function of Age and Sex

Activity in Swiss-Webster mice peaked at a higher level and decreased
more rapidly with age in males (Figure 1) than in females (Figure 2).
At ten days of age both male and female offspring exposed in utero to
3-methylcholanthrene had aryl hydrocarbon hydroxylase levels four
to five times greater than those of age and sex-matched controls. At
20 days this difference was no longer statistically significant.

B. Response to Induction by 3-Methylcholanthrene and Phenobarbital

The magnitude of the responses to induction by 3-methylcholanthrene
pretreatment (300 - 600%) did not differ significantly from controls
compared to 3-methylcholanthrene exposed mice of either sex
(Figure 3). The relative lack of response of lung aryl hydrocarbon
hydroxylase to induction by phenobarbital is in agreement with earlier
studies on extrahepatic tissues (Conney, 1967). Adult females showed a
greater response to induction by phenobarbital than did males of the
same age (100% versus a 25% for control males and a 55% decrease in the
experimental males).

C. Strain Differences

A study has been initiated to compare lung aryl hydrocarbon hydroxylase levels of Swiss-Webster mice at various ages with those of highly
inducible (with respect to hepatic aryl hydrocarbon levels) hybrid strains

and their (C57 Bl/6J x C3H/HeJ) F_1 cross and a non-inducible hybrid (DBA/
1J x SWR/J) F_1. Preliminary data comparing these strains at 20 days and
at 10 weeks of age, as well as their response to induction by 3-methyl-
cholanthrene at these ages, are shown in Table I. Basal levels at 20 days
of age were lower for DBA/1J x SWR/J than for the other three strains.
Females had higher basal levels than did males at 10 weeks in the same
SWR/J and C57Bl/6J x C3HeJ strains and lower levels than males in the
C57Bl/6J mice. The induction ratio was greater for all strains in the
10-week-old mice than for neonates, although absolute levels at these
two ages were virtually identical. The aryl hydrocarbon hydroxylase
activity in males from the inducible hybrid cross was increased to a
greater degree by 3-methylcholanthrene pretreatment than in females at
both ages studied.

D. Kinetic Studies

Lung aryl hydrocarbon hydroxylase activity measured at benzo(a)-
pyrene final concentrations of 1.2 to 50 µM resulted in Lineweaver-Burk
plots which despite some discrepant values, perhaps because crude
homogenates were used, had correlation coefficients (r) of 0.95 or
greater. Linear regression analysis indicated a significant age difference between males at 9, 12 and 16 weeks, and females at 12, 18 and
67 weeks of age. There was a decrease in rate of substrate metabolism
with increasing age (Figures 4 and 5). Comparison of control and experimental offspring found a significant difference only in the 9-week-old
males.

E. Transplacental vs. Suckling Exposure

Foster studies were done to determine whether the extremely elevated
lung aryl hydrocarbon hydroxylase levels found in 10-day-old mice (Figures
1 and 2) were due to prenatal, postnatal or combined exposure to 3-methyl-
cholanthrene. Analysis of the results (Table II) were marred by the
aberrant value for the 20-day-old male controls, which was higher than
found in eight similar groups in other studies. Use of the Newman-Keuls
analysis of variance permitted comparison of each group with one another
(Table III). The results indicate that prenatal exposure resulted in
levels of activity which were lower than controls, except in the afore-
mentioned 20-day-old male group. Despite this trend the magnitude of
the depression was not statistically significant. Conversely, postnatal
exposure caused significant increases in both sexes at both ages, again
except for the aberrant male 20-day-old group. Postnatal exposure after
prenatal resulted in a lesser increase than postnatal exposure alone,
consistent with the observation of lowered levels of activity in groups
exposed only prenatally.

IV. DISCUSSION

Aryl hydrocarbon hydroxylase activity was extremely elevated in
ten-day-old male and female 3-methylcholanthrene exposed offspring. At
later ages there were generally no significant differences in enzyme

activities between sex-matched controls and offspring exposed to 3-methylcholanthrene.

Induction with 3-methylcholanthrene did not result in differences between sex-matched controls and exposed offspring. Significant differences were seen in response to phenobarbital induction at 75 weeks of age. There were sex differences in the direction and magnitude of response between control and experimental offspring.

We queried whether the source of 3-methylcholanthrene or its metabolites that caused the marked elevation in hydroxylase activity in 10-day-old lungs was transplacental or via suckling. There is evidence supporting both routes.

Administration of 3-methylcholanthrene to pregnant females can affect aryl hydrocarbon hydroxylase levels directly by 3-methylcholanthrene delivered transplacentally to the fetus. Tomatis et al. (1971) have shown that exposure to 3-methylcholanthrene in utero without postnatal exposure via suckling was sufficient to induce a high incidence of tumors in several species of mice. Studies done using ^{14}C-3-methylcholanthrene administered intragastrically to pregnant mice showed that from 0.26% (Turusov et al., 1973) to 10% (Takahashi and Yasuhira, 1973) of the maternal dose of 3-methylcholanthrene reached the fetuses as unmetabolized 3-methylcholanthrene. As little as 2 ng 3-methylcholanthrene/mg of lung tissue was sufficient to produce a 75% incidence of pulmonary tumors in the offspring.

Another route of 3-methylcholanthrene exposure is through the milk. Methylcholanthrene and/or its metabolites have been shown to be highly concentrated in mammary glands, particularly when administered in a lipid vehicle (Dao, 1969), and were still concentrated in mammary glands eight days after a single oral administration (Dao et al., 1959). These rats, receiving 3-methylcholanthrene in some form only through the milk, had an increased incidence of tumors.

The foster study data indicate that lung aryl hydrocarbon hydroxylase levels in neonates were elevated by exposure to 3-methylcholanthrene and/ or metabolites in the milk without prior transplacental exposure, and actually lowered by prenatal exposure. The possibility of manipulating aryl hydrocarbon hydroxylase levels in specific tissues according to the route of exposure to the carcinogen could be useful in studies correlating hydroxylase levels and tumor formation in target tissues.

Elevated lung aryl hydrocarbon hydroxylase levels peaked at ten days of age. Studies have indicated that the highest mean lung tumor count was found in mice injected with 3-methylcholanthrene at two weeks of age (O'Gara et al., 1963). This possible correlation requires further investigation.

Pre- and/or postnatal exposure to carcinogens could influence the manner in which adults respond to re-exposure to the same or related compounds. Studies of factors affecting the metabolic or inductive mechanisms in target tissues are important in this respect. We have found some subtle differences between control and 3-methylcholanthrene exposed mice which are being further studied from this perspective.

V. SUMMARY

Studies were done to determine whether perinatal exposure to 3-methylcholanthrene produced any changes in the lung's ability to metabolize or detoxify polycyclic hydrocarbons. Pregnant outbred Swiss-Webster mice were treated with 4 mg 3-methylcholanthrene in oil s.c. on two successive days prior to delivery. Lung aryl hydrocarbon hydroxylase activity in the offspring was studied as a function of age, sex, strain and inducibility. Activity varied with age and strain and was induced in offspring of mothers injected with 3-methylcholanthrene prior to delivery. Aryl hydrocarbon hydroxylase activity of mice exposed to 3-methylcholanthrene in utero was about four times greater than controls at ten days of age but only slightly elevated at twenty days. Lung aryl hydrocarbon hydroxylase levels were elevated more by exposure to 3-methylcholanthrene and metabolites in the milk than via the transplacental route.

Perinatal exposure to carcinogens, using lung aryl hydrocarbon hydroxylase as a measure of that exposure, may influence the manner in which the adult handles re-exposure to the same or related carcinogens.

TABLE I. Comparison of Lung Aryl Hydrocarbon Hydroxylase Activity of Swiss-Webster Mice With That of Strains and Hybrids in Which Hepatic Aryl Hydrocarbon Hydroxylase Activity is (C57 B1 and its hybrid) or is not (DBA x SWR/J)F_1 Responsive to Induction by 3-Methylcholanthrene

Condition	Age	Swiss-Webster		C57 B1/6J		(C57 B1/6J X C3H/HeJ)F_1		(DBA/1J X SWR)F_1	
		Male	Female	Male	Female	Male	Female	Male	Female
Basal	20d	1.54±.17[a]	1.17±.3	1.32±.5	1.05±.05	1.69±.12	1.81±.09	0.84±.07	0.83±.05
3-MC Induced	20d		3.04±.4			3.61±.01	3.10±.07		
Induced/Basal			2.6			2.1	1.7		
Basal	10wk	0.85±.04	1.41±.11	1.33±.07	0.67±.09	0.88±.07	1.15±.09	1.43±1.5	
3MC Induced	10wk	3.03±.5			5.02±.3	3.50±.4	3.10±.4		
Induced/Basal		3.5			7.5	4.0	2.7		

a AHH activity is expressed as fluorescent units/mg protein/30 min, mean ± SEM, N = 5.

TABLE II. Cross-Fostering Study of Aryl Hydrocarbon Hydroxylase Activity in Lungs of Young Swiss-Webster Mice Exposed Pre- and/or Postnatally to 3-Methylcholanthrene

Group 3-MC Exposure	A Control	B Prenatal	C Postnatal	D Both	A Control	B Prenatal	C Postnatal	D Both
			Male				Female	
10 d/o	1.37±.52	0.83±.12	2.67±.30	2.95±.36	0.96±.24	0.56±.12	3.70±.6	3.06±.17
		NS[a]	NS	P < .05		NS	P < .01	P < .01
20 d/o	3.39±.4[a]	1.78±.17	2.86±.27	2.38±.23	1.97±.22	2.18±.31	2.93±.18	2.86±.20
						NS	P < .01	P < .05

Groups A, B, C, D are defined in the Methods. Values are mean fluorescent units/mg protein/30' ± SEM; N = 5.
[a] This value was 1½ times higher than means from eight other studies of mice of this age.

TABLE III. Newman-Keuls Analysis of Variance of Data from Foster Nursing Study

Age	Sex	Order of Activity	A Control	B Prenatal	C Postnatal	D Both
				Experimental Group		
10 d	M	Prenatal	NS	--	*	*
		Control	--	NS	*	*
		Postnatal	--	--	--	NS
10 d	F	Prenatal	NS	--	*	*
		Control	--	NS	*	*
		Both	--	--	*	--
20 d	M	Prenatal	*	--	*	NS
		Both	*	NS	NS	--
		Postnatal	NS	--	--	--
20 d	F	Control	--	NS	*	*
		Prenatal	NS	--	NS	NS
		Both	--	--	--	--

*P < 0.05

NS = not significant

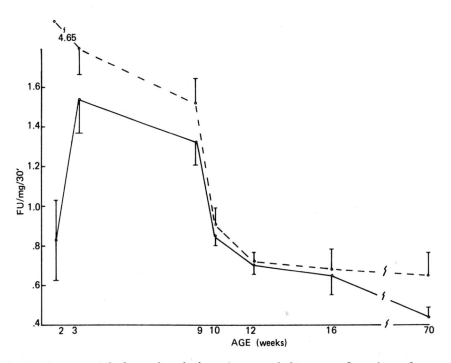

FIG. 1. Lung aryl hydrocarbon hydroxylase activity as a function of age
in male Swiss Webster mice. Activity in control mice (solid line) was
compared to that of 3-methylcholanthrene exposed offspring (dashed line).
Values are means ± S.E.M., N = 5.

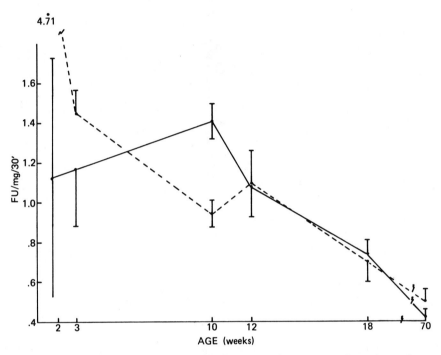

FIG. 2. Lung aryl hydrocarbon hydroxylase activity as a function of age in female Swiss Webster mice. Activity in control mice (solid line) was compared to that of 3-methylcholanthrene exposed offspring (dashed line).

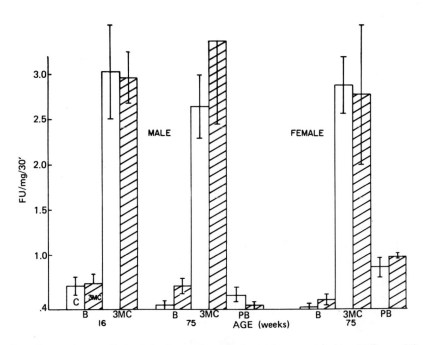

FIG. 3. Comparison of aryl hydrocarbon hydroxylase activity before (B) and after treatment with 3-methylcholanthrene (3-MC) or phenobarbital (PB). Values are means ± S.E.M., N = 5.

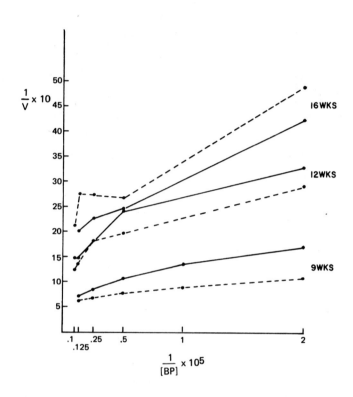

FIG. 4. Lineweaver-Burk plot of benzo(a)pyrene metabolism in lung homogenates of male Swiss-Webster mice. Control mice (solid line) were compared to 3-methylcholanthrene exposed mice (dashed line).

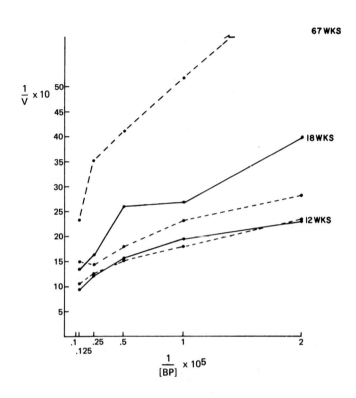

FIG. 5. Lineweaver-Burk plot of benzo(a)pyrene by lung homogenates of
female Swiss Webster mice. Control mice (solid line) were compared to
3-methylcholanthrene exposed mice (dashed line).

REFERENCES

1. Burki, K., Liebelt, A. and Bresnick, E. Expression of Aryl Hydrocarbon Hydroxylase Induction in Mouse Tissue in vivo and in Organ Culture. Arch. Biochem. Biophys. 158: 641-649, 1973.

2. Conney, A. Pharmacological Implications of Microsomal Enzyme Induction. Pharmacol. Rev. 19: 317-366, 1967.

3. Dao, T., Bock, F. and Crouch, S. Level of 3-Methylcholanthrene in Mammary Glands of Rats after Intragastric Instillation of Carcinogen. Proc. Soc. Exp. Biol. Med. 102: 635-638, 1959.

4. Dao, T. Studies on Mechanism of Carcinogenesis in the Mammary Gland. Prog. Exp. Tumor Res. 11: 235-261, 1969.

5. Gelboin, H., Nadao, K., and Wiebel, F. Microsomal Hydroxylases: Induction and its Role in Polycyclic Hydrocarbon Carcinogenesis and Toxicity. Fed. Proc. 31: 1298-1309, 1972.

6. Lowry, O., Rosebrough, N., Farr, A., and Randall, R. Protein Measurement with the Folin Phenol Reagent. J. Biol. Chem. 193: 265-275, 1951.

7. Nebert, D., and Gelboin, H., Substrate-inducible Microsomal Aryl Hydroxylase in Mammalian Cell Culture. J. Biol. Chem. 243: 6250-6261, 1968.

8. Nebert, D., and Gelboin, H. The in vivo and in vitro Induction of Aryl Hydrocarbon Hydroxylase in Mammalian Cells of Different Species, Tissues, Strains, and Developmental and Hormonal States. Arch. Biochem. Biophys. 134: 76-89, 1969.

9. Nettesheim, P., and Hammons, A. Induction of Squamous Cell Carcinoma in the Respiratory Tract of Mice. J. Nat. Cancer Inst. 47: 697-701, 1971.

10. O'Gara, R., Kelly, M., Brown, J., and Mantel, N. Induction of Tumors in Mice Given a Minute Single Dose of Dibenz(a,h)anthracene or 3-Methylcholanthrene as Newborns. A Dose-Response Study. J. Natl. Cancer Inst. 35: 1027-1042, 1963.

11. Shimkin, M. Pulmonary Tumors in Experimental Animals. Advances in Cancer Res. 3: 223-266, 1955.

12. Soyka, L., Knight, S., and Hunt, W. Effect of in utero Exposure to 3-Methylcholanthrene on Hepatic Microsomal Drug Metabolizing Enzyme Activity of Mice. Proc. Third Int. Symp. Detection and Prevention of Cancer. In press.

13. Takahashi, G., and Yasuhira, K. Macroautoradiographic and Radiometric Studies on the Distribution of 3-Methylcholanthrene in Mice and their Fetuses. Cancer Res. 33: 23-28, 1973.

14. Tomatis, L., Turusov, V., Guibbert, D., Duperray, B., Malaveille, C., and Pacheco, H. Transplacental Carcinogenic Effect of 3-methylcholanthrene in mice and Its Quantitation in Fetal Tissues. J. Natl. Cancer Inst. 47: 645-651, 1971.

15. Turusov, V., Tomatis, L., Guibbert, D., Duperray, D., and Pacheco, H. The Effect of Prenatal Exposure of Mice to Methylcholanthrene Combined With the Neonatal Administration of Diethylnitrosamine. In:Transplacental Carcinogenesis. Ed.: L. Tomatis and U. Mohr. IARC Scientific Publication #4. Lyon, 84-91, 1973.

16. Wiebel, F., Lentz, J., and Gelboin, H. Aryl Hydrocarbon Hydroxylase: Inducible in Extrahepatic Tissues of Mouse Strains Not Inducible in Liver. Arch. Biochem. Biophys. 154: 292-294, 1973.

EPITHELIAL DIFFERENTIATION OF THE EMBRYONIC HAMSTER TRACHEA
AND ITS SIGNIFICANCE FOR STUDIES ON DIETHYLNITROSAMINE
TRANSPLACENTAL CARCINOGENESIS

Makito Emura

Laboratory of Cell Biology
Aichi Cancer Center Research Institute
Nagoya 464
Japan

Ulrich Mohr

Abteilung fuer Experimentelle Pathologie
Medizinische Hochschule Hannover
3000 Hannover 61
Karl-Wiechert-Allee 9
Federal Republic of Germany

INTRODUCTION

The prenatal tracheal epithelium of the Syrian golden hamster is one of the most suitable experimental systems for
studying transplacental carcinogenesis with diethylnitrosamine
(Mohr, Althoff, Wrba, 1965; Mohr, Althoff, Authaler, 1966;
Mohr, 1973; Mohr, Reznik-Schueller, Reznik, et al., 1975).   In
this system, the susceptibility of cells to diethylnitrosamine
might be closely correlated to a certain differentiated state
of the epithelia (Mohr, Reznik-Schueller, Reznik,et al.,
1975). The present study was undertaken to establish whether
there is any evidence to support this assumption. Hence,
transplacental carcinogenesis experiments, in conjunction with
morphological investigations of differentiation, were performed on this system, and the results compared.

PROCEDURES AND MATERIALS USED

Transplacental Carcinogenesis Experiment

One hundred and five female Syrian golden hamsters (Cent-
raal Proefdierenbedrijf TNO, Zeist, Holland) were hand-mated
and individually housed in Makrolon cages Type II (polyacryl,
400 cm^2; Becker and Co. GmbH, Castrop-Rauxel, West Germany).
The day after mating was counted as day 1. The animals were
kept under standard laboratory conditions (room temperature
22 $\pm$ 2°C; relative humidity 55 $\pm$ 5%; air exchange 8 times per
hour) and given a pelleted diet (Hope Farms, RMH-TMB, Woerden,
Holland) and water ad libitum. Fifteen groups, each consisting
of 6 pregnant females, were given a single subcutaneous injection of 45 mg diethylnitrosamine/kg body weight in solution
with physiologic saline on one of the 15 days of pregnancy. An
equivalent group treated on day 15 of pregnancy with the solvent alone served as a vehicle control. (Diethylnitrosamine
was synthesized by Dr. F.W. Krueger, Krebsforschungszentrum,
Heidelberg, West Germany; it had a purity of 99.5%.) The litters were weaned on the 25th day after birth, separated from
their mother and housed according to sex and litter in Makrolon cages, Type III (900 cm^2). Both mother and offspring were
observed until spontaneous death. Thereafter, complete autopsies were performed; all organs were fixed in 4% buffered formalin. Skulls were decalcified with Decal (Scientific Products,
Evanston, Ill., U.S.A.) and all tissues were embedded in Parap-
last. The larynx, cranial and middle and caudal parts of the
trachea, as well as its bifurcation, were embedded separately
and cut into graded sections. Histological sections were routinely stained with hematoxylin and eosin and those of the
respiratory system were also stained with alcian blue and
periodic acid-Schiff. Only those offspring and their respective mothers surviving the weaning period were evaluated.
Since cannibalism of litters by their treated mothers was high,
the actual numbers available for analysis were rather low in
several groups.

Morphological Examination of the Tracheal Differentiation

Under the same laboratory conditions as above, seventy four
Syrian golden hamsters were hand-mated and sacrificed on the
different days of pregnancy. Days of fetal development were
calculated with the day following mating as the 1st prenatal
day. The mothers were anaesthetized with ether and the young
fixed either in Bouin's solution or in utero by means of perfusion with 2% cacodylate buffered glutaraldehyde (pH=7.4).
The tissues were routinely stained with hematoxylin and eosin
for histological examination. For electron microscopy the tissues were cut into small pieces and post-fixed in 1% osmium
tetroxide. After dehydration through an ascending series of
ethanols they were embedded in Epon 812. Ultrathin sections
were cut with an LKB Ultrotome III, stained with uranyl acetate and lead citrate, and observed on a Philips EM 201 electron microscope at 60 KV.

RESULTS

Development of Respiratory Tract Tumors in the Offspring and
the Mother

The offspring of mothers injected with a single dose of
diethylnitrosamine on one of the fifteen gestation days developed tumors in various organs. The incidence of tumors in the
respiratory organs is summrized in Table I. It is noteworthy
in this table that the respiratory tract tumors were developed
only in the offspring of mothers treated with diethylnitrosamine on one of the last four (12th to 15th) gestation days.
Their incidence finally reached a rate of 95% in those animals
treated on the 15th prenatal day. The tumors in the larynx and
trachea were most frequent, and histologically squamous cell
papillomas and papillary polyps. Particularly, the incidence
of tumors in the trachea increased the later the carcinogen
was administered. A few adenocarcinomas and one squamous cell
carcinoma additionally developed in the nasal cavities. All
pulmonary tumors were bronchogenic adenomas. The mother also

developed high incidence of respiratory tract tumors (Mohr, Reznik-Schueller, Reznik, et al., 1975).

Differentiation of the Tracheal Epithelium

In the prenatal Syrian golden hamster the tracheo-bronchial rudiment separated from the embryonal esophageal duct between the 9th and 10th prenatal day. The tracheal epithelium of up to the 12th prenatal day mainly consisted of one layer of columnar cells. Thereafter, primitive luminal and basal cells first appeared, then multiplication of ciliary basal bodies began and finally ciliated and mucous progenitor cells occurred towards the 14th prenatal day (Emura, Mohr, 1975).

Ultrastructural examination of the developing tracheal epithelia revealed marked changes in both the nuclear chromatin and the endoplasmic reticulum of interphase cells. The chromatin in most of these cells on the 10th and 11th prenatal day was dispersed almost homogeneously (Fig. 1a). On the 12th prenatal day, however, condensation of chromatin (heterochromatization) occurred to a moderate degree in 20 to 30% of these cells (Fig. 1b). On the 13th prenatal day, the chromatin condensed extensively in 80 to 95% of both luminal and basal cells (Fig. 1c). Thereafter, an increasing amount of chromatin was involved with progressively stronger condensation up to the 1st postnatal day, when ciliated and mucous cells showed markedly higher degree of chromatin condensation than the basal cells.

Most of the endoplasmic reticulum cisternae in the epithelial cells of the 10th and 11th prenatal day (Fig. 2) possessed wide and short profiles with a few ribosomes attached. On the 12th prenatal day (Fig. 3), however, these cisternae became considerably elongated and narrower with more ribosomes attached. This suggests conformational change of rough endoplasmic reticulum from the primitive to the functionally competent form. Very frequent encounter of obliquely cut narrow profiles seem to indicate the endoplasmic reticulum cisternae at this stage to be tubular in shape. On the 13th prenatal (Fig. 4) and later days, more of the narrow and long cisternal profiles with many ribosomes prevailed. The obliquely cut narrow profiles became gradually rare. This suggests that the endoplasmic reticulum cisternae at these stages were expanding into flattened saccular forms. In this way the total volume of endoplasmic reticulum as well as its functional competence increased with time. A certain amount of the rudimentary endoplasmic reticulum seemed to develop from small vesicles originating in the outer nuclear membrane (Fig. 5).

The mitotic activity of the tracheal epithelial cells was highest (about 4.5%) on the 11th prenatal day, sharply decreased towards the 12th prenatal day (about 2.3%), and declined rather gradually thereafter (Fig. 6). In the meantime, the area showing more dividing cells shifted from the luminal to the basal layer of the epithelium. Interestingly, the mitotic activity went with a reverse relation to both the incidence of tracheal tumors (Table I) and the degree of epithelial differentiation.

DISCUSSION

The development of respiratory tract tumors is characteristic of the Syrian golden hamsters treated with diethylnitrosamine in their prenatal as well as postnatal life. The occurrence of susceptibility to the diethylnitrosamine carcinogenicity in the prenatal tracheal epithelia of this animal species was confined to the last four (12th to 15th) gestation days, during which period the epithelia underwent gradual differentiation. Prior to this no respiratory tract tumors can be induced. This would indicate either a metabolic insufficiency of the target cells, or the inability of these cells to respond neoplastically to the carcinogen. With progress of differentiation, the mitotic activity of the tracheal epithelia devreased and the incidence of tracheal tumors inversely increased. It is general opinion that embryonic cells possessing a high mitotic activity are particularly susceptible to the effects of carcinogens. However, our results on this point seem to indicate that the susceptibility of the prenatal tracheal epithelial cells of the Syrian golden hamster to the

transplacental carcinogenicity of diethylnitrosamine has no
direct relation to their mitotic activity; rather, it occurs
with the advance of epithelial differentiation. From the present ultrastructural examination, it is evident that the earliest phase of this differentiation resides in the conformational change of such subcellular entities as the nuclear chromatin and endoplasmic reticulum of the epithelial cells around
the 12th prenatal day.

The condensed heterochromatin, in contrast to the loosened
euchromatin, is virtually inactive in deoxyribo- and ribonucleic acid synthesis (Frenster, 1969a; Milner, 1969). The great
increase in chromatin condensation (Kernell, Bolund, Ringertz,
1971) and the final cessation of mitotic cycle before marked
hemoglobin synthesis (Holtzer, Weintraub, Mayne, et al., 1972)
have been well known in the erythroid cell differentiation.
Thus, the increasingly stronger chromatin condensaton (heterochromatization) in the differentiating tracheal epithelial
cells may cause steady decrease in their mitotic activity,
while only the basal cells with less condensed heterochromatin
retaining this activity to some extent.

The nuclear peripheral heterochromatin in the tracheal epithelia of the Syrian golden hamster was reported to be a preferential binding site for ^{3}H-benzo(a)pyrene (Harris, Kaufman,
Sporn, et al., 1973). Phytohemagglutinin (Stanley, Frenster,
Rigas, 1971), mercuric chloride (Frenster, 1969b) and cupric
chloride (Hardy, Bryan, 1975) are also reported to bind pref-
erentially the heterochromatin. In addition, the developing
tracheal epithelia of the Syrian golden hamster became first
susceptible to the transplacental effects of diethylnitrosamine around the 12th prenatal day. It is assumable, therefore,
that in these epithelia the chromatin condensation initiated
also around the same prenatal time and continued progressively
may provide similar binding sites for various carcinogens.

Differentiation of rough and smooth endoplasmic reticulum
has been mainly studied in the fetal livers of various animals
and man. In chick and some other embryonic tissues the rudimentary endoplasmic reticulum is known to develop from small
vesicles originating from the outer nuclear membrane (Birge,

Doolin, 1974). The distinct conformational change of the rough endoplasmic reticulum initiated around the 12th prenatal day in the developing tracheal epithelia of the Syrian golden hamster can be considered to morphologically indicate its differentiation into functionally competent state (Dallner, Siekevitz, Palade, 1966a,b). The endoplasmic reticulum in these prenatal tracheal epithelia was almost all rough surfaced throughout the prenatal period. The main source of the enzyme activity for drug metabolism has been attributed to the smooth endoplasmic reticulum. However, it was recently found that in the liver of fetal rats and rabbits some enzymes of mixed function oxidase system were already weakly active before the recognizable development of the smooth endoplasmic reticulum (Gillete, Stripp, 1975). Further, the activation of diethylnitrosamine into its ultimate carcinogen takes place in the trachea of adult Syrian golden hamster (Montesano, Magee, 1974). It is thus very likely that among various enzymes which would become operative in the rough endoplasmic reticulum assuming a functionally competent shape in the tracheal epithelial cells of the 12th prenatal and later days the enzymes responsible for the conversion of diethylnitrosamine into its ultimate carcinogen be included. The differentiating tracheal epithelia of the Syrian golden hamster, again, became first susceptible to the transplacental effects of diethylnitrosamine around the 12th prenatal day. In view of these, the observed prenatal age dependent susceptibility of the tracheal epithelial cells to the transplacental carcinogenicity of diethylnitrosamine may be due to the acquisition by their endoplasmic reticulum of an ability to activate diethylnitrosamine after such definite stage of ontogenesis.

Our present investigations demonstrate a valid correlation between the ultrastructural features of the developing tracheal epithelial cells and their biochemical capacity for the intracellular metabolism of diethylnitrosamine. However, with this interpretation of our results the pronounced organotropism of diethylnitrosamine remains unexplained. Further, it might be possible that the metabolic influence from the pla-

centa and the fetal liver should modify the above presumed
activation of diethylnitrosamine by the fetal tracheal tissue.

SUMMARY

Using embryonic tracheal epithelia of the Syrian golden
hamster, a question was studied whether the prenatal age dependency of the diethylnitrosamine transplacental carcinogenesis was correlated with the process of tissue differentiation.
In the transplacental carcinogenesis experiments, pregnant
Syrian golden hamsters were treated with diethylnitrosamine at
a single subcutaneous dose of 45 mg/kg body weight on one of
the 15 days of pregnancy. Normal differentiation of the epithelia was examined by light and electron microscopy. The offspring of mothers treated on one of the last four days (12th-
15th prenatal day) of pregnancy developed respiratory tract
tumors. During the same period of pregnancy both nuclear
heterochromatization and formation of rough endoplasmic reticulum were progressively prominent in normally differentiating
epithelial cells. The nuclear heterochromatization may provide
possible binding sites for various carcinogens. Also, the formation of rough endoplasmic reticulum in its functionally competent shape may indicate the appearance in this organelle of
an enzyme activity necessary for the conversion of diethylnitrosamine to its ultimate carcinogen. Thus, the present
results demonstrate a valid correlation between the transplacental carcinogenicity of diethylnitrosamine and the tissue
differentiation.

TABLE I. Respiratory Tract Tumors of Offspring on Different Prenatal Days with a Single Dose of Diethylnitrosamine and in NaCl Control Group

Treatment	Day of treatment	Nasal cavity	Larynx	Trachea	Lung	Total number of animals	Tumor bearing animals
Diethyl-nitrosamine	1-11	0	0	0	0	174	0
	12	1	2	1	0	10	4
	13	1	5	2	0	20	8
	14	0	8	8	1	24	17
	15	3	5	10	3	20	19
NaCl	15	0	0	0	0	36	0

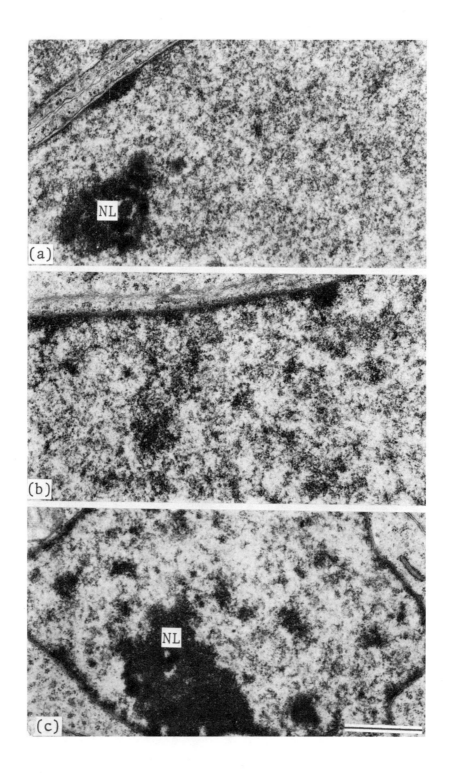

FIG. 1. Electron micrographs showing various degrees of nuclear chromatin
condensation in the differentiating tracheal epithelial cells on the 11th
(a), 12th (b), and 13th (c) prenatal days; (c) shows the nucleus of a basal
cell. The fine granular structures, except those in the nucleoli, represent the crosscut profiles of chromatin fibrils. The chromatin fibrils in
(a) are dispersed uniformly, while in (b) and (c) they are coming together
more closely to form localized clumps. The condensation is more extensive
in (c) than in (b). Note that the areas free from the chromatin fibrils
(light areas in the picture) are increasingly larger with the progression
of developmental day. NL, nucleolus. X 21,000.

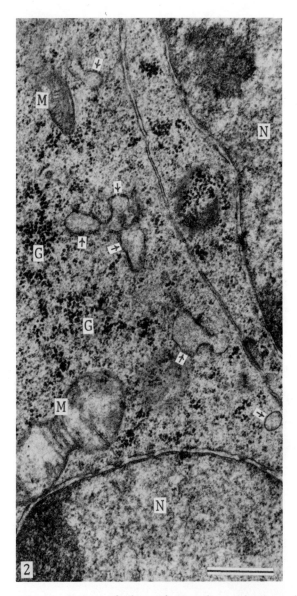

FIG. 2. Conformational change of the endoplasmic reticulum cisternae in
cells of the developing tracheal epithelia of the Syrian golden hamster.
G, glycogen granules; N, nucleus; NL, nucleolus; M, mitochondrion;
V, cytoplasmic vesicle. X 18,000. A cell on the 11th prenatal day, in
which wide and short cisternal profiles (arrows) are prominent. Relatively
few ribosomes are attached.

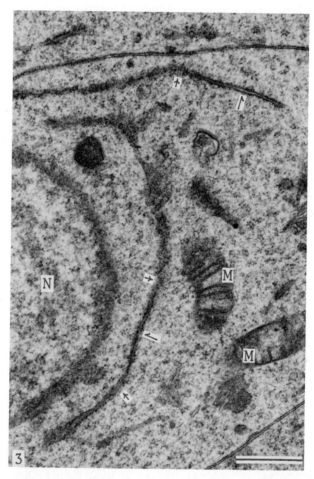

FIG. 3. Conformational change of the endoplasmic reticulum cisternae in cells of the developing tracheal epithelia of the Syrian golden hamster. G, glycogen granules; N, nucleus; NL, nucleolus; M, mitochondrion; V, cytoplasmic vesicle. X 18,000. A representative cell of the 12th pre-natal day. Some cisternae (long arrows) show considerably long and narrow profiles cut obliquely at places (short arrows).

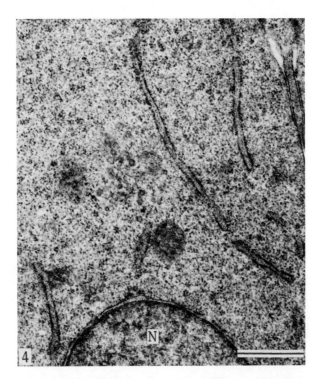

FIG. 4. Conformational change of the endoplasmic reticulum cisternae in
cells of the developing tracheal epithelia of the Syrian golden hamster.
G, glycogen granules; N, nucleus; NL, nucleolus; M, mitochondrion;
V, cytoplasmic vesicle. X 18,000. A cell on the 13th prenatal day.

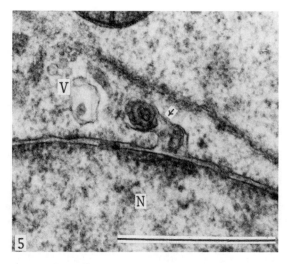

FIG. 5. A vesicle and a bleb (arrow) formed from the outer nuclear
membrane in a cell of the developing epithelium of Syrian golden hamster
trachea on the 12th prenatal day. V, cytoplasmic vesicle. X 43,000.

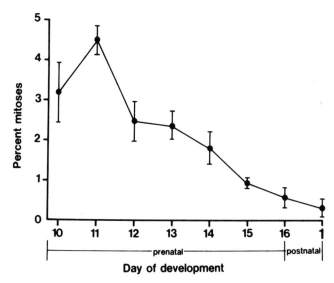

FIG. 6. Change of the mitotic activity in developing tracheal epithelia
of the Syrian golden hamster expressed in percent of mitoses. Cells of
more than 2,000 were counted along the whole length of sections of both
dorsal and ventral side epithelia. Determinations were made for at least
6 animals from 4 different litters on each developmental day except for
the 1st postnatal day, for which they were made on 4 animals from 2 litters. Each point represents a mean of the determinations. Vertical lines
indicate the range of confidence limits at 95% coefficient.

REFERENCES

1. Birge, W.J., and Doolin, P.F. The Ultrastructural Differentiation Of The Endoplasmic Reticulum In Choroidal Epithelial Cells Of The Chick Embryo. Tissue Cell, 6:335-360, 1974.

2. Dallner, G., Siekevitz, P., and Palade, G.E. Biogenesis Of Endoplasmic Reticulum Membranes. I. Structural And Chemical Differentiation In Developing Rat Hepatocyte. J. Cell Biol., 30:73-96, 1966a.

3. Dallner, G., Siekevitz, P., and Palade, G.E. Biogenesis Of Endoplasmic Reticulum Membranes. II. Synthesis Of Constitutive Microsomal Enzymes In Developing Rat Hepatocyte. J. Cell Biol., 30:97-117, 1966b.

4. Emura, M., and Mohr, U. Morphological Studies On The Development Of Tracheal Epithelium In The Syrian Golden Hamster. I. Light Microscopy. Z. Versuchstierk., 17:14-26, 1975.

5. Frenster, J.H. Biochemistry And Molecular Biophysics Of Heterochromatin And Euchromatin. In: Handbook Of Molecular Cytology. Frontiers of Biology. Ed.: A. Lima-De-Faria. North-Holland, Pub. Co., Amsterdam, 15:251-276, 1969a.

6. Frenster, J.H. Ultrastructural Effects Of Mercuric Chloride On Nuclear Heterochromatin Within Human Lymphocytes. Abstr. J. Cell Biol., 43:39-40, 1969b.

7. Gillete, J.R., and Stripp, B. Pre- And Postnatal Enzyme Capacity For Drug Metabolite Production. Fed. Proc., 34: 172-178, 1975.

8. Hardy, K.J., and Bryan, S.E. Localization And Uptake Of Copper Into Chromatin. Toxicol. Appl. Pharmacol., 33:62-69, 1975.

9. Harris, C.C., Kaufman, D.G., Sporn, M.B., Boren, H., Jackson, F., Smith, J.M., Pauley, J., Dedick, P., and Saffiotti, U. Localization Of Benzo(a)pyrene-^{3}H And Alterations In Nuclear Chromatin Caused By Benzo(a)pyrene-Ferric Oxide In The Hamster Respiratory Epithelium. Cancer Res., 33:2842-2848, 1973.

10. Holtzer, H., Weintraub, H., Mayne, R., and Mochan, B. The Cell Cycle, Cell Lineages, And Cell Differentiation. In: Current Topics in Developmental Biology. Ed.: A.A. Moscona, and Alberto Monroy. Academic Press, Inc., London, 7:229-256, 1972.

11. Kernell, A.M., Bolund, L., and Ringertz, N.R. Chromatin Changes During Erythropoiesis. Exptl. Cell Res., 65:1-6, 1971.

12. Milner, G.R. Nuclear Morphology And The Ultrastructural Localization Of Deoxyribonucleic Acid Synthesis During Interphase. J. Cell Sci., 4:569-582, 1969.

13. Mohr, U., Althoff, J., and Wrba, H. Diaplacentare Wirkung Des Carcinogens Diaethylnitrosamin Beim Goldhamster. Z. Krebsforsch., 66:536-540, 1965.

14. Mohr, U., Althoff, J., and Authaler, A. Diaplacental Effect Of The Carcinogen Diethylnitrosamine In The Golden Hamster. Cancer Res., 26:2349-2352, 1966.

15. Mohr, U. Effects Of Diethylnitrosamine On Fetal And Suckling Syrian Golden Hamsters. In: Transplacental Carcinogenesis. Ed.: L. Tomatis and U. Mohr. IARC Scientific Pub., 4:65-70, 1973.
16. Mohr, U., Reznik-Schueller, H., Reznik, G., and Hilfrich, J. Transplacental Effects Of Diethylnitrosamine In Syrian Hamsters As Related To Different Days Of Administration During Pregnancy. J. Natl. Cancer Inst., 55:681-683, 1975.
17. Montesano, R., and Magee, P.N. Comparative Metabolism In Vitro Of Nitrosamines In Various Animal Species Including Man. In: Chemical Carcinogenesis Essays. Ed.: R. Montesano and L. Tomatis. IARC Scientific Pub., 10:39-56, 1974.
18. Stanley, D.A., Frenster, J.H., and Rigas, D.A. Localization Of H³-Phytohemagglutinin Within Human Lymphocytes And Monocytes. Proceedings of the Fourth Annual Leucocyte Culture Conference. Ed.: O.R. McIntyre. Appleton-Century-Crofts, New York, 4:1-9, 1971.

A NEW ANIMAL MODEL FOR THE DIRECT INDUCTION OF NEOPLASMS DURING EMBRYONIC AND FETAL DEVELOPMENT

William Jurgelski, Jr., Ph.D., M.D., Pearlie M. Hudson, B.S., Ronnie L. Dunn, and Hans L. Falk, Ph.D.

National Institute of Environmental Health Sciences
Research Triangle Park, North Carolina

INTRODUCTION

In experiments conducted over the past 30 years (1-8), transplacental exposure of traditional eutherian laboratory animals to a variety of carcinogens has failed to reproduce the wide spectrum of neoplasms theoretically to be expected when carcinogenesis is initiated in actively differentiating tissues. With rare exceptions transplacentally induced tumors in the usual laboratory animals do not differ either in latency or morphology from tumors induced during adulthood in the same species and they are analogous to only a narrow portion of the spectrum of neoplasms observed in the human adult from the perinatal period to senility (2-4,6,7). In particular, the diversity of human tumor types and behavior, ranging from tumors of infancy and childhood (embryonal forms) with short latencies and occasional spontaneous regression, to neoplasms of adult life with varying degrees of malignancy and with latencies often approximating the life span of the host, has not been approached experimentally by the transplacental route. Conditions which prevent the carcinogen from reaching the fetus in full concentration or activity, such as short biological half life and/or placental and maternal alteration, may account in part for this failure. Additional considerations especially for those neoplasms susceptible to endocrine inhibition and immunological suppression, may be the short interval, in most eutherian laboratory mammals and particularly in rodents, between the completion of organogenesis and the functional maturation of the reproductive and lymphoid systems. In such species, the growth of a transplacentally induced tumor would have to be explosive to achieve detectable size before onset of endogenous sex hormone secretion and lymphoid activity (6). While the above factors may be involved to varying degrees in determining the tumor types that are induced by a given carcinogen in a particular species or strain, genetic factors may in fact play the dominant role (9).

The postnatal completion of embryonic and fetal development in the opossum (Didelphis virginiana Kerr) suggested to us that this species might offer certain advantages over the typical eutherian fetus in utero for experimental oncogenesis and especially for the induction of embryonal tumors (10, 11). At birth after a 13 day ± 6 hr gestation (12), the opossum represents an amalgam of fetal and embryonic tissue; while determination is largely complete, differentiation has only progressed to the level necessary for extrauterine survival (13). The components of the endocrine system are still in the anlage state (13), the gonads are just beginning to differentiate (14), the lymphoid system is largely unformed (15), and there is no immunologic competence (16-18). Thus, the first 2 1/2 months of postnatal development in the opossum is roughly equivalent to the last 7-8 months of intrauterine development in the human and to the final 8-9 days of gestation in the typical rodent (13-18). During this period, the young opossum is involuntarily attached to the maternal teat within the marsupium or pouch, where maternal influence is limited to constituents of maternal milk (19) and the pouch environment (20). Accordingly, there is the opportunity in the opossum, beginning in some tissues at the anlage state, to expose developing embryonic and fetal tissue to carcinogens (a) in the absence of placental interference, (b) under minimal maternal influence (10,11), (c) in the absence of full endocrine and immunologic function at the target tissue level and (d) without toxicity to the mother.

Furthermore, the opossum matures slowly in relation to its short life span (about 2 1/2 years) and relatively small body size (about 1.5 to 3 kg). For example, maturation of the lymphoid system requires about 60 days post partum (15,18) and full sexual development is not attained for at least nine months after birth (12). Demonstrated immunologic consequences of the lymphoid maturation rate in the opossum are the absence of circulating antibody production before 7 days of age (18), an inability to reject skin allografts prior to 12 days of age (16), and an acquired tolerance to soluble and particulate antigens administered earlier than 2 weeks of age (17). There is, thus, a longer period in the opossum than in the typical eutherian laboratory mammal for the oncogenic process to proceed prior to full functional maturation of several factors which may influence or inhibit the oncogenic influence.

In an initial experiment to explore the opossum's susceptibility to cancer induction early in postnatal development, opossums of known age were exposed orally to ethyl nitrosourea (ENU) at several stages of post partum development. Embryonal tumors induced in this study have been described in a preliminary report (11), and the relationship between susceptibility to embryonal tumor induction and the stage of morphologic maturation of the presumed target tissues has been considered for four of these neoplasms (21). In this paper, we present a preliminary survey of the entire spectrum of neoplasms induced postnatally with ENU in the opossum in order to demonstrate the potential of the opossum model for carcinogenesis.

PROCEDURES AND MATERIAL USED

In two separate experiments performed in successive years, 532 opossums from 72 litters bred in captivity (22-24) and obtained within 17 hours of birth (24) were divided by litter into ten groups according to age; (<1 day old and 1, 2, 3, 4, 6, 8, 10, 12, and 16 weeks of age). In the first experiment, animals were orally exposed (22,25) to approximately (22,25) 100 mg/kg ethyl nitrosourea (ENU) (26) as a single dose. In the second study, the same total oral dose of ENU was administered in increments of 25 mg/kg each given every other day. The ENU was administered within one hour of solution in pH 4.0 saline phosphate buffer. One or two animals in each litter were controls given saline phosphate buffer only. Opossums with visible tumors were killed at various ages as determined by animal and tumor condition. Animals without grossly manifest tumors were killed either when moribund or two years after drug administration.

RESULTS

A spectrum of mesenchymal and epithelial neoplasms comprising 43 different tumors distributed among 21 different sites developed in the ENU treated opossums. Fifty-four percent of the treated opossums had one or more primary neoplasms. Seventy-three percent of the tumor bearing animals

had more than one primary neoplasm. Neoplasms (small nephroblastomas) were
found in two control animals.

Seven types of embryonal tumors were induced in six different sites
(Table I). These tumors were closely analagous in morphology and biology
to their counterparts in the human. With the exception of the ameloblastoma, (Fig. 5), one of two odontogenic tumors, a correlation was apparent
to a varying degree between susceptibility to the embryonal tumors and the
state of morphologic maturation of the presumed target tissues (21). Three
of these neoplasms, an intraocular neoplasm (teratoid medulloepithelioma)
(Fig. 1), a tumor of the neuron (ganglioglioma) (Fig. 2), and a tumor of
the jaw (odontogenic myxoma) (Fig. 3) are of interest because they have not
to our knowledge been previously induced experimentally. These neoplasms
as well as the embryonal tumor of the kidney (nephroblastoma) (Fig. 4) and
a second type of embryonal jaw tumor (ameloblastoma) (Fig. 5) were notable
for their morphologic similarity to analagous human cancers.

One teratoma and several types of hamartomas and malformations
developed in opossums given ENU prior to three weeks post partum (Table
II). These lesions were frequently present in tumor bearing animals. A
single teratoma of the neck was found in an animal given ENU at birth.
Two types of hamartomas were found. Hemangiomas were present in 11 different sites and osteomas were seen in 3 different skeletal locations. Malformations in the form of cysts of the kidney and of hypoplasia of the
genetalia were also found in high incidence in the ENU treated opossums.

In the kidney an embryonal neoplasm was occasionally present at the
same site as a malformation. Thus, in two animals given ENU every other
day from day 7 to 13, neoplastic and teratologic changes were found in the
same kidney. Such a coincidence of tumor and malformation has not been
previously reported under experimental conditions despite its occasional
occurrence in the human (27).

Thirty-six different tumors (12 benign and 24 malignant types) analogous in varying degrees to tumors which normally appear during adult life
in man were induced in 20 different sites (Table III). The incidence of
most of these tumors was too low to determine whether there was a correlation between susceptibility and age of the host at time of tumors induction.
However, a number of the neoplasms with high incidence such as the benign
tumors of the thyroid, liver, stomach, and the malignant tumors of the jaw,
liver, and lung were induced throughout the 16 week period of exposure.
Several of the "adult type" tumors were of particular interest because of

their malignancy. Thus, the adenocarcinoma of the lung (Fig. 6), the hepatocellular carcinoma of the liver (Fig. 7), the cholangiocarcinoma of the
bile ducts (Fig. 8), the melanoma of the skin, and the adenocarcinoma of
the large and small intestines metastasized to various sites. The pulmonary adenocarcinoma, and the melanoma of the skin showed the most widespread metastases. A granulocytic leukemia was also highly malignant with
massive infiltrates of tumor cells in liver, lymph nodes, kidney, and lung.

"Adult type" tumors of special interest because of their rarity in
eutherian laboratory species or because their target sites appear resistant
to neoplastic transformation in these species, were the basal cell carcinoma of the skin (1 case) (Fig. 9), the cystadenocarcinoma of the liver
(4 cases) (Fig. 10), the ductal adenoma of the pancreas (3 cases) (Fig. 11),
the adenocarcinoma of the prostate (2 cases) (Fig. 12), and the cutaneous
papilloma (35 cases).

DISCUSSION

The induction of embryonal tumors in the opossum may be explained in
part by the unique opportunity in this marsupial for the direct exposure of
slowly maturing fetal and embryonic tissue to carcinogens in the absence of
interference attributable, in the eutherian mammal, to the mother, the
placenta, and the fetoplacental unit. A more important factor facilitating
the induction of such tumors in the opossum may be the slow postnatal
maturation characteristic of the marsupial. In particular, the late
development of sexual and lymphoid function in the opossum may provide a
longer period than that in the typical eutherian laboratory mammal for the
initiation and development of the oncogenic process in the absence of inhibition often associated with full endocrine and immunologic function. The
possibility that the opossum has a specific innate susceptibility either to
the types of tumors induced or to the carcinogen or to both must also be
considered. A number of spontaneous neoplasms have been reported in the
opossum, including renal adenoma (28), carcinoma of urinary bladder (29),
adenocarcinoma of the mammary gland (28), osteosarcoma of the skull and
ribs (28), lymphosarcoma (30), adenocarcinoma of the lungs (30), bronchial
papillary adenomas (31,32), multiple papillary adenomas of the urinary
bladder (32), squamous cell carcinoma (33), cutaneous papilloma (34), and
carcinosarcoma of the oral cavity (35). Sarcomas with various degrees of
differentiation as well as melanomas have been induced in opossums

approximately 19 days old with methyl-cholanthrene given subcutaneously (36). While these data are inadequate to support a genetic predisposition of the opossum to the tumors induced by ENU, a hereditary predisposition to certain types of neoplasms in other species including man (9,37-49) and well established species and strain specific responses to carcinogens suggest such a possibility. Pertinent to any genetic explanation for the susceptibility of the opossum to the tumors reported may be a recent taxonomic study which shows that the opossum is karyotypically, and possibly in other ways as well, an aberrant form by comparison to other marsupials (50). Perhaps also relevant to any explanation for the opossums unique susceptibility to certain tumors like those in man, particularly embryonal neoplasms, are experiments which show that the order of effectiveness of three alkylating agents in inducing DNA repair in opossum lymphocytes *in vitro* is comparable to that in human lymphocytes (51).

Our results indicate that the opossum early in postnatal life is a useful model for the induction and characterization of certain of the major dysontogenetic neoplasms which have been difficult or impossible to reproduce in the traditional laboratory species. The induction of one of the embryonal tumors, the teratoid medulloepithelioma, in an intraocular site, is of particular interest because intraocular tumors have not previously been reported under experimental conditions in any species following systemic exposure to a carcinogen. The opossum would also appear to have potential as an animal model for several tumors of adult life, particularly for malignant neoplasms of lung, liver, intestine, and skin and possibly of pancreas and prostate as well.

The opossum model permits developing embryonic and fetal tissue to be exposed directly to carcinogens in the absence of indirect effects resulting from reactions, which, *in utero* may occur between the carcinogen and the interposed maternal and placental tissues. Accordingly, the model may be especially useful in exploring the relationships between susceptibility to tumor induction and differentiation of the target tissue under conditions where extra-fetal activation or inactivation or a short biological half life of the carcinogen may obscure or prevent the response of the target tissue per se (21). The opossum model may also be of value in clarifying the apparent interrelationship of carcinogenesis, teratogenesis, and mutagenesis *in vivo* since it permits direct carcinogen induced teratologic or mutagenic changes to be distinguished from identical lesions which may be the indirect result, under in utero conditions, of physical and/or physiologic reactions between the carcinogen and the maternal and/or fetoplacental units.

The experiments reported here utilized a single chemical carcinogen administered orally in single or multiple doses to opossums at several different ages. A higher yield for specific tumor types and perhaps for the associated malformations as well may reasonably be anticipated with establishment of the optimum combination of carcinogen, dosage, route, treatment schedule and age. In view of the heterogenous nature of the opossums currently available to the laboratory (22), selection and breeding for susceptibility to specific tumors would probably also offer considerable potential.

Chemical induction in the opossum, at stages of development comparable to in utero stages in man and other eutherian species, of a broad spectrum of tumors with a wide range of latencies and malignancies, supports the emerging concept that in utero exposure to carcinogens in humans may account for a greater proportion of tumors than previously believed. This concept is fueled by experimental evidence that transplacental exposure to a carcinogen tends to enhance the effect of subsequent exposures during postnatal life to the same or some other carcinogen (52) and by the recent discovery of "adult type" neoplasms (clear cell adenocarcinomas) in the vaginas of adolescent girls born to mothers given diethylstilbestrol during pregnancy (53).

SUMMARY

Opossums orally exposed to 100 mg/kg of ethyl nitrosourea at stages of development from birth to 16 weeks of age developed a spectrum of both epithelial and mesenchymal embryonal and "adult type" neoplasms with diverse latencies and a range of malignancies. Several of the induced tumors have not previously been induced in laboratory species by systemic administration of a carcinogen. The opossum model may be of special value in experimental perinatal carcinogenesis under conditions where extra-fetal activation or inactivation or a short biological half life of the carcinogen may obscure or prevent the response of the target organ.

TABLE I. Embryonal Neoplasms Induced Postnatally in the Developing Opossum with Ethyl Nitrosourea

Site	Neoplasm	Age at ENU Treatment in Days Postpartum	Tumor Incidence*	%
Eye	Teratoid Medulloepithelioma	7-28	5/166	3%
Kidney	Nephroblastoma[1,2]	<1-56	66/245	27%
Liver	Hepatoblastoma	<1	1/35	3%
Brain	Ganglioglioma	<1-56	12/245	5%
Muscle	Rhabdomyosarcoma[3]	<1-42	1/226	.5%
Jaw	Ameloblastoma	7-84	15/247	6%
	Myxoma	<1-42	2/226	1%

[1]Metastatic to liver and lymph nodes.

[2]Small nephroblastomas were found in two control animals.

[3]Metastatic to lung, liver, adrenal, and lymph nodes.

*Number of tumor bearing opossums
 Number of susceptible opossums at risk

TABLE II. Teratomas, Hamartomas and Malformations Induced Postnatally
in the Developing Opossum with Ethyl Nitrosourea

Lesion	Site	Age at ENU Treatment in Days Postpartum	Incidence*	%
Teratoma	Neck	<1	1/35	3%
Hamartoma				
Hemangioma	Liver	<1-7	2/71	3%
	Lung	7	1/53	2%
	Spleen	<1	1/35	3%
	Brain	<1-14	3/140	2%
	Skin	<1-56	14/245	6%
	Left Atrium	<1-56	10/245	4%
	Jaw	7-42	3/196	2%
	Epididymis	7-21	5/68	7%
	Glans, Penis	7	1/24	4%
	Stomach	56	1/19	5%
	Small Intestine	<1	1/35	3%
Osteoma	Mandible	7-70	14/233	6%
	Calvarium	14	1/57	2%
	Vertebral Column	<1-42	2/226	1%
Malformations				
Cysts	Kidney	<1-14	10/140	7%
Hypoplasia	Kidney	<1-14	2/140	1%
	Female Genitalia	<1-28	80/110	73%
	Male Genitalia	<1-28	80/110	73%

*Number of tumor bearing opossums
 Number of susceptible opossums at risk

TABLE III. "Adult Type" Neoplasms Induced Postnatally in the Developing Opossum with Ethyl Nitrosourea

Site	Neoplasm	Age at ENU Treatment in Days Postpartum	Tumor Incidence*	%
Thyroid	Colloid Nodule	<1-84	35/277	13%
	Follicular Adenoma	<1-56	3/245	1%
Lung	Adenoma	<1-112	78/291	27%
	Adenocarcinoma[1]	<1-112	7/291	2%
	Fibrosarcoma	42	1/30	3%
Liver	Bile Duct Adenoma[2]	<1-70	12/263	5%
	Cholangiocarcinoma[2]	<1-112	22/291	8%
	Hepatocellular Carcinoma[2]	7-84	3/247	1%
	Cystadenocarcinoma	<1-84	4/277	1%
Kidney	Renal Cell Carcinoma	<1-84	4/277	1%
Stomach	Gastric Polyp[3]	<1-56	21/245	9%
	Adenocarcinoma	56	1/19	5%
	Fibrous Histiocytoma	56	1/19	5%
Small Intestine	Adenocarcinoma[3]	<1	1/35	3%
Brain	Malignant Glioma	<1-7	2/71	3%
Pituitary	Adenoma	<1-84	2/277	1%
	Craniopharangioma	<1	1/35	1%
Colon	Adenocarcinoma	42-70	2/67	3%
Pancreas	Islet Cell Adenoma	7-56	4/210	2%
	Duct Adenoma	42	1/30	3%
Ovary	Granulosa Cell Tumor	7	1/29	3%

[1]Metastatic to liver, lymph nodes, kidney, tongue, heart, brain, muscle, and spleen.

[2]Metastatic to lymph nodes and kidney.

[3]Metastatic to liver

*Number of tumor bearing opossums
Number of susceptible opossums at risk

TABLE III. "Adult Type" Neoplasms Induced Postnatally in the Developing
Opossum with Ethyl Nitrosourea (Cont'd)

Site	Neoplasm	Age at ENU Treatment in Days Postpartum	Incidence*	%
Bladder	Adenocarcinoma	7	1/53	2%
Prostate	Adenoma	7-14	2/58	3%
	Adenocarcinoma	7	1/24	4%
Jaw	Squamous Cell Carcinoma	14-84	21/194	11%
	Fibrosarcoma	42-84	3/81	4%
Lymph Node	Lymphoma[1]	7-14	2/110	2%
Skin	Melanoma[3]	<1-7	3/71	4%
	Basal Cell Carcinoma	<1	1/35	3%
	Squamous Cell Carcinoma	<1	2/35	6%
	Cylindroma	<1	1/35	3%
	Cutaneous Papilloma	<1-112	35/291	12%
	Lipoma	7-112	4/261	2%
Bone	Chondrosarcoma	7-42	2/196	1%
Pinna	Fibrosarcoma	7-14	2/110	2%
Blood	Granulocytic Leukemia[2]	7-84	13/247	5%

[1]Neoplastic infiltrate in kidney.

[2]Neoplastic infiltrate in liver, kidney, lungs, and lymph nodes.

[3]Metastatic to brain and bone marrow.

*Number of tumor bearing opossums
 Number of susceptible opossums at risk

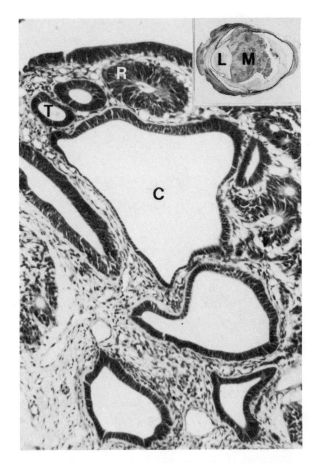

FIG. 1. Intraocular teratoid medulloepithelioma: C, cyst; T, tubule;
R, rosette, Hematoxylin & Eosin. H&E x170. Inset: Section of calotte
of an opossum eye containing a teratoid medulloepithelioma: M, tumor;
L, lens; H&E X 2.2.

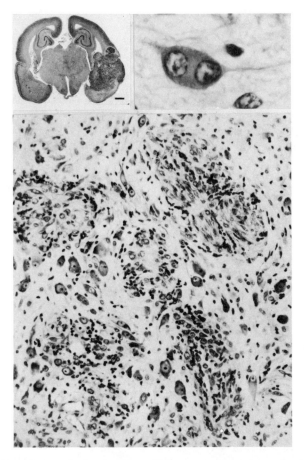

FIG. 2. Ganglioglioma of the brain. The tumor is composed of neoplastic neurons showing a spectrum of development H&E x 160. Inset upper left: low power appearance of a cross section of an opossum brain containing a ganglioglioma. Scale bar = 1 cm. Inset upper, right: binucleate neoplastic neuron from the ganglioglioma shown in Fig. 2. H&E x860.

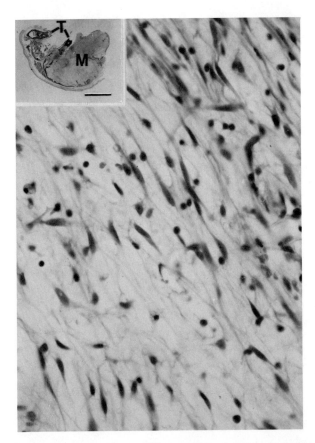

FIG. 3. Myxoma of the jaw. The tumor is composed of stellate cells in a mucinous matrix. H&E x400. Inset: Low power appearance of a cross section of a mandible containing a myxoma. T, teeth; M, tumor. H&E. Scale bar = 1 cm.

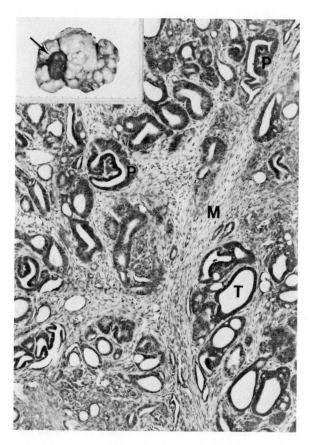

FIG. 4. Nephroblastoma. M, mesenchyme, T, neoplastic tubules; P, pseudo-
glomerulus. Inset: gross appearance of a nephroblastoma; arrow, kidney.
H&E x85. Scale division = 1 mm.

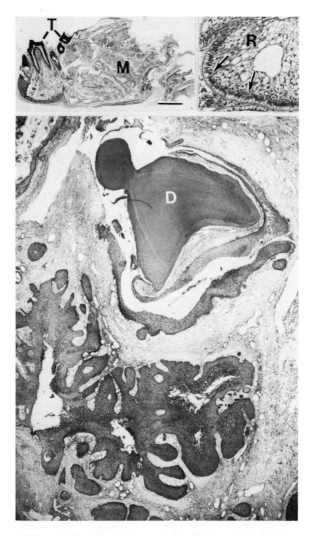

FIG. 5. Odontogenic ameloblastoma. The tumor is composed of epithelial
elements with a resemblance to the internal dental epithelium and the
spindle cells of the dental lamina. Dentine, D, is being formed. H&E x33.
Inset upper left: low power appearance of a longitudinal section through
a mandible containing an ameloblastoma, T, teeth; M, tumor H&E scale bar
= 1 cm. Inset upper right: high power appearance of the ameloblastoma.
R, stellate reticulum; arrows, palasade cells. H&E x90.

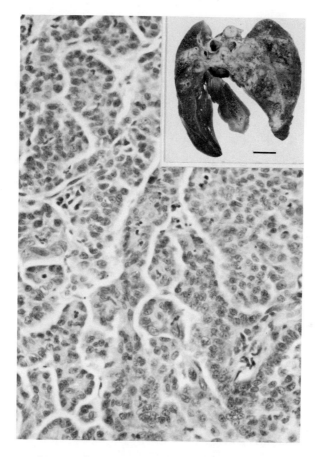

FIG. 6.   Adenocarcinoma of the lung with neoplastic cells in glandlike
configurations. H&E x100. Inset: gross appearance of the tumor in
FIG. 6.   Scale bar = 1 cm.

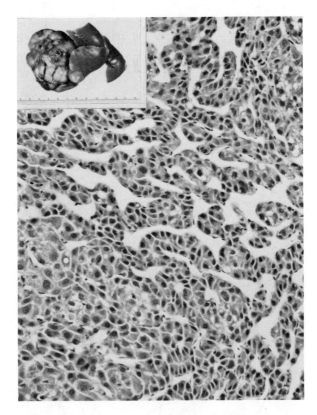

FIG. 7. Hepatocellular carcinoma composed of neoplastic cells in a
trabecular pattern. H&E X105. Inset: Gross appearance of the tumor
shown in FIG. 7. Scale division = 1 mm.

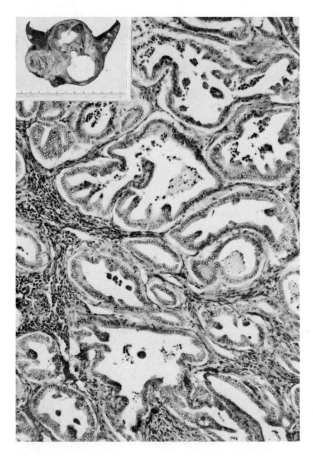

FIG. 8. Cholangiocarcinoma of the liver. The tumor cells form large cysts and tubules. H&E x100. Inset: Gross appearance of a section through a liver largely replaced by a cholangiocarcinoma. Scale division = 1 mm.

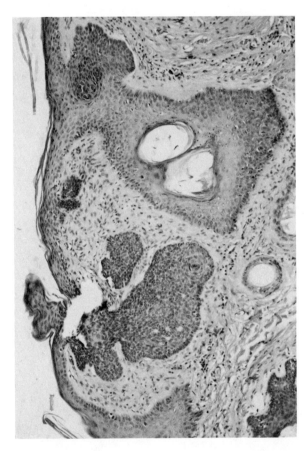

FIG. 9. Basal cell carcinoma of the skin showing keratocystic differentiation. H&E x44.

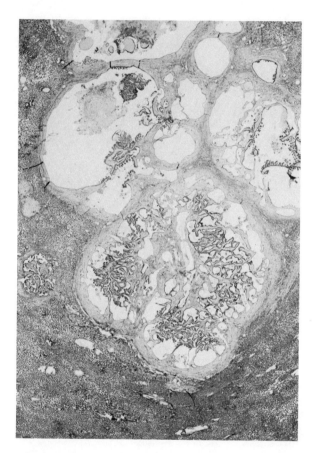

FIG. 10. Cyst adenocarcinoma of the liver. Large cysts containing complex
papillary formations are present. H&E x11.5.

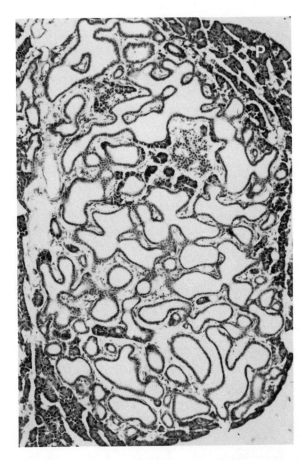

FIG. 11. Ductal adenoma of the pancreas. P, normal pancreatic acini. H&E x100.

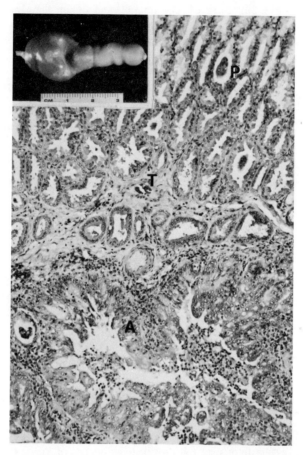

FIG. 12. Adenocarcinoma of the prostate. P, normal prostate, T, transition zone, A, adenocarcinoma. H&E x100. Inset: Gross appearance of an opossum prostate gland containing an adenocarcinoma. Scale division = 1 mm.

REFERENCES

1. Larsen, C. D. Pulmonary Tumor Induction by Transplacental Exposure to Urethane. J. Natl. Cancer Inst., 8: 63-69, 1947.

2. Vesselinovitch, S. D., and Mihailovick, N. The Development of Neurogenic Neoplasms, Embryonal Kidney Tumors, Harderian Gland Adenomas, Anitschkow Cell Sarcomas of the Heart, and Other Neoplams in Urethane-Treated Newborn Rats. Cancer Res., 28: 888-897, 1968.

3. Della Porta, G., and Terracini, B. Chemical Carcinogenesis in Infant Animals. Progr. Exp. Tumor Res., 11: 334-353, 1969.

4. Toth, B. A Critical Review of Experiments in Chemical Carcinogenesis Using Newborn Animals. Cancer Res., 28: 727-738, 1968.

5. Druckrey, H. Specific Carcinogenic and Teratogenic Effects of "Indirect" Alkylating Methyl and Ethyl Compounds and Their Dependency on Stages of Ontogenic Developments. Xenobiotica, 3: 271-303, 1973.

6. Rice, J. M. An Overview of Transplacental Carcinogenesis. Teratology, 8: 113-125, 1973.

7. Transplacental Carcinogenesis (Tomatis, L., and Mohr, V., eds.) IARC Scientific Publication No. 4. Lyon, Internat. Agency for Res. in Cancer, WHO, 181 pp., 1973.

8. Koestner, A. Transplacental Carcinogenesis. In Proc. 10th Canadian Cancer Research Conference, Toronto Press, pp. 65-82, 1974.

9. Schlumberger, H. G. Tumors Characteristic for Certain Animal Species, A Review. Cancer Res., 17: 823-832, 1957.

10. Jurgelski, W., Jr., Hudson, P. M., Falk, H. L., and Kotin, P. Ethylnitrosourea Carcinogenesis in the Neonatal Marsupial (Didelphys Marsupialis Virginiana Kerr) - A New Model for Oncogenesis. Abstr. Proc. Amer. Assoc. Cancer Res., 13: 93, 1972.

11. Jurgelski, W., Jr., Hudson, P. M., Falk, H. L., and Kotin, P. Embryonal Neoplasms in the Opossum: A New Model for Solid Tumors of Infancy and Childhood. Science, 193: 328, 1976.

12. Reynolds, H. D. Studies on Reproduction in the Opossum (Didelphis virginiana). Univ. Calif. Publ. Zool., 52: 223-284, 1952.

13. McCrady, E., Jr. The Embryology of the Opossum. Amer. Anat. Mem., No. 16, Philadelphia, Wistar Instit. Anat. Biol., 233 pp., 1938.

14. Burns, R. K. Hormones Versus Constitution Factors in the Growth of Embryonic Sex Primordia in the Opossum. Amer. J. Anat., 98: 35-67, 1956.

15. Block, M. The Blood Forming Tissues and Blood of the Newborn Opossum (<u>Didelphys</u> <u>virginiana</u>) I. Normal Development Through About the One Hundredth Day of Life. Ergeb. Anat. Entwicklungsgesch., <u>37</u>: 237-366, 1964.

16. La Plante, E. S., Burrell, R. G., and Watne, A. L. Skin Allograft Studies in the Pouch Young of the Opossum. Transplantation, <u>7</u>: 67-72, 1969.

17. Major, P. C. and Burrell, R. Induction of Acquired Tolerance in Neonatal Opossums. J. Immunol., <u>106</u>: 1690-1691, 1971.

18. Rowlands, D. T., Jr., Blakeslee, D., and Lin, H. The Early Immune Response and Immunoglobulins of Opossum Embryos. J. Immunol. <u>108</u>: 941-946, 1972.

19. Bergman, H. C. and Housley, C. Chemical Analyses of American Opossum Milk. Comp. Biochem. Physiol., <u>25</u>: 213-218, 1968.

20. Farber, J. P., and Honsley, C. The Pouch Gas of the Virginiana Opossum (<u>Didelphis</u> <u>virginiana</u>) Resp. Physiol <u>11</u>: 335-345, 1971.

21. Jurgelski, W., Jr., Hudson, P. M., and Falk, H. L. Tissue Differentiation and Susceptibility to Embryonal Tumor Induction by Ethylnitrosourea in the Opossum. Proc. of the Conf. on Perinatal Carcinogenesis. Rice, J. M., ed.) U. S. Gov. Printing Office (In press).

22. Jurgelski, W., Jr. The opossum (<u>Didelphis</u> <u>virginiana</u> <u>Kerr</u>) as a Biomedical Model. I. Research Perspective, Husbandry, and Laboratory Technics. Lab. Anim. Sci., <u>24</u>: 375-403, 1974.

23. Jurgelski, W., Jr., Forsythe, W., Dahl, D., Thomas, L. D., Moore, J. A., Kotin, P., Falk, H. L., and Vogel, F. S. The Opossum (<u>Didelphis</u> <u>virginiana</u> <u>Kerr</u>) as a Biomedical Model. II. Breeding the Opossum in Captivity: Facility Design. Lab. Anim. Sci., <u>24</u>: 404-412, 1974.

24. Jurgelski, W., Jr., and Porter, M. E. The Opossum (<u>Didelphis</u> <u>virginiana</u> <u>Kerr</u>) as a Biomedical Model. III. Breeding the Opossum in Captivity: Methods. Lab. Anim. Sci., <u>24</u>: 412-425, 1974.

25. Jurgelski, W., Jr. A Method for Administering Test Materials to the Newborn Opossum. Lab. Anim. Sci., <u>21</u>: 748-751, 1971.

26. Schuchardt, GMBH and Co., Chemische Fabric, Munich, Germany.

27. Teter, J., and Boczkowski, K. Occurrence of Tumors in Dysgenetic Gonads. Cancer, <u>20</u>: 1301-1310, 1967.

28. Fox, H. Disease in Captive Wild Mammals and Birds. J. B. Lippincott Co., Philadelphia, Pa., 1923.

29. Fox, H. Subjects of Pathological Interest. Report Penrose Lab. Mus. Comp. Path. Zool. Soc., Philadelphia, Pa., 16-22, 1933.

30. Lombard, L. S., and Witte, E. J. Frequency and Types of Tumors in Mammals and Birds of the Philadelphia Zoological Garden. Cancer Res., 19: 127-141, 1959.

31. Sherwood, B. F., Rowlands, D. T., and Hackel, D. B. Pulmonary Adenomatosis in Opossums Didelphis virginiana J. Amer. Vet. Med. Assoc., 155: 1102-1107, 1969.

32. Sherwood, B. F., Rowlands, D. T., Hackel, D. B., and Le May, J. C. The Opossum Didelphis virginiana as a Laboratory Animal. Lab. Animal Care., 19: 494-499, 1969.

33. Synder, R. L., and Ratcliffe, H. L. Primary Lung Cancers in Birds and Mammals of the Philadelphia Zoo. Cancer Res., 26: 514-518, 1966.

34. Koller, L. D. Cutaneous Papillomas on an Opossum. J. Nat. Cancer Inst., 49: 309-313, 1972.

35. Gupta, B. N. Carcinosarcoma in an Opossum. J. Amer. Vet. Med. Assoc. 163: 586-588, 1973.

36. Andrews, E. J. Methylcholanthrene Carcinogenesis in the North American Opossum (Didelphis virginiana) J. Nat. Cancer Inst., 51: 1217-1225, 1973.

37. Fox, R. R., Devan, B. A., and Meir, H. Transplacental Induction of Primary Renal Tumors in Rabbits Treated with 1-ethyl-1-nitrosourea. J. Natl. Cancer Inst., 54: 1439-1448, 1975.

38. Reese, A. B. Heredity and Retinoblastoma. Arch. Ophthalmol., 42: 119-122, 1949.

39. Falls, H. F., and Neel, J. V. Genetics of Retinoblastoma. Arch. Ophthalmol., 46: 367-389, 1951.

40. Knudson, A. G., Jr. Mutation and Cancer: Structural Study of Retinoblastoma. Proc. Natl. Acad. Sci., 68: 810-823, 1971.

41. Knudson, A. G., Jr. Genetics and the Etiology of Childhood Cancer. Pediat. Res., 10: 513-517, 1976.

42. Macklin, M. T. Inheritance of Retinoblastoma. Arch. Ophthalmol., 62: 842-851, 1959.

43. Anderson, D. E. Genetic Varieties of Neoplasia. In Genetic Concepts and Neoplasia, 23rd Annual Symposium on Fundamental Cancer Research Baltimore, Williams and Wilkins Co., pp. 85-111, 1970.

44. Fraumeni, J. F. Genetic Factors. In Cancer Medicine (Holland, J. F. and Frei, F., III, eds.) Philadelphia, Lea and Febiger, pp. 7-15, 1973.

45. Maslow, L. A. Wilms' Tumor. Report of Three Cases and a Possible Fourth One in the Same Family. J. Urol., 43: 75-81, 1940.

46. Brown, W. T., Puranik, S. R., Altman, D. H., et al. Wilms' Tumor in Three Successive Generations. Surgery, 72: 756-761, 1972.

47. Chapian, M. A. Wilms' Tumor: Report of Two Cases in the Same Family. Rhode Island Med. J., 31: 105-114, 1948.

48. Gaulin, E. Simultaneous Wilms' Tumors in Identical Twins. J. Urol. 66: 547-550, 1951.

49. Cochran, W., and Froggatt, P. Bilateral Nephroblastoma in Two Sisters. J. Urol., 97: 216-220, 1967.

50. Gardner, A. L. The Systematics of the Genus Didelphis (Marsupialia): Didelphidae in North and Middle America. Lubbock, Mus. Texas Tech. Univ., 1973.

51. Meneghini, R. Repair Replication of Opossum Lymphocyte DNA: Effect of Compounds that Bind to DNA. Chem.-Biol. Interactions, 8: 113-126, 1974.

52. Napalkov, N. P. Some General Considerations on the Problem of Transplacental Carcinogenesis in Transplacental Carcinogenesis (Tomatis, L. and Mohr, V., eds.) IARC Scientific Publication No. 4. Lyon, Internat. Agency for Research in Cancer, WHO pp. 1-13, 1973.

53. Herbst, A. L., Oldfelder, H., and Poskanzer, D. C. Adenocarcinoma of the Vagina. Association of Maternal Stilbestrol. N. Eng. J. Med., 284: 878-881, 1971.

Chapter 12

CHRONOBIOLOGY

CAN CHRONOBIOLOGY BE IGNORED WHEN
CONSIDERING THE CANCER PROBLEM?

L. E. Scheving, E. R. Burns and J. E. Pauly

Department of Anatomy, College of Medicine
University of Arkansas for Medical Sciences
Little Rock, Arkansas

I. INTRODUCTION

An important consideration in cancer chemotherapy is the cell cycle which is a series of sequential steps a cell must pass through before it can divide. The cell cycle has been partitioned into four separate time periods: the pre-DNA synthetic phase (G_1), the period of DNA replication (S), the post-DNA synthetic or pre-mitotic phase (G_2), and the actual mitosis (M).

A prominent feature of the cell cycle is the circadian variation that has been demonstrated for the synthetic (S) and mitotic (M) stages. With few exceptions (to be cited throughout the paper), this variation has been ignored in cytokinetic studies and in cancer chemotherapy.

Conceivably the circadian variation in DNA synthesis and in the mitotic index is related to the high-amplitude susceptibility-resistance rhythms known to characterize cell-cycle-specific drugs such as cytosine arabinoside (ara-C). It is our contention that the circadian variation in the S and M stages, as well as the rhythmic nature of drug effectiveness, can be exploited to optimize cancer chemotherapy. Experimental data to support the rationale for the above statement are presented in this paper.

II. PROCEDURES AND MATERIALS

The Materials and Methods previously have been published in detail (see Burns et al., 1976) and will not be repeated here. It should be kept in mind that, unless specifically noted, all studies were performed on male mice fed ad libitum and subjected to 12 hours of artificial fluorescent light (0600 to 1800) alternating with 12 hours of darkness. When speaking of incorporation of tritiated thymidine (^{3}HTdR) into DNA, we stress that we have isolated and quantified the DNA unless otherwise noted. Also for another laboratory to replicate our data, it would be essential that the animals be subjected to the same standardized conditions.

III. RESULTS AND DISCUSSION

A. Cell Proliferation

Figure 1 serves to introduce the concept of rhythmicity for this presentation. Each datum point represents the mean level (and SE) of the incorporation of ^{3}HTdR into the DNA of tissue obtained from animals that
were injected intraperitoneally (i.p.) with the isotope one-half hour prior
to sacrifice. The lowest levels occur around the time of transition of
light to dark; the ascending limb is associated primarily with the dark
span (active time for animals), and the descending limb is associated with
the light span (inactive time for animals). The profile of the rhythm on
the second day is not exactly that of the first day since DNA synthesis is
still high at the third 0800 point. In our opinion this does not suggest
that the rhythms are longer than 24 hours. Instead we believe, from many
other rhythmic studies done by us, that on the third day the descending
limb would be steeper and the trough would be reached at approximately the
same time on the third day as on the previous two days. Each subgroup of
animals was maintained in separate isolation chambers and was not, to the
best of our knowledge, disturbed in any way immediately prior to or during
the entire sampling span. Therefore, it is not likely in this case that
the higher levels of DNA synthesis seen at the third 0800 time point were
due to the so-called "serial effect" described by Halberg (1959). A serial effect implies that the values obtained from animals at the end of the
study may be significantly higher or lower (depending on the variable)
than those at the beginning of the study because of the repeated stimuli to
the animals caused by entering the animal room to fetch them for sampling.

From a number of light-dark synchronized studies on rodents, we have
found that the trough of a rhythm is the most fixed point in relation to
local clock time. It is important for anyone entering the field of chronobiology research to recognize that the profile of the rhythm can vary
somewhat from day to day. Because of such variation, one must be extremely careful in experimental work not to attach too much significance to
minor changes in phasing, amplitude or level; such changes may represent
little more than normal biological variation. Also a glimpse at the
chronograms in figure 1 reveals the fallacy of assuming that rhythmicity
is merely a "day-night" phenomenon. Such an assumption must have been
made by some workers because many studies have been reported in the literature showing two data-sampling points - one during the day and one during
the night. A not-uncommon practice has been to cite such data as evidence
for or against rhythmicity - often without pointing out the deficiency in
sampling. Such data as presented in figure 1 irrevocably refute the concept that circadian variation represents no more than minor fluctuation
around a 24-hour mean and hence is of no major significance in experimental design or perhaps deserves no more consideration than to sample at the
same time each day (Scheving, 1973).

The reliability of our method for estimating the DNA pattern of fluctuation is good (in a number of cases we have compared such data with
autoradiographic analysis and found almost identical phasing with the two
methods). The same rhythmic pattern was obtained for the lateral edge of
the tongue as for the tip (fig. 1), but here the level was significantly
lower. This latter conclusion would not have been noted, however, if we
had sampled at only 1400 and 1700. Examination of tissue obtained at

different circadian phases is necessary to establish what actually is going on in a particular tissue. It is obvious that single-time-point sampling may lead one into pitfalls.

We have repeatedly reported a similar rhythmic phenomenon for the corneal epithelium (Scheving and Pauly, 1967). The phasing of the rhythm for both tissues is practically identical. We emphasize that for both tissues (as well as for others) the peak and trough of the S and M stages do not occur each day at a precise, fixed clock time, but either one may vary between 2 or 3 hours.

Figure 2 illustrates the rhythm in DNA synthesis for the thymus and spleen. The data are plotted as percent change in the 24-hour mean in order to facilitate comparison because the absolute levels of DNA synthesis in these two tissues is quite different. Note that the ascending limb of the curve is associated with activity, and the descending limb with the rest span of the animals. The details of the studies on the spleen and thymus have been reported by Burns et al. (1976) and Pauly et al. (1976), respectively.

Figure 3 shows the same rhythmic variable (DNA synthesis) in the bone marrow and duodenum of mice. The phasing of the two rhythms is similar. It should be noted that in the bone marrow and gut, unlike many other tissues, there always is a relatively high degree of synthesis going on; but still many cells are synchronized and proceed in a rhythmic manner with essentially the same phasing pattern as other tissues. In the cornea, cell division drops to practically zero at certain circadian phases.

It is still being reported in the literature that cell division in the gut undergoes no circadian change. The data presented in a 1976 reference source ("Cell Biology, Biological Handbook," Eds., P. L. Altman and D. D. Katz, Fed. Amer. Socs. Exper. Biol., 1976) would lead one to believe that cell division in the entire gut is devoid of a circadian rhythm. It is difficult to understand why the compiler of the extensive mitotic-index table in this reference completely ignored, in the case of both the gut and cornea, all the existing data which does document circadian variation. The reasons for the perpetuation of the steady-state or non-rhythmic concept of proliferation in the gut were discussed critically in detail (Scheving, Burns and Pauly, 1972) and will not be repeated here; rather we shall present data to further document its rhythmic nature. It should be kept in mind that what we claim for the gut is essentially true for the pattern of fluctuation in DNA of bone marrow.

The chronograms on the left in figure 4 represent data expressed as absolute values and those in the middle as percent change from the 24-hour mean. Since these studies were not designed to test for reproducibility of the data, one should not be surprised to find that the over-all 24-hour means of the amount of ^{3}HTdR incorporated into DNA are quite different. The differences seen in these mean levels represent many things, including different specific activities of the radioisotopes injected, different age of the animals, etc. What is relevant to this presentation and what can logically be compared is the phasing of the rhythms, and they are best illustrated as percent change of the mean. A summary of all six studies is shown in the chronogram on the right of figure 4; this shows that a rhythm in DNA synthesis in the duodenum does exist and that its phasing is very similar to that for DNA synthesis in the tongue (fig. 1) as well as in the cornea (Scheving and Pauly, 1967). In fact, the phasing is remark-ably similar to that seen in data on regenerating mouse liver (Barnum et al., 1957); the method used by these investigators was the incorporation of radioactive phosphorus into the tissue.

Our concept of normal in vivo DNA synthesis in rodents is that many of the cells that are dividing in a particular tissue are doing so in synchrony. The total number of all the dividing cells involved in this synchrony for each tissue varies. In the case of the cornea most of the dividing cells are synchronized; for the gut some are not and this accounts for the fact that we always find some dividing cells. The one thing that most tissues have in common is that the cells in synchrony with each other are characterized by rhythms with similar phasings. These tissues include urinary bladder, epidermis, various oral tissues, connective tissues, bone marrow and gut; the supporting evidence for this hypothesis has been re-viewed previously (Scheving and Pauly, 1973). In the present paper, the spleen and thymus have been added to the above list; and it can be induced from recently published data (Krueger, Bo and Hoopes, 1975) that the uter-ine epithelium can also be added.

Halberg and associates (Luce, 1970) have reported that different types of mouse pancreatic cells divide rhythmically; but when the mitotic index rhythms are compared, the different cell types have different phas-ings. This would suggest that cell division in the pancreas is under less of a systemic control mechanism than that we visualize for many of the tissues we have analyzed.

DNA synthesis has been similarly analyzed in four different tumor models (L1210, adenocarcinoma, Lewis lung and Ehrlich ascites). This was done by sampling at 3-hour intervals along a 24-hour time scale at differ-ent intervals after tumor inoculation - for example, on the second, fourth and sixth days for the L1210 leukemia. One thing is certain in neoplastic populations: the fluctuation in DNA synthesis along the 24-hour time scale is dramatic but its phasing is unpredictable. The rhythm is dramatically different on each day, especially while the cells are in their exponential phase of growth. The presence of the tumor also causes the phasing of rhythms in some tissues to become unpredictable. Our impression (data to be presented elsewhere) is that those tumors in the stationary phase would have a tendency to be more circadian and to have the least effect on the host rhythms of the bone marrow and gut.

From extensive studies done on the rat corneal epithelium, Scheving and Pauly (1967) reported that there was a remarkable similarity in phas-ing between the mitotic-index and DNA-synthesis rhythms. This was sur-prising because the duration of DNA synthesis (transit time) has been cal-culated to be about 8 to 10 hours which would suggest that the peak and trough of DNA synthesis and mitosis in synchronized, dividing cells should be separated in time by approximately the same interval. We offered two possible explanations: (1) that there were two cohorts of cells, one syn-thesizing and one mitosing, and the group synthesizing today would repre-sent the mitotic peak of tomorrow; and (2) (the explanation we favor) that the G_2 phase may be very short and the transit time of DNA synthesis in the cornea may vary a great deal (Burns and Scheving, 1975; also this sym-posium). Figure 5 shows this phenomenon for both the duodenum and corneal epithelium. Sigdestad and Lesher (1972) reported a similar finding for the mouse gut, as did Chumak (1963) for the cornea.

More recently Scheving et al. (1975) reported a similar phasing for the mitotic index and DNA-synthesis rhythms in the livers of mice bearing an i.p. 8-day Ehrlich ascites carcinoma. This finding was surprising because Nash and Echave-Llanos (1971) reported that there was an 8-hour lag between the peaks of the DNA-synthesis and mitosis rhythms in the livers of mice bearing a fast-growing hepatoma. Also, Barnum et al. (1957) reported that the synthesis and mitotic-index rhythms in mouse regenerating liver were separated in time by 6 to 12 hours. It is probable that in the case of the adult regenerating liver, where a G_0 or non-cycling population of cells is induced to enter the cell cycle, the peak in DNA synthesis of the wave of cells that began synthesizing DNA after partial hepatectomy would preceed the mitotic-index peak by 6 to 12 hours as claimed by Barnum et al. (1957). However, we cannot explain the findings of Nash and Echave-Llanos (1971) in light of our own data - the two studies should be comparable. A Shortcoming of their data is that the mitotic-index and DNA-synthesis rhythms were determined separately on two different groups of animals and were done at least one year apart.

We emphasize that we do not claim that the two rhythms (S and M) are identical, but they are generally similar. In fact we suspect, but cannot prove as yet, that the DNA-synthesis rhythm does begin its increase before the mitotic-index rhythm begins to increase; and if we obtain data at frequent enough intervals this might be resolved. The practical point to be made in light of these findings is that one should not determine a mitotic circadian curve and then, from published data on transit times for synthesis, extrapolate back and assume that the phasing of the synthesis curve will be advanced by a fixed number of hours; unfortunately this practice has not been uncommon. Another practical point is that there is one phase of the rat's circadian system when synthesis (S) and division (M) activities are minimal. From our repeated studies on DNA-synthesis rhythms, we find that the upswing may be abrupt in one instance but less abrupt in a comparable study. Nevertheless, the upswing usually does start at the beginning or during the early part of the nocturnal phase.

B. Susceptibility-Resistance Rhythms

Since it is well established that the biological system is rhythmically changing, it follows that the organism is biochemically a different entity at different circadian phases. Therefore, it reacts differently to an identical stimulus at different circadian times. This variation has been documented many times using a variety of stimuli which have included carcinogens, immunizing agents and physical agents as well as toxic agents such as drugs, chemicals and poisons. Several reviews of this phenomenon have appeared (Reinberg and Halberg, 1971; Moore Ede, 1973; Scheving, Mayersbach and Pauly, 1974).

Within the past few years a series of studies, which largely has been a collaborative effort of three laboratories (Universities of Arkansas, Minnesota and Tennessee), has shown that by applying chronobiological methods and concepts to the treatment of leukemia-bearing mice, host tolerance to a carcinostatic drug could be improved. Figure 6 illustrates the results of the first in this series of studies. The data clearly show that there is a rhythm in susceptibility to cytosine arabinoside (ara-C) (Scheving et al., 1974; Cardoso, Scheving and Halberg, 1970). Since this drug is cell-cycle specific in that it specifically inhibits DNA synthe-

1067

sis, it was of interest to compare its susceptibility (mortality) rhythm to the rhythm characterizing DNA synthesis in the gut (fig. 7). In this case the peak in mortality is associated with that phase of the circadian system when DNA synthesis is lowest. Does this imply that ara-C is having its greatest effect at the time of conversion of the cells from G_1 to S? It has been claimed that this is the most vulnerable part of the cycle. If so, we must conclude that cells are most sensitive to this drug at a time when we actually find the lowest level of DNA synthesis (percentage of labeled cells) for a tissue. Of course one must keep in mind that the variation in toxicity we are witnessing may be due primarily to other factors such as absorption, distribution, elimination and variation in rate of metabolism.

The question asked in 1971 was what could be done with such chronobiologically determined toxicity data in the area of chemotherapy. To explore such a question, it is ideal to have some accepted reference data which have been determined without chronobiological considerations with which to compare. Fortunately the excellent work of Skipper et al. (1967) involving the treatment of L1210 leukemic mice with ara-C seemed to offer an ideal reference. Skipper and his co-workers consistently were able to eradicate 10^5 leukemic cells (sometimes 10^6) without animal deaths due to toxicity; this was accomplished by giving four treatment courses of 120 mg of ara-C per kg body weight in equal doses spaced at 3-hour intervals over a 24-hour span. Between each course was a 3-day rest span. Courses of 240 mg/kg of ara-C given on the same schedule were so toxic that they killed all the animals.

An experiment was designed by Haus et al. (1972) to determine if the tolerance of BDF_1 mice to the 240 mg/kg dose could be improved by applying chronobiological methods and concepts. This was done by inoculating BDF_1 with L1210 leukemic cells and administering the 240 mg/kg of the ara-C in a special manner. Instead of giving the drug in 8 equal doses at 3-hour intervals, it was given in sinusoidally increasing and decreasing amounts over the 24-hour span. A number of different sinusoidal treatment schedules were designed (fig. 8). The "best" (most effective) sinusoidal treatment schedules resulted when the largest amount of the drug was given at the times of peak host resistance to the drug, and the smallest dose was administered when the animal was most susceptible. The application of this technique resulted in statistically significant increases in survival time when compared to the reference (Skipper) schedule of equal doses (Haus et al., 1972). Hence it was reported that a carcinostatic drug extensively used by clinicians is tolerated better when timed according to the host's circadian system than when it is administered on a conventional or unchanging schedule. Later, after a series of studies, it was reported that by applying this technique the cure rate could be doubled (Kuhl et al., 1974). A comprehensive review of these studies and their implications to chronotherapy has been published (Halberg et al., 1973). More recently toxicity data have been published which demonstrate clearly that studies of this nature are remarkably reproducible from one laboratory to another (fig. 9) (Scheving et al., 1976).

We are reporting at this meeting (details to be published elsewhere) data which show that by using one of the best ara-C schedules in combination with cyclophosphamide, one can optimize treatment of mice bearing an inoculum of 10^6 leukemic cells. This was done by giving all animals the conventional four courses of the "best" ara-C sinusoid (120 mg/kg/course).

The mice were subdivided into groups of 25 animals and each of eight groups received, at a different circadian phase, 50 mg/kg of cyclophosphamide once per course of ara-C. The response to treatment was strongly circadian-phase dependent with as many as 94% of the animals within a group cured at one circadian phase and as few as 44% cured at another (cure implies that an animal was apparently healthy at 70 days after inoculation of tumor).

When the inoculum was increased to 4.4 x 10^6, the dosage of ara-C to 150 mg/kg/course, and the dosage of cyclophosphamide to 62.5 mg/kg (with the protocol otherwise remaining the same as above), the chronobiological approach significantly enhanced the effectiveness of the treatment over that obtained with the conventional treatment schedule. For example, with the chronobiological approach there was: (1) more than double survival time, (2) a seven-fold increase in numbers of cured animals (at certain stages of the mouse circadian system), and (3) as little as one-half the weight loss during the course of drug treatment.

We conclude that one should not ignore the circadian variation in dealing with any aspect of the cancer problem. The evidence is compelling that the temporal organization carries with it significant implications for cancer chemotherapy as well as for basic cancer research. Perhaps we can come to better grips with the mechanism if we consider the rhythmic nature that characterizes all cell division in the first place. More researchers working in this important area are urgently needed.

Acknowledgements

This work was supported in part by grant #5RO1 CA 14388 from the National Institutes of Health.

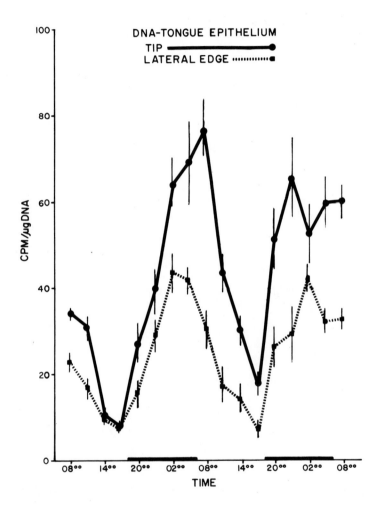

FIG. 1. The two chronograms represent studies done on the same BDF$_1$ male mice (N = 8 per time point) (see text).

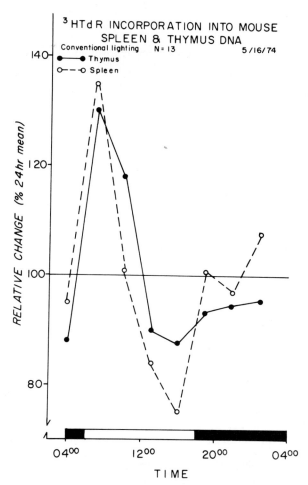

FIG. 2. A comparison of the phasing of the circadian rhythms in the uptake of [3]HTdR into DNA of the spleen and thymus of Swiss Webster mice. The two chronograms represent the same mice. For details of these studies, see Burns et al. (1976) and Pauly et al. (1975).

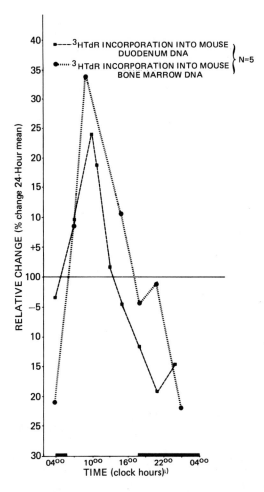

FIG. 3. Chronograms showing the similarity in phasing of DNA synthesis rhythms between bone marrow and duodenum in Swiss Webster mice. Study performed 2/28/74.

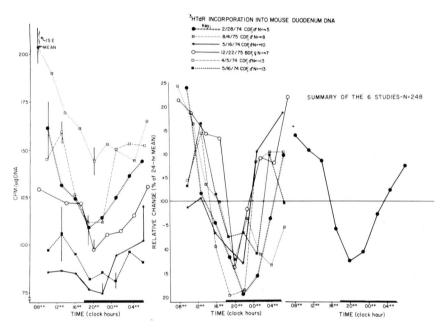

FIG. 4. A composite of chronograms obtained from control animals in several studies performed by us for diverse reasons. The point emphasized is that in all cases there was a rhythm in DNA synthesis and the phasing was quite reproducible. For explanation of the variation seen in the overall mean, see text. For the sake of clarity, standard errors are shown only for the high and low points of each chronogram.

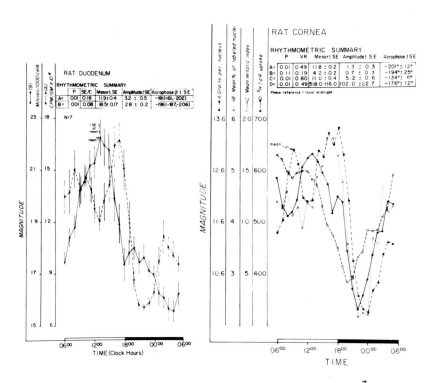

FIG. 5. Significant fluctuation in the mitotic index and in ^{3}H-thymidine
uptake into the duodenum of the rat is shown on the left side. On the
right, the chronograms show the pattern of fluctuation in ^{3}H-thymidine uptake, percentage of labeled cells, numbers of grains per labeled nucleus
and mitotic rate in rat corneal epithelium. Note that in both cases we
were measuring only the uptake of the isotope into the tissue; we did not,
as in later studies, quantify DNA. Also demonstrated is the rhythmometric
summary of the data. For a more detailed account of the conditions of
both these studies, see Scheving et al. (1972) for the duodenum and Scheving
and Pauly (1967) for the cornea.

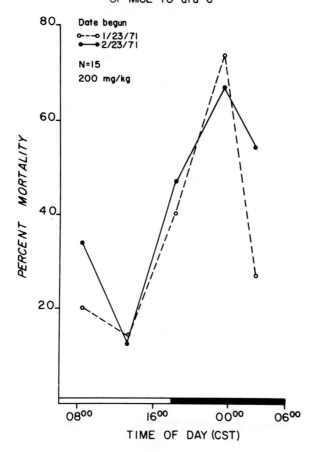

FIG. 6. Circadian susceptibility rhythm of BDF$_1$ mice to arabinosyl cytosine (ara-C) given on five consecutive days at single, defined, circadian
system phases (Scheving et al., 1974).

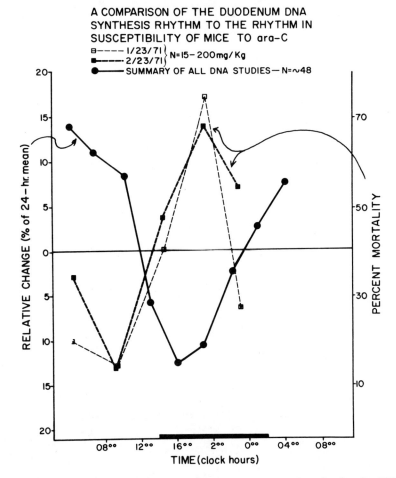

FIG. 7. Comparison of the ara-C toxicity rhythm to the rhythm in DNA synthesis in the duodenum (see text).

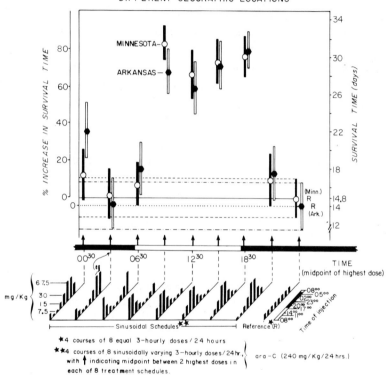

FIG. 8. Survival time of CD2F$_1$ mice on different drug administration schedules (top); and timing of doses of ara-C (bottom) in sinusoidal and reference (R) schedules. All treatment schedules comprise four courses, each consisting of a total of 240 mg/kg/24 hr. When the same total dose of ara-C is given, certain sinusoidal drug-administration schedules are definitely better tolerated by mice than are other sinusoids or than is a currently conventional reference treatment schedule of 8 equal doses over a 24-hr span. Also note unequivocal reproducibility of chronotoxicity to ara-C in experiments done on the same days in different laboratories in different geographic locations. For details, see Scheving et al. (1976).

REFERENCES

1. Barnum, C. P., Jardetzky, C. D., and Halberg, F. Nucleic Acid Synthesis In Regenerating Liver. Texas Rept. Biol. Med., 15: 134-147, 1957.
2. Burns, E. R., and Scheving, L. E. Circadian Influence On The Wave Form Of The Frequency Of Labeled Mitoses In Mouse Corneal Epithelium. Cell Tissue Kinet., 8: 61-66, 1975.
3. Burns, E. R., Scheving, L. E., Pauly, J. E., and Tsai, T. H. Effect Of Altered Lighting Regimens, Time Limited Feeding And Presence Of Ehrlich Ascites Carcinoma On The Circadian Rhythm In DNA Synthesis Of Mouse Spleen. Cancer Res., 36: 1538-1544, 1976.
4. Cardoso, S. S., Scheving, L. E., and Halberg, F. Mortality Of Mice As Influenced By The Hour Of Day Of Drug (Ara-C) Administration. Pharmacologist, 12: 302, 1970.
5. Chumak, M. G. Mitotic Cycle Of Epithelium Cells Of Cornea In Mice. Studied By Means Of Thymidine Tagged With Tritium. Dokl. Akad. Nauk SSSR, 149: 960-962, 1963.
6. Haus, E., Halberg, F., Scheving, L. E., Cardoso, S., Kühl, J., Sothern, R., Shiotsuka, R., Hwang, D. S., and Pauly, J. E. Increased Tolerance Of Leukemic Mice To Arabinosyl Cytosine With Schedule Adjusted To Circadian System. Science, 177: 80-82, 1972.
7. Halberg, F. Lighting Regimen And Experimental Method; Light-Synchronized Periodicity Analysis. 12th Ann. Conf. Elect. Tech. In Med. & Biol., Digest Of Technical Papers, pp. 78-79, 1959.
8. Halberg, F., Haus, E., Cardoso, S. S., Scheving, L. E., Kühl, J. F. W., Shiotsuka, R., Rosene, G., Pauly, J. E., Runge, W., Spalding, J. F., Lee, J. K., and Good, R. A. Toward A Chronotherapy Of Neoplasia: Tolerance Of Treatment Depends Upon Host Rhythms. Experientia, 29: 909-1044, 1973.
9. Krueger, W. A., Bo, W. J., and Hoopes, P. C. A Circadian Rhythm On Mitotic Activity In The Uterine Luminal Epithelium Of The Rat: Effect Of Estrogen. Anat. Rec., 183: 563-566, 1975.
10. Kühl, J. F. W., Haus, E., Halberg, F., Scheving, L. E., Pauly, J. E., Cardoso, S. S., and Rosene, G. Experimental Chronotherapy With Ara-C: Comparison Of Murine Ara-C Tolerance On Differently Timed Treatment Schedules. Chronobiologia, 1: 316-317, 1974.
11. Luce, G. G. Biological Rhythms In Psychiatry And Medicine. Public Health Service Pub. #2088, U. S. Dept. Health, Education and Welfare, 1970.
12. Moore Ede, M. C. Circadian Rhythms Of Drug Effectiveness And Toxicity. Clin. Pharmacol. Ther., 14: 925-935, 1973.
13. Nash, R. E., and Echave Llanos, J. M. Twenty-Four Hour Variations In DNA Synthesis Of A Fast-Growing And A Slow-Growing Hepatoma: DNA Synthesis Rhythm In Hepatoma. J. Nat. Cancer Inst., 47: 1007-1012, 1971.
14. Pauly, J. E., Scheving, L. E., Burns, E. R., and Tsai, T. H. Circadian Rhythm In DNA Syntheses Of Mouse Thymus: Effect Of Altered Lighting Regimens, Restricted Feeding And Presence Of Ehrlich Ascites Tumor. Anat. Rec., 184: 275-284, 1976.
15. Reinberg, A., and Halberg, F. Circadian Chronopharmacology. Ann Rev. Pharmacol., 2: 455-492, 1971.
16. Scheving, L. E. Some Ideas Associated With Chronobiology. Int. J. Chronobiology, 1: 17-18, 1973.
17. Scheving, L. E., Burns, E. R., and Pauly, J. E. Circadian Rhythms In Mitotic Activity and ^{3}H-Thymidine Uptake In The Duodenum: Effect Of Isoproterenol On The Mitotic Rhythm. Amer. J. Anat., 135: 311-317, 1972.

18. Scheving, L. E., Burns, E. R., and Pauly, J. E. Coincidence In Timing Between The S And M Stages Of The Cell Cycle In Liver Parenchymal Cells In Mice Bearing An 8-Day Ehrlich Ascites Tumor (EAT). Chronobiologia, Suppl. 1, pp. 61-62, 1975.
19. Scheving, L. E., Haus, E., Kühl, J. F. W., Pauly, J. E., Halberg, F., and Cardoso, S. Different Laboratories Closely Reproduce Characteristics Of Circadian Rhythm In Ara-C Tolerance By Mice. Cancer Res., 36: 1133-1137, 1976.
20. Scheving, L. E., Mayersbach, H. v., and Pauly, J. E. An Overview Of Chronopharmacology. Europ. J. Toxicology, 7: 203-227, 1974.
21. Scheving, L. E. and Pauly, J. E. Circadian Phase Relationships Of Thymidine-H^3 Uptake, Labeled Nuclei, Grain Counts And Cell Division Rate In Rat Corneal Epithelium. J. Cell Biol., 32: 677-683, 1967.
22. Scheving, L. E. and Pauly, J. E. Cellular Mechanisms Involving Biorhythms With Emphasis On Those Rhythms Associated With The S And M Stages Of The Cell Cycle. Int. J. Chronobiology, 1: 269-286, 1973.
23. Sigdestad, C. P. and Lesher, S. Circadian Rhythm In The Cell Cycle Time Of The Mouse Intestinal Epithelium. J. Interdisp. Cycle Res., 3: 39-46, 1972.
24. Skipper, H. E., Schabel, F. M., Jr., and Wilcox, W. S. Experimental Evaluation Of Potential Anticancer Agents. XXI. Scheduling Of Arabinosyl Cytosine To Take Advantage Of Its S Phase Specificity Against Leukemia Cells. Cancer Chemotherap. Res., 51: 125-165, 1967.

1079

THE INFLUENCE OF CIRCADIAN VARIATION

ON IN VIVO CELL KINETIC STUDIES

E. Robert Burns and Lawrence E. Scheving

Department of Anatomy, College of Medicine
University of Arkansas for Medical Sciences
Little Rock, Arkansas 72201

I. INTRODUCTION

The use of the mitotic index and the uptake of tritiated thymidine (TdR) in basic cell kinetic work on normal and neoplastic populations of cells has been of paramount importance in cancer research (see DeVita, 1971; Skipper, 1971). Such cell kinetic data have been the basis for many specific therapeutic protocols, e.g., giving cytosine arabinoside (ara-C) every three hours during one 24-hour period to assure that every L1210 leukemia cell which entered S phase was exposed to ara-C (Skipper, 1967). It seems logical that anything which can be learned about the uptake of TdR in relation to cell kinetics would be of importance to basic cancer research including cell kinetic studies and the use of cell kinetics in the design of therapeutic protocols.

When sampling intervals have been every 3-4 hours or more frequently in one 24-hour period, chronobiological investigations have repeatedly demonstrated that the mitotic index (MI), the labeling index (LI), the grain count and the liquid scintillation determination of the uptake of TdR are characterized by statistically significant circadian fluctuation. The first report of a circadian rhythm in DNA synthesis was that of Barnum, Jardetzky and Halberg (1958). Circadian variation in the mitotic index was noted even earlier (for a review see Scheving and Pauly, 1973). The well-documented circadian rhythms in these growth-related variables have been and are still essentially unnoticed or actively ignored. In fact, a 1976 reference source ("Cell Biology", edited by Altman and Katz) presents several tables on mitotic indices and cell kinetic data with no reference to published chronobiological data in this area. Such data gathered without chronobiological consideration are unreliable.

The objectives of this paper are (1) to restate the phenomenon of circadian rhythmicity in MI, LI, DNA synthesis, etc. (see above) and (2) to demonstrate specifically how the circadian system of the host can influence cell kinetic data obtained with the frequently employed FLM or frequency of labeled mitoses method.

The question asked is, "What influence does the circadian system have on the determination of cell cycle variables with the FLM technique?"

II. PROCEDURES AND MATERIALS USED

Male mice (CDF_1 and Swiss-Webster) were standardized to a light-dark cycle (light from 0600-1800, CST) for at least two weeks prior to and throughout the duration of the experiments. One large group of CDF_1 mice was injected i.p. with 25 μCi TdR at 0900 and a second large group was injected with 25 μCi TdR at 2100. TdR was also injected (25 μCi/mouse) into a large group of Swiss-Webster mice bearing an 8-day-old Ehrlich Ascites Carcinoma (EAC) at 0900 and into a second large group of EAC-bearing mice at 2100. After the injection of the TdR at 0900 or 2100, subgroups of three mice each were killed at 1, 2, 3, 5, 7, 9, 11, 13, 17, 21, 23, 25, 27, 29, 31, 33 and 35 hours. Autoradiographs were prepared of the cornea, esophagus and the EAC. Thirty mitotic figures/mouse were counted for each tissue at each time point and classified as labeled or unlabeled. This resulted in a minimum of 90 mitotic figures/time point. FLM curves were constructed from these data. The transit times through S (T_S), $G_2 + \frac{1}{2}M$ ($T_{G_2} + \frac{1}{2}M$), etc., were calculated according to established procedures (Lala, 1971).

III. RESULTS

Figures 1 (cornea) and 2 (esophagus) clearly demonstrate that there are substantial differences in the FLM curves not only between the two organs, but more importantly between the 0900 and 2100 groups for each organ. For the cornea (Fig. 1), no second wave of labeled mitoses was seen in either the 0900 or the 2100 group. When TdR was injected at 0900 (dashed line), T_S was 12.2 hours and $T_{G_2} + \frac{1}{2}M$ was 4.0 hours. However, when TdR was injected at 2100 (solid line, T_S was 5.4 hours and $T_{G_2} + \frac{1}{2}M$ was 8.0 hours.

In the esophagus (Fig. 2), the only group which demonstrated a second wave of labeled mitoses was the group injected with TdR at 0900 (dashed line); no second wave of labeled mitoses was observed in the 2100 group (solid line). When TdR was injected at 0900, T_S for the esophagus was 5.3 hours and $T_{G_2} + \frac{1}{2}M$ was 2.5 hours. When TdR was injected at 2100, T_S was 3.5 hours and $TG_2 + \frac{1}{2}M$ was 4.5 hours.

Figure 3 demonstrates the FLM curves obtained at two different points in the circadian system (0900 and 2100) for the 8-day-old EAC. In the TdR at 2100 group (solid line), T_S was 20.3 hours and $T_{G_2} + \frac{1}{2}M$ was 5.8 hours. In the TdR at 0900 group (dashed line), T_S was 28.5 hours and $T_{G_2} + \frac{1}{2}M$ was 4.3 hours.

IV. DISCUSSION

One would expect that significant circadian fluctuation in such growth-related variables as MI, LI and the uptake of TdR (grain count and liquid scintillation counts) (see Scheving and Pauly, 1967) would result in a significant variation in the data obtained with the FLM technique; this is obviously the case. The FLM curves initiated at 0900 and 2100 probably demonstrate the extreme differences simply because 0900 and 2100 are, in general, the times of peak and trough activity, respectively in the MI, LI, grain count, and DNA synthesis rhythms (see Scheving and

Pauly, 1973). The data strongly suggest that T_S and $T_{G2 + \frac{1}{2}M}$, as well as the other components of the cell cycle, are characterized by circadian rhythmicity. Support for this statement can be found in the work of Tvermyr (1972) who reported that T_S varied from 5 to 12 hours depending on the point in the circadian system when the experiment was initiated. Sigdestad and Lesher (1972) initiated FLM curves for mouse intestine at 1500 and 0300 and found that T_{G1} varied by two hours. More recently, Møller, Larsen and Faber (1974) initiated FLM curves for the hamster cheek pouch at 1100, 1500, 1700, 2400 and 0500 and reported a circadian variation in T_S of 8.0 to 13.5 hours; $T_{G2 + \frac{1}{2}M}$ varied from 1.8 to 2.8 hours. The details of the work presented in this paper can be found in Burns and Scheving, 1975; Burns et al., 1976a; and Burns et al., 1976b.

Chronobiology, therefore, has broadened the general field of cell kinetics by demonstrating the circadian nature of several growth-related variables. Most, if not all, in vivo populations of renewing cells are not totally asynchronous, but are characterized by some degree of synchrony as evidenced by the significant circadian rhythms in mitosis and DNA synthesis. These observations should not be ignored in any kind of cell kinetic work. Consideration of them will serve to refine our knowledge of normal and neoplastic growth and therefore lead to more precise therapeutic protocols in the treatment of the tumor-bearing host.

V. SUMMARY

Cell kinetics is important for a complete understanding of both normal and neoplastic growth. Cell kinetics plays a major role in the design of effective therapeutic protocols. The chronobiological aspects of cell kinetic experiments have revealed prominent circadian fluctuation in all measurable variables, such as the mitotic index, the labeling index, grain counts, liquid scintillation counting of the incorporation of tritiated thymidine, the length of the S phase, the length of the $G_2 + \frac{1}{2}M$ phase, etc. Such data will eventually lead (1) to a more complete understanding of normal and neoplastic cell growth and, consequently, (2) to more refined and biologically effective therapeutic protocols for the treatment of cancer.

Acknowledgements

This work has been supported by a grant from the National Cancer Institute (RI1-CA-14388). Dr. Burns is the recipient of a Research Career Development award (1KO4-CA-70594) from the National Cancer Institute.

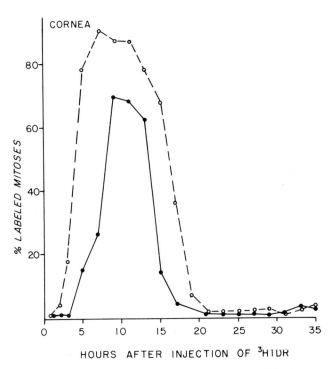

FIG. 1. FLM curves obtained from the mouse cornea. TdR injected at 0900 (dashed line). TdR injected at 2100 (solid line). (Reprinted from Burns et al., 1976b, courtesy of _Chronobiologia_.)

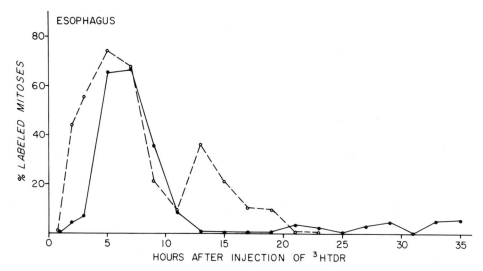

FIG. 2. FLM curves obtained from the mouse esophagus. TdR injected at 0900 (dashed line). TdR injected at 2100 (solid line). (Reprinted from Burns et al., 1976b, courtesy of *Chronobiologia*.)

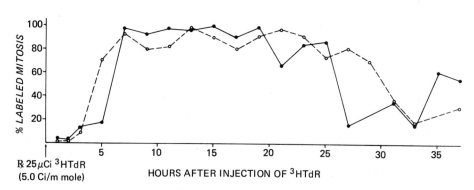

FIG. 3. FLM curves obtained from an 8-day-old Ehrlich Ascites Carcinoma. TdR injected at 0900 (dashed line). TdR injected at 2100 (solid line). (Reprinted from Burns et al., 1976b, courtesy of *Chronobiologia*.)

References

1. Barnum, C. P., Jardetzky, C. D., and Halberg, F. Time Relations Among Metabolic and Morphologic 24-Hour Changes in Mouse Liver. Am. J. Physiology, 195: 301-310, 1958.
2. Burns, E. R., and Scheving, L. E. Circadian Influence on the Wave Form of the Frequency of Labeled Mitoses in Mouse Corneal Epithelium. Cell Tiss. Kinet., 8: 61-66, 1975.
3. Burns, E. R., Scheving, L. E., Fawcett, D. F., Gibbs, W. M., and Galatzan, R. E. Circadian Influence on the Frequency of Labeled Mitoses Method in the Stratified Squamous Epithelium of the Mouse Esophagus and Tongue. Anat. Rec., 184: 265-274, 1976a.
4. Burns, E. R., Scheving, L. E., Gibbs, W. M., Fawcett, D. F., and Galatzan, R. E. Circadian Influence on the Wave Form of the Frequency of Labeled Mitoses Curve. Chronobiologia (in press), 1976b.
5. DeVita, V. T. Cell Kinetics and the Chemotherapy of Cancer. Cancer Chemotherap. Rept., 2: 23-33, 1971.
6. Lala, P. Studies on Tumor Cell Population Kinetics. In: Methods in Cancer Research. Ed.: H. Busch. Academic Press Inc., New York, pp. 3-95, 1971.
7. Moller, U., Larsen, J. K., and Faber, M. The Influence of Injected Tritiated Thymidine on the Mitotic Circadian Rhythm in the Epithelium of the Hamster Cheek Pouch. Cell Tiss. Kinet., 7: 231-239, 1974.
8. Scheving, L. E., and Pauly, J. E. Circadian Phase Relationships of Thymidine-^{3}H Uptake, Labeled Nuclei, Grain Counts and Cell Division Rate in Rat Corneal Epithelium. J. Cell Biol., 32: 677-683, 1967.
9. Scheving, L. E., and Pauly, J. E. Cellular Mechanisms Involving Biorhythms With Emphasis on Those Rhythms Associated With the S and M Stages of the Cell Cycle. Int. J. Chronobiology, 1: 269-286, 1973.
10. Sigdestad, C. P., and Lesher, S. Circadian Rhythm in the Cell Cycle Time of the Mouse Intestinal Epithelium. J. Interdispl. Cycle Res., 3: 39-46, 1972.
11. Skipper, H. H., Schabel, F. M., and Wilcox, W. S. Experimental Evaluation of Potential Anticancer Agents. XXI. Scheduling of Arabinosyl Cytosine to Take Advantage of Its S-Phase Specificity Against Leukemia Cells. Cancer Chemotherap. Rept., 51: 125-141, 1967.
12. Skipper, H. E. The Cell Cycle and Chemotherapy of Cancer. In: The Cell Cycle and Cancer. Ed.: R. Baserga. Marcel Dekker, New York, pp. 358-387, 1971.
13. Tvermyr, E. M. Circadian Rhythms in Hairless Mouse Epidermal DNA Synthesis as Measured by Double Labeling with H^3-Thymidine. Virchows Arch. Abt. B. Zellpath., 11: 43-54, 1972.

CHRONOBIOLOGICAL APPROACH
TO THE
THERAPEUTICS AND PATHOGENESIS
OF NEOPLASIA

S. S. Cardoso*, K. Philippens, T. Avery,
C. King, P. Cruze, C. Eastridge and
H. Von Mayersbach

The Department of Pharmacology, University of Tennessee Center
for the Health Sciences; St. Jude's Children Research Hospital;
Veterans Administration Hospital, Memphis, Tennessee and
Department fur Anatomie Medizinische Hochschule, Hannover, Germany

Supported in part by USPHS Grant CA-11332-04 and Alexander Von
Humboldt Foundation (*Senior U.S. Scientist Award)

The toxic as well as the therapeutic responses to drugs have been
shown to depend, to a significant degree, upon the time of the day
(circadian phase) of drug administration (18). While these circadian
dependent responses do not appear to represent a matter of either death
or survival of the recipient for the great majority of therapeutic agents,
such is not the case in cancer chemotherapy (3,5,8).

In cancer chemotherapy, one exploits narrow quantitative differences
between normal and tumor cells with therapeutic doses which often approach
lethal doses. Thus, the identification and use of circadian phases of
minimum host susceptibility (for drug administration) might conceivably
lead to improved chemotherapy. Evidence supporting this approach to
cancer chemotherapy has been presented (5,13,20,21).

Empirical explorations of circadian phases of drug administration
have initially led to the identification of circadian phases of greater
mitotic inhibitory effect upon experimental tumors by cyclophosphamide (2).

Subsequent studies were made with primary consideration toward
avoiding or decreasing host toxicity. For this purpose, the host's
biochemical cytokinetical and circadian mitotic rhythms data served as a
guide in the design of circadian schedules of drug administration
(chronotherapy). The corneal epithelium of the rat was chosen as the
target tissue for the antimitotic effect of the cell cycle phase-specific
agent cytosine arabinoside (ARA-C). The schedules (circadian phases)
chosen for the administration of ARA-C were those that should elicit
either maximum or minimum mitotic inhibitory effect upon mitoses in the
corneal epithelium (3,5).

The results obtained strongly suggested that host toxicity was
indeed a controllable response through chronotherapy. Subsequently,

these results were confirmed with the use of normal and tumor bearing mice in studies in which death served as the end point to measure toxicity (6,20). More significantly, these studies showed that ARA-C's therapeutic effect was maintained at the circadian phase in which its administration elicited a minimum of toxicity (5,12,13,21).

More recent and extensive work, conducted independently in different laboratories, clearly demonstrated a circadian dependent effect for cyclophosphamide both with the use of tumor bearing (1,8) and non-tumor bearing animals (14). As based on these results, a clinical protocol has just been started (11). On the other hand, these cyclophosphamide studies also revealed a significant variation in the overall levels of toxicity and of therapeutic effects, when comparing 3 successive experiments (1). Furthermore, the variations were of such magnitude as to interfere with the predictability of results.

To circumvent and/or control this variable, attempts were made to obtain a greater degree of "standardization" of the animals for periodicity studies. This was done with either pharmacological and/or physical (drug and/or light induced phase shifts) conditioning of the animals prior to the experiments (9). Clearly, if obtained, this increased standardization of the animals (response to drugs) could be therapeutically meaningful if achieved with: 1) maintained or increased circadian dependent responses to the given drug; 2) phase-shifts of circadian systems of the host not paralleled by phase-shifts of critical systems of the tumor tissue (7).

The results obtained with some of these attempts at improving chronotherapy are reported in this communication.

METHODS AND MATERIAL

Animals used: the mice used were BDF$_1$ of either sex with weights ranging from 15 to 22 grams; the rats used were of the Holtzman strain, of either sex, with weights ranging from 110 to 250 grams for the entire series of experiments. On the other hand, the weight of the animals (rats) did not differ by more than 30 grams in each single experiment. All animals were standardized for periodicity studies with alternating periods of light and darkness in which artificial lights were kept on from 0600 to 1800 hours of the day. The temperature in the animal quarters was kept at 23° C ± 2. Transplant of L1210 tumor to BDF$_1$ mice was always carried out from 0900 to 1100 hours of the day. The tumor innoculum (1x10^6 cells) was administered by the I.P. route. Treatment was begun at 24 hours post transplantation of the tumor. Some groups of tumor bearing mice were treated later, as indicated under the results.

Animal deaths resulted from the effects produced by either the drug or the tumor and post mortem examinations were frequently required to establish the actual cause. Treated animals surviving 60 days post-transplantation of the tumor were considered cured.

For the purpose of determining the effect of drug upon mitoses, control and treated animals were sacrificed at the times indicated under results, the eyes collected, fixed, stained and counted as previously described (4,5).

The treatment with either ARA-C, cyclophosphamide or dexamethasone, was carried out at the times indicated under results. Each animal received a single dose of the carcinostatic agent (dose under results) by the I.P. route.

RESULTS

Circadian dependent effect of cancer chemotherapy agents upon mitoses in the corneal epithelium.

Cytosine arabinoside.

Shown in Figure 1 are the results obtained with the administration of 30 mg/kg of body weight of ARA-C by the intraperitoneal route (IP) at either 1400 or at 2300 hours of the day. The rats were sacrificed at the times shown in the abscissa. The sacrifice for the 1400 and 2300 hours treatment groups started, respectively, 9 and 4 hours post ARA-C administration. As shown, a depression of the overall levels of cell division along with an apparent phase-shift (peak displaced from 0700 to 1100 hours of the day) follows the administration of ARA-C at 2300 hours. On the other hand, neither effect was apparent when drug administration was made at 1400 hours of the day.

Cyclophosphamide.

Figure 2 presents the results obtained with the administration of a single 360 mg/kg dose of cyclophosphamide at either 0900 or at 1630 hours of the day. When compared with untreated controls, the levels of mitoses in the corneal epithelium of mice treated at 0900 hours were inhibited to a greater degree than those which were observed in mice treated at 1630 hours.

Circadian dependency of cyclophosphamide's toxic and therapeutic effects.

Figure 3 presents the pooled percentages of cures and mortalities (from 3 experiments) observed for each of 8 treatment-time subgroups of L1210 bearing mice. In addition to pooling the data from 3 experiments, we also pooled (means in the figure) the results obtained with the administration of cyclophosphamide at 2 dose levels, i.e., at 300 and 360 mg/kg. Thus, in fact, each of the different time points shown in Figure 3 depicts the percent cures or deaths (mortality axis) observed with the treatment of a total of 60 mice. As shown in the Figure, both mortality and cure rates showed a significant circadian dependence; i.e.; varying degrees of response related to the time of drug administration. In addition, the comparison of the 2 curves clearly indicates an inverse relationship to exist between cures and toxic deaths.

Table I and Table II.

The data in these Tables present an overall view of dose-responses to cyclophosphamide as well as the variations in response observed from experiment to experiment. For the purpose of evaluating the dose-response curves (from 3 experiments), the data obtained with the administration of the agent at all circadian phases were pooled. The data thus prepared, and presented in Table I, indicate a direct relationship to exist between dose and response for both the toxic and the therapeutic effects of the drug. Table II focuses upon the variation of results which occurred from experiment to experiment. It shows that this variation ranged from 12 to 55 percent in terms of toxic deaths and from 9 to 20 percent for cure rates.

Attempts to curb drug toxicity, through drug-induced phase shifts.

Figure 4.

Figure 4 presents the results obtained in one experiment in which the circadian peak levels of cell division in the cornea of untreated control rats were compared with those observed in the cornea of animals treated with Dexamethasone, or ARA-C, or Dexamethasone plus ARA-C. As indicated in the graph, ARA-C was administered at 2300 hours of the day before sacrifice to rats pretreated or not with 400 µg of dexamethasone at 1500 hours of the day (8 hours prior to ARA-C administration). Comparison of the experimental groups with controls reveals: a) displacement of the high levels of mitoses from 0700 to 0900 hours in the dexamethasone group of rats; b) a significant inhibition of the overall levels of mitoses in the cornea of rats treated with ARA-C alone. c) the absence of ARA-C's mitotic inhibitory effects in dexamethasone pretreated rats.

Drug induced alterations of circadian mitotic rhythms in normal and tumor tissue: the response to dexamethasone.

Table III presents the mitotic counts observed in two tumors (Ehrlich carcinoma and Morris 7777 hepatoma) and the respective corneas of the tumor bearing animals. In these experiments, the tumor bearing animals were subdivided into two groups, control and dexamethasone treated animals. The experimental group received a single 400 µg dose of dexamethasone at 2300 hours of the day. Sacrifice of both control and experimental animals was done at either 32, 36, or 44 hours after dexamethasone administration (respectively at 0700, 1100 or 1900 hours of the day). Immediately after sacrifice, samples of the tumor as well as the eyes of these animals were harvested for the mitotic determinations. As shown in the Table, dexamethasone produced a profound depression of mitoses in the corneas but not in the tumor tissues of these animals.

DISCUSSION

Biological rhythms have for a long time been recognized as an adaptation-response by living organisms to natural oscillations of environmental parameters such as light, temperature and the availability of food. More recent studies in this field of biology have identified: a) disturbances of biological rhythms which are characteristic of certain neoplastic diseases (10,15); and b) the influence which circadian rhythms exert upon drug effect (2,17).

These findings led us to initiate studies which eventually were extended to cover the following 3 distinct areas of chronobiology:

I)   Determinations of circadian dependent effects of cancer chemo-
     therapy agents.
II) Modulation of circadian rhythms in attempts to modify the
     toxicity of subsequently administered chemotherapeutic agents.
III) Study of the circadian dependent effects of drugs in normal
     and tumor tissues.

To facilitate the discussion, the results obtained in each of the above
areas will be dealt with separately.

I. Circadian dependent effect of cancer chemotherapy agents.

Initially, the corneal epithelium of rats and mice served as a
target tissue for our determinations of the circadian dependent mitotic
inhibitory effect of carcinostatic agents. We felt that with a homogenous
population of cells, high rates of cell division, and a high amplitude of
circadian mitotic rhythm, this particular tissue would constitute a very
appropriate and practical system (4,5) for studying and tentatively
identifying circadian phases of maximum and minimum susceptibility to
the antimitotic effect of carcinostatic agents. Furthermore, the data
obtained with the use of ARA-C and cyclophosphamide in the cornea, were
subsequently confirmed in studies done with BDF_1 control and L1210 bearing
mice (8,12). Shown in Figures 1, 2, 3 and Tables I and II, are the results obtained in a series of experiments with either ARA-C or
cyclophosphamide. The data above demonstrate a clear circadian dependency
for both drugs and a classical dose-response relationship for cyclophosphamide. They demonstrate, as well, that this pronounced circadian
dependency makes it mandatory, we believe, to avoid drug administration
at hours of increased host susceptibility. On the other hand, the data
in Tables I and II point out that toxicity, along with the large
variations of results observed from experiment to experiment, still limit
the full potential of chronotherapy.

II. Modulation of circadian rhythms and drug interaction. Attempts to curtail toxicity.

Toxicity, as well as the above variation of experimental results,
could in part be related to spontaneous time displacements (phase-shifts)
of the circadian mitotic peaks and troughs. Therefore, attempts were
made to develop methods with which to control or limit these spontaneous
phase-shifts. We felt, for instance, that with the use of these drug
induced phase-shifts we could override the normal control mechanisms
operating in the host and thus overcome or limit experimental variation
(9). These drug-induced phase-shifts would hopefully work as a
"resetting pharmacological cue", to be applied at specific circadian
phases, in preparation for chronotherapeutic experiments. The results,
obtained in one of these experiments in which the animals were pretreated
with dexamethasone, are presented in Figure 4. The time span shown
covers only the circadian phase of maximum mitotic activity as dexamethasone, when administered at 1500 hours, exerts its preponderant
effect at this particular phse of the circadian mitotic rhythm (4).

In this experiment (Figure 4), the dexamethasone treated group of
animals had maximum levels of cell division at 0900 hours while, in

other experiments, the circadian mitotic peak occurred between 0700 and 0900 hours. In contrast, the control mitotic peak occurred at 0700 hours in this experiment and from 0500 to 1000 hours in the entire series of experiments. These results indicated that we had at hand a method with which to enhance the standardization of the animals for periodicity studies. Thus, in subsequent studies, some of the experimental groups were pretreated with dexamethasone and subsequently with ARA-C. In one experiment, in which 180 rats were used, the mitotic rates were determined in the corneas of animals treated with dexamethasone, with ARA-C, or with ARA-C in combination with dexamethasone. The results obtained are presented in Figure 4. They demonstrate: a) The pronounced mitotic inhibitory effect of ARA-C; b) A phase shifting effect by dexamethasone; c) The remarkable interaction between ARA-C and dexamethasone in which dexamethasone, administered at 1500 hours, rendered the animals completely resistant to the mitotic inhibitory effects of ARA-C administered subsequently at 2300 hours.

The demonstration that this drug interaction might be of practical value in terms of curbing host toxicity remains as a task for the future. Although preliminary experiments have been carried out with these "drug standardized" animals, the results obtained thus far are not conclusive (9).

III. <u>Circadian dependent drug effects in normal and tumor tissues.</u>

This series of experiments was designed to obtain and compare the responses (7,16,19,22) of normal and tumor tissue to drugs known to produce phase-shifts (4,16). Exploitable differences in the responses of normal and tumor tissue should lead to improved chronotherapeutics and to further understanding of the defective mechanisms which have been described in some types of neoplasia (22). One could for instance pretreat the tumor bearing animals and separate critical phases of drug susceptibility of tumor tissue from those of normal tissues. Subsequently one could administer the therapeutic agent at the "proper time", i.e., at times known to elicit maximum effect upon the tumor and minimum effect upon the normal tissues of the host.

The data obtained in two of these experiments are presented in Table III (7,19). The two tumors investigated differ significantly from normal tissue in their response to dexamethasone, as illustrated by the profound suppression of mitoses found in the corneas but not in the tumor tissues. These differences in response suggest: a) that continuing efforts in this area of chronobiology should ultimately result in significantly improved schedules of drug administration for cancer chemotherapy; b) that drug induced phase-shifts may serve as a tool in studies focusing on the pathogenesis of neoplasia.

SUMMARY AND CONCLUSION

The results presented in this communication indicate:
A) That a significant improvement in the therapeutic effectiveness of at least two cancer chemotherapeutic agents, cytosine arabinoside and cyclophosphamide, can currently be obtained by their administration at circadian phases of maximum drug tolerance by the host.

B) That foreseeable progress will bring to our hands additional knowledge that will insure therapeutic exploitation of the critical differences between normal and tumor tissue to circadian phases of susceptibility for numerous other established antineoplastic agents.

C) Attainment of the latter will herald the establishment of chronotherapy as a major consideration in the preparation of chemo-therapeutic protocols for the treatment of cancer.

TABLE I. The Therapeutic and Toxic Effects of Cyclophosphamide Upon BDF_1 Mice Bearing L_{1210} Leukemia

Effect	Cyclophosphamide mg/kg of body weight			
	180*	240	300	360
Toxic deaths	26 (10.8%)	53 (22%)	90 (37.5%)	144 (60%)
Cures (60 days	20 (8.3%)	36 (15%)	43 (17.9%)	44 (18.3%)

* Total of 240 mice/dose

TABLE II. The Therapeutic and Toxic Effects of Cyclophosphamide Upon BDF_1 Mice Bearing L_{1210} Leukemia

Experiment	Toxicity Deaths	Cures
#3 (320)	40 mice (12.5%)	65 (20%)
#1 (320)	94 mice (29.3%)	49 (15%)
#2 (320)	179 mice (55.9%)	31 (9.6%)

( ) number of mice/experiment

TABLE III. The Effect of Dexamethasone Upon Mitoses of Normal and Tumor Tissues

Tissue	Treatment	Mitoses/100 fields ± SE*			C/D**
		0700h	1100h	1900h	
Ehrlich*** Carcinoma	CONTROL DEXAMETHASONE	70±10 62±11	86±18 61± 5	65± 4 103±16	0.97
MORRIS 7777 Hepatoma	CONTROL DEXAMETHASONE	70±11 72± 5	104±10 84±11	64± 5 65±11	1
CORNEA (rats)	CONTROL DEXAMETHASONE	148±11 2.4± 2	107±10 4.4± 1	37±11 14± 5	14

		Mitoses/1000 cells ± SE			
		0700h	1100h	1900h	
CORNEA*** (mice)	CONTROL DEXAMETHASONE	7.4±1.8 1 ± .04	10 ±1.1 2.7±0.8	0.74±0.25 1.7 ±0.4	3.3

*   Standard error of the mean values (3 or more animals).

** C/D =   Mean (0700 + 1100 + 1900) of control/mean of values in Dexamethasone treated animals.

***   G. Rosene, L. Scheving and S. S. Cardoso (19).

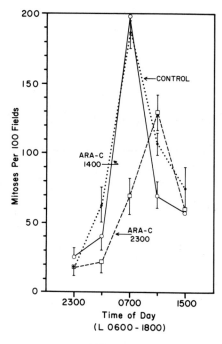

FIG. 1

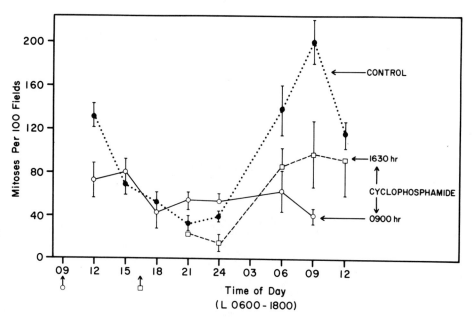

FIG. 2

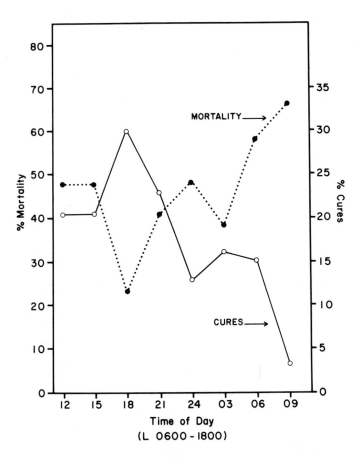

FIG. 3

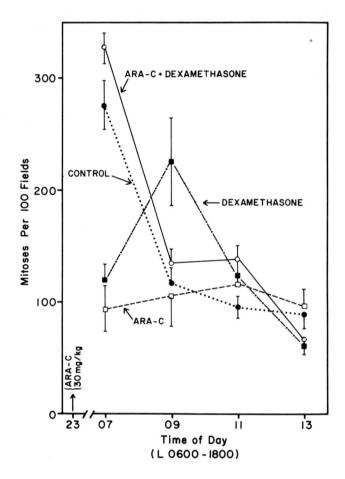

FIG. 4

REFERENCES

1. Avery, T., Cardoso, S. S., Venditti, J. and Goldin, A. Investigation of circadian dependence of host and tumor responses to cyclophosphamide. In preparation for publication.

2. Badran, A. F. and Echave Llanos, J. M. Persistence of mitotic circadian rhythm of transplantable mammary carcinoma after 35 generations: its bearing on the success of treatment with endoxan. J. National Cancer Institute 35, 285-290, 1965.

3. Cardoso, S. S. and Carter, R. Circadian mitotic rhythm as a time table guide for the administration of antimetabolites. Federation Proceedings 27, 659, 1968.

4. Cardoso, S. S. and J. G. Sowell. Control of cell division in the cornea of rats. I. Interaction between Isoproterenol and Dexamethasone. Proc. Soc. Exptl. Biology and Medicine 147, 309-313, 1974.

5. Cardoso, S. S. and Carter, R. E. Circadian mitotic rhythm as a guide for the administration of antimetabolites. Proc. Soc. Exptl. Biology and Medicine 131, 1403-1406, 1969.

6. Cardoso, S. S., Scheving, L. E. and Halberg, F. Mortality of mice as influenced by the hour of the day of drug (ARA-C) administration. Pharmacologist 12, 302, 1970.

7. Cardoso, S. S., Blatteis, C. M., Fuste, F. J. and Morris, H. P. Sensitivity of Morris Hepatoma 7777 circadian mitotic rhythm to dexamethasone. Fifth International Congress of Pharmacology Proceedings, Page 37, San Francisco, 1972.

8. Cardoso, S. S., Avery, T., Venditti, J. and Goldin, A. Investigation of circadian dependence of host and tumor responses to cyclophosphamide. Sixth Intern. Congress of Pharmacology Abstract p. 1334 Helsinki, Finland, 1975.

9. Cardoso, S. S., Philippens, K. M. H., Sauerbier, I., Bhattacharya, R., Avery, T. and H. von Mayersbach. Standardization of chronotherapeutics through light and isoproterenol induced circadian phase-shifts Federation Proceedings 35, 724, 1976.

10. Doe, R. P., Vennes, J. A. and Flink, E. B. Diurnal variation of 17-hydroxy corticosteroids, sodium potassium, magnesium and creatinine in normal subjects and in cases of treated adrenal insufficiency and Cushing's syndrome. J. Clinical Endocrinology 20, 253-265, 1960.

11. Eastridge, C. and Cardoso, S. S. unpublished observations.

12. Halberg, F., Haus, E., Cardoso, S. S., Scheving, L. E., Kuhl, J. F. W., Shiotsuka, R., Rosene, G., Pauly, J. E., Runge, W., Spalding, J. E., Lee, J. E. and Good, R. E. Towards a chronotherapy of neoplasia: Tolerance of Treatment Depends Upon Host Rhythms. Experientia 29, 909-934, 1973.

13. Haus, E., Halberg, F., Scheving, L. E., Cardoso, S. S., Kuhl, J. F. W., Sothern, R., Shiotsuka, R., Hwang, D. S. and Pauly, J. E. Increased tolerance of leukemic mice arabinosyl cytosine with schedule adjusted to circadian system. Science 177, 80-82, 1972.

14. Haus, E., Fernandes, G., Kuhl, J. F. W., Yunis, E. J., Lee, J. E. and Halberg, F. Murine circadian susceptibility rhythm to cyclophosphamide. Chronobiologia 1, 270-277, 1974.

15. Hymes, A. C. and Doe, R. P. Adrenal function in cancer of the lung with and without Cushing's syndrome. American Journal of Medicine 33, 398-407, 1962.

16. King, C. D., Kauker, M. L. and Cardoso, S. S. Control of cell division in the cornea of rats III. Mitogenic effect of isoproterenol and theophylline. Proc. Soc. Exptl. Biology and Medicine 149, 840-844, 1975.

17. Radzialowski, F. M. and Bousquet, W. F. Daily rhythmic variation in hepatic drug metabolism in the rat and mouse. Journal Pharmacol. Exptl. Therapeutics 163, 229-238, 1968.

18. Reinberg, A. and Halberg, F. Circadian Pharmacology. Annual Review of Pharmacology 455-492, 1971.

19. Rosene G., Scheving, L. E. and Cardoso, S. S. In preparation for publication.

20. Scheving, L. E., Cardoso, S. S., Pauly, J. E., Halberg, F. and Haus, E. Variations in susceptibility of mice to the carcinostatic agent arabinosyl cytosine. In Chronobiology pp 213-217. L. E. Scheving, J. E. Pauly and F. Halberg (eds). Tokio, Igaku Shoin Ltd, 1974.

21. Scheving, L. E., Haus, E., Kuhl, J. F. W., Halberg, F. and Cardoso, S. S. Close Reproduction by Different Laboratories of Characteristics of Circadian Rhythm in 1-D-Arabinofuranosylcytosine Tolerance by Mice. Cancer Research 36, 1133-1137, 1976.

22. Sharma, R. K. (In Press) Modified Cellular and Molecular Controls in Neoplasia. Japanese-Australian-American Cancer Symposium, Raven Press, New York.

THE ONCOGENIC IMPLICATIONS OF CHRONOBIOTICS IN THE SYNCHRONIZATION
OF MAMMALIAN CIRCADIAN RHYTHMS: BARBITURATES AND METHYLATED XANTHINES

Charles F. Ehret and Kenneth W. Dobra

Division of Biological and Medical Research
Argonne National Laboratory
Argonne, Illinois 60439

INTRODUCTION

This paper gives cause to raise seriously the question "Are circadian
dyschronics a new high-risk group in cancer epidemiology?" By the term
circadian dyschronic we mean an individual whose circadian temporal organization is sufficiently disordered as to make difficult or ambiguous diagnosis of the circadian phases at which characteristic chronotypic functions
occur. The question is an important one in preventive medicine, because if
there is a positive correlation between circadian dyschronism and high cancer risk (as present evidence cited below suggests), then systematic measures designed to guard against environmental inputs and lifestyles that
tend to cause dyschronism should have the concomitant value of reducing
tumor incidence. Because contemporary urban societies are heavily contaminated with chronobiotics and other circadian zeitgebers that alter the
biological time structure by rephasing circadian rhythms, dyschronics and
marginal or "minimal deviation dyschronics" probably constitute a significant fraction of the population.

The methylated xanthines and barbiturates recently implicated as carcinogens or as cocarcinogens (32,33,34,38,40) have long been known for
their effects upon wakefulness and sleep. These effects are undoubtedly
due at least in part to their chronobiotic action: that is to say, they
are clearly capable of altering biological time structure by rephasing a
circadian rhythm. The action appears to be a general one, since theophylline and pentobarbital have been shown to phase-shift chronotypically the
circadian rhythm of deep body temperature in the rat (11), and theophylline
and caffeine similarly influence circadian leaf movements in a higher plant,
Phaseolus (27). Correlated with the phase-shifting effect of theophylline
in the mammal is its well-known influence upon enzyme induction and glycogen depletion. This influence has more recently been shown to be strikingly chronotypic: theophylline administered shortly before and during the
early active phase causes a maximum phase delay in the circadian temperature rhythm, and maximally induces the regulatory enzyme tyrosine aminotransferase (TAT) at about the same time (10). The chronobiotic action of
pentobarbital is similar: it causes maximum phase delay when administered
in the hours shortly before and during the early active phase (Figures 1
and 2). On the other hand, when theophylline is given in the early

1101

inactive phase, when TAT is at a minimum and glycogen levels are high, a maximum in both glycogen depletion and in phase shift is seen, but during this phase of the circadian cycle the chronobiotic induces phase advance (Figure 2A). In noting the efficacy of pentobarbital and the methylated xanthines as chronobiotics, the present study shows that dosage levels of phenobarbital in the diet at and near those that are cocarcinogenic also induce circadian dyschronism.

PROCEDURES AND MATERIALS USED

Male Charles River rats (200-250 g) were housed singly in two controlled environment rooms at Argonne National Laboratory, and their deep-body temperatures were monitored continually by means of intraperitoneally implanted temperature telemeters; temperature recordings were made at 15-minute intervals by means of a data acquisition system previously described (11). During the 9 days preceding the administration of phenobarbital in the diet, rats were entrained by programmed feeding cycles (feeding followed by "starvation," FS), and by programmed light-dark cycles (LD cycles). The feeding phase of the FS cycle consisted of presenting a complete diet containing 30% casein and free of phenobarbital, which coincided with the first 7 hours of the dark (D) phase of the LD cycle. The starvation (S) phase (absence of food) occurred at the eighth hour of the dark phase and continued for the next 10 hours of the dark and during all of the light phase of the LD cycle. The irradiance levels during the daily DL 17:7 cycle were for D $\sim$ 40 lux (for 17 hours) and for L $\sim$ 600 lux (for 7 hours) at cage level from 15-watt daylight fluorescent lamps. Entrainment on the control diet was followed first by a 2 day starvation-interval (SS) still on DL, and then by ad libitum free access (FF) to the new diet which consisted of the control diet supplemented with phenobarbital. During the period following entrainment and on FF, the rats thus received no further entraining clues and remained in "free run" (FF and continuous darkness, DD) for 7 days.

The efficacy of the entrainment protocols, as well as the drug effects, were observed as oscillations in the deep-body temperature as monitored by the telemeters. The telemetry data, a series of frequencies which have a polynomial relationship to temperature, were collected in a digital format. The digital frequencies were first transformed to the equivalent temperature in °C by a second degree polynomial with unique coefficients for each transmitter. Following plotting and visual inspection of the temperature data, an animal in each of the phenobarbital dosage categories was selected for statistical analysis. The dosage categories were control (no phenobarbital) and 0.05%, 0.2%, and 0.3% phenobarbital added to the diet. The autocovariance and power spectral estimates were computed on each series in a manner similar to the methods of Panofsky and Halberg (30,31), except that the raw data were not transformed initially, to determine the frequency composition of the series and the variance associated with each frequency. The program used for this computation was selected from the Biomedical Programs (5).

RESULTS

Figure 3 contains the raw temperature data from eight rats that were given varying doses of phenobarbital in the diet for 7 days, ranging from 0.05% to 0.3%. The control animal maintained a strong circadian rhythm of deep body temperature through free-run (FF, DD). With increasing dosage of phenobarbital in the diet two responses are observed. First, the mean body temperature remains nearly a constant with only minor trends or drifts observable for individual animals during the period of observation. Second, the circadian oscillation becomes less evident with increased dosage. This seems to be due to a decrease in the overall range of the temperatures from the mean, thus reducing the amplitude of the oscillations. There is also an increase in random transient changes in deep-body temperatures which tend to further obscure the circadian oscillations. In the extreme case (0.3%), where the circadian component of the deep-body temperature is nearly obscured, there appears to be an absence of any other dominant oscillation.

Power spectral analysis was used first to determine if there was a decrease in the variance of the circadian component of the frequency spectrum; and second, to determine if the transient frequencies were randomly distributed or if a dominant frequency with period less than 24 hours became evident.

Figure 4 contains the raw variance spectral estimates of the four time series in °C/cycle/96 hours. The abscissa has been converted to period (τ), the reciprocal of frequency. The analysis shows that as the percent of phenobarbital in the diet increases, the variance of the 24-hour component diminishes, and there is no significant increase in any other component of the frequency spectrum. Figure 4, inset, shows the variance of the power spectral estimates at a frequency of 0.042 cycles/hour ($\tau = 24$ hours) as a function of the percent phenobarbital in the diet. Again, the 24-hour component diminishes very strongly with increases in phenobarbital in the diet.

Two additional comments should be made. First, the amount of phenobarbital actually ingested by each animal was not known, and therefore the data could not be normalized for percent phenobarbital ingested per unit time. Since animals in the higher dosage categories probably consumed less food per unit time, the amount of phenobarbital in the animal was probably not as high as the proportional increase of percent phenobarbital in the diet would suggest. Therefore, the suppression of the 24-hour component of the frequency spectrum is potentially much greater with increases in phenobarbital than the data suggest. In addition, differences in phase of the deep-body temperature following resumption of free-run on a diet free of phenobarbital was not studied. These variables are presently under investigation in our laboratory.

DISCUSSION

In a mammal, several days are required after administration of a single dose of a chronobiotic, given during some phase of the circadian cycle that is responsive to resetting, before one can resolve distinctly whether or not a phase-shift has occurred. For example in Figure 1, when pentobarbital was given at 0408 on the seventh day after entrainment had begun (third record from the top of the figure) there is clear evidence of a phase delay of about 12 hours on days 11 and 12 when compared with free-running controls (e.g., top and bottom of the figure). However, during the first few days following injection, irregular "phase-transients" are seen in the oscillations. These irregularities make it difficult or impossible to predict at what phase angle the oscillation may ultimately stabilize. Since every infradian-mode eukaryotic cell in the body is a circadian oscillator (8), one may best regard the phase-response transients seen in a metazoan organism (composed of billions of cells), as representing cohorts of cells in the various tissues and organs that remain somewhat out of synchrony with one another following the stimulus, until they are finally brought together into circadian synchrony once again by intercellular coordinating mechanisms (also composed of cells in disarray during the transient). The continual delivery of chronobiotics to such a metazoan system would tend to keep it in a constant state of disarray. Even if individual cells, or cohorts of cells, that are members of the coordinating system retain their singular integrity as functional circadian oscillators, the system as a whole would probably appear to be dyschronic if the cells were not in synchrony with one another. One might expect the number of cells in disarray in such a system to be a function of the dose (below saturation levels) of the chronobiotic given (Figures 3 and 4). However, even at the lowest dosages administered, producing only a "minimal deviation dyschronic," it is probable that very large numbers of cells in the body receive and act upon the signal to reset their circadian oscillators.

Although the molecular basis for the circadian clock is not generally agreed upon (16), there is a great deal of evidence that many of the chronotypic properties of circadian systems are remarkably similar at cellular and organismic levels. Some of these properties are included in the schematic for a circadian oscillator given in Figure 5. Fundamental to the present thesis that chronobiotics are carcinogens is the observation that gene action is a circadian chronotypic property (8). Any circadian phase-response in a nucleated, multicellular system requires a corresponding re-setting of the ongoing phases of transcription and of replication (or of replication-probability in infradian cells, whose cell-division probability is low) in all cells of the body. It is difficult to conceive of how such intervention, either directly or indirectly, into the mechanisms of ongoing nucleic acid synthesis on single strands of DNA could occur without some associated increase in risk of mutational damage. Indeed, evidence from prokaryotic systems indicates that increased spontaneous mutagenesis occurs during transcription (18); furthermore, evidence from protistans has shown that heat synchronized cells in the course of synchronization become over-charged with an excess of DNA (19) of unique sequences (41), which is then cast out of the nucleus by what could be interpreted today as an excision and repair mechanism on a massive scale. The chronobiotic role of the bar-biturates is probably a broad one, not only in affecting nucleic acid synthesis (32), but also as strongly competitive base analogs (23) influencing all aspects of purine and pyrimidine metabolism. The experimental and theoretical bases for associating circadian energy-reserve utilization with gene action, as schematized in Figure 5, and with the basic molecular mechanism of the circadian clock have been already described extensively elsewhere (6,19). Briefly stated, the circadian oscillation occurs only during infradian growth (when cell-division probability is low); at the start of the infradian mode, energy reserves (such as glycogen) are at their highest, and during their course of depletion and synthesis, the intracellular levels of energy reserves show a marked circadian rhythm, the regulation of which by the catecholamine and indoleamine pathways are chronotypically similar in protistans (6,9) and in higher organisms (2,4). The circadian regulation of energy, mediated through the biogenic amines, therefore appears to be a general property of the circadian biological oscillator at the cellular level, which has been exploited by the higher organisms in the course of their neurophysiological and neuroendocrinological integrative evolution. These pathways should, therefore, represent not only universally applicable foci for chronobiotic control of the circadian clock, but, if chronobiotics are carcinogens, then the same pathways should also represent the sites of increase in tumor incidence wherever blockage or perversion of a function is induced by a genetic deficiency disease, or a drug, or by a dietary habit.

Consistent with this thesis is the apparent correlation observed between patients with neuroblastoma (21,25), or ganglioneuroma (26) and disturbed catecholamine metabolism; the concurrences between childhood leukemia and phenylketonuria (28); the association between hepatic cancer and a variety of liver diseases, including glycogen-storage and other non-malignant metabolic disorders (14,29,39); the apparent association between leukoplakia and abnormal tryptophan metabolism (37); and the apparently high cancer mortality among diabetics (39). Widely prescribed drugs that interfere with catecholamine metabolism include some associated with human cancer, such as reserpine, which is associated with breast cancer. Other drugs that look highly suspicious are amphetamine (correlated with Hodgkins disease), diphenylhydantoin, chlorpromazine, and other phenothiazines (20). An interesting drug-like carcinogen is the bracken fern, capable of causing bladder cancer in cattle (3) and prevalent in human nutrition, in Japan. One of the carcinogens involved, present in bracken fern is shikimic acid, an intermediate in the pathway of phenylalanine and tyrosine metabolism. Also of importance in human nutrition are the methylated xanthines mentioned earlier for their chronotypic inductive effect on TAT (10) and chronobiotic action (11); however, epidemiologic studies have associated coffee drinking, but not tea drinking with cancer of the lower urinary tract (38). It is conceivable that the average habitual time of day for drinking these two beverages differs in the population studied. If one recalls that the chronobiotic action of a methylated xanthine is chronotypically significant, causing phase delay, no phase change, or phase advance (Figure 2) depending upon when the methylated xanthine is given, then one should also expect that mutagenicity and oncogenic sequelae are also chronotypic and a function of the magnitude of the induced phase change. Hence, if one extrapolates from rodent to man, coffee or tea consumed in the mid-to-late afternoon may be less oncogenic than the same beverages taken in the early morning or late evening hours. Similar considerations of the possible influence of the habitual temporal patterns in ones lifestyle on cancer-risk must be given to the many nutritional studies that claim a reduced incidence of tumors for rodents (12,35,36) and cattle (1) on long-term caloric restriction. As pointed out earlier (7) in each of these studies the food-restricted animals were actually favored because programmed-feeding gave them circadian cues, whereas the non-restricted ones were fed ad libitum, a protocol that generally leads to dyschronism in old isolated animals (personal communication, George A. Sacher). Other drug-like effects of diet are known that are of potentially large chronobiotic significance, such as the tendency of a high-protein meal to stimulate the catecholamines, and of a high-carbohydrate meal to stimulate serotonin-biogenic amines that are normally chronotypically elevated half a day apart from one another, during active and inactive phases respectively (13,15,22). Finally, one can point out that if circadian dyschronism is an etiologically significant clue that oncogenic damage has occurred and is occurring, then rhythmic infradian functions, such as menstruation and ovulation, that depend upon the circadian oscillation to measure the days faithfully should also be adversely affected in dyschronic individuals. It is well documented that irregular menses are one of the factors common to human populations at high risk of breast cancer, ovarian cancer, and cancer of the corpus uteri (17). In conclusion, we concur with Ernst Wynder's view, in considering persons at high risk in cancer (42), that "the leading causes of death today are the result of lifestyle," but we add that it is now our burden to define the biophysical and temporal boundaries of "style."

SUMMARY

Methylated xanthines and barbiturates are not only chronobiotics, but are also oncogens or cocarcinogens. Low levels of phenobarbital in the diet induce circadian dyschronism in rats: conversely, ad libitum dietary regimens that tend to favor dyschronism in old rats also correlate with high tumor incidence. Epidemiological evidence shows that persons at high risk of cancer include those who have had genetic deficiency diseases or who have taken drugs that are known to interfere with the putative molecular-genetic pathways for circadian regulation: those interfering especially with the storage and regulation of energy reserves, and the regulation of the catecholamine and indoleamine synthetic pathways. It is suggested that each time that the circadian biological oscillator in a cell is reset by a chronobiotic, or by any other circadian zeitgeber, there is increased risk of oncogenic damage to the gene-action machinery of the cell; for this reason all chronobiotics may be oncogenic when taken at a vulnerable phase of the circadian cycle.

ACKNOWLEDGMENTS

We thank John C. Meinert, Kenneth R. Groh, and Jay L. Schlabach for their excellent technical assistance, and acknowledge fruitful discussions with Drs. Carl Peraino and R. J. M. Fry. This work was supported by the U.S. Energy Research and Development Administration.

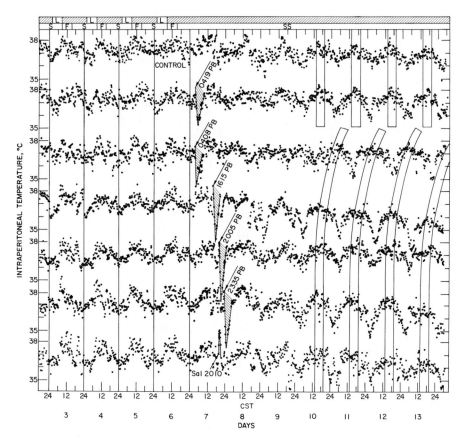

FIG. 1. Telemetry plot of deep-body temperatures measured every 15 minutes
in seven rats over 11 days. During days 1 through 6 (days 1 and 2 not
shown), the animals were entrained by daily programs of feeding (FS 7:17)
and i-lumination (DL 17:7). During days 7 through 13, the animals free-ran
in constant dim light (DD) and starvation (SS, top bars). Pentobarbital
(PB, 40 mg/kg) was injected at times shown by arrows on day 7. The rat at
the top (control) was uninjected; the rat at the bottom received saline
only (at 0814 hours). The induced phase shifts are highlighted by bars
drawn through the thermal peaks on days 10 through 13 (after Ehret, Potter,
and Dobra, 11).

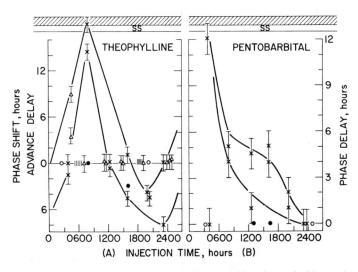

FIG. 2. A. Phase response curve, relating magnitude and direction of theophylline-induced phase shift in thermal peaks of the rat to the time of injection of the drug. The results from three separate experiments are shown. The injections were given during free-run under conditions of SSDD. Crosses and triangles are for a dosage of 75 mg/kg body weight. Open and closed circles represent uninjected and saline injected controls, respectively. The short vertical bars represent a dosage of 30 mg/kg body weight, in which, in ten rats, no phase shifts were induced. The vertical brackets are the ranges of ± 1 hour for thermal peaks (from Ehret et al., Ref. 11). B. As in A, but for pentobarbital at 40 mg/kg, injected during free-run SSDD. For complete experimental details see Ehret et al. (11).

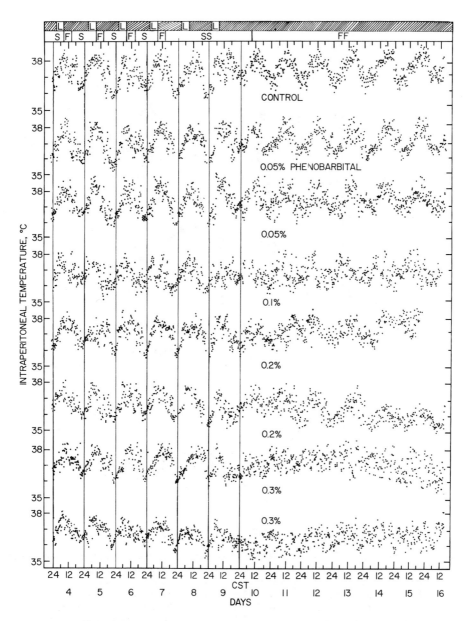

FIG. 3. Telemetry plot of deep-body temperatures measured every 15 minutes in eight rats over 13 days. During days 1 to 7 (days 1 to 3 not shown), the animals were entrained by daily programs of feeding (FS 7:17) and illumination (DL 17:7). During days 8 and 9, the animals continued on LD entrainment but were not fed. During days 10 through 16, the rats "free-ran" in constant dim light (DD) with food continuously present (FF). The rat at the top (control) received a 30% protein diet free of phenobarbital, while the remaining rats received a 30% protein diet with the given percentage of the dry weight as phenobarbital.

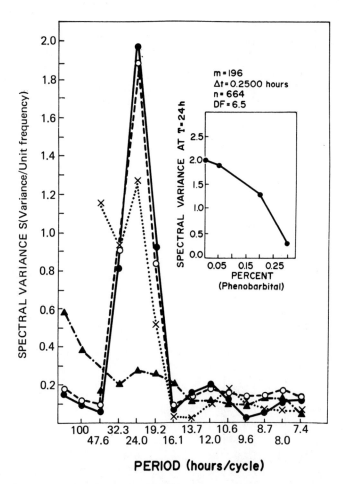

FIG. 4. Power spectral estimates of four rats over a period of 7 days with data points every 15 minutes. The ordinate is variance of power spectral estimates in units of $(°C)^2/cycle/96$ hours; the abscissa shows the periods at which spectral estimates were calculated in units of hours. There were 664 data points/rat, and the total number of lags was 196. The dotted line (-.-), control diet; open circles (--0--), 0.05% phenobarbital diet; X's (...X...), 0.2% phenobarbital diet; filled triangles (-.-▲-.-), 0.3% phenobarbital diet. Inset: Power spectral estimates at τ = 24 hours for the same 4 rats plotted as a function of the percent phenobarbital in the diet.

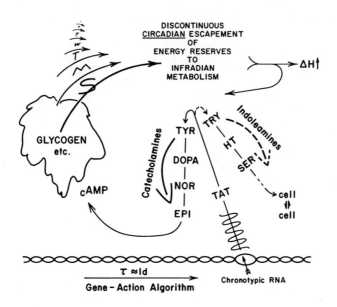

FIG. 5. An energy-reserve escapement with alternate path options (the one choice being if catecholamines, then "release"; vs. if indoleamines, then "hold") is coupled to a gene-action circadian oscillator that generates chronotypic enzymes (such as TAT) that control the path of choice. This scheme results in long-term conservation of energy reserves through circadian metering during infradian growth. During diurnal entrainment, glycogen depletion occurs daily, represented by the arrows and days-of-the-week (upper left) (from Ehret and Dobra, Ref. 9).

REFERENCES

1. Anderson, D.E., Pope, L.S., and Stephens, D. Nutrition And Eye Cancer In Cattle. Journal Natl. Cancer Inst. 45: 697-707, 1970.

2. Axelrod, J. The Pineal Gland: A Neurochemical Transducer. Science 184: 1341-1348, 1974.

3. Berg, J.W. Diet. In: Persons At High Risk Of Cancer. Ed.: Joseph F. Fraumeni, Jr., Academic Press, New York, pp. 201-224, 1975.

4. Black, I.B., and Axelrod, J. The Regulation Of Some Biochemical Circadian Rhythms. In: Biochemical Actions Of Hormones. Ed.: G. Litwack, Academic Press, New York, pp. 135-155, 1970.

5. Dixon, W. BMD Biomedical Computer Programs, University of California Press, Berkeley, pp. 459-482, 1970.

6. Dobra, K.W., and Ehret, C.F. Circadian Regulation Of Glycogen, Tyrosine Aminotransferase, And Several Respiratory Parameters In Solid Agar Cultures Of Tetrahymena pyriformis. Chronobiologia (in press) 1976.

7. Ehret, C.F. Significance Of Circadian Rhythms. In: Ageing And Levels Of Biological Organization. Ed.: Austin M. Brues and George A. Sacher, University of Chicago Press, Chicago and London, pp. 209-217, 1965.

8. Ehret, C.F. The Sense Of Time: Evidence For Its Molecular Basis In The Eukaryotic Gene-action System. Adv. Biol. Med. Phys. 15: 47-77, 1974.

9. Ehret, C.F., and Dobra, K.W. The Infradian Eukaryotic Cell: A Circadian Energy-reserve Escapement. Chronobiologia, (in press) 1976.

10. Ehret, C.F., and Potter, V.R. Circadian Chronotypic Induction of Tyrosine Aminotransferase And Depletion Of Glycogen By Theophylline In The Rat. Int. J. Chronobiol. 2: 321-326, 1974.

11. Ehret, C.F., Potter, V.R., and Dobra, K.W. Chronotypic Action Of Theophylline And Pentobarbital As Circadian Zeitgebers In The Rat. Science 188: 1212-1215, 1975.

12. Ershoff, B.H., Bajwa, G.S., Field, J.B., and Baretta, L.A. Comparative Effects Of Purified Diets And A Natural Food Stock Ration On The Tumor Incidence Of Mice Exposed To Multiple Sublethal Doses Of Total-body X-Irradiation. Cancer Research 29: 780-788, 1969.

13. Fernstrom, J.D., and Wurtman, R.J. Nutrition And The Brain. Science 230: 84-91, 1974.

14. Fraumeni, J.F., Jr., Miller, R.W., and Hill, J.A. Primary Carcinoma Of The Liver In Childhood: An Epidemiologic Study. Journal of the National Cancer Institute 40: 1087-1099, 1968.

15. Halberg, F. Protection BY Timing Treatment According To Bodily Rhythms - An Analogy To Protection By Scrubbing Before Surgery. Chrono-Biologia 1 (Suppl. 1): 27-67, 1974.

16. Hastings, J.W., and Schweiger, H.G. The Molecular Basis Of Circadian Rhythms. Dahlem Konferenzen, Berlin (in press), 1976.

17. Henderson, B.E., Gerkins, V.R., and Pike, M.C. Sexual Factors And Pregnancy. In: Persons At High Risk Of Cancer. Ed.: Joseph F. Fraumeni, Jr., Academic Press, New York, pp. 267-284, 1975.

18. Herman, Robert K. Effect Of Gene Induction On Frequency Of Intragenic Recombination Of Chromosome And F-merogenote In Escherichia coli K-12. Genetics 58: 55-67, 1968.

19. Hjelm, K.K., and Zeuthen, E. Synchronous DNA-synthesis Induced By Synchronous Cell Division In Tetrahymena. Compt. Rend. Trav. Lab. Carlsberg 36: 127-160, 1967.

20. Hoover, R., and Fraumeni, J.F. Drugs. In: Persons At High Risk Of Cancer. Ed.: Joseph F. Fraumeni, Jr., Academic Press, New York, pp. 185-199, 1975.

21. Imashuka, S., and LaBrosse, E.H. Metabolism of 1-3,4-Dihydroxyphenyl-alanine-2,5,6-^{3}H And 3,4-Dihydroxyphenylethylamine-2-^{14}C In A Patient With Neuroblastoma. Journal of Clinical Endocrinology and Metabolism 32: 241-253, 1971.

22. Kolata, G.B. Brain Biochemistry: Effects Of Diet. Science 192: 41-42, 1976.

23. Kyogoku, Y., Lord, R.C., and Rich, A. Specific Hydrogen Bonding Of Barbiturates To Adenine Derivatives. Nature 218: 69-72, 1968.

24. Kuntzman, R. Drugs And Enzyme Induction. Ann. Rev. Pharmacol. 9: 21-36, 1969.

25. LaBrosse, E.H. Catecholamine Metabolism In Neuroblastoma: Kinetics Of Conversion Of ^{3}H-Methoxy-4-hydroxyphenylglycol To ^{3}H-Methoxy-4-hydroxymandelic Acid. Journals of Clinical Endocrinology and Metabolism 30: 580-589, 1970.

26. LaBrosse, E.H., Imashuku, S., and Fineberg, S.E. Distribution And Turnover Of 7-^{3}H-Methoxy-4-hydroxymandelic Acid In A Patient With Ganglioneuroma. Journal of Clinical Endocrinology and Metabolism 35: 753-761, 1972.

27. Mayer, W., and Scherer, I. Phase-shifting Effect Of Caffeine In The Circadian Rhythm Of Phaseolus coccineus L. Z. Naturforschung 30C: 855-856, 1975.

28. Miller, R.W. Childhood Cancer And Congenital Defects: A Study Of Death Certificates During The Period 1960-1966. Pediat. Res. 3: 389-397, 1969.

29. Mulvihill, J.J. Congenital And Genetic Diseases. In: Persons At High Risk Of Cancer. Ed.: Joseph F. Fraumeni, Jr., Academic Press, New York, pp. 3-37, 1975.

30. Panofsky, H. and Halberg, F. I. Thermo-variance Spectra: Method And Clinical Illustrations. Exp. Med. and Surgery 19: 284-309, 1961.

31. Panofsky, H., and Halberg, F. II. Thermo-variance Spectra: Simplified Computational Example And Other Methodology. Experimental Medicine and Surgery 19: 323-338, 1961.

32. Peraino, C., Fry, R.J.M., and Staffeldt, E. Reduction And Enhancement By Phenobarbital Of Hepatocarcinogenesis Induced In The Rat By 2-Acetylaminofluorene. Cancer Res. 31: 1506-1512, 1971.

33. Peraino, C., Fry, R.J.M., and Staffeldt, E. Enhancement Of Spontaneous Hepatic Tumorigenesis In C3H Mice By Dietary Phenobarbital. J. Natl. Cancer Inst. 51: 1349-1350, 1973.

34. Peraino, C., Fry, R.J.M., Staffeldt, E., and Kisieleski, W.E. Effects Of Varying The Exposure To Phenobarbital On Its Enhancement Of 2-Acetylaminofluorene-induced Hepatic Tumorigenesis In The Rat. Cancer Res. 33: 2701-2705, 1973.

35. Ross, M.H., and Bras, G. Tumor Incidence Patterns And Nutrition In The Rat. Journal of Nutrition 87: 245-260, 1965.

36. Ross, M.H., and Bras, G. Lasting Influence Of Early Caloric Restriction On Prevalence Of Neoplasms In The Rat. Journal Natl. Cancer Inst. 47: 1095-1113, 1971.

37. Shimkin, M.B. Overview: Preventive Oncology. In: Persons At High Risk Of Cancer. Ed.: Joseph F. Fraumeni, Jr., Academic Press, New York, pp. 435-448, 1975.

38. Simon, D., Yen, S., and Cole, P. Coffee Drinking And Cancer Of The Lower Urinary Tract. Journal of the National Cancer Institute 54: 587-591, 1975.

39. Templeton, A.C. Acquired Diseases. In: Persons At High Risk Of Cancer. Ed.: Joseph F. Fraumeni, Jr., Academic Press, New York, pp. 69-84, 1975.

40. Thorpe, E., and Walker, A.I.T. The Toxicology Of Dieldrin (HEOD). II. Comparative Long-term Oral Toxicity Studies In Mice And Dieldrin, DDT, Phenobarbitone, β-BHC, and γ-BHC. Food Cosmet. Toxicol. 11: 433-442, 1973.

41. Wille, J.J. Selective Amplification Of Repetitive DNA In The Eukaryote, Tetrahymena. Biochem. Biophys. Res. Commun. 46: 692-699, 1972.

42. Wynder, E.L. Discussion Following Overview: Preventive Oncology by Michael B. Shimkin. In: Persons At High Risk Of Cancer. Ed.: Joseph F. Fraumeni, Jr., Academic Press, New York, p. 448, 1975.

CIRCADIAN RHYTHM WITH LARGE AMPLITUDE
IN MURINE TOLERANCE OF VINCRISTINE

Devendra P. Dubey, Franz Halberg, Shamsul Huq, Shahid Rahman,
Henry Fink, Robert B. Sothern, Lee Anne Wallach, Erhard Haus,
Mark E. Nesbit, Athanasios Theologides and Lawrence E. Scheving

Chronobiology Laboratories, Department of Laboratory Medicine
and Pathology, University of Minnesota, Minneapolis, Minn.
55455; Department of Medicine, University of Minnesota, Mpls.,
Minn. 55455; Department of Clinical and Anatomic Pathology,
St. Paul-Ramsey Hospital, St. Paul, Minn. 55105 and Department of Anatomy, Medical Center, University of Arkansas,
Little Rock, Arkansas 72201.

I. INTRODUCTION

The experimental basis for improving the tolerance of
oncotherapy by adjustment of timing of treatment according to
circadian rhythms--i.e., a chronotolerance--has been documented in mice and rats for the LD_{50} of whole body x-irradiation
(1-3) and the following chemotherapeutic agents: adriamycin
(4,5), daunomycin (6), arabinosyl cytosine (4,7-9), and cyclophosphamide (10). Thus, treatment according to host rhythms
can reduce undesired side effects, while treatment according
to any tumor rhythms may serve, further, for optimizing desired therapeutic effects; when rhythms are ignored in a giv-
en treatment schedule unwarranted toxicity or even death may
result (11-14).

Vincristine, the salt of an alkaloid obtained from a
common flowering herb, the periwinkle plant (Vinca rosea
Linn.) is a useful cancer chemotherapeutic agent, especially
in certain acute leukemias. In combination with other agents,

it has been used in treating neuroblastoma, Hodgkin's disease, lymphosarcoma, reticulum-cell sarcoma, rhabdomyosarcoma, Wilm's tumor and others. In vitro application of vincristine to neoplastic cells may cause an arrest of mitotic division at the stage of metaphase. The drug's manufacturers recommend treatment at weekly intervals. There is no mention of the stage of rhythm when administration of vincristine may be optimized to produce the maximal desired effect while minimizing unwanted deleterious effects, such as damage to healthy cells undergoing their own circadian cell cycle. Not even a time of day of administration is recommended, and in fact such a statement without added specification(s) of a synchronizer routine would constitute an insufficient precaution in itself (15).

II. PROCEDURES AND MATERIALS USED

Mortality from vincristine was tested in two separate studies, each on nearly 120 approximately 10-week old, male hybrid (CDF_1) mice, singly housed in cages measuring 29 x 18 x 12 cm, with food and water freely available.

For one week or longer, these animals remained in a sound-dampened rhythmometry room at $24 \pm 1^{\circ}C$ in light from 06^{00} to 18^{00} CST alternating with darkness. In one study (I), the cages housing the mice were on open shelves, side by side, while in another study (II), each cage was in its own compartment in so-called "hives" (16). For each study, animals were assigned (with stratification by shelf or "hive" location) to injection at one of six timepoints (00^{00}, 04^{00}, 08^{00}, 12^{00}, 16^{00}, 20^{00}). Each mouse in a group (n = 19 or 20/group) received a single intraperitoneal injection of vincristine, either 5.2 mg/kg (study I) or 5.1 mg/kg (study II). For each series of injections covering 24 hours the drug solution was prepared at the start of study and was stored in an amber-colored bottle in a refrigerator at $4^{\circ}C$; aliquots from this bottle were drawn at four-hour intervals from this stock solution for injection at a given circadian stage.

For study II, a fresh solution was made just before the last (16^{00}) timepoint and administered to a subgroup of 20

1116

mice, to check on stability of the drug in solution. Mice
were returned in their cages to their appropriate locations in
the rhythmometry room where they remained undisturbed for 10
days except for the frequent (several times daily) checking
and recording of mortality. After 10 days post-injection no
more deaths occurred.

III. RESULTS

Figure I summarizes the two studies when overall mortality, irrespective of circadian state at injection, approached
50% (45% for study I and 48% for study II). Numbers of surviving mice per timepoint are expressed as percent of the total
group (19 or 20) treated at that timepoint and are presented
separately for each study and also as the mean of the two
studies.

When 45% of the animals had died in study I, summarized
irrespective of circadian stage, one finds at one timepoint
only 25% of the animals surviving; at another 85% are alive--
a 340% difference in survival rate. For study II the difference in survival rates ranges from 30% to 63%--a 210% difference.

In study II, at the last (6th) timepoint, one group of
mice received a dose from a drug solution made up at the start
of the study, whereas another group received a fresh solution
of vincristine. Survival rates are 63% and 60%, respectively,
a finding which renders it unlikely that the drug deteriorated
during the timespan of the study.

The fit of a 24-hour cosine curve by the method of least
squares to the data on the percentage survival in the two
studies described a statistically significant circadian rhythm,
summarized in Figure 2. Estimates of some rhythm parameters,
all derived from the fitted curves are: Mesor = 51% (the
rhythm-adjusted overall average percentage survival), Amplitude = 23.5% (extent of predictable change, i.e., one-half the
peak-trough difference). The timing of the rhythm or Acrophase, ϕ, described by the lag of the peak after lights-on

1117

(in degrees) was at -193° (with 24 hours $\equiv 360^{\circ}$ and hence $15^{\circ} = 1$ hour).

Table I shows for each study survival times (in hours) computed at 10 days post-R_x; all mice surviving at that time are assigned a survival time of 10 days rather than the longer actual survival times. A statistically significant circadian rhythm can be described for both series of survival times by the fit of a 24-hour cosine curve. This finding agrees with the results obtained by summarizing the percentage of survivors. In study I, the acrophase is at -223° $(-194,-252)$ $(P < .01)$ and in study II, it is at -198° $(-153,-243)$ $(P < .05)$ from light-on (used as zero time)--in close agreement with the acrophase for % survivors: -193° which has 95% confidence limits between -150 and -235.

IV. DISCUSSION

A circadian rhythm in susceptibility of mice to the antineoplastic drug vincristine is described by analyses of 1) the percentage of survivors/timepoint, summarized when overall mortality nears 50% or 2) the survival times/timepoint summarized at 10 days post-injection. High tolerance is found late during the light span and in early-to mid-dark. Low tolerance occurs toward the end of the dark span and at the beginning of the light span for these nocturnally active rodents. These results on mammalian tolerance to vincristine indicate that the right circadian time is as important as the right dose. Work toward an optimization of the the circadian timing in the clinical administration of vincristine is mandatory. As a working hypothesis, one may anticipate best human tolerance during the habitual late-resting span and early or in the middle of the activity span.

V. SUMMARY

In each of 2 studies, 120 male CDF$_1$ mice, 10 weeks of age, were standardized singly housed at $24 \pm 1^{\circ}$C with food and water freely available, in 12 hours of daily artificial light alternating with darkness. In both studies every 4 hours during a 24-hour span a separate subgroup of mice received a single i.p. injection of vincristine either 5.2 (I) or 5.1 (II) mg/kg. Percent survivors per timepoint were evaluated when overall mortality was near 50%. Differences along the 24-hour scale in survival ranged from as low as 21% to as high as 85% in study I, and from 30% to 63% in study II. The least squares fit of a 24-hour cosine curve described a circadian rhythm with a double amplitude of 47% and an acrophase about 1 hour after lights-out. Results indicate the urgency of optimizing the circadian time for clinical administration of this drug. The right time is as important as the right dose for the case of mammalian tolerance to vincristine treatment.

Supported by U.S. Public Health Service (5-K06-GM-13981-14) (CA-07306) (CA-15548) (CA-08832), National Cancer Institute (1R01-CA-14445-01), Masonic Memorial Research Fund, and the St. Paul-Ramsey Medical Education and Research Foundation.

TABLE I. Circadian State Dependence of i.p. Vincristine Gauged in Groups of CDF_1 Mice by Mean Survival Time* with Standard Error**

Study No.	Test Time in Clock Hours (Hours After Light-Onset)					
	08^{00}	12^{00}	16^{00}	20^{00}	00^{00}	04^{00}
	(02)	(06)	(10)	(14)	(18)	(22)
I *	155 ± 12	139 ± 14	176 ± 11 [19]	191 ± 13	191 ± 12	143 ± 8 [19]
II *	133 ± 11	136 ± 14	163 ± 14	164 ± 15	153 ± 13	133 ± 11

*In hours elapsed from injection to recording of death(checks at ~12-hourly intervals). 20 mice/timepoint, unless other number is given in brackets, standardized in light from 06^{00} to 18^{00} alternating with darkness. Note that the three longest survival times (underlined) coincide in the two experiments, as supported by results of cosinor analyses.

**Circadian system stages being gauged by reference to the presumably synchronizing cycle of light and darkness.

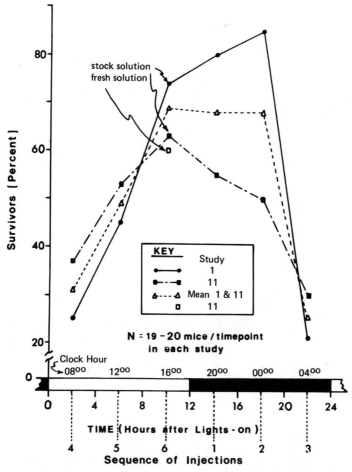

FIG. 1. Circadian rhythym in susceptibility of intact male CDF$_1$ mice to the antineoplastic drug vincristine. The percent survivors per timepoint in each of two studies when overall mortality approached 50% following a single dose of drug administered i.p. (5.2 and 5.1 mg/kg in experiments I and II, respectively). Shielding in time enhances tolerance of vincristine if one can extrapolate from murine data here shown to human patients.

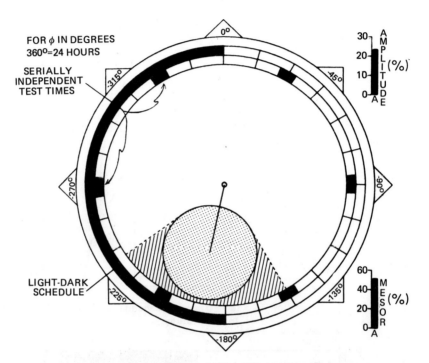

FIG. 2. Circadian rhythm susceptibility of mice to vincristine. The percent survivors per timepoint, summarized when overall mortality was approximately 50%. Results from two separate studies (237 intact male CDF$_1$ mice) with single i.p. injection of vincristine sulfate at one of six timepoints, 4 hr apart (shown on inner circular scale as black bars. The so-called cosinor method represents a first step toward obtaining estimates of extent of benefit associated with treatment timed according to rhythms. It assesses circadian and other rhythms with yet lower frequency, just as the EEG and ECG assess rhythms in action potentials of brain or heart.

REFERENCES

1. Halberg, F. Temporal Coordination of Physiologic Function. Cold Spring Harbor Symposium Quant. Biol., 25: 289-310, 1960, cf p. 310.
2. Haus, E., Halberg, F., and Loken, M.K. Circadian Susceptibility-Resistance Cycle of Bone Marrow Cells To Whole Body X-Irradiation In BALB/c Mice. In: Chronobiology, Eds.: L. E. Scheving, F. Halberg and J.E. Pauly. Igaku Shoin Ltd., Tokyo, 115-122, 1974.
3. Haus, E., Halberg, F., Loken, M.K., and Kim,U.S. Circadian Rhythmometry Of Mammalian Radiosensitivity. In: Space Radiation Biology. Eds.: A. Tobias and P. Todd. Academic Press, New York, 435-474, 1973.
4. Halberg, F., Haus, E., Cardoso, S.S., Scheving, L.E., Kühl, J.F.W., Shiotsuka, R., Rosene G., Pauly, J.E., Runge, W., Spalding, J.F., Lee, J.K., and Good, R.A. Toward A Chronotherapy Of Neoplasia: Tolerance Of Treatment Depends Upon Host Rhythms. Experientia, 29: 909-934, 1973.
5. Kühl, J.F.W., Grage, T.B., Halberg, F., Rosene, G., Scheving, L., and Haus, E. Ellen-Effect: Tolerance of Adriamycin By Bagg Albino Mice and Fisher Rats Depends On Circadian Timing Of Injection. International Journal of Chronobiology, 1: 335 , 1973.
6. Davies, G., MacDonald, J., Halberg, F., and Simpson, H. Circadian Rhythm In Murine Tolerance Of Daunomycin. J. Lancet, 2: 779, 1974.
7. Haus, E., Halberg, F., Scheving, L., Cardoso, S., Kühl, J. F.W., Sothern, R., Shiotsuka, R., Hwang, S., and Pauly, J. E. Increased Tolerance Of Leukemic Mice To Arabinosyl Cytosine Given On Schedule Adjusted To Circadian System. Science, 177: 80-82,1972.
8. Scheving, L.E., Cardoso, S.S., Pauly, J.E., Halberg, F., and Haus, E. Variations In Susceptibility Of Mice To The Carcinostatic Agent Arabinosyl Cytosine. In: Chronobiology. Eds: L.E. Scheving, F. Halberg, and J.E. Pauly, Igaku Shoin Ltd., Tokyo, 213-220, 1974.
9. Scheving, L.E., Haus, E., Kühl, J.F.W., Pauly, J.E., and Cardoso, S.S. Close Reproduction By Different Laboratories Of Characteristics Of Circadian Rhythm In 1-D-Arabinofuranosylcytosine Tolerance By Mice. Cancer Research, 36: 1133-1137, 1976.
10. Haus, E., Fernandes, G., Kühl, J.F.W., Yunis, E.J., and Halberg, F. Murine Circadian Susceptibility Rhythm To Cyclophosphamide. Chronobiologia, 1: 270-280, 1974.
11. Halberg, F. When To Treat. Indian J. Cancer, 12: 1-20, 1975.
12. Halberg, F. When To Treat. Haematologica, 60: 1-30,1975.
13. Halberg, F. Protection By Timing Treatment According To Bodily Rhythms-- An Analogy To Protection By Scrubbing Before Surgery. Chronobiologia, 1(Supplement): 27-68,1974.
14. Haus, E., Halberg, F., Kühl, J.F.W., and Lakatua, D.J. Chronopharmacology In Animals. Chronobiologia, 1(Supplement): 122-156, 1974.

15. Halberg, F. Physiologic 24-Hour Periodicity; General And Procedural Considerations With Reference To The Adrenal Cycle. Z. Vitamin-Hormon-u. Fermentforsch., 10: 225-296, 1959.
16. Runge, W., Lange, K., and Halberg, F. Some Instruments For Chronobiologists Developed At The University of Minnesota. Int. J. Chronobiology, 2: 327-341, 1974.

Chapter 13

EPIDEMIOLOGY

VARIATIONS IN CANCER DEATH RATES

Edward A. Lew

Department of Epidemiology and Statistics
American Cancer Society, Inc.
New York, New York

It is now essential to be cautious in interpreting variations in cancer death rates because of the inherent fluctuations in these mortality rates from year to year, the multiplicity of factors, some known, some suspected, and some unknown, affecting cancer, the diversity of the populations in which cancer has been observed, and the limitations on the accuracy and completeness in the reporting of cancer by site.

Unless there is evidence both internal and extraneous that a variation has biological meaning and the numbers observed have statistical validity, we need time out for critical analysis and vigilance about the shortcomings of the figures before us.

All of you, I am sure, will recall the widespread publicity given last fall to the preliminary finding that the cancer death rate in the United States had jumped 5.2 percent during the first seven months of 1975 over the rate for comparable period of 1974. This promptly gave rise to the speculation that some new forms of man made pollution hitherto unsuspected were finally producing an upsurge in cancer death rates that might portend an epidemic of neoplastic disease.

The sharp increase in reported deaths from cancer in the early months of 1975 could be corroborated by the increased cancer mortality computed and independently coded by at least two large life insurance companies. For instance, the death rate from all forms of cancer among the fifteen million ordinary policyholders of the Metropolitan Life Insurance Company rose by 6 percent during the first half of 1974. Another life insurance company reflecting the experience of a different segment of the population recorded a similar increase.

By the end of 1975 the cancer death rate for the entire calendar year was estimated to have increased by something less than 3 percent. The corresponding age-adjusted death rate for the general population was estimated to be only about 1 percent higher. This is consistent with the finding that the ordinary policyholders of the Metropolitan Life Insurance Company actually registered a lower age-adjusted cancer death rate in 1975 than in 1974 as did several other insurance companies.

It should therefore be manifest that we must not jump at conclusions

1127

about short time changes in the cancer death rate. Some perspective on the variability of this death rate from year to year can be gained by considering the course of cancer death rates since 1939. Figure 1 shows percent increase in cancer mortality – all forms for all ages combined – by decades since 1930 and indicates also the maximum increase in the death rate during the decade in any one year.

During the 1930's and the 1940's the cancer death rates increased by 23.5 percent and 16.2 percent respectively. This was the period when lung cancer was being diagnosed more accurately and the diagnosis of lung cancer came into its own. During these two decades annual increases of about 4 percent a year in the overall cancer death rates were recorded several times. During the 1950's the increase in mortality from all forms of cancer slowed down to about 6.7 percent, with a maximum rise in any one year of about 2 percent. In the 1960's the death rate from all forms of cancer continued to increase at a slightly greater rate, but the maximum rise in any one year was only about 1.5 percent. Extrapolating from the experience during 1970-1974, and increase of about 10% in the overall cancer death rate might have been anticipated, but the higher death rate registered in 1975 suggests that a rise of about 12 percent in the overall cancer death rate for the decade is more likely, with a maximum increase of about 3 percent in any one year.

A substantial portion of the increase in the overall cancer death rate unadjusted for age represents the effects of aging and more generally of a changing age composition. It is difficult to forecast the effects of a changing age composition on the overall cancer death rate because the shape of the cancer mortality curve at the advanced ages is not adequately known.

The preceding remarks were intended to lead to the conclusion that over the past three or four decades there have been a number of sharp increases in the overall cancer death rate during the first half of the year – exceeding 5 percent on several occasions. This is manifest not only in the mortality experience of the general population of the United States but also in the mortality experience of large groups of insured lives. In a few instances changes in codes contributed to this phenomenon, but it would have still been true that sizable fluctuations for no apparent reason have occurred. There appears to be no significant correlation between large increases in the overall cancer death rate and influenza epidemics in the early months of the year.

A very much broader range of variability in cancer death rates is exhibited in comparisons of cancer mortality between different countries. This is particularly so when we consider the extreme variability of cancer death rates by site.

We need, nevertheless, to be more circumspect than many publicists have been in making comparisons between cancer death rates of different countries. For instance, most people fail to see the fundamental objection to comparing the cancer death rates for the United States as a whole with the cancer death rates of small nations such as Norway, Denmark, Sweden, Holland, Israel or New Zealand. Some overzealous spokesmen for the public health movement have tried to present health conditions in the United States in an unfavorable light by ranking mortality rates for the United States as a whole alongside of those for selected small countries with relatively low death rates from some particular cause or causes. Such improper comparisons have attracted a great deal of attention without eliciting the criticism that it doesn't make much sense to rank the average for a continent with more than 200 million people alongside the figures for nations of 2 to 10 million people. It should be obvious that in an aggregate of over 200 million people there are bound to be numerous subgroups or regions that have been subject to mortality distinctly higher and distinctly lower than the average for the aggregate. To rank the mortality rates for selected portions of one continent-Western Europe - such as the Scandinavian countries and Holland alongside of the average for another continent - the United States - merely proves that one can select small portions of a large aggregate that will show markedly more favorable characteristics than the average for another aggregate - even though the two large aggregates involved may both exhibit similar characteristics overall.

In order to present more meaningful comparisons between countries, it is desirable to select regions with approximately equal populations, similar degrees of industrialization and heavy industry in particular, and some common cultural patterns.

I have tried to emphasize this by the figures in Figure 2 which presents the variations in cancer death rates for males and females in the age range 45-75 for whites in the United States, for the block of industrialized countries of Western Europe and for Japan.

This slide indicates that for a number of cancer sites there has been very little difference in death rates between whites in the United States and the inhabitants of the block of industrialized nations of Western Europe. These sites include cancer of the intestines and rectum, cancer of the breast, cancer of the prostate and respiratory cancer in the case of females. It shows, however, that both males and females in this part of Western Europe have experienced distinctly higher mortality from cancer of the stomach and that males in this part of Western Europe have been subject to higher death rates from respiratory cancer.

Furthermore this slide brings out that the death rates from cancer of the stomach has been at a very much higher level in Japan than in the United States or Western Europe. On the other hand Japan has reported very much lower mortality from cancer of the breast, prostate, intestines and rectum and respiratory cancer.

It is probably more instructive to focus attention on the areas with relatively high and low cancer mortality in North America and Western Europe. Such comparisons indicate similar ranges of variability in cancer death rates on both continents, as shown in Figure 3.

In North America we find the highest levels of cancer - all forms at attained ages 45-74 - in the Middle Atlantic and New England states and the lowest levels in the West North Central and Mountain States. It is noteworthy that the corresponding level of cancer mortality in Canada is about intermediate between the highest and the lowest found in the United States.

In Western Europe the highest levels of cancer - all forms at attained

ages 45-74 - occur in England and Germany, with male cancer death
rates significantly greater than those reported from the Middle Atlantic
and New England States. The lowest levels of cancer mortality in
Western Europe have been recorded in Spain, but there is some question
as to how much credibility should be given to these figures. The level
of cancer death rates in the Scandinavian countries and Holland closely
resembles that of Canada.

The very wide variations in cancer mortality for particular sites of
cancer in different parts of the world have been scrutinized for clues
about the etiology of diverse forms of cancer. This examination has
had to bear in mind at all times the varying accuracy and styles of
reporting causes of death in different countries and the relative
degrees of completeness of death registration in different regions.
There are grounds for believing that the quality of the information of
death certificates in Canada and many countries of Western Europe is
reasonably comparable to that in the United States.

Because of the real difficulties in making comparative studies of cancer
mortality by site between different countries, it would appear that we
could probably learn much more from intensive studies of the accuracy
and completeness of cancer diagnoses in different parts of the United
States. There is, in my judgement, a fertile field for research in the
diagnoses of cancer between the more medically backward areas of the
United States and the areas where more sophisticated appraisals prevail.

When we engage in studies of regional variations in cancer mortality
within the United States, we will of course be expected to keep a
watchful eye on the environmental factors suspected of causing or
contributing to the causation of cancer.

In planning such studies we must therefore make sure to allow for effects
associated with socio-economic, educational and endogenous influences
before ascribing any striking differentials in cancer mortality to
environmental factors.

The classic investigations conducted for many years by the Registrars
General of England and Wales as well as of Scotland provide us with
a methodology of weighing the separate effects of occupational hazards
and those associated with different modes of living. This has been
done by considering the extra mortality of men in particular occupations
involving occupational hazards with the extra mortality of their wives.
The latest studies of the Registrar General for England and Wales,
covering the period 1959-1963, show that the level of cancer death rates
for men aged 15-64 has been twice as high for men in the lowest social
class as for men in the highest social class. For cancers of the digestive
system the differential has been of about the same order, but the cancer
death rates for the respiratory system have been three times as high for
the lowest as for the highest social class. In the case of married women
aged 15-64 the differential between the lowest and the highest social
class was about 1-1/2 times for cancer of the respiratory tract. No
significant difference by social class was noted for leukemia in either
sex.

The most nearly comparable study for the United States was one developed
for men only by Guralnick from the experience during 1950. It showed a

forty percent greater death rate from cancer of the digestive system in the lowest social class as compared with that in the highest social class. For respiratory cancer the corresponding differential was sixty percent. An inverse relationship appeared to hold for cancer of the prostate and leukemia.

Guralnick also investigated the mortality of men in the United States in 1950 by occupation. Figure 4 presents her findings by broad occupational categories. It shows that professional workers experienced cancer death rates of the digestive system 10 percent below the average for all occupations, whereas laborers were subject to cancer death rates from this cause 25 percent above the average for all occupations. Professional workers experienced mortality from respiratory cancer 25 percent below the average for all occupations, whereas laborers had cancer death rates from this cause 25 percent above the average for all occupations. There was no significant relationship observed by occupational categories for cancer of the prostate or leukemia.

A more recent study of cancer mortality in the United States by social class is given in Figure 5. It compares the mortality rates from cancer by site among male and female policyholders of the Metropolitan Life Insurance Company, separately for the so-called industrial policyholders who were predominantly industrial or service workers and their wives and separately for ordinary policyholders who were drawn largely from the middle and better to do segments of the population. This comparison indicates a differential in favor of male ordinary policyholders as compared to male industrial policyholders of 75 percent for cancer of the respiratory tract, 70 percent for cancer of the kidney, 35 percent for cancer of the prostate and 25 percent for cancer of the digestive system. Female ordinary policyholders recorded significantly lower mortality than female industrial policyholders only for cancer of the digestive system and cancer of the uterus, the differential for both sites being of the order of 20 percent.

Another significant bit of evidence as to the effect of social class on cancer death rates was developed from a series of mortality studies of the salaried personnel of large corporations. In two very large corporations the personnel in the two highest salary classes experienced mortality from all forms of cancer that was about 20 percent below that in the lowest salary classes. The corresponding differential for cancer of the respiratory tract was of the order of 50 percent.

A notable study by Kitagawa and Hauser of the effects of education on mortality, based on the 1960 experience in the general population of the United States, suggests that educational attainment is a better prognostic indicator of mortality than either occupation or income - during the working years of life. A summary of the Kitagawa-Hauser findings is shown in Figure 6. It brings out that college men experienced a 30 percent lower mortality from all forms of cancer than did those with less than 8 years of schooling and that the corresponding differential for college women was of the order of 25 percent. College men experienced cancer death rates of the lung and stomach that were approximately half of those of men with less than 8 years of schooling. College women experienced cancer death rates of the uterus that were less than half those of women with less than 8 years of schooling. The college women's death rates from cancer of the lung were only 70 percent of those for women with less than 8 years of schooling. Cancer of the prostate among college men was distinctly higher than that for men with less education, while cancer of the breast among college women was about 30 percent higher than for women with less than 8 years schooling; the death rate from cancer of the breast rose progressively with greater educational attainment.

Some light on the endogeneous factors affecting cancer death rates is shed by the differentials in cancer mortality among whites and non-whites as well as by the differential between the native-born whites and white migrants from various countries. The key study in this area was made by Haenszel in 1960 based on the experience in 1950; its principal findings are presented in Figure 7. It is noteworthy that in 1950 the reported death rates among non-whites were similar to those for foreign-born whites for cancer of the digestive system, both being about 50 percent higher than for native-born whites. Virtually all groups of foreign-born whites exhibited excess mortality from cancer of the digestive organs as compared with the native-born. The cancer death rates for the foreign-born whites varied widely, but their mortality from cancer of the prostate was uniformly lower than that of native-born whites. The foreign-born whites showed similar patterns of cancer mortality irrespective of their place of residence. More recent data suggest that the cancer mortality of foreign-born whites has drawn much closer to that of the native-born, but some differentials which are probably significant remain. Furthermore, the character of recent migrants has changed radically, very many more recently coming from Asia and Central or South America.

It is difficult to separate the endogenous factors from the effects of low economic living standards in the case of non-whites, as was many years ago the case of foreign-born whites. The quality of reporting of cancer deaths among non-whites in 1950 left much to be desired and current cancer death rates among whites and non-whites present quite a different picture from that twenty five years ago. Generally speaking the differentials between white and non-white cancer death rates have widened and much of this can be attributed to improved cancer diagnoses among non-whites.

Better medical care facilities have produced a much higher proportion of microscopically confirmed cancer diagnoses for both whites and non-whites. But despite the more sophisticated methods of arriving at cancer diagnoses, there are still many areas of the United States - particularly the rural regions - which do not show up well on the proportion of microscopic confirmation of cancer. This is indicated in Figure 8, which shows that in some parts of this country only 60 percent of the cases certified as cancer of the pancreas have been so confirmed; only 70 percent of the cases certified as cancer of the stomach and less than 80 percent of the cases certified as cancer of the lung have been microscopically confirmed in a few areas.

I can perhaps best sum up the message I want to convey by an anecdote. An epidemiologist revisits the university he graduated from after many years and talks to the professor under whom he studied. He is surprised to find that the professor is still asking the same questions of his students as he did when the epidemiologist was in his class. He inquires why the questions asked are virtually identical and is informed that

although the questions have remained unchanged the answers are currently
quite different. This is the position we find ourselves in. The
questions about variations in cancer death rates are much the same as
those raised in the past, but the answers we seek today are different.
The explanations we are looking for must take account of the natural
variability of cancer which has now been well documented, the diverse
characteristics of the populations studied, the multiplicity of the
factors known to affect cancer, the effects of rapidly changing demographic and social trends, and the dubious validity and incompleteness
of some of the statistics on cancer. If we are to avoid premature false
conclusions, we must examine our data more rigorously, check their
accuracy and representativeness, try to secure extraneous corroborative
evidence, and above all consider the plausibility of the variations
observed from a biological viewpoint.

VARIATION IN CANCER DEATH RATES
UNITED STATES, 1930-74

Percent Increase in Death Rates for All Forms of Cancer (All ages combined)

Percent Increase Over Decade

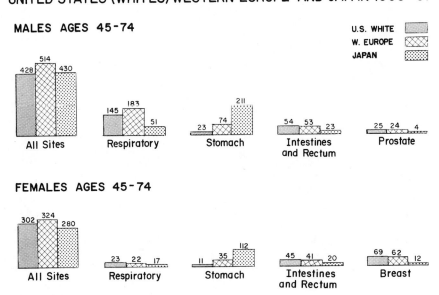

23.5   16.2   6.7   8.4   10.0

1930-40   1940-50   1950-60   1960-70   1970-80

Maximum Increase in One Year

4.0   4.0   2.0   1.5   1.8

1970-80 ESTIMATED ON BASIS OF 1970-74 INCREASE

FIG. 1

VARIATION IN CANCER DEATH RATES
UNITED STATES (WHITES) WESTERN EUROPE*AND JAPAN 1966-67

MALES AGES 45-74

U.S. WHITE
W. EUROPE
JAPAN

All Sites: 428, 514, 430
Respiratory: 145, 183, 51
Stomach: 23, 74, 211
Intestines and Rectum: 54, 53, 23
Prostate: 25, 24, 4

FEMALES AGES 45-74

All Sites: 302, 324, 280
Respiratory: 23, 22, 17
Stomach: 11, 35, 112
Intestines and Rectum: 45, 41, 20
Breast: 69, 62, 12

*UNITED KINGDOM, IRELAND, BELGIUM, FRANCE, WESTERN GERMANY AND SWITZERLAND

FIG. 2

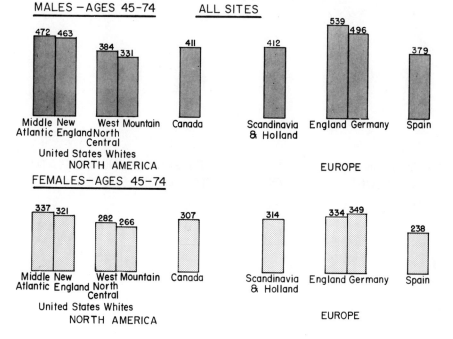

VARIATIONS IN CANCER DEATH RATES
NORTH AMERICA AND EUROPE REGIONAL COMPARISONS 1966-67

MALES — AGES 45-74   ALL SITES

FIG. 3

VARIATIONS IN CANCER DEATH RATES BY OCCUPATIONAL LEVEL
WHITE MEN AGED 20-64, U.S., 1950

Site of Cancer	All Occupations	Professional Workers	Technical Administrative Managerial	Clerical Workers	Semi Skilled	Laborers
Digestive Organs	96%	86%	85%	102%	103%	120%
Stomach	92	56	69	93	103	122
Intestines & Rectum	102	114	102	113	103	110
Respiratory	101	78	90	114	115	126
Prostate	87	116	92	84	85	94
Leukemia	102	117	101	107	92	99

FIG. 4

VARIATION IN CANCER DEATH RATES BY SOCIOECONOMIC STATUS
INSURED LIVES AND U.S. POPULATION 1963-64

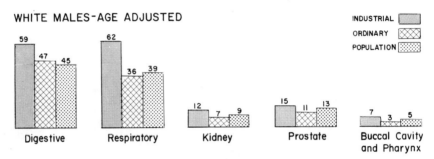

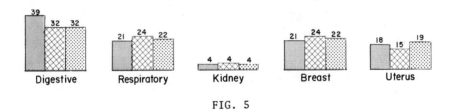

FIG. 5

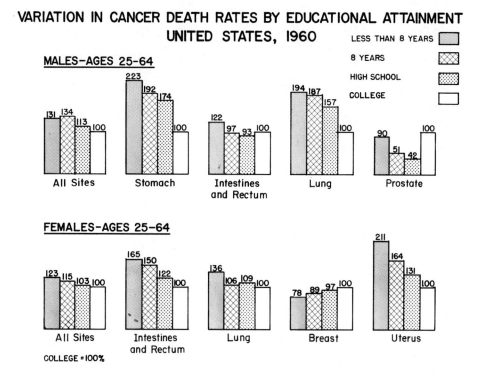

VARIATION IN CANCER DEATH RATES BY EDUCATIONAL ATTAINMENT
UNITED STATES, 1960

FIG. 6

VARIATION IN CANCER DEATH RATES BY RACE AND ETHNIC ORIGIN
WHITE MEN – AGE STANDARDIZED– U.S., 1950

Ethnic Origin	Digestive Organs	Stomach	Intestines & Rectum	Respiratory	Prostate	Leukemia
Native Born White	100%	100%	100%	100%	100%	100%
Non White	154	212	92	95	300	79
Foreign Born White	145	179	120	133	89	107
Born England & Wales	136	151	120	131	97	81
Born Germany	148	182	128	112	96	101
Born Poland	166	225	108	188	79	108
Born Russia	152	187	136	155	68	145
Born Italy	124	123	119	90	64	106

MORTALITY RATIOS TO NATIVE BORN WHITE

FIG. 7

VARIATION IN CANCER DEATH RATES
Proportion of Cases Microscopically Confirmed

Third National Cancer Survey 1969–71

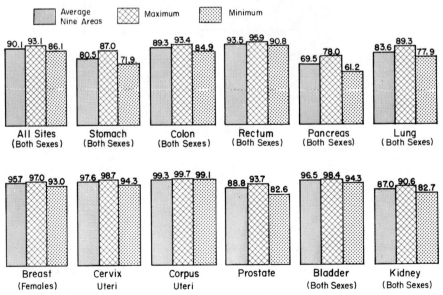

FIG. 8

PROSPECTIVE STUDIES ON CANCER EPIDEMIOLOGY
BASED ON CENSUS POPULATION IN JAPAN

Takeshi Hirayama, M.D.

Chief, Epidemiology Division
National Cancer Center
Research Institute, Tokyo

INTRODUCTION

A population prospective study on the health consequences of selected risk factors including cigarette smoking
and alcohol drinking has been in progress in Japan since the
fall of 1965.
The result of 9 years follow-up will be presented focussing
on the role of cigarette smoking and alcohol drinking.(1.2.3)

PROCEDURES AND MATERIALS USED

Some 265,118 adults, 122,261 males and 142,857 females,
aged 40 years and above, 91-99% of the census population in
the study area in 29 Health Center Districts in Japan, interviewed from Oct. 1 to Dec. 31, 1965, have been followed by
establishing a record linkage system between the risk factor
records, a current residence list obtained by specially plann-
ed annual census, and death certificates. This investigation
is the first of its kind conducted in Asian population.

RESULTS

A total of 24,668 deaths including 6,485 cancers
occurred during the 9 year period. Number of death by each
site of cancer is shown in Table 1. Age specicic death rates
for each cause of death in the study population were similar
to those for the whole country.

(1) Cigarette smoking:

Both men and women who smoked cigarettes daily experienced highest death rates from cancers of all sites.   The

habit of daily smoking of cigarettes was noted to enhance the standardized mortality ratio for cancer of all sites far higher (SMR 1.67 for males and 1.35 for females) than any of other habits.

The risk was noted particularly high when the habit was initiated at teen-age period. A significantly higher risk in daily cigarette smokers was observed with cancer of following selected sites: mouth (SMR 3.32) pharynx (4.22) esophagus (1.83) stomach (1.54) liver (1.67) pancreas (1.50) larynx (16.99) lung (3.75) in males and cancer of all sites (1.35) mouth (1.88) stomach (1.34) liver (1.65) larynx (3.65) lung (1.83) in females. Liver cirrhosis was noted also in higher risk in daily smokers, SMR being 1.30 in males and 1.91 in females. (Fig. 1)(Table II)

(2) Alcohol drinking:

Compared to smoking, alcohol drinking is less related to cancer of all sites, SMR being 1.07 for males and 1.10 for females, but is significantly associated to cancer of selected sites. Risk in daily smokers is noted to be significantly higher in following cancers: mouth (2.45) pharynx (2.42) esophagus (1.86) liver (1.22) lung (1.20) liver cirrhosis (1.74) in males and esophagus (3.61) lung (2.99) and liver cirrhosis (3.81) in females.(Fig. 1)(Table III)

It is of interest to observe that the risk in occasional drinkers is almost same as that in non drinkers. (Fig.2) Therefore it appeared that if one only drinks occasionally, alcohol drinking carries no elevated risk to any type of cancer.

(3) Combined habit of cigarette smoking and alcohol drinking:

Risk for various cancers was compared between those who smokes daily but do not drink and those with combined habit of smoking and drinking. (Fig. 3) Cancers of larynx and lung showed highly elevated risk in smoking only group. Risk appeared not going up when habit of daily alcohol drinking was added. These two cancers could therefore be considerd as belonging to absolute cigarette diseases. Cancers of stomach and pancreas also showed significantly higher risk in daily smokers. The risk did not go up higher when habit of daily drinking was added.

Most of other digestive tract cancers showed higher risk when habits of smoking and drinking are combined. These include cancer of the mouth, pharynx, esophagus, and liver. Liver cirrhosis also showed similar pattern.

(4) Analysis in progress:

A far more detailed analysis on the role of cigarette smoking and alcohol drinking is in progress for both men and women based on ten years follow-up material taking into con-

sideration other factors such as occupation, dietary habits,
medical and reproductive history etc. Life style dependent
risk for cancer and other major diseases is expected to reveal
by such analysis.

DISCUSSION

Nine year follow-up results of a large prospective
epidemiologcal study of 265,118 men and women currently in
progress in Japan is thus providing evidence for selected risk
factors closely linked with life style of present day society
such as cigarette smoking and alcohol drinking. Certain
cancers, such as larynx and lung, showed elevated risk in
cigarette smokers regardless of presence or absence of drinking habit, while the risk for most of digestive tract cancers
was observed selectively high when habits of cigarette smoking and alcohol drinking are combined.
Most probably mechanism of oncogenic action of cigarette smoking of larynx and lung cancer must be different from that of
digestive tract cancers, the former being of contact carcinogenesis and the latter of metabolic carcinogenesis.
Occasional drinkers of alcohol showed almost same risk as non
alcohol drinkers. Spacing in drinking habit is, therefore,
strongly recommended.

SUMMARY

Nine year follow-up results of a large prospective
studies for 265,118 adults on cancer epidemiology in Japan was
presented. A total of 24,668 deaths including 6,485 cancers
took place during observed period.
A significantly elevated risk was observed with cancer of all
sites, mouth, pharynx, esophagus, stomach, liver, pancreas,
larynx, and lung in males and cancer of all sites, mouth,
stomach, liver, larynx, and lung in females. Daily alcohol
drinking was observed to enhance the risk for following
cancers; mouth, pharynx, esophagus, liver and lung in males
and esophagus and lung in females.
The risk in occasional drinkers was noted almost same as that
in non drinkers.
From the observation of the effect of combined habit of smoking and drinking the mechanism of carcinogenesis due to
cigarette smoking was discussed for each site of cancer.

TABLE I

NUMBER OF DEATH FROM CANCER BY EACH SITE
AND PERCENTAGE TO CANCER OF ALL SITES

PROSPECTIVE STUDY 1966-74

	Male			Female		
		%	Japan*		%	Japan*
Total	3830	100.0	100.0	2655	100.0	100.0
Lip	1	0.0	0.0	1	0.0	0.0
Tongue	15	0.4	0.4	10	0.4	0.3
Salivary gland	2	0.1	0.1	4	0.1	0.1
Other mouth	8	0.2	0.1	1	0.0	0.1
Oropharynx	1	0.0	0.1	0	-	-
Nasopharynx	5	0.1	0.1	2	0.1	0.0
Hypopharynx	3	0.1	0.1	2	0.1	0.1
Other pharynx	5	0.1	0.1	1	0.0	0.1
Esophagus	197	5.2	5.8	64	2.4	2.3
Stomach	1713	44.7	45.4	887	33.4	36.9
Small intestine	3	0.1	0.2	5	0.2	0.2
Large intestine	85	2.2	2.5	106	4.0	4.0
Rectum	133	3.5	3.7	122	4.6	4.1
Liver	424	11.0	9.1	299	11.3	7.2
Pancreas	156	4.1	3.9	95	3.6	3.7
Peritoneum	56	1.5	0.3	58	2.2	0.6
Nose, nasal cavities	39	1.0	1.1	24	0.9	0.9
Larynx	38	1.0	1.2	8	0.3	0.3
Lung	502	12.8	11.8	174	6.5	6.0
Other respiratory	38	0.7	0.5	12	0.4	0.5
Bone	24	0.6	0.6	21	0.8	0.6
Soft tissue	4	0.1	0.1	4	0.2	0.1
Melanoma of skin	7	0.2	0.1	3	0.1	0.1
Other skin	13	0.3	0.5	21	0.8	0.5
Breast	1	0.0	0.0	118	4.5	4.6
Cervix				323	12.3	11.8
Other uterus				4	0.1	0.5
Ovary				44	1.7	1.9
Other female genital				18	0.7	0.3
Prostate	50	1.3	1.4			
Testis	-	-	-			
Other male genital	2	0.1	0.1			
Urinary bladder	61	1.6	1.6	33	1.2	1.1
Kidney, other urinary	21	0.5	0.7	12	0.5	0.5
Eye	2	0.1	0.0	0	-	-
Brain and nerve	35	0.9	0.2	25	0.9	0.2
Thyroid	9	0.2	0.2	13	0.5	0.7
Other endocrine	2	0.1	0.0	2	0.1	0.0
Lymphosarco,a	45	1.2	0.9	17	0.6	0.8
Hodgkin	13	0.3	0.3	14	0.5	0.2
Other lymphoma	2	0.1	0.4	8	0.3	0.4
Multiple mydoma	23	0.6	0.4	10	0.4	0.5
Leukemia	42	1.1	1.4	39	1.5	1.5

* Japan total,age 40 and over,cancer of all sites
  male 62,571 female 48,305, 1970

TABLE II   NUMBER OF ACTUAL AND EXPECTED DEATH FROM CANCER
BY SITE IN DAILY CIGARETTE SMOKERS (RISK IN NON SMOKERS=1.00)

	MALES				FEMALES			
	Obs.	Exp.	Ratio	X^2	Obs.	Exp.	Ratio	X^2
ALL TYPES	3043	1819.4	1.67	822.90***	410	302.9	1.35	37.86***
MOUTH	23	6.91	3.32	37.46***	3	1.59	1.88	1.25
PHARYNX	12	2.84	4.22	29.54***	0	0.66	0	0.66
ESOPHAGUS	172	65.9	2.61	170.82***	8	7.5	1.06	0.03
STOMACH	1332	862.7	1.54	255.29***	137	102.1	1.34	11.92***
COLON	65	46.41	1.40	7.44**	17	12.19	1.39	1.89
RECTUM	94	98.51	0.95	0.20	14	14.88	0.94	0.05
LIVER	332	198.4	1.67	89.96***	56	33.8	1.65	14.58***
PANCREAS	127	84.3	1.50	21.62***	16	10.6	1.50	2.75
LARYNX	35	2.06	16.99	526.72***	3	0.82	3.65	5.79*
LUNG	444	118.4	3.75	895.40***	34	18.5	1.83	12.98***
PROSTATE	36	32.56	1.10	0.36	-	-	-	-
CIRRHOSIS	299	229.19	1.30	21.26***	38	19.84	1.91	16.62***

PROSPECTIVE STUDY 1966-74 JAPAN

SIGNIFICANT AT * 5 % LEVEL
** 1 % LEVEL
*** 0.1% LEVEL

TABLE III NUMBER OF ACTUAL AND EXPECTED DEATH FROM CANCER
BY SITE IN ALCOHOL DRINKERS (RISK IN NON DRINKERS=1.00) MALES

	DAILY				OCCASIONAL			
	OBS.	EXP.	RATIO	X^2	OBS.	EXP.	RATIO	X^2
ALL TYPES	1336	1243.31	1.07	6.89**	908	973.13	0.93	4.38*
MOUTH	15	6.10	2.45	12.98****	4	5.12	0.78	0.24
PHARYNX	8	3.30	2.42	6.69**	2	2.47	0.80	0.08
ESOPHAGUS	93	49.94	1.86	37.12****	39	38.50	1.01	0.00
STOMACH	570	581.07	0.98	0.21	403	454.08	0.88	5.74*
COLON	31	24.53	1.26	1.70	22	18.93	1.16	0.49
RECTUM	38	46.26	0.82	1.47	36	35.28	1.02	0.01
LIVER	158	128.77	1.22	6.63	103	102.63	1.00	0.00
PANCREAS	50	52.64	0.94	0.13	38	41.04	0.92	0.22
LARYNX	12	11.24	1.06	0.05	9	8.35	1.07	0.05
LUNG	189	156.29	1.20	6.84***	113	122.13	0.92	0.68
PROSTATE	18	16.57	1.08	0.12	11	12.04	0.91	0.08
CIRRHOSIS	181	103.67	1.74	57.68***	77	84.18	0.91	0.61

PROSPECTIVE STUDY 1966-74 JAPAN

SIGNIFICANT AT * 5% LEVEL
** 1% LEVEL
*** 0.1% LEVEL

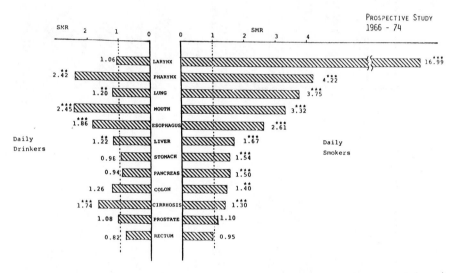

FIG. 1. Standardized mortality ratio for cancer of selected sites in daily smokers and in daily drinkers (males). Prospective study 1966-1974.

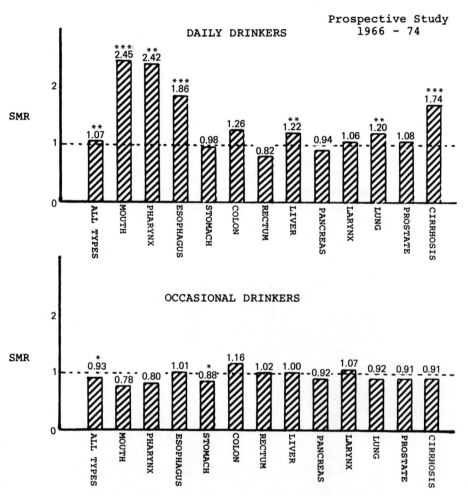

FIG. 2. Standardized mortality ratio for cancer of selected sites in daily drinkers and occasional drinkers (males). Prospective study 1966-1974.

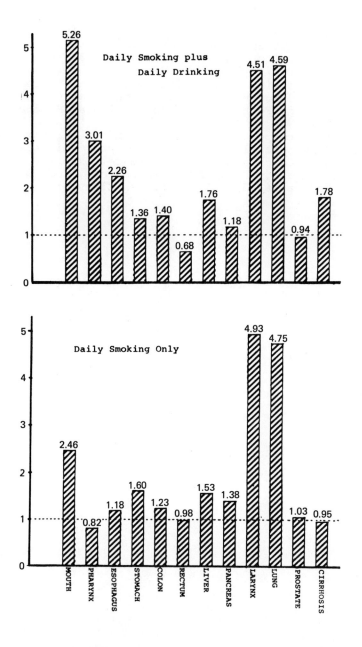

Unit = Risk in those neither smoke nor drink daily

FIG. 3. Standardized mortality ratio for cancer of selected sites in those with habit of daily smoking only.

REFERENCES

1. T. Hirayama; A prospective study on the influence of
   cigarette smoking and alcohol drinking on the death rates
   for total and selected causes of death in Japan.
   Smoke Signals 16(7): 1-8 July 1970
2. T. Hirayama; Smoking in relation to the death rates of
   265,118 men and women in Japan. Presented at the American
   Cancer Society's Fourteenth Science Writers' Seminar.
   March27, 1972.
3. T. Hirayama; Prospective studies on cancer epidemiology
   based on census population in Japan. Proceedings XI
   International Cancer Congress, Florence, 1974.)
   Cancer Epidemiology, Environmental Factors, Vol. 3,
   Excerpta Medica 26-35, 1975, American Elsevier

NEGLIGIBLE ROLE OF ALCOHOL AND TOBACCO
IN THE ETIOLOGY OF ESOPHAGEAL CANCER
IN IRAN--A CASE CONTROL STUDY

E. Mahboubi, N.E. Day, P. Ghadirian
and S. Salmasizadeh

Eppley Institute for Research in Cancer
University of Nebraska Medical Center
Omaha, Nebraska (E.M.)

The International Agency for Research
on Cancer
Lyon, France (N.E.D.)

Institute of Public Health Research
University of Teheran, Iran (P.G., S.S.)

INTRODUCTION

Esophageal cancer is a form of cancer in which death rates vary dramatically from one locale to another. In some areas the rate differential consists of a 100-fold variance between the highest and the lowest rates (2, 6, 7, 10).

Among the areas of high esophageal cancer incidence in the world, one of the most interesting is the northeastern corner of Iran, where the incidence of the disease is among the highest ever recorded (7). This area is populated by central Asian Turkomans and is a semi-desert region. However, unusually high rates (although lower than in the Turkoman group) are also found among the Turkic-speaking (Ghizilbash Turks) and Persian-speaking populations to the southeast of the Caspian Sea. Esophageal cancer has been known to exist in this area for several hundred years (3), and its incidence varies strikingly from east to west, by as much as 30-fold for women and 6-fold for men.

It has been suggested that at least 80% of cancer in general is caused by environmental factors (4), and studies conducted in Africa (1), France (11), Puerto Rico (8) and the United States (12) have shown that alcohol and tobacco play important roles in the etiology of esophageal cancer. However, these factors seem unlikely to be of much significance in the high incidence area of Iran for two reasons. Firstly, the Islamic religion forbids its members to consume alcohol, and though some urban dwellers are not rigidly orthodox and may use it sparingly, villagers would consume almost none. Secondly, in high incidence areas, where the disease is more common among females than males, it is known that women practically never consume alcohol or use tobacco.

To confirm these impressions by sound epidemiological methods, a case control study was conducted from 1969-72. In the study, a group of 151 esophageal cancer victims and 301 healthy controls were interviewed. Investigations were made of personal habits to ascertain consumption rates of alcohol, tobacco and opium in esophageal cancer patients and healthy controls. Particular emphasis was placed on high incidence areas where esophageal cancer was most common in females.

PROCEDURES AND MATERIALS USED

This case control study is based on data obtained by the authors from 1969-1972 through interviews of esophageal cancer patients and controls in villages of the Caspian Littoral. The study was conducted in the patients' homes, while patients were hospitalized, or at Babol Medical Research Station, where they came for consultation and to have arrangements made for free hospitalization and treatment (i.e., surgery, radiation or both).

Controls were randomly chosen from healthy individuals in the patients' village or a neighboring village, and were matched by age and sex with patients. The questionnaire for interviews was developed through consultations with a gastroenterologist, the late Dr. U. de Jong of the International Agency for Research on Cancer, Lyon, France. The questionnaire was tested, revised and retested before use. Information obtained included occupation, education, history of drinking, smoking, and eating habits, and detailed data on nutritional factors.

Only 28% of the patients in the study had a histological confirmation of squamous cell carcinoma of the esophagus. The diagnosis for the remaining 72% was based on X-rays only, although a followup of interviewed cases showed that all had died within a year.

A total of 169 patients and 318 controls were contacted and interviewed. Of these cases, 151 patients and 301 controls were included in the present study; the remainder were not used in data analysis because they were from areas outside the Caspian Littoral.

RESULTS

The distribution of the cases and controls by age, sex and ethnic group is given in Table I. Turkomans and Turkish-speaking groups are listed together. The effects of alcohol, tobacco smoking, chewing of nass (a mixture of tobacco, lime and ash) and opium use were analyzed by sex, age and ethnic group.

I. ALCOHOL

Among Turkomans and Turks, only two patients had consumed alcohol, and then in moderation (once monthly or so, as compared to three controls). Among males speaking Persian, there was a slightly higher alcohol consumption. Of 67 Persian male esophageal patients, 15 had consumed alcohol, nine drank moderately, while only two said they used alcohol on a regular basis. In matching these patients with controls, there was no significant difference between the two groups and clearly no association with esophageal cancer. Table II gives detailed information regarding alcohol consumption.

II. TOBACCO

Table III shows the distribution by age, sex and ethnic group of cigarette smoking for cases and controls. In Turkomans and Turks, smoking was clearly not associated with the disease, while in Persian-speaking patients, there was a small excess of heavy smokers (i.e., those smoking more than 20 cigarettes per day). A total of 46% of all patients smoked, as opposed to 53% of the controls. Heavy smokers totaled 34% of all patients and 29% of controls. These figures, however, did not approach

statistical significance, and clearly indicate cigarette smoking is of
no significance in the etiology of this disease.

III. NASS USE

Nass (a tobacco and lime mixture) is commonly chewed by the Central
Asian populations at high risk for esophageal cancer (9,13), and thus it
was a suspected causative agent. However, Table IV clearly shows that
nass was not associated with the disease among Turkomans and Turks. In
Persian-speaking groups, there is an indication that nass may have increased the risk; however, less than 6% of the patients chewed nass.
Thus, this factor makes little, if any, contribution to the overall incidence. Table IV clearly indicates that there was no "moderate" use of
nass or tobacco among patients or controls, i.e., subjects chewed daily
or not at all.

IV. OPIUM USE

Table V gives data on opium use among cases and controls, by age,
sex and language group. The findings should be treated with caution, as
opium is often taken as a pain killer by the sick. Although particular
attention was paid to obtaining a history of opium use before the onset
of the disease, a positive response would be more likely to come from
those with esophageal cancer, as it is generally accepted that they do
use opium, while a healthy person, may not readily admit to opium use.
In view of these caveats, calculated values of the relative risks and of
significance levels are of little interest. Nevertheless, there is an
indication that regular opium use did increase the risk for esophageal
cancer. It is clearly not the factor responsible for the very high rates
among Turkomans, as this factor must affect females at least as much as
males, whereas the effect of opium was inappreciable among women, especially in Turkoman women with their very high incidence.

DISCUSSION

The results of this study, in which nearly 500 patients and healthy
individuals were interviewed, confirmed initial observations that neither
alcohol, tobacco, nor their combinations contributed appreciably to
esophageal cancer risk in northeastern Iran.

Opium use may be a risk factor for the disease but further work is needed to obtain more objective measures of opium intake, especially from the healthy population. However, opium is clearly not the factor underlying the very high risk among the Turkoman people.

Further studies in the Caspian Littoral have shown that in this region, long-term nutritional deficiencies exist and this may be related to the increased risk of esophageal cancer, without the added influence of either tobacco or alcohol (5). These deficiencies appear particularly severe among Turkomans and since the present studies failed to pinpoint any specific factor or known carcinogen, it seems that the combination and/or interaction of several factors are indicated as a possible cause. These factors include: nutritional deficiency, trauma to esophageal mucosa through ingestion of dust and silica particles, consumption of hot beverages, and dietary constituents deriving from typical central Asian climatic and soil types. The latter would include mycotoxins produced by fungi favored by the special environmental conditions, and possibly extraneous carcinogenic seeds in the wheat.

Thus, elimination of alcohol and tobacco as prime suspects in the causation of esophageal cancer calls for further study of other factors. The investigations are presently underway.

ACKNOWLEDGEMENT: This work was supported by the Institute of Public Health Research, University of Teheran, Iran and the International Agency for Research on Cancer, Lyon, France. The writing of this paper was financed by contract NO1 CP33278 from the National Cancer Institute, NIH, PHS. The authors thank Mardelle Susman for editorial assistance.

SUMMARY

A case control study was conducted to determine the influence of alcohol, tobacco and opium use in esophageal cancer. The study focused on an area of high esophageal cancer incidence, the Caspian Littoral of Iran. In interviews with 151 patients and 301 healthy controls, alcohol and tobacco were found to play negligible roles in the disease, and other possible causative agents are suggested. The data showed that opium may play a role in the disease's etiology, but the possibility of bias in response could not be excluded.

TABLE I. Distribution of 151 Cases of Esophageal Cancer by Age, Sex and Language Groups, with 301 Controls

Ages of Subjects

Number of cases/Number of controls

First Language	< 35		36 – 44		45 – 54		55 – 64		65 and Over		Total Cases		Total Controls	
	M[a]	F	M	F	M	F	M	F	M	F	M	F	M	F
Turkoman or Turkic	1/2	5/14	1/19	1/10	3/9	8/8	5/15	1/7	7/7	1/3	17	16	52	42
Persian	3/15	6/17	5/40	7/21	16/36	16/19	18/27	14/10	25/17	8/5	67	51	135	72
Total in each age group	4/17	11/31	6/59	8/31	19/45	24/27	23/42	15/17	32/24	9/8	84	67	187	114

[a] M = Males; F = Females.

1154

TABLE II. Frequency of Consumption of Alcoholic Drinks in 151 Cases of Esophageal Cancer Patients and in 301 Controls

First Language	Frequency[a]	Ages of Subjects											Total of Cases and Controls			
		< 35		35 – 44		45 – 54		55 – 64		65 and Over		Cases		Controls		
		M[b]	F	M	F	M	F	M	F	M	F	M	F	M	F
		Number of cases/Number of controls													
Turkoman and Turkic	0	1/2	5/14	1/17	1/10	2/9	8/8	5/14	1/7	6/7	1/3	15	16	49	42
	1	0/0	0/0	0/2	0/0	1/0	0/0	0/0	0/0	0/0	0/0	2	0	2	0
	2	0/0	0/0	0/0	0/0	0/0	0/0	0/0	0/0	0/0	0/0	0	0	0	0
	3	0/0	0/0	0/0	0/0	0/0	0/0	0/0	0/0	0/0	0/0	0	0	0	0
Persian	0	2/13	6/17	2/32	7/21	12/24	16/19	16/22	14/10	20/16	7/5	52	50	107	72
	1	1/1	0/0	2/6	0/0	1/6	0/0	1/4	0/0	4/1	0/0	9	0	18	0
	2	0/1	0/0	1/2	0/0	2/5	0/0	1/0	0/0	0/0	0/0	4	1	8	0
	3	0/0	0/0	0/0	0/0	1/1	0/0	0/1	0/0	1/0	0/0	2	1	2	0
Total, according to frequency of consumption	0	3/15	11/31	3/49	8/31	14/33	24/27	21/36	15/17	26/23	8/8	67	66	156	114
	1	1/1	0/0	2/8	0/0	2/6	0/0	1/0	0/0	5/1	0/0	11	0	20	0
	2	0/1	0/0	1/2	0/0	2/5	0/0	1/0	0/0	0/0	0/0	4	0	8	1
	3	0/0	0/0	1/1	0/0	1/1	0/0	0/2	0/0	1/0	1/0	2	1	3	0

[a] 0 = Never drink
1 = Occasionally, i.e., once a month
2 = Up to twice or three times a week
3 = One drink per day or more

[b] M = Males; F = Females.

1155

TABLE III. Number of Cigarette Smokers among 151 Esophageal Cancer Patients and 301 Controls

First Language	Frequency[a]	< 35 M[b]	< 35 F	35 - 44 M	35 - 44 F	45 - 54 M	45 - 54 F	55 - 64 M	55 - 64 F	65 and Over M	65 and Over F	Total Cases M	Total Cases F	Total Controls M	Total Controls F
		Number of cases/Number of controls										Total of Cases and Controls			
Turkoman and Turkic	0	0/2	5/14	0/10	1/10	2/8	8/8	4/11	1/7	6/6	1/3	12	16	37	42
	1	0/0	0/0	0/3	0/0	0/1	0/0	0/2	0/0	0/1	0/0	0	0	7	0
	2	0/0	0/0	1/2	0/0	0/0	0/0	0/0	0/0	0/0	0/0	1	0	2	0
	3	1/0	0/0	0/4	0/0	1/0	0/0	1/2	0/0	1/0	0/0	4	0	6	0
Persian	0	2/12	6/17	5/20	7/21	4/12	14/19	10/15	14/10	15/4	7/5	36	48	63	72
	1	1/0	0/0	0/0	0/0	1/1	0/0	2/4	0/0	3/1	0/0	7	0	6	0
	2	0/1	0/0	0/9	0/0	0/6	0/0	0/3	0/0	1/8	0/0	1	0	27	0
	3	0/2	0/0	0/11	0/0	11/17	2/0	6/5	0/0	6/4	1/0	23	3	39	0
Total by frequency of use	0	2/14	11/31	5/30	8/31	6/20	22/27	14/26	15/17	21/10	8/8	48	64	100	114
	1	1/0	0/0	0/3	0/0	1/2	0/0	2/6	0/0	3/2	0/0	7	0	13	0
	2	0/1	0/0	1/11	0/0	0/6	0/0	0/3	0/0	1/8	0/0	2	0	29	0
	3	1/2	0/0	0/15	0/0	12/17	2/0	7/7	0/0	7/4	1/0	27	3	45	0

[a] 0 = Never smoke
1 = Less than 10 cigarettes per day
2 = 10-19 cigarettes per day
3 = 20 or more cigarettes per day

[b] M = Males; F = Females.

TABLE IV. Use of Nass in 151 Cases of Esophageal Cancer Patients and in 301 Controls[a]

First Language	Frequency[b]	< 35 M[c]	< 35 F	35 - 44 M	35 - 44 F	45 - 54 M	45 - 54 F	55 - 64 M	55 - 64 F	65 and Over M	65 and Over F	Total of Cases and Controls M	F	M	F
		Number of cases/Number of controls													
Turkoman and Turkic	0	1/2	5/14	1/18	1/10	2/4	8/8	4/13	1/17	4/4	1/3	12	16	41	42
	1	0/0	0/0	0/0	0/0	0/0	0/0	0/0	0/0	0/0	0/0	0	0	0	0
	2	0/0	0/0	0/1	0/0	1/5	0/0	1/2	0/0	3/3	0/0	5	0	11	0
Persian	0	3/14	6/17	5/40	7/21	15/35	16/19	17/27	13/10	22/17	8/5	62	50	133	72
	1	0/0	0/0	0/0	0/0	0/0	0/0	0/0	0/0	0/0	0/0	0	0	0	0
	2	0/1	0/0	0/0	0/0	1/1	0/0	1/0	1/0	3/0	0/0	5	1	2	0
Total Nass users by frequency	0	4/16	11/31	6/58	8/31	17/39	24/27	21/40	14/17	26/21	9/8	74	66	174	114
	1	0/0	0/0	0/0	0/0	0/0	0/0	0/0	0/0	0/0	0/0	0	0	0	0
	2	0/1	0/0	0/1	0/0	2/6	0/0	2/2	1/0	6/3	0/0	10	1	13	0

[a]Nass = Mixture of tobacco with ashes and lime which is chewed.

[b]Frequency: 0 = Never

1 = Occasionally

2 = Every day

[c]M = Males; F = Females.

1157

TABLE V. Use of Opium by 151 Esophageal Cancer Patients and in 301 Controls

Number of cases/Number of controls

First Language	Frequency[a]	< 35 M[b]	< 35 F	35–44 M	35–44 F	45–54 M	45–54 F	55–64 M	55–64 F	65 and Over M	65 and Over F	Total Cases M	Total Cases F	Total Controls M	Total Controls F
Turkoman and Turkic	0	0/2	5/14	0/17	1/10	1/7	7/8	4/14	1/7	5/6	1/3	10	15	46	42
	1	0/0	0/0	0/1	0/0	0/0	0/0	0/0	0/0	0/0	0/0	0	0	1	0
	2	0/0	0/0	0/1	0/0	0/1	0/0	0/1	0/0	1/1	0/0	1	0	4	0
	3	1/0	0/0	1/0	0/0	2/1	1/0	1/0	0/0	1/0	0/0	6	1	1	0
Persian	0	3/15	6/17	3/39	7/21	8/31	10/19	13/22	13/10	11/16	5/5	38	41	123	72
	1	0/0	0/0	0/0	0/0	0/2	0/0	0/0	0/0	1/0	0/0	1	0	2	0
	2	0/0	0/0	0/0	0/0	1/0	4/0	0/1	0/0	3/0	0/0	4	4	1	0
	3	0/0	0/0	2/1	0/0	7/3	2/0	5/4	1/0	10/1	3/0	24	6	9	0
Total by frequency of use	0	3/17	11/31	3/56	8/31	9/38	17/27	17/36	14/17	16/22	6/8	48	56	169	114
	1	0/0	0/0	0/1	0/0	0/2	0/0	0/0	0/0	1/0	0/0	1	0	3	0
	2	0/0	0/0	0/1	0/0	1/1	4/0	0/2	0/0	4/1	0/0	5	4	5	0
	3	1/0	0/0	3/1	0/0	9/4	3/0	6/4	1/0	11/1	3/0	30	7	10	0

[a]Frequency: 0 = Never used
1 = Occasionally, less than once a week
2 = Once a week to once a day
3 = More than once a day

[b]M = Males; F = Females.

REFERENCES

1. Cook, P. Cancer of the Oesophagus in Africa. Br. J. Cancer, 25: 853-878, 1971.

2. Doll, R., Muir, C., and Waterhouse, J. Cancer Incidence in Five Continents, Vol. II. International Union Against Cancer, 1970.

3. Hakim, S.E.A. National Cancer Conference. Bangalor, Nov. 3-6, 1971. Tata Press, Ltd., Bombay-25, 1971.

4. Higginson, J., and Muir, C.S. Epidemiology. In: Cancer Medicine. Eds.: J.F. Holland and E. Frei III. Lea and Febiger, Philadelphia, p. 249, 1973.

5. Hormozdiari, H., Day, N.E., Aramesh, B., and Mahboubi, E. Dietary Factors and Esophageal Cancer in the Caspian Littoral of Iran. Cancer Res. 35:3493-3498, 1975.

6. Kmet, H., and Mahboubi, E. Esophageal Cancer in the Caspian Littoral of Iran: Initial Studies. Science, 1975:846, 1972.

7. Mahboubi, E., Kmet, J., Cook, P.J., Day, E., Ghadirian, P., and Salmasizadeh, S. Oesophageal Cancer Studies in the Caspian Littoral of Iran: The Caspian Cancer Registry. Br. J. Cancer, 28:197-214, 1973.

8. Martinez, I. Factors Associated with Cancer of the Esophagus, Mouth, and Pharynx in Puerto Rico. J. Natl. Cancer Inst., 42:1069-1077, 1969.

9. Rahmatian, H., and Mojtabai, A. Experimental Carcinoma of Esophagus. Acta Medica Iranica, 8:11-18, 1965.

10. Segi, M., and Kurihara, M. Cancer Mortality for Selected Sites in 24 Countries, no. 6, 1966-1967. Japan Cancer Society, 1972.

11. Tuyns, A.J. Cancer of the Oesophagus: Further Evidence of the Relation to Drinking Habits in France. Int. J. Cancer, 5:152-156, 1972.

12. Wynder, W.E., and Bross, I.J. A Study of Etiological Factors in Cancer of the Esophagus. Cancer, 14:389-412, 1961.

13. Warwick, G.P., and Harington, J.S. Some Aspects of the Epidemiology and Etiology of Esophageal Cancer with Particular Emphasis on the Transkei, South Africa. In: Advances in Cancer Research. Eds.: G. Klein, S. Weinhouse, and A. Haddow. Academic Press Inc., New York, 17:81-229, 1973.

GEOGRAPHICAL DISTRIBUTION OF GASTROINTESTINAL
CANCER AND BREAST CANCER AND ITS RELATION
TO SELENIUM DEFICIENCY

Birger Jansson, Mary Anne Malahy and G. Burton Seibert [1]

National Large Bowel Cancer Project
The University of Texas System Cancer Center
M.D. Anderson Hospital and Tumor Institute
Houston, Texas

I. INTRODUCTION

Most cancers are caused by environmental agents, natural or man-made, according to the general conviction of researchers in cancer epidemiology and carcinogenesis. Much effort has been directed towards finding the carcinogens and describing their action. Less effort has been directed towards finding and explaining the action of agents that inhibit the effects of carcinogens. From a conceptual point of view, the probability for a person to get cancer during a time unit, for example during a year, may be illustrated as in Figure 1. For any given level of the amount of carcinogens to which a person is exposed, the incidence probability may be reduced by increasing the amount of inhibitors (protecting agents, anti-carcinogens). In order to decrease the probability to get cancer, one can thus either decrease the amount of carcinogens or increase the amount of inhibitors or - most effectively - simultaneously decrease the carcinogens and increase the inhibitors. Even if for some cancers the carcinogens remain unknown, it might be possible to find means to reduce their effects, thereby reducing incidence probabilities.

During a person's life span the amount of carcinogens to which he or she is exposed will change, e.g. due to a change of diet, a change of habits, or a change of place of living. For similar reasons the amount of protection may change. The amount of protection may also decrease with growing age or increase during special time periods, such as pregnancies, which are observed

The authors gratefully acknowledge the support, interest, and encouragement given by the Project Director of the National Large Bowel Cancer Project, Dr. Murray M. Copeland, and by the Project's Associate Director for Scientific Operations, Dr. Rulon W. Rawson.

1) Presently at Penrose Cancer Hospital, Colorado Springs, Colorado.

to decrease breast cancer rates. Knowing the incidence probabilities for each time unit, one might calculate the probability to get cancer during some arbitrary time interval, which is equivalent to determining the cancer rates.

A group of compounds which are antioxidants or have antioxidant properties have drawn special interest as cancer inhibitors. Wattenberg (ref. 32) reported no evidence of large bowel neoplasia in mice given the antioxidant disulfiram compared to a control group in which all mice showed multiple tumors. Both groups of mice were given the carcinogen dimethylhydrazine (DMH). Other examples are the inhibition of transplantable murine melanoma by vitamin A as reported by Felix et al. (ref. 10) and the increase in colon tumors in rats that are deficient in vitamin A when challenged with the carcinogen aflatoxin B (Newberne-Rogers, ref. 22). Vitamin E has also been mentioned as an inhibitor either alone or together with the trace element selenium, which also has antioxidant properties.

In this paper we discuss different indications that point at selenium as a cancer inhibitor. We begin with comparisons between the geographical distribution of colorectal cancer rates and breast cancer rates on one hand and the distribution of selenium on the other hand. The following section contains some results from the literature on selenium as a cancer inhibitor where two animal experiments are of great interest.

Since experimental evidence on the relationship between human cancers and the prevalence of selenium is difficult to obtain, to a great extent one must lean on indirect evidences. In the last two sections, two relationships of this indirect nature are discussed. Firstly, it is shown that there seems to be a positive correlation between breast cancer rates and age at diagnosis - low rates thus correspond to early onset of the disease and high rates to late onset of the disease, which is analogous to findings in an animal experiment. There does not seem to be any similar relationship for colon cancer, rectum cancer, or stomach cancer. Secondly, by using U.S. mortality data and natality statistics, it is shown that there is a negative correlation between the rates for colon, rectum, breast and stomach cancer on one hand, and the birth rates on the other hand. This is expected since it is known that selenium deficiency reduces the fertility for some animal species.

II. GEOGRAPHICAL DISTRIBUTION

In the paper by Jansson et al. (ref. 14) maps are presented that show high and low mortality rate areas for the counties in the continental U.S. It is also pointed out in the same paper that for this geographical area there is a high correlation between the geographical distributions of colon cancer and breast cancer ($\rho = .93$) and rectum cancer and breast cancer ($\rho = .95$). The corresponding breast cancer map has been constructed, but not yet published. The data for this study was taken from Mason-McKay (ref. 18). A number of similar maps using the same source have been published in an atlas by Mason et al. (ref. 19).

In order to reduce some of the statistical variations, that, above all, depend on small populations in many of the counties, and in order to be able to compare cancers with different rates on an equal basis, a ranking procedure has been used. The counties have been ranked according to cancer rates from the county with highest rate (rank = 1) to the county with lowest rate (rank = 3055). This has been done for:

Male colon cancer
Female colon cancer
Male rectum cancer
Female rectum cancer
Male breast cancer
Female breast cancer
Male stomach cancer, and
Female stomach cancer.

In all cases the white population only has been considered. Since colon cancer and rectum cancer have very similar geographical distributions, the sum of the ranks for male and female colon cancer and male and female rectum cancer has been calculated for each county. These sums have been reranked from the county with the lowest sum of ranks (highest rates) to the one with the highest sum of ranks (lowest rates). Thus, for each county we have calculated

Rank [Rank (colon, male) + Rank (colon, female) + Rank (rectum, male) + Rank (rectum, female)].

After locating the 300 counties with the highest ranks, the 300 counties next highest, the 300 counties lowest and the 300 counties next lowest, we find the result confirms and refines previous findings that the high colorectal cancer area is found in the Northeast and the low colorectal cancer area is found in the South and in the Rocky Mountains area. A finer structure has been obtained by dividing the 300 counties in the U.S. with high colorectal cancer rates into groups of 100 counties. In Figure 2 the distribution of these high colorectal cancer areas in the Northeast is displayed. The result is interesting, for it shows clearly that the Atlantic coast from Canada to and including New Jersey is the most dominating area for colorectal cancer. In a similar study of low colorectal cancer areas no dominating areas were found.

In a similar study the differences in the distributions of colon cancer and rectum cancer have been studied by determining for each county

Rank [Rank (colon, male)+Rank (colon, female)-Rank (rectum, male) -Rank (rectum, female)].

The distribution is mainly random indicating no geographical difference in the prevalence of colon cancer and rectum cancer. There is, however, a tendency to rectum cancer dominance in the Pacific area.

Most large bowel cancer epidemiologists agree on the hypothesis that the carcinogen causing this cancer is to be found in the diet, especially in beef and animal fat (ref. 4, 13, 36, 37). Objecting opinions have been brought forward, however; an example is a recent paper by Enstrom (ref. 9).

Since the diet is rather homogenous over the U.S., the distribution maps with their clearly marked high rate and low rate areas indicate that some factors besides the carcinogens in the diet influence the cancer rates. One such factor may be the trace element selenium, that is deficient in areas with high colorectal cancer rates and high breast cancer rates.

III. SOME INDICATIONS OF SELENIUM ACTING AS AN INHIBITOR

In this section we present a number of evidences which indicate that selenium acts as an inhibitor or a protector against cancer.

A. Geographic Correspondence Between Selenium-Deficient Areas and High Cancer Rate Areas

The distribution in the U.S. of the selenium concentration in crops, soil, water, etc. is presented in a number of articles; we refer to Kubota et al. (ref. 17), Kubota, and Allaway (ref. 16), and Allaway et al. (ref. 1). Besides discussing the prevalence of selenium in U.S.A., these papers present maps showing the selenium distribution. There is good agreement between the areas low in selenium and the areas high in colon, rectum, and breast cancer. This is particularly evident in the northeastern region of the country. Unfortunately, the maps are not detailed enough to reveal if there is a difference in the selenium concentration in the coastal regions of New England and its inland regions.

A detailed global distribution of selenium is not known. A few observations may be noted. Japan, which has very low rates for colon and breast cancer, has the highest production of selenium per unit of area of all countries (29 pounds / sq. mile). A table of world production of selenium is given in Zingaro-Cooper (ref. 38).

New Zealand is a country in which the selenium concentration in the soil has been thoroughly studied due to the selenium - responsive diseases that occur in animals in this country, Wells (ref. 34), Andrews et al. (ref. 3), Hartley - Grant (ref. 12). New Zealand has been shown to have large selenium deficient areas; it also has very high rates for colon, rectum, and breast cancer.

B. An Observation of a New Zealand Veterinarian

The late Dr. Wedderburn, a veterinarian in New Zealand, has in a brief communication (ref. 33) noted his observation that since the introduction of selenium drenching of the sheep in New Zealand, the incidence of intestinal adenocarcinomas and other neoplasms of these animals has been reduced almost to zero. In a personal communication Dr. Money, Ministry of Agriculture and Fisheries, New Zealand, recalled that Dr. Wedderburn had observed before the drenching period small intestinal carcinoma in about 2% of ewes between 4 and 7 years in age. After the use of selenium became common, it was rare to see carcinoma cases with Dr. Wedderburn concluding that they had virtually disappeared.

C. Observations of Cancer Rate Differences in Areas Low and Areas High in Selenium in the U.S. and in Canada

In a series of papers Shamberger and his coworkers have discussed the role of antioxidants and especially selenium as inhibitors of cancer (ref. 24, 25, 26, 27). From Shamberger et al. (ref. 28) we extract the data in Tables I and II. Table I gives the ratio of the observed to the expected cancer death rates in 17 pairwise matched large cities in the U.S., with one city of the pair in a high selenium area and its matched city in a low selenium area. Table II is a similar table for some Canadian areas, but in this case the age-adjusted mortality rates are given.

For the organs listed, the cancer incidence is higher in areas low in selenium than in areas high in selenium in the U.S.A. as well as in Canada.

D. Induced Cancer in Rats Inhibited by Selenium

Harr et al. (ref. 11) report an experiment in which they fed rats diets containing selenium in varying concentrations as well as a known carcinogen. Eighty female OSU-brown rats were used. These rats were divided into four groups with twenty rats per group. The rats, which were vitamin E-supplemented and selenium-deficient were fed the carcinogen N-2 fluorenyl acetanide (FAA) and varying amounts of selenite. The results, extracted from the paper by Harr et al., are shown in Table III. There is a dramatic decrease in the rates of induced hepatic and mammary cancers following increased additions of selenium.

E. Spontaneous Mammary Tumors in Mice Inhibited by Selenium

Schrauzer and Ishmael (ref. 23) report an experiment in which they used female virgin C3H-mice. These mice develop mammary carcinoma with 85% incidence at an age between 12 and 16 months. Sixty mice were divided into two groups of 30 mice each. One group was given 2 ppm selenium in the drinking water, the other group no selenium. The results presented in Table IV are extracted from Schrauzer and Ishmael's paper. There is again a very dramatic reduction in the incidence rate of mammary cancer for the mice given selenium.

Moreover the morbidity of the disease was changed - the survival time for the selenium fed mice being considerably longer. Very interesting and quite unexpected was the finding that the incidence age was lowered for those mice in the selenium group that developed mammary cancer compared to the cases in the control group. One would expect the opposite, namely that a higher incidence rate should be accompanied by an earlier onset of the disease. The selenium thus seems to have an effect similar to a natural immunization - it reduces the incidence age, but most animals will overcome the disease and remain protected against further inductions.

IV. STUDY OF THE RELATION BETWEEN INCIDENCE RATE AND AGE AT DIAGNOSIS FOR HUMAN BREAST CANCER

The finding by Schrauzer and Ishmael that there is a positive correlation between age at diagnosis and incidence rate for some mice mammary tumors, interested us since it contradicted our belief that one would expect a negative correlation between these two entities. From the international incidence data published by UICC and edited by Doll et al. (ref. 8), we extracted incidence rates, age - adjusted by a world standard population, for some low rate, middle rate and high rate regions. Using data from the same sources, we calculated the conditional distribution function for the age at diagnosis for persons with the disease, and displayed the relationship in diagrams. The study was performed for cancer of the colon, rectum, stomach, and breast. For colon cancer, rectum cancer, and stomach cancer, this material did not show any obvious relations; for breast cancer, however, we retrieved Schrauzer and Ishmael's finding. The results are presented in the upper diagram in Figure 3. On the median level, where the distribution function is 0.5, there is a difference in age at diagnosis of approximately 15 years between the low rate areas, represented by Japan and Singapore, and the medium and high rate areas, represented by Connecticut in their extreme. There is a monotonically increasing age at diagnosis for increasing incidence rates. The only exception is Singapore. For this area, however, the statistics are only given for women below age 75, compared to age 85+ for the other regions, which means that Singapore, at least for high ages, is not comparable with the others. The lower diagram in Figure 3 is a transformation of the upper one, giving the relation between age at diagnosis and incidence rate for the first quintile, the median, and the third quintile of the distribution. One may note that above rate 30/100,000/ year there is only a small difference in age at diagnosis, while the difference is considerable when we move towards lower incidence rates.

A similar study was performed using data from the 3rd National Cancer Survey (Cutler and Young, ref. 7; Cutler et al., ref. 6). The results for the nine regions for which data is reported in this survey are shown in Figure 4. There is a clear tendency pointing at a positive correlation here also between age at diagnosis and incidence rate. Since all the rates are high, we can, however, not expect a clear-cut result in this case. The greatest exception for the rule is the San Francisco - Oakland area. This area together with the counties in the Great Valley is an exceptional area for breast cancer with very high rates.

V. RELATION BETWEEN BIRTH RATES AND CANCER MORTALITY RATES

In order to get indirect evidences for the role of selenium as an inhibitor of carcinogens, one can choose to study known properties of selenium for animals and try to retrieve the same properties among humans. Since it is known that a deficiency of selenium - like a deficiency of vitamin E - reduces the fertility of animals, see e.g. Buchanan-Smith et al. (ref. 5), one may expect a similar effect for humans. In low selenium areas one would thus expect low birth rates and high colorectal and breast cancer rates and in high selenium areas, high birth rates and low cancer rates. This has been studied by using natality statistics for the 48 continental states in U.S.A. (ref. 31) and mortality statistics for the same states (Mason - McKay, ref. 18). The results for colon, rectum, stomach, and breast cancer are shown in scattergrams in Figures 5 - 8. The results support the hypothesis of a negative correlation between birth rates and mortality rates for colon cancer, rectum cancer, and for female breast cancer, with correlation coefficients between - 0.73 and - 0.83. The relation is much less obvious for stomach cancer.

Birth rates are affected by many different phenomena of biological, cultural, or religious nature. Nevertheless, the finding of a negative correlation between birth rates and colon, rectum, and breast cancer rates for human data is support for the hypothesis that selenium - or some other agent - acts as an inhibitor of these cancers.

VI. DISCUSSION

We have in this paper delineated evidences, taken from reports of other researchers and from our own studies, indicating that selenium may act as an inhibitor of cancer of the colon, rectum, and breast. It may share this property with other antioxidants such as vitamin E. It is known that vitamin E alone, or selenium alone, or sometimes combination of both can cure some cattle diseases even if given in trace amounts only.

The way the antioxidants act as cancer inhibitors is unclear. It has been suggested that the antioxidants suppress the peroxidation of polyunsaturated lipids thereby reducing the production of malonaldehyde, which is known to be both mutagenic and carcinogenic (Shamberger - Willis, ref. 29; Tappel, ref. 30; Mukai - Goldstein, ref. 21).

If it can be definitely established that selenium or vitamin E or some other antioxidant - can reduce the incidence of some human cancers, it might be given in non-toxic amounts as a food additive. This would be a more profitable way to reduce cancer rates than attempts to change persons' eating habits.

Table I   Mean values of observed/expected cancer rates in pairs of matched cities. From Shamberger et al., (ref. 28).

OBSERVED/EXPECTED CA RATE (U.S.A.)

	AREA THAT IS	
	LOW IN SE	HIGH IN SE
STOMACH	1.68	.99
COLON	1.08	.80
RECTUM	1.39	.89

Table II   Age-adjusted death rates in Canadian areas low and high in selenium. From Shamberger et al., (ref. 28).

AGE-ADJUSTED DEATH RATE (CANADA)

	AREA THAT IS	
	LOW IN SE	HIGH IN SE
INTESTINE	18.4	11.6
STOMACH	19.1	16.6
RECTUM	8.6	6.0
BREAST	24.2	21.7

Talbe III   Relation between incidence rates of FAA-induced cancers in rats and amount of selenium added to the food. Each group contained 20 rats. From Harr et al., (ref. 11).

GROUP	ADDITION OF SE	RATS WITH HEPATIC OR MAMMARY CANCER
I	2.5 ppm	0 %
II	.5 ppm	10 %
III	.1 ppm	60 %
IV	0	60 %

Table IV   The incidence rate of spontaneous mammary tumors for mice is reduced by adding 2 ppm selenium to the drinking water - 30 mice in each group. From Schrauzer-Ishmael (ref. 23).

SE IN DR-WATER	INCIDENCE RATE	AGE AT INCIDENCE	SURVIVAL TIME
2 ppm	10 %	9 months	5-7 months
0 ppm	82 %	12-16 months	4 months

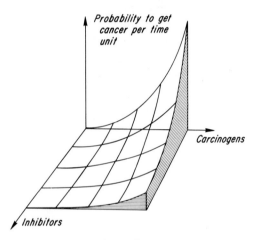

FIG. 1. A conceptual representation of the probability of getting cancer
as a function of the independent variables "amount of carcinogen" and
"amount of inhibitors" to which a person has been exposed.

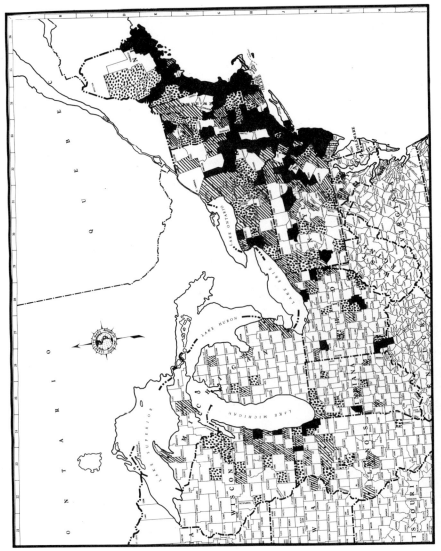

FIG. 2. A more detailed presentation of the U.S. counties highest in colorectal cancer. The high rates along the New England coast are most striking. Solid: highest 100 counties. Striped: second highest 100 counties. Dotted: third highest counties.

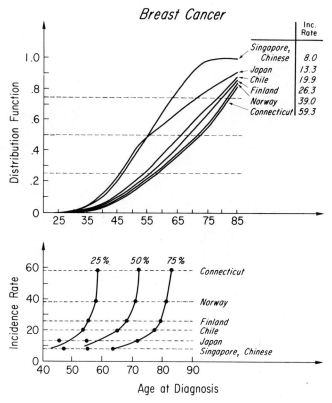

FIG. 3. Relation between age at diagnosis and incidence rate for breast cancer. International data.

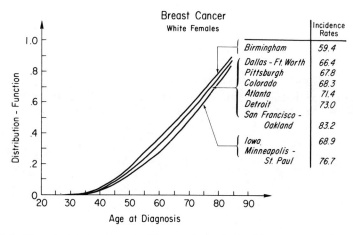

FIG. 4. Relation between age at diagnosis and incidence rate for breast cancer of whites in ine regions in U.S.A.

1171

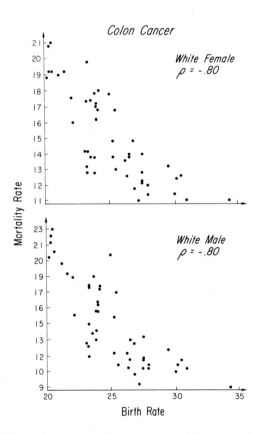

FIG. 5. Relation between birth rate and mortality rate in colon cancer for whites in the continental states of the U.S.A.

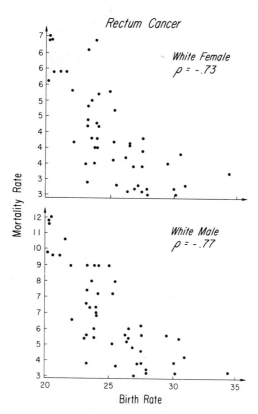

FIG. 6. Relation between birth rate and mortality rate in rectum cancer for whites in the continental states of the U.S.A.

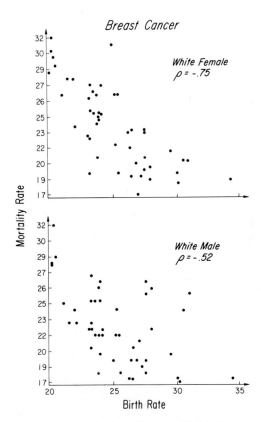

FIG. 7. Relation between birth rate and mortality rate in breast cancer for whites in the continental states of the U.S.A.

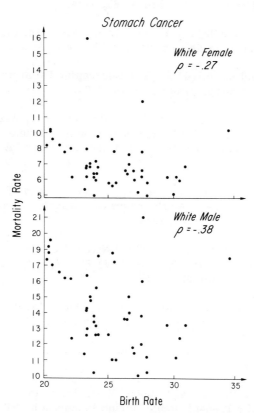

FIG. 8.   Relation between birth rate and mortality rate in stomach cancer for whites in the continental states of the U.S.A.

REFERENCES

1. Allaway, W.H. Selenium in the Food Chain. Cornell Vet., 63; 151-170, 1973.

2. Allaway, W.H., Laitinen, H.A., Lakin, H.W., Muth, O.H., and Oldfield, J.E. Selenium. Geochemistry and the Environment, Vol. I: The Relation of Selected Trace Elements to Health and Disease. National Academy of Sciences, Washington, D.C., pp. 57-63, 1974.

3. Andrews, E.D., Hartley, W.J., and Grant, A.B. Selenium-Responsive Diseases of Animals in New Zealand. NZ Vet J., 16: 3-17, 1968.

4. Berg, J.W., and Howell, M.A. The Geographic Pathology of Bowel Cancer. Cancer (Suppl.), 34: 807-814, 1974.

5. Buchanan-Smith, J.G., Nelson, E.C., Osburn, B.I., Wells, M.E., and Tillman, A.D. Effects of Vitamin E and Selenium Deficiencies in Sheep Fed a Purified Diet during Growth and Reproduction. J Anim Sci., 29: 808-815, 1969.

6. Cutler, S.J., Scotto, J., Devesa, S.S., and Connelly, R.R. Third National Cancer Survey - An Overview of Available Information. J Natl Cancer Inst., 53: 1565-1575, 1974.

7. Cutler, S.J., and Young, J.L. Third National Cancer Survey: Incidence Data, 1975. DHEW Publication No. (NIH) 75-787, U.S. Government Printing Office, Washington, D.C.

8. Doll, R., Payne, P., and Waterhouse, J. Cancer Incidence in Five Continents, A Technical Report. UICC, Switzerland, 1966.

9. Enstrom, J.E. Colorectal Cancer and Consumption of Beef and Fat. Br J Cancer, 32: 432-439, 1975.

10. Felix, E. L., Loyd, B., and Cohen, M.H. Inhibition of the Growth and Development of a Transplantable Murine Melanoma by Vitamin A. Science, 189: 886-888, 1975.

11. Harr, J.R., Exon, J.H., Wesivig, P.H., and Whanger, P.D. Relationship of Dietary Selenium Concentration; Chemical Cancer Induction; and Tissue Concentration of Selenium in Rats. Clin Toxicol, 6: 487-495, 1973.

12. Hartley, W.J., and Grant, A.B. A Review of Selenium Responsive Diseases of New Zealand Livestock. Fed Proc., 20: 679-688, 1961.

13. Hill, M.J. Bacteria and the Etiology of Colonic Cancer. Cancer (Suppl.) 34: 815-818, 1974.

14. Jansson, B. J., Seibert, G.B., and Speer, J.F. Gastrointestinal Cancer-its Geographical Distribution, and its Correlation to Breast Cancer. Cancer (Suppl.), 36: 2373-2384, 1975.

15. Klayman, D.L, and Gunther, W.H.H. Organic Selenium Compounds: Their Chemistry and Biology. John Wiley and Sons, Inc., New York,1973.

16. Kubota, J., and Allaway, W.H. Geographic Distribution of Trace Element Problems in the United States. Micronutrients in Agriculture. Soil Science Society of America, Inc., Madison, Wisconsin, pp. 525-554, 1972.

17. Kubota, J., Allaway, W.H., Carter, D.L., Cary, E.E., and Lazar, V.A. Selenium in Crops in the United States in Relation to Selenium - Responsive Diseases of Livestock. J Agric Food Chem., 15: 448-453, 1967.

18. Mason, T.J., and McKay, F.W. U.S. Cancer Mortality by County: 1950-1969, 1974. DHEW Publication No. (NIH) 74-615, U.S. Government Printing Office, Washington, D.C.

19. Mason, T.J., McKay, F.W., Hoover, R., Blot, W.J., and Fraumeni, J.R., Jr. Atlas of Cancer Mortality for U.S. Counties: 1950-1969,1975. DHEW Publication No. (NIH) 75-780, U.S. Government Printing Office, Washington, D.C.

20. Maugh, F.H.,II. Vitamin A: Potential Protection for Carcinogens. Science, 136: 1198, 1974.

21. Mukai, F.H., and Goldstein, B.D. Mutagenicity of Malonaldehyde, a Decomposition Product of Peroxidized Polyunsaturated Fatty Acids. Science, 191: 868-869, 1976.

22. Newberne, P.M., and Rogers, A.E. Rat Colon Carcinomas Associated with Aflatoxin and Marginal Vitamin A. J Natl Cancer Inst. 50: 439-448, 1973.

23. Schrauzer, G.N., and Ishmael, D. Effects of Selenium and of Arsenic on the Genesis of Spontaneous Mammary Tumors in Inbred C_3H Mice. Ann Clin Lab Sci., 4: 441-447, 1974.

24. Shamberger, R.J. Relationship of Selenium to Cancer. I. Inhibitory Effect of Selenium on Carcinogensis. J Natl Cancer Inst., 44: 931-936, 1970.

25. Shamberger, R.J. Increase of Peroxidation in Carcinogenesis. J Natl Cancer Inst., 48: 1491-1497, 1972.

26. Shamberger, R.J., and Rudolph, G. Protection against Cocarcinogenesis by Antioxidants. Experientia, 22: 116, 1966.

27. Shamberger, R.J., Tytko, S., and Willis, C.E. Antioxidants in Cereals and in Food Preservatives and Declining Gastric Cancer Mortality. Cleve. Clin. Q., 39: 119-124, 1972.

28. Shamberger, R.J., Tytko, S., and Willis, C. Antioxidants and Cancer: Selenium Distribution and Human Cancer Mortality in the United States, Canada and New Zealand. Trace Substances in Environmental Health - VII. University of Missouri, Columbia ,pp. 31-34, 1974.

29. Shamberger, R.J., and Willis, C.E. A New Carcinogen is Present in Beef and Other Meats. Proc. of the AACR and ASCO, AACR Abstracts, Abstract No. 269, 1975.

30. Tappel, A.L. Vitamin E and Free Radical Peroxidation of Lipids. Annals of the New York Academy of Sciences, 203: 12-28, 1972.

31. Vital Statistics of the United States, 1968. Live Births per 1000 Population/Year, Vol. I, Natality.

32. Wattenberg, L.W. Inhibition of Dimethylhydrazine - Induced Neoplasia of the Large Intestine by Disulfiram. J Natl Cancer Inst., 54: 1005-1006, 1975.

33. Wedderburn, J.F. Selenium and Cancer. NZ Vet J., 20: 56-57, 1972.

34. Wells, N. Selenium in Horizons of Soil Profiles. NZ J Sci., 10: 142-179, 1967.

35. Wolf, E., Kollonitsch, V., and Kline, C.H. A Survey of Selenium in Livestock Production. J Agric Food Chem., 11: 355-360, 1963.

36. Wynder, E.L., and Reddy, B.S. The Epidemiology of Cancer of the Large Bowel. Digestive Diseases, 19: 937-946, 1974.

37. Wynder, E.L., and Shigematsu, T. Environmental Factors of Cancer of the Colon and Rectum. Cancer, 20: 1520-1561, 1967.

38. Zingaro, R.A., and Cooper, W.C. Selenium. Van Nostrand Reinhold Company, New York, 1974.

THE BALKAN ENDEMIC NEPHROPATHY
AND CANCER OF THE URINARY TRACT

Markovic B. and Lebedev S.

Medical Center
Gnjilane, Yugoslavia

SUMMARY

A chronic kidney disease - Balkan endemic nephropathy is followed
by a high percentage of malignant urothelial tumors. These malignant diseases of the urinary tract are caused by unhealthy drinking water, which is from time to time penetrated by eroded silicate minerals, containing heavy, blastomogenic metals: Ni, Cr and
the others.

In order to induce these diseases of the urinary tract in experimental animals we crushed silicate minerals to obtain particles 1-
3 microns in size. The particles of silicate minerals, containing
blastomogenic metals, were added to the clean drinking water with
which animals were watered, under physiological conditions, for several months. In such a way silicates were applied in laboratory
work under the same conditions which naturally exist and influence
the occurrence of EN and the urinary tract tumors in human subjects.

The chronic interstitial (endemic) nephritis and tumors of the urinary tract urothelium were simultaneously induced in experimental
animals after twelve months.

In human subjects the urinary tract could be affected by these diseases in early childhood, so that persons who had left the foci
of disease died of EN and cancer of the urinary tract several decades after they had left the endangered regions. The full preventive effect of the "clean" drinking water introduction can be expected only many decades after it had been introduced into the foci
of disease.

INTRODUCTION

Nephrotoxicity of silicate minerals is caused by desintegration of
eroded silicate particles along with the release of silicic acid.
They become nephrotoxic under pH conditions in the human kidneys
(Markovic B. and Arambasic M., 1971). The blastomogenic effect of
silicate minerals is conditioned by the presence of heavy blastomogenic metals in them (Markovic B., 1974). All silicate minerals
are not nephrotoxic. Quartz is the most toxic silicate. Some gra-
nits are toxic too. If the silicate rocks are caught by a metamor-
phic process they remain non-toxic or only slightly toxic.

The assumption of some authors, relating to the nephrotoxicity of
SiO_2 from industrial waste waters, produced by technological pro-

1179

cesses or chemically stable and inactive silicate compounds (Duancic V., 1960), could not be experimentally proved (Newberne P. and Wilson R., 1970).

Under the pathogenic effect of unhealthy drinking water, which contains eroded silicate minerals and heavy blastomogenic metals, two processes are taking place in the urinary tract: one on the kidneys, which under the effect of silicic acid become fibrotic, athrophic, necrotic and contracted, and the other on the urothelium under the blastomogenic effect of heavy metals during their excretion through the urinary canals (Markovic B., 1974).

PROCEDURE AND MATERIALS USED

a. Toxic Properties of the Noxa

Quartz is the most toxic of all silicate minerals regarding its effect upon the kidneys. Besides its inflammatory-proliferative activity quartz also acts upon the coagulation of proteins (Milius F. and Groschuff N., 1906), dehydration and necrosis of the renal tissue (Markovic B. and Arambasic M., 1971).

In this pathogenic process a portion of silicic acid, released from a quartz particle, forms a silico-protein complex, which is further eliminated with the urin, while the other portion is polymerized in the renal tissue (Markovic B., 1974). When the renal pH index changes from acid into alkaline, the recrystallization of silicic acid becomes possible.

b. The Blastomogenic Property of the Noxa

Of heavy, blastomogenic metals, contained in the acid and basic silicate volcanic rocks, nickel has a strong blastomogenic effect, because of its penetrability and affinity to nitrogen in amino acids. The imino groups of the polypeptide series wind round Ni-ions and thus new protein structures are created. A disturbed protein synthesis, in a part of cell responsible for reproduction, leads to a

loss of further normal cellular reproduction.

Of the other carcinogens some heavy metals like molibdenum, wolfram and vanadium form stable organic compounds of phosphoric acid.Dephosphorization of nucleic acids, which are carriers of genetic information (desoxyribonucleic acids), disturbs the gene structure and along with it the normal regulating mechanism of the cellular growth and development (Jakov F. and Monod I., 1961).

Chromium, tin, uranium can also be important in this malignant process in the urothelium, where a slightly acid effect of the polymerized silicic acid during excretion is another significant moment as well.

MATERIAL AND METHODS

We took silicate minerals, used in our experimental work, directly from the rocks in the regions affected by these diseases. The material was chemically analysed for the content of microelements by means of spectral emission analysis; while quartz did not contain microelements (traces only), basic quartzit contained them in the following concentrations: Ni - 0.012, Cr - 0.058, Al - 0.360, Mg - 0.100, Ba - 0.043, Fe - 0.260, Ca - 0.520, Ti - 0.010 (per cent values). Quartz and quartzit were ground in a mortar and the size of particles was microscopically measured. They were added to the clean

drinking water as follows: 50 mg of quartz + 100 mg of quartzit per liter. The water from the waterworks was used. Throughout the entire experiment the water was bacteriologically safe and did not show any significant change in the chemical content or in pH (7.2 - 7.8). White experimental mice, over six months old, were used as experimental animals.

a. Controls

Twenty mice were fed with oats and were given plain bread from time to time. They were watered with the water from the waterworks.

b. Experimental Group

The number of animals was the same as for the controls. Their feeding was also identical. They were watered with the water containing quartz and quartzit silicate suspension. Quartz and quartzite were finely ground into particles 1-3 microns in size and were added to the water in the following concentration: 50 mg of quartz + 100 mg of quartzit per liter.

The animals were deprived of all food for six hours and after that they were watered and allowed to drink water with silicate suspension "ad libitum" for one hour. Their feeding continued after the watering.

The silicate suspension, shaken before use, was given to the mice from hanging bottles. Prepared and kept in the dark, the suspension was used several days at the most.

Two months after the beginning of experiment the animals showed clinical signs of disease. They lost weight and suffered from polydipsia and polyuria. Every fourth month they were deprived of quartzit during the first fifteen days, being watered only with the quartz suspension (50 mg/ l). During the next fifteen days they were deprived of the quartz suspension too, being given only the bread soaked in clean water, instead in the noxious agents.

During that interval the animals recovered and the experiment was carried on with the silicate suspension again.

To obtain better results the exposure to the influence of noxious agents should be reduced and interrupted every fourth month. Thus natural conditions of long-term, but temporary intoxication are imitated.

Chronic interstitial (endemic) nephritis and tumors of the urinary tract urothelium were simultaneously induced in experimental animals after twelve months.

RESULTS

a. The Kidney – On the Cellular Level

Under the toxic effect of silicic acid upon the kidneys of experimental animals two simultaneous pathogenic processes take place:inflammatory-proliferative in the interstice and dystrophic, atrophic and necrotic in the parenchyma. Atrophic and necrotic lesions can affect the interstice too. The initial inflammatory infiltration by lymphocytes and plasma cells begins focally, in the interstice around the blood vessels, glomeruli and tubules. It develops, through further growth of fibroblasts and fibrocytes, into sclerosis of the interstice.

The focal periglomerular inflammatory-proliferative infiltration leads to a fibrotic thickening of the Bowman capsule.

The proliferative process affects the intercapillary mesangium of the glomerular capillary ball as well. In such a way the majority of glomeruli end up in this sclerogenic process with sclerosis and hyalinization.

The parenchymal lesions start as dystrophic-hypertrophic, atrophic or necrotic ones.

While the endothelium of the capillary ball is hypertrophic in some glomeruli, the number of the endothelial nuclei in the other glomeruli is reduced and the endothelium is atrophic.

The glomeruli of necrotic endothelium and the capillary ball were noticed too.

The main changes in the tubules start in their proximal convoluted parts. The initial changes of the tubular epithelium may be dystrophyc-hypertrophic. They develop more often than atrophic or necrotic changes. When necrosis affects the tubular epithelium, tubular basement membrane and interstitial stroma, the tubular lumina join together and microcystic formations are seen.

The larger blood vessels are passable. The secondary sclerotic changes are marked in the middle of the blood vessels' wall. Some of the smallest blood vessels may be sclerotically changed and their lumina obturated.

b. On the Subcellular Level

The kidney samples were taken from sacrificed animals nine months after the beginning of experiment and from that time onward till the end of experiment. The samples were fixated in 1% OsO_4 and embeded in Epon 812. The slices were cut on Sjöstrand Om U_2 ultramicrotome and stained with uranyl acetate and lead hydroxide. The samples were examined under Philips EM 300 electron microscope at 80 100 kv.

The renal tissue was analysed for ultrastructural abnormalities on the interstitial glomeruli, the tubules and blood vessels. The most striking changes included the focal mesenchymal proliferation of the interstice of the kidney cortex and medulla with multiplication of the collagenic fibres.

The glomerular changes were of the focal nature. The Bowman capsule was thickened because of the mesenchymal hypertrophy between the visceral and parietal sheets. In some glomeruli periglomerular proliferation of the fixed connective cells was noted, particularly around the vascular pole of the Malphigian corpuscule. Atrophy of the macula densa cell-elements was observed. In the intercapillary mesangium of the capillary ball proliferation of the mesangial cells , associated with the increased secretion of the mesangial matrix, was seen. The mesangial axis was thickened (axial glomerulitis).

The capillary basement showed irregular thickenings. Mesangial hypertrophy, thickening of the capillary basement membrane and swelling (hypertrophy) of the endothelial cells of the capillary ball cause the capillary lumina´s narrowing up to their partial or complete obstruction.

The podocytes show a generalized swelling. Their foot processes may be well preserved. They are somewhere deformed.

In some glomeruli the endothelial cells of the capillary ball were atrophic or necrotic. Instead of a capillary ball in some glomeruli a non-structural, amorhpous "detritus" was seen.

Pathological changes in the tubules almost exclusively affect the proximal convoluted tubules. The basement membrane of some tubules is thickened, the epithelium atrophic. Fine spherical osmiophilic grains 0.05 to 0.1 mcr in diameter were observed in the basement membrane of some tubules. In some epithelial cells large osmiophilic inclusions were situated close to the basement membrane of the tubules.

The fine spherical granular osmiophilic inclusions, "electron dense bodies", 0.1 to 0.5 mcr in diameter were seen in the mitochondria of the proximal tubular epithelium of all studied kidney samples (Fig. 1).

In some cases "electron dense bodies" increase in size with the reduction of density of the mitochondrial matrix up to the point of resembling large vacuoles, filled up with osmiophilic inclusions.

Atrophic changes of the larger blood vessels mostly affect the middle of the wall (media). The smallest arteries show focal or diffuse initial fibrosis and collagenization.

c. The Results Obtained on the Urothelium of the Urinary Canals

Neoplastic proliferation of the urothelium was found in more than 50% of the animals used for the experimental group. In some cases this proliferation was benign (Fig. 2) and in the other cases with the signs of malignancy (Figs. 3 and 4).

Multiplicity of tumors was noted in the urinary tract of some animals. Two or three tumors with or without the signs of malignancy could be found on the same renal pelvis.

DISCUSSION

In human subjects this pathogenic process of the urinary tract develops in natural conditions under the influence of much smaller quantities of noxious agents than the quantities we used in our experiments.

The human kidney is more susceptible to a toxic effect of the noxa in lower concetrations because of acid pH of the kidney interstice and urine, compared with pH of the alkaline kidney interstice and urine of experimental animals (Markovic B. and Arambasic M.,1971). In this regard some domestic animals, belonging to the group of carnivora (dog, cat, swine), would be more suitable for experimental work (Newberne B. and Wilson R., 1970).

Now more facts are known about pathogenic processes in children as well. Bulgarian investigators performed renal biopsies in children originating from the families affected by EN and concluded that pathogenic processes can develop in children in a latent form (Jurukova Z. and Dimitrov Z., 1972).

In the course of previous experiments with quartz we sacrificed young mice aged 10-12 weeks. They were exposed to the influence of noxious agent during intra-uterine and lactation period. The pathological process in their kidneys showed specific dissemination in the early phase of disease, involving all parenchymal structures, as well as the mesenchyma. The focal interstitial lesions largely involved the external cortical zone with a triangular form, the basis facing the capsule. The triangular apex was turned towards the middle of the cortex.

The interstitial lesions consisted predominantly of acellular sclerosis without inflammatory cells.

Compared with these sclerogenic changes of the interstice glomerular findings were of somewhat different nature.

The small glomeruli, resembling the "foetal glomeruli", with few capillaries deficient in mesangial and endothelial cells, were covered, along their external surface, with densely arranged hyperchronic endothelial nuclei.

Contrary to the "foetal glomeruli" another their type was also seen. The cystic glomeruli, with largely widened capsular space and reduced hyalinized capillary ball, compressed to the vascular pole of the Bowman capsule, were very often noticed.

The structural "simplification" of some glomeruli and tubular changes, consisting of pronounced atrophy of the proximal tubules, was very often seen. Many of the lesions found in the substratum of the young mice were due to a disturbed intra-uterine kidney development.

The latent, clinically asymptomatic period of disease lasts in adults, as well as in children, many years. The pathological process which develops in the kidneys during that period affects them to a point when they become impaired to such extent that functional-clinical signs are brought along.

By chemical analysis of the kidneys of the patients who died of EN and cancer of the urinary tract considerable concentrations of heavy metals were discovered (Ni, Cr and the others), as well as high concentrations of silicon (Makarov V. et al., 1966, 1967).

The high concentrations of SiO_2 in the kidneys were related to the patients who died of EN, having lived all the time prior to their death in endemic areas where they had been exposed to the toxic effect of the noxious agents.

Further chemical analyses of the kidneys of the patients who died of EN in non-endemic regions might show whether silicon in high, abnormal concentrations could be found in their kidneys. EN will continue to progress after the patient leaves the endangered region. The hydrolytic property of silicic acid accounts for a protraction of pathogenic process. When separated from its organic compounds in the kidneys silicic acid is capable of repeating its effect. It is not known whether silicic acid is during its pathogenic activity finally fixed in the kidneys or extracted owing to its hydrolytic property.

In this connection it is illusory to expect immediate preventive effects from the introduction of "clean" drinking water into the foci of EN. The urinary tract could be affected by these diseases in early childhood. There were cases, reported by field investigators, that patients who moved away from the foci of disease, died of EN and cancer of the urinary tract, several decades after they had left the endemic areas.

The full preventive effect of the "clean" drinking water could be expected only many decades after such water is brought to the foci of disease.

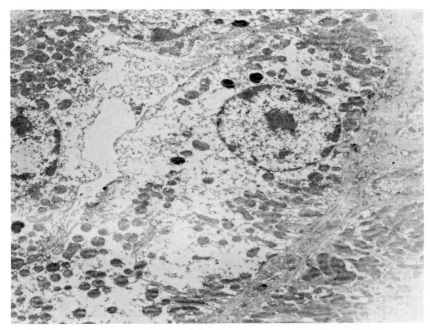

FIG. 1. The kidneys of experimental animals - mice (photographs 1-4).
Twelve months exposure: quartz 50 mg + quartzit 100 mg/l. Electron
microscopy x 7,000. The epithelial cells of the proximal convoluted
tubules hypertrophically swollen. Hydropic and vacuolar degeneration of
the cells. Osmiophilic inclusions, electron dense bodies, present in some
mitochondria.

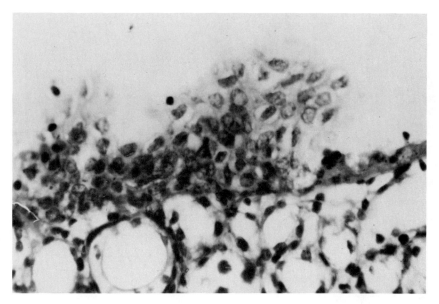

FIG. 2. The kidneys of experimental animals - mice (photographs 1-4).
Twelve months exposure: quartz 50 mg + quartzit 100 mg/l. HE 10 x 40.
The benign neoplasmatic proliferation of the renal pelvis.

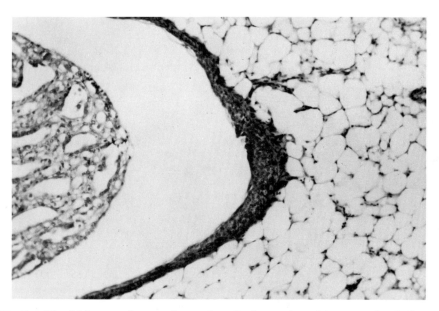

FIG. 3. The kidneys of experimental animals - mice (photographs 1-4).
Twelve months exposure: quartz 50 mg + quartzit 100 mg/l. HE 10 x 40.
The neoplastic proliferation of the renal pelvis with signs of malignancy.

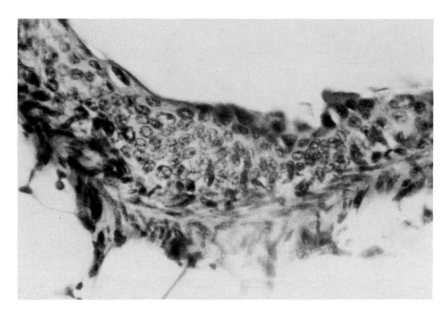

FIG. 4. The kidneys of experimental animals - mice (photographs 1-4).
Twelve months exposure: quartz 50 mg + quartzit 100 mg/1. HE 10 x 40.
A detail of Fig. 3.

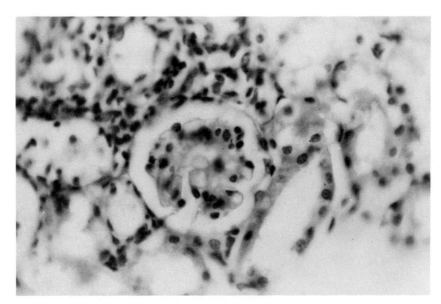

FIG. 5. The kidneys of experimental animals - mice (photographs 1-4).
Twelve months exposure: quartz 50 mg + quartzit 100 mg/1. HE 10 x 40.
The glomeruli resembling "foetal" glomeruli.

REFERENCES

1. Duancic V. Essai d'explication de la manifestation de l'affection renale de masse a Slavonski Kobas. Bioloski glasnik, **3** : 43 - 45 1960.

2. Jakov F. and Monod J. Genetic Regulatory Mechanism in the Synthesis of Proteins. J. Mol. Biol., 3: 318-355, 1963.

3. Jurukova Z. and Dimitrov Z. Electron Microscopic Study of Kidney Biopsy of Clinically Healthy Children, Familially Burdened With Endemic Nephropathy. Abstr. Second Symposium on Endemic Nephropathy, Sofia, 203-207, 1972.

4. Makarov V., Topakbasan S., Dinev I. and Topusov R. Research Into Biological Materials for the Anomalous Contents of Microelements in the Organs of the Dead Due to Endemic Nephropathy. Symposium on Endemic Nephropathy, Nis, Yugoslavia, 150-163, 1966.

5. Makarov V., Topakbasan S. and Dinev I. Research Into Biological Materials for the Anomalous Contents of Microelements in the Kidneys of the Dead Due to Endemic Nephropathy. Symposium on Endemic Nephropathy, Nis, Yugoslavia, 30-31, 1967.

6. Markovic B. and Arambasic M. Experimental Chronic Interstitial Nephritis Compared With Human Endemic Nephropathy. J. Path.,103: 35-41, 1971.

7. Markovic B. Experimental Chronic Interstitial Nephropathy Followed by Tumors of the Urinary Tract. Acta Urol. Japon. 20: 63-67, 1974.

8. Mylius F. and Groschuff H. Alfa und Beta Kiesselsaure in Lösung. Berichte d. Deutsch. chemisch. Gesellschaft, 39: 116-120, 1906.

9. Newberne P. and Wilson R. Renal Dammages Associated With Silicon Compounds in Dogs. Proceed. of the National Academy of Sciences, 65, 4: 872-875, 1970.

INDEX OF CONTRIBUTORS

7632477

3 1378 00763 2477